TEXTBOOK OF ORAL AND MAXILLOFACIAL SURGERY

TEXTBOOK OF ORAL AND MAXILLOFACIAL SURGERY

Edited by

GUSTAV O. KRUGER, B.S., A.M., D.D.S., D.Sc., F.A.C.D., F.I.C.D.

Professor of Oral Surgery and Associate Dean for Graduate Studies, Georgetown University School of Dentistry, Washington, D.C.; Chief of Dental Staff, Georgetown University Hospital, Washington, D.C.; Senior Consultant, District of Columbia General Hospital, Washington, D.C.; Consultant to Veterans Administration Hospitals in Martinsburg, W.Va., and Washington, D.C., United States Naval Dental School, Bethesda, Md., and Walter Reed Army Hospital, Washington, D.C.; Past Chairman, United States Public Health Service Clinical Cancer Training Committee (Dental), National Cancer Institute; Past Chairman, Review Commission on Advanced Education in Oral Surgery, Council on Dental Education; Past President, Middle Atlantic Society of Oral Surgeons; Diplomate and Past President, American Board of Oral and Maxillofacial Surgery

Art editor

B. JOHN MELLONI

FIFTH EDITION

with **1,557** illustrations and **3** color plates

THE C. V. MOSBY COMPANY

ST. LOUIS • TORONTO • LONDON   1979

FIFTH EDITION

Copyright © 1979 by The C. V. Mosby Company

All rights reserved. No part of this book may be reproduced in any manner without written permission of the publisher.

Previous editions copyrighted 1959, 1964, 1968, 1974

Printed in the United States of America

The C. V. Mosby Company
11830 Westline Industrial Drive, St. Louis, Missouri 63141

Library of Congress Cataloging in Publication Data
Main entry under title:

Textbook of oral and maxillofacial surgery.

   Fourth ed. (1974) by G. O. Kruger, published
under title: Textbook of oral surgery.
   Bibliography: p.
   Includes index.
   1. Mouth—Surgery. 2. Maxilla—Surgery.
3. Face—Surgery. I. Kruger, Gustav O. Textbook of
oral surgery. [DNLM: 1. Surgery, Oral. WU600.3 T354]
RK529.K78 1979   617′.522   78-26118
ISBN   0-8016-2792-3

CB/CB/B 9 8 7 6 5 4 3 2 1   03/A/300

Contributors

CHARLES C. ALLING III, D.D.S., M.S., F.A.C.D., F.A.D.S.A.

Professor and Chairman, Department of Oral and Maxillofacial Surgery, University of Alabama School of Dentistry; Chairman, Oral Surgery Service, Eye Foundation Hospital, Birmingham, Ala.; Consultant, United States Army, United States Veterans Administration, American Cancer Society; Colonel, United States Army (Retired); Past Officer, Board of Directors, American Association of Oral and Maxillofacial Surgeons; Diplomate and Member of the Board of Directors, American Board of Oral and Maxillofacial Surgery

S. ELMER BEAR, D.D.S., F.A.C.D.

Professor and Chairman, Department of Oral and Maxillofacial Surgery, School of Dentistry; Professor of Surgery, School of Medicine, Medical College of Virginia, Virginia Commonwealth University; Consultant, United States Naval Hospital, Portsmouth, Va., and McGuire Veterans Hospital, Richmond, Va.; Diplomate, American Board of Oral and Maxillofacial Surgery; formerly Speaker, House of Delegates and Past President of American Association of Oral and Maxillofacial Surgeons; Director, OSPAC; Chairman, Educational Foundation, American Association of Oral and Maxillofacial Surgeons

PHILIP J. BOYNE, D.M.D., M.S., D.Sc.(Hon.), F.A.C.D., F.I.C.D.

Professor of Oral Surgery, School of Medicine and School of Dentistry, Loma Linda University, Loma Linda, Calif.; Director of Graduate Program in Oral and Maxillofacial Surgery, Loma Linda University; Chief of the Oral Surgery Service, Loma Linda University Hospital; Research Professor of Surgery, School of Medicine, University of Miami, Miami, Fla.; Director of Graduate Research Studies in Oral and Maxillofacial Surgery, School of Medicine, University of Miami; formerly Dean and Professor of Oral Surgery, University of Texas Dental School, San Antonio, Tex.; formerly Assistant Dean and Chairman of the Section of Oral Surgery, U.C.L.A. School of Dentistry, Los Angeles, Calif.; formerly Professor of Oral Surgery, U.C.L.A. School of Dentistry and U.C.L.A. School of Medicine, Los Angeles, Calif.; President, American Institute of Oral Biology; Captain, United States Navy Dental Corps (Retired); Diplomate and Member of the Board of Directors of the American Board of Oral and Maxillofacial Surgery; Secretary-Treasurer of the American Board of Oral and Maxillofacial Surgery; Consultant to the American Dental Association Councils on Dental Education and Hospital Dental Services; Consultant to the Veterans Administration Central Office and Veterans Administration Hospitals, Loma Linda and Long Beach, Calif.; Member, Merit Review Board in Oral Biology for the Veterans Administration; Consultant, United States Naval Hospitals in Long Beach and San Diego, Calif.; Research Section Editor, Journal of Oral Surgery; Member of the Editorial Board of International Journal of Oral Surgery; and Member of the Editorial Board, Postgraduate Medicine

JACK B. CALDWELL, D.D.S., M.Sc., F.A.C.D., F.I.C.D.

Colonel, United States Army Dental Corps (Retired); Consultant in Oral Surgery, Fitzsimons General Hospital, Denver, Colo.; formerly Chief of Dental Service, Second General Hospital, and Oral Surgery Consultant to the Chief Surgeon, United States Army, Europe; formerly Visiting Professor, College of Physicians and Surgeons, School of Dentistry, San Francisco, Calif.; formerly Staff Member, Army Medical Service Graduate School, Walter Reed Army Medical Center, Washington, D.C.; formerly Chief of Oral Surgery, Walter Reed General Hospital, Washington, D.C., Fitzsimons General Hospital, Denver, Colo., and Letterman General Hospital, San Francisco, Calif.;

Member, American Society of Oral and Maxillofacial Surgeons; Diplomate and Past President, American Board of Oral and Maxillofacial Surgery

DONALD E. COOKSEY, D.D.S., M.S., F.A.C.D.

Professor of Oral Surgery, University of Southern California School of Dentistry, Los Angeles, Calif.; Captain, United States Navy Dental Corps (Retired); formerly Commanding Officer, United States Naval Dental Clinic, Yokosuka, Japan; Chief of Clinical Services, Head of Oral Surgery Division, and Consultant-Instructor in Oral Surgery, United States Naval Dental School, National Naval Medical Center, Bethesda, Md.; Guest Lecturer, University of Pennsylvania, Philadelphia, Pa., and Georgetown University, Washington, D.C.; Diplomate and Past President, American Board of Oral and Maxillofacial Surgery

ROY C. GERHARD, B.S., D.D.S., F.A.C.D.

Colonel, United States Army Dental Corps (Retired); formerly Chief, Oral Surgery, and Director, Residency Training Program, Walter Reed Army Hospital; formerly Consultant in Oral Surgery, First United States Army; formerly Guest Lecturer, Graduate School of Dentistry, Howard University; formerly Chief, Dental Service, 102nd Medical Detachment, Munich, Germany; formerly Consultant in Oral Surgery, Munich Medical Service Area, Munich, Germany; formerly Assistant, Zahnaertzliches Institut, Zurich, Switzerland; Diplomate and Member, Advisory Committee, American Board of Oral and Maxillofacial Surgery; Member, American Society of Oral and Maxillofacial Surgeons

JOHN M. GREGG, D.D.S., M.S., Ph.D.

Professor of Oral and Maxillofacial Surgery; Principal Investigator, Dental Research Center, University of North Carolina; Diplomate, American Board of Oral and Maxillofacial Surgery; Director, Post-Doctoral Program, Craniofacial Pain Mechanisms and Control

LOUIS H. GUERNSEY, B.S., D.D.S., M.S.D., F.A.C.D., F.I.C.D.

Professor and Chairman, Oral and Maxillofacial Surgery Department, Director, Postgraduate Oral Surgery Program, The Affiliated Hospitals, School of Dental Medicine, University of Pennsylvania; Consulting Staff, Children's Hospital of Pennsylvania; Presbyterian–University of Pennsylvania Medical Center; Medical College of Pennsylvania Hospital; Pennsylvania Hospital; Chief, Oral Surgery Section, Hospital of the University of Pennsylvania, Philadelphia, Pa.; Colonel, United States Army (Retired); Diplomate, American Board of Oral and Maxillofacial Surgery

MERLE L. HALE, B.A., D.D.S., M.S., F.A.C.D.

Professor and Head, Department of Oral Surgery, Head, Department of Dentistry, University Hospitals and Clinics, University of Iowa College of Dentistry; Clinical Professor, Oral Surgery, College of Medicine, Iowa City, Ia.; Consultant in Oral Surgery, Veterans Administration Hospital, Iowa City, Ia.; Editor, Oral Surgery Section of Year Book of Dentistry; Diplomate, American Board of Oral and Maxillofacial Surgery; National Consultant in Oral Surgery to the Surgeon General, United States Air Force

H. DAVID HALL, D.M.D., M.D.

Professor and Chairman, Department of Oral Surgery, Vanderbilt University Medical Center, Nashville, Tenn.; Diplomate, American Board of Oral and Maxillofacial Surgery

JAMES R. HAYWARD, D.D.S., M.S., F.A.C.D.

Professor of Oral Surgery, University of Michigan School of Dentistry and Medical School and Director, Section of Oral Surgery, University of Michigan Hospital, Ann Arbor, Mich.; Diplomate and Past President, American Board of Oral and Maxillofacial Surgery; Past President, American Association of Oral and Maxillofacial Surgeons; Past Editor, Journal of Oral Surgery

FRED A. HENNY, D.D.S., F.D.S.R.C.S.(Eng.), F.A.C.D.

Diplomate and Past President, American Board of Oral and Maxillofacial Surgery; formerly Chief of Division of Dentistry and Oral Surgery, Henry Ford Hospital, Detroit, Mich.; Past Associate Chairman, Department of Oral Surgery, Sinai Hospital of Detroit, Detroit, Mich.; Past President, International Association of Oral Surgeons; Past Editor, Journal of Oral Surgery; Past President, American Association of Oral and Maxillofacial Surgeons; Honorary Member, International Association of Oral Surgeons, British Association of Oral Surgeons, Australian, New Zealand Association of Oral Surgeons, Greek Society of Oral Surgeons; Consultant, Council on Hospital Dental Service, American Dental Association

EDWARD C. HINDS, B.A., D.D.S., M.D., F.A.C.S., F.A.C.D.

Professor of Surgery, The University of Texas Dental Branch, Houston, Tex.; Chief, Dental Service, Ben Taub General Hospital and The Methodist Hospital, Houston, Tex.; National Consultant to the Surgeon General, United States Air Force, 1964-1969; Consultant, Veterans Administration Hospital, Houston, Tex., William Beaumont Army Hospital, El Paso, Tex., and Wilford Hall Air Force Hospital, San Antonio, Tex.; Consultant in Oral Surgery to the Central Office, Veterans Administration; Diplomate, American Board of Oral and Maxillofacial Surgery; Diplomate, American Board of Surgery

GUSTAV O. KRUGER, B.S., A.M., D.D.S., D.Sc., F.A.C.D., F.I.C.D.

Professor of Oral Surgery and Associate Dean for Graduate Studies, Georgetown University School of Dentistry, Washington, D.C.; Chief of Dental Staff, Georgetown University Hospital, Washington, D.C.; Senior Consultant, District of Columbia General Hospital, Washington, D.C.; Consultant to Veterans Administration Hospitals in Martinsburg, W.Va., and Washington, D.C., United States Naval Dental School, Bethesda, Md., and Walter Reed Army Hospital, Washington, D.C.; Past Chairman, United States Public Health Service Clinical Cancer Training Committee (Dental), National Cancer Institute; Past Chairman, Review Commission on Advanced Education in Oral Surgery, Council on Dental Education; Past President, Middle Atlantic Society of Oral Surgeons; Diplomate and Past President, American Board of Oral and Maxillofacial Surgery

CLAUDE S. La DOW, D.D.S., M.Sc.(Dent.)

Clinical Professor, Department of Oral Surgery, University of Pennsylvania School of Dental Medicine, Philadelphia, Pa.; Senior Attending Oral Surgeon, Presbyterian–University of Pennsylvania Medical Center; Chief of Dentistry and Oral Surgery, Lankenau Hospital, Philadelphia, Pa.; Consultant to Paoli Memorial Hospital, Paoli, Pa., Veterans Administration Hospital, Coatesville, Pa., Veterans Administration Hospital, Philadelphia, Pa., and Mercy Catholic Medical Center, Philadelphia, Pa.; Diplomate and Past President, American Board of Oral and Maxillofacial Surgery

THEODORE A. LESNEY, D.D.S., F.A.C.D.

Captain, Dental Corps, United States Navy (Retired); formerly Chief of the Dental Service, Head of Oral Surgery, and Consultant-Instructor to Dental Intern and Residency Training Programs at the following naval hospitals: Great Lakes, Ill., Portsmouth, Va., San Diego, Calif., and the Naval Dental School, National Naval Medical Center, Bethesda, Md.; Diplomate, American Board of Oral and Maxillofacial Surgery

KEITH J. MARSHALL, D.D.S.

Chief, Oral Surgery, Director, Postgraduate Course in Oral Surgery, and Director, Oral Surgery Residency Training, Letterman Army Medical Center, San Francisco, California; Diplomate, American Board of Oral and Maxillofacial Surgery

SANFORD M. MOOSE, D.D.S., F.A.C.D.

Clinical Professor of Oral Surgery Emeritus, School of Dentistry, University of the Pacific, San Francisco, Calif.; Special Civilian Consultant in Maxillofacial Surgery to the Surgeon General, United States Army; formerly Consultant to the Central Office, Veterans Administration; Consultant in Oral Surgery and Faculty Member, Graduate Training Programs, Letterman Army Medical Center, San Francisco, Calif.; formerly Member of California State Board of Public Health; formerly Consultant in Oral Surgery, Veterans Administration Hospital, Palo Alto, Calif., Veterans Hospital, Livermore, Calif., and United States Public Health Service Hospital, San Francisco, Calif.; Honorary Staff Member of Sequoia Hospital, Redwood City, Calif.; formerly Chief of Oral Surgery, Mount Zion Hospital, San Francisco, Calif.; Oral Surgery Staff, Peninsula Hospital, Burlingame, Calif.; Oral Surgery Staff, Mills Memorial Hospital, San Mateo, Calif.; Fellow, International Association of Oral Surgeons; Diplomate and Former Director, American Board of Oral and Maxillofacial Surgery

EDWARD R. MOPSIK, B.S., D.M.D., M.S.

Formerly Associate Professor of Oral Surgery, Georgetown University School of Dentistry, Washington, D.C.; formerly Consultant, District of Columbia General Hospital, Washington, D.C.; Diplomate, American Board of Oral and Maxillofacial Surgery

JAMES A. O'BRIEN, B.S., D.D.S., F.A.C.D.

Diplomate and former Member, Advisory Committee, American Board of Oral and Maxillofacial Surgery

LEROY W. PETERSON, D.D.S., F.A.C.D.

Professor of Oral Surgery, Washington University School of Dental Medicine, St. Louis, Mo.; Consultant in Oral Surgery, Veterans Administration Hospital, St. Louis, Mo.; Consultant to the Journal of the American Dental Association; Founder and Fellow, International Association of Oral Surgeons; Past President, American Association of Oral and Maxillofacial Surgeons; Diplomate, American Board of Oral and Maxillofacial Surgery

DONALD C. REYNOLDS, D.D.S., M.S., F.A.C.D., F.I.C.D.

Professor of Oral Surgery, Georgetown University School of Dentistry, Washington, D.C.; Consultant, District of Columbia General Hospital, Washington, D.C., and Veterans Administration Hospital, Martinsburg, W.Va.; Diplomate, American Board of Oral and Maxillofacial Surgery

ROBERT B. SHIRA, D.D.S., F.A.C.D., F.I.C.D., D.Sc.

Dean and Professor of Oral Surgery, Tufts University School of Dental Medicine, Boston, Mass.; formerly Major General, United States Army, and Chief, Army Dental Corps; formerly Chief of Dental Service and Chief of Oral Surgery, Walter Reed General Hospital, Washington, D.C.; Past President, American Dental Association; Past President, American Association of Oral and Maxillofacial Surgeons; Diplomate and Past

President, American Board of Oral and Maxillofacial Surgery; Editor, Journal of Oral Surgery, Oral Medicine and Oral Pathology; Advisory Board, American Dental Society of Anesthesiology; Consultant, Dental Advisory Panel, Food and Drug Administration; Member, Advisory Panel, United States Army Medical Research and Development Command; Past Chairman, Council on Dental Therapeutics and currently Consultant to Council of Dental Therapeutics and Council, Scientific Sessions, American Dental Association

DANIEL GORDON WALKER, A.B., D.D.S., M.Sc., M.D.

Clinical Associate Professor of Surgery, Division of Oral and Maxillofacial Surgery, University of Texas Medical Branch, Houston, Tex.; Clinical Associate Professor of Surgery, University of Texas Dental Branch, Houston, Tex.; Attending Surgeon, The Methodist Hospital, Hermann Hospital, and Diagnostic Hospital, Houston, Tex.; Consultant, Veterans Administration Hospital, Houston, Tex.; Consultant, Texas Children's Hospital, Houston, Tex.; Section

Editor, Journal of Oral Surgery; formerly Chief of Oral Surgery, 3380 United States Air Force Hospital, Keesler Air Force Base, Ala.; formerly Chief of Oral Surgery, Memorial Hospital System, Houston, Tex.; Past President, Southwest Society of Oral Surgeons; formerly Consultant to Council on Dental Education, American Dental Association; Diplomate and formerly Member of Advisory Committee, American Board of Oral and Maxillofacial Surgery

PHILLIP EARLE WILLIAMS, B.S., D.D.S., M.S., F.A.C.D.

Retired Faculty Member, Baylor Dental College and South-Western Medical School of the University of Texas, Dallas, Tex.; formerly First Vice-President, American Dental Association; Past Director, American Association of Oral and Maxillofacial Surgeons; Past President, American College of Dentists; Diplomate and Past President of the American Board of Oral and Maxillofacial Surgery; Past President of Texas Dental Association; Past President of South-West Society of Oral Surgeons

TO
SIMON P. HULLIHEN
1810-1857

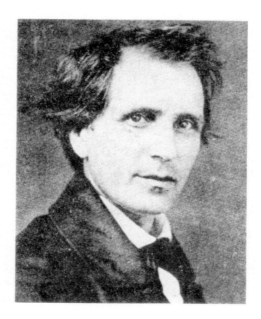

The first oral surgeon in
the United States

Preface

This text was written to provide a concise description of principles and procedures in each important aspect of oral and maxillofacial surgery in a logical sequence, as it may be presented to students in the lecture course.

The book is designed to fit the needs of the undergraduate student, but general practitioners, residents, oral surgeons, and other specialists will also find it useful. Emphasis has been placed on the fundamentals of judgment and technique. Even if the reader does not perform all the procedures described, he or she should have a clear idea of what is done, how it is done, and why it is done.

The first edition was published in 1959. In the four revisions since then considerable change in philosophy, materials, and technique reflects the progress that the specialty of oral surgery has achieved. The health sciences in general, and oral surgery in particular, have made rapid and substantial advances based on basic research, clinical investigation, and worldwide clinical experience.

Comprehensive review has been undertaken in this fifth edition. Major revision has been completed in many chapters, and many new photographs and drawings have been added. I welcome two new authors in this edition, one writing on principles of surgery and the other on hemorrhage and shock. Both chapters have been rewritten completely.

The contributors have been selected because of their competence in the field. Each has devoted his efforts to one chapter. It is to them that any credit for this work is due. Without exception, they have been generous with their time and efforts.

I should like to thank B. John Melloni, Director of Medical-Dental Communications, Georgetown University Medical Center, for his generous guidance and supervision of the art work. Peter Stone of his department made the new drawings and put together the photographs for this edition in a superb manner. He is a meticulous illustrator, a talented artist, and a most cooperative collaborator.

Gustav O. Kruger

Contents

COLOR PLATES

TEXTBOOK OF ORAL AND MAXILLOFACIAL SURGERY

CHAPTER 1

Principles of surgery

H. David Hall

Oral surgery is unique among surgical specialties in that it identifies strongly with dentistry. This is a proper relationship since a thorough knowledge of dentistry is a prerequisite for the well-qualified oral surgeon. But oral surgery is no less a surgical specialty than urology, for example. The common link between oral surgery and other surgical specialties is that the same surgical principles apply to therapy. Thus the principles that guide the general surgeon in treating appendicitis are the same as those that guide the oral surgeon in treatment of an odontogenic cellulitis. The fact that details of application of surgical principles may differ to accommodate local peculiarities sometimes obscures this relationship.

However, the casual observer may think that some surgical principles do not apply to a particular surgical specialty such as oral surgery. An example is the principle of asepsis, because aseptic technique clearly is different for abdominal operations and oral operations. Aseptic technique has been modified to take into account differences in the response of a wound in each area; the general principle of asepsis is the same. Thus the challenge for each surgical specialist is not only to know surgical principles but also to know how they apply to a particular area of interest.

ASEPSIS

Prior to the mid-nineteenth century, surgeons made no specific efforts to reduce bacterial contamination of the wound. Yet wounds often healed after primary closure. As hospitals became more prevalent, patients with septic conditions were housed with other patients, since isolation procedures had not been developed. With increased opportunities for wound contamination, especially from these patients, wound infection became commonplace. Even before Lister made his contribution to antisepsis, Semmelweis and O. W. Holmes observed that puerperal fever was spread from infected to uninfected parturient women in the obstetrical wards by their doctors. The simple act of washing hands between patients, thereby reducing the number of virulent bacteria introduced into wounds, greatly reduced puerperal sepsis. Although these doctors did not know what it was that caused the infections, they clearly understood the nature of the transfer. A few years later Pasteur developed the germ theory of disease. This concept provided a basis for understanding wound sepsis. Lister grasped the significance of Pasteur's work and began development of aseptic surgical technique.

Even with modern aseptic surgical technique, some bacteria get into wounds. But wounds are able to tolerate a limited number of bacteria without becoming infected. Several factors determine the maximum number of bacteria that a wound will tolerate. One very important factor is local immunity, and this varies with the area of the body. The oral and maxillofacial region and perineum, for example, have a greater resistance to infection than other regions of the body. Relatively large numbers of indigenous bacteria can be introduced into oral or perineal wounds and rarely cause infection. This is fortunate since it is virtually impossible to reduce bacterial contamination in the mouth or perineum to levels common for other areas of the body. The current aseptic techniques for the oral and maxillofacial area rely principally on prevention of wound contamination by foreign and especially more virulent bacteria.

There are also other factors that determine the maximum number of bacteria with which wounds can become contaminated before developing infection. The body's general resistance to infection is clearly an important factor. Diabetes is an example of a common condition in which there is an increase in susceptibility to infection. Other less common but by no means rare examples are suppression of immunity by corticosteroids or other drugs, leukemia, and uremia. Local wound factors also influence susceptibility to infection. Wound infection is more common after devitalization of tissue, as can occur with accidental injury or careless surgical technique. Thus although aseptic technique is an important factor in reducing wound infections, other factors also have an important influence on the problem. The surgeon who understands these interrelationships is able to make appropriate adjustments in patient management and maintain a low infection rate in most circumstances.

ANALYTICAL APPROACH TO SURGICAL CARE

One of the more important contributions to the care of the surgical patient was appreciation of the value of an analytical approach. The essence of an analytical approach to a clinical puzzle is separation of the various problems and establishment of the relationships of the individual problems to each other. The solution often is evident at this point, or a possible solution is suggested that can be tested.

The first step in the analysis of any situation is to obtain accurate data. The traditional means of establishing these data is by historical, physical, and laboratory examination of the patient. Skill in application of examination technique is essential in order to obtain accurate data. For example, a common tendency of the less experienced clinician is to establish a tentative diagnosis early in the historical evaluation of a patient and then to ask leading questions in an effort to support the diagnosis. Open-ended questions would clearly provide more accurate information even if they might cause some discomfort to the clinician looking for support for an early impression. Similarly, a thorough, careful physical examination of a patient will often yield information missed by a more hurried, less orderly examination. Detection of a small sinus tract in the sulcus overlying a fracture site in a patient with delayed union is an easily missed but very important finding. In particularly difficult diagnostic problems, the more famous surgeons have been noted for the unhurried, careful, and thoughtful examinations they perform.

In addition to being accurate, the information must also be pertinent. This aspect of patient evaluation probably requires the greatest amount of experience for perfection. With increased knowledge of a condition, one begins to recognize which information is particularly pertinent for its diagnosis and treatment. The practitioner can then probe the more relevant areas with greater care. For example, determining that a patient with bleeding from the gingival crevice recently began taking quinidine, which can cause thrombocytopenia, has greater significance in this patient than in a patient who has an infected tooth. Thus skill in patient evaluation requires not only a knowledge of the technique of evaluation but also a knowledge of specific conditions.

Analysis of the information obtained from patient evaluation may readily yield a diagnosis but often does not. A system that lists problems based on the level of information available has a clear advantage over a system that tends to force a premature diagnosis. The problem-oriented medical record is an example of the former system. This method of recording data, which allows identification of discrete problems and their relationships to one another, is especially useful in sorting out complex situations. It also has the advantage of reducing the chances that some problems will be ignored in developing a coordinated treatment plan. For example, a patient with an open bite may also be found to have increased lower facial height, retruded chin, lip incompetence, increased nasolabial

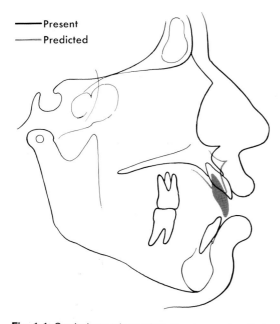

—— Present
—— Predicted

Fig. 1-1. Cephalometric tracing showing a plan that corrects only one of several problems—the open bite.

angle, increased maxillary-alveolar bone height, increased backward rotation of the mandible, minor crowding of the dental arch, and increased curve of Spee in the maxilla (Fig. 1-1). Without a listing of all of the problems, it is easy to focus only on the chief complaint of open bite or perhaps some, but not all, of the other problems. In this example, attention only to the open bite could result in a surgical procedure to close the bite by inferior movement of the anterior maxilla to permit occlusion of the maxillary incisors with the mandibular incisors. This approach to treatment, while providing a good occlusion, would fail to correct other problems and would even create a new one—changing a normal maxillary lip-to-tooth ratio to one with excessive exposure of the teeth (Fig. 1-1). On the other hand, recognition of the various problems and their relationships to each other would more likely lead to another treatment plan. A better plan would be developed if there was recognition that vertical increase in the maxillary bone rotates the mandible, creating a secondary deficiency of the chin, increasing lower facial height, and causing lip incompetence. Thus segmental maxillary osteotomy, with intrusion of the posterior segments and rearrangement of the anterior segments, would also close the open bite. In contrast to the anterior maxillary osteotomy alone for closure of the open bite, this plan would address the other coexisting problems. Thus the combination of a segmental maxillary osteotomy with intrusion to retain the present adequate lip-to-tooth relationship could correct the open bite as well as other important abnormalities (Fig. 1-2). Specifically the procedure would correct the occlusion and provide some correction for the deficient chin, increased lower facial height, and lip incompetence by allowing the mandible to rotate forward. The need for an orthodontist to align the teeth also would be more obvious with this problem-oriented approach. Thus the competent surgeon not only exercises care and

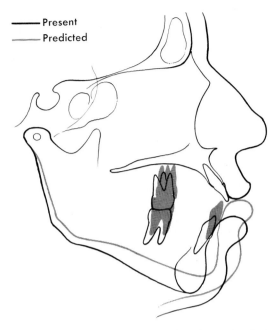

——— Present
——— Predicted

Fig. 1-2. Cephalometric tracing showing a plan that corrects the open bite as well as other problems.

thoroughness in collecting data through the patient evaluation but also organizes these data in a way that encourages an analytical evaluation of problems and, thereby, a more rational approach to surgical therapy.

The analytical approach is also applicable to other aspects of surgical care. Careful assessment of a patient's problems and meticulous planning for the surgical procedure usually eliminate any significant surprises during the operation. But occasional unanticipated findings or events are unavoidable. A few moments of analysis of the situation usually suggest the best course of action. A careful, thorough approach is more important than speed.

Surgeons have an obligation to improve therapy by advancing surgical knowledge. If we do not advance surgical knowledge, our patients will pay the price for our failure to do so. Testing carefully posed hypotheses in the laboratory and evaluating the results of treatment are the two chief means of advancing surgical knowledge. While not all surgeons will have the opportunity or skills required for testing hypotheses in the laboratory, all of us do have the opportunity to learn from the care given our patients. When we evaluate or compare methods of therapy, it is important to make accurate observations. The history of surgery is replete with examples of new operations that, after their initial enthusiastic reception, were found to be ineffective and were therefore discarded. This disservice to patients largely can be avoided by utilizing a study design that minimizes the chances for error in interpretation. Observer bias, placebo effect, individual variability, and comparison of treatment groups with inappropriate controls are well known for their ability to obscure the real effects of therapy.

RESPONSE OF THE BODY TO INJURY

Surgeons, unlike other practitioners, treat patients who have injuries. The injury may be caused by such diverse means as the surgeon's scalpel or a motor vehicle. Francis D. Moore and others have elucidated the major features of the metabolic response of the body to an operation. Knowledge of the characteristics of this response provides the surgeon with a means of assessing the patient's progress after an operation and provides clues for therapy.

The body's response to a surgical procedure, in general, seems to be directed toward maintenance of the internal environment by a process termed homeostasis. That is, an operation activates autoregulatory mechanisms that enhance the ability of a person to withstand the injury. One insult causing this response is hemorrhage. Loss of about 15% of blood volume by venous hemorrhage causes characteristic changes. Typical early changes include increased blood levels of epinephrine, norepinephrine, aldosterone, angiotensin, renin, and antidiuretic hormone. These mechanisms promote conservation of body water and sodium and especially intravascular volume. The depression of urine and sodium excretion by hemorrhage is shown in

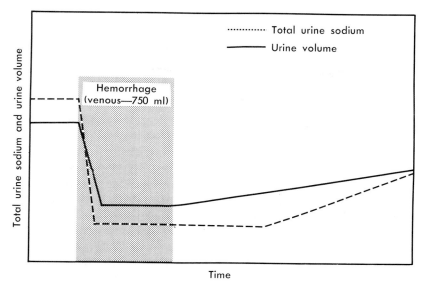

Fig. 1-3. Depression of urine and sodium excretion caused by hemorrhage.

Fig. 1-3. These and other responses restore the intravascular water, electrolyte, and protein content. In fact, the transcapillary filling begins almost immediately after onset of hemorrhage, and volume restoration is complete 18 to 24 hours later.

The response of the patient to an operation may be divided into four phases of convalescence. The first phase is acute injury, and it is characterized by a catabolic state. This phase lasts for 2 to 5 days, depending primarily on the magnitude of the surgical procedure, the quality of care after operation, and the health status of the patient. During this time the patient is apathetic and generally wishes to be left alone. The metabolic response includes negative nitrogen and potassium balances and increased catecholamine and corticosteroid production. Most of the studies concerning the response to injury have been concerned with this first phase. The catabolic phase ends rather abruptly with the "turning point." During this brief phase, the patient begins to expand his concerns from his own small world to the larger events of life. He becomes more active and alert, his appetite increases, and diuresis begins. The major

metabolic alterations of the acute injury phase are reversed. The "turning point" phase then passes into an anabolic phase. In this phase the patient experiences a further gain in appetite, gains strength, increases activity, and has a return of sexual function. A positive nitrogen balance continues until the nitrogen losses are restored. The anabolic phase lasts for about 2 to 3 weeks, during which time lean muscle mass is restored. The last phase is characterized by a gain in fat.

There are two chief ways to design surgical care based on these predictable responses to injury. One approach is to alter responses that seem to be at odds with attempts to help patients recover from injury. Excessive amounts of edema, for example can be reduced by appropriate use of corticosteroids. But, there are other responses that are not modified to any appreciable extent by active treatment. The negative nitrogen balance that follows injury has resisted, with some success, numerous efforts to reverse it. A second and more common way to utilize knowledge of the response to injury is to design therapy to work in concert with these changes. Knowing that for about 2 days after an operation there is significant water and sodium retention is obviously useful in administering intravenous fluids properly during this period. Another factor concerns the severalfold rise in corticosteroid production after an injury (Fig. 1-4). Blood levels become elevated almost immediately and persist for 2 to 3 days after an operation of mild to moderate severity. However, when the adrenal-pituitary axis has been suppressed by the long-term use of corticosteroids, the patient's adrenal gland is unable to respond to increased demands for several months after cessation of steroid therapy. Extraction of teeth in such a patient requires replacement therapy during this period of increased corticosteroid need to avoid the profound shock and death that otherwise can occur. A final factor concerns diet. During the acute injury phase, diet, in contrast to fluid balance, is relatively unimportant. The body shifts to a catabolic state for production of energy during this transient phase of starvation. With the later anabolic phase, however, diet assumes a key role. A nutritious diet rich in protein and calories is needed for restoration of lean muscle mass.

Management of wounds is a fundamental skill of the surgeon. Wounds, like the body, respond in a predictable manner. While the general status of a patient clearly has an influence on wound response, more often local factors are the major determinants. Nonetheless, a fairly serious derangement of a patient's health can affect the wound response perceptibly. Such factors as poor nutritional status can retard wound healing. In the scorbutic individual, for example, wounds heal poorly and have little tensile strength.

For the majority of patients, the manner in which wounds are made and cared for largely determines how they heal. Even in patients in whom the wound is appreciably influenced by their general status, good operative technique and postoperative care permit optimal healing under the circumstances.

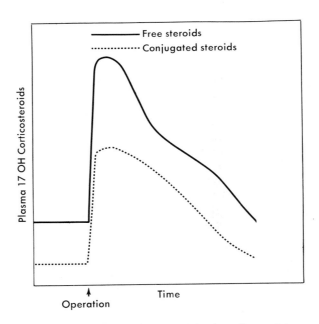

Fig. 1-4. Rise in corticosteroid production after an injury.

Understanding how different wounds heal is important in planning wound management. An open, soft tissue wound, for example, displays remarkable contraction during healing. The epithelial edges move toward one another with marked diminution in size of a wound scar (Fig. 1-5). This contracture phenomenon can virtually eliminate a sulcus created by a vestibuloplasty procedure that leaves an open wound. The contracture is especially great on the labial side of the mandible but can be inhibited by several methods. One of the most effective ways is to cover the raw surface with an epithelial graft, especially a full-thickness graft (Fig. 1-6). In fact, truly effective vestibuloplasty techniques did not evolve until these methods guided development of the operative procedures.

After the wound has been closed, the care

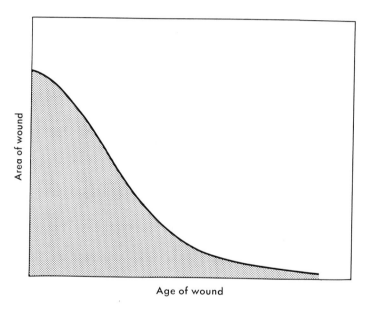

Fig. 1-5. Wound contraction during healing.

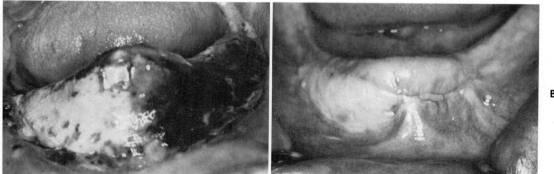

Fig. 1-6. A, Wound on the labial side of the mandible at 1 week. A palatal graft covers right half of wound. **B,** Same wound at 4 weeks. Note prevention of wound contracture by palatal graft (patient's right) and marked contraction of nongraft-covered wound (patient's left).

administered until healing has progressed to a scar can greatly influence the course of events. The dressing of wounds and timing of removal of drains or sutures influence the rate of healing as well as the nature of the ultimate scar. For example, improper dressing care that allows a secondary wound infection delays healing and creates a more prominent scar. Immobilization of wounds, such as by use of a stent or sutures for graft immobilization in vestibuloplasty procedures, is another instance in which the predictable response of a wound is utilized in planning for optimal care.

SUMMARY

Surgical principles can be grouped into three major areas: asepsis, the analytical approach to surgical care, and the formulation of surgical care based on the response of the body to injury. The best surgeons not only base surgical therapy on these principles but leaven them with a generous portion of humane, compassionate concern for the patient.

REFERENCES

1. Billingham, R. E., and Russell, P. S.: Studies on wound healing, with special reference to contracture in experimental wounds in rabbit's skin, Ann. Surg. **144:**961, 1956.
2. Donoff, R. B.: Biological basis for vestibuloplasty procedures, J. Oral Surg. **34:**890, 1976.
3. Sabiston, D. C., Jr., editor: Textbook of surgery, ed. 10, Philadelphia, 1972, W. B. Saunders Co., pp. 1-424.
4. Skillman, J. J., Lauler, D. P., Hickler, R. B., Lyons, J. H., Olson, J. E., Ball, M. R., and Moore, F. D.: Hemorrhage in normal man, Ann. Surg. **166:**865, 1967.
5. Smith, L. L., Steenburg, R. W., Gruber, U. F., Kaalstad, A. J., and Moore, F. D.: The effect of testosterone on corticosteroids in surgical trauma: studies in man, J. Clin. Endocrinol. **20:**919, 1960.
6. Weed, L. L.: Medical records, medical education, and patient care, Cleveland, 1970, Year Book Medical Publishers, Inc., pp. 3-60.

CHAPTER 2

Principles of surgical technique

Theodore A. Lesney

STERILIZATION OF ARMAMENTARIUM
Introduction

The prevention of infection is surely the mandatory requirement of surgical practice and is thereby foundational in the establishment of sound surgical techniques. Infection control is certainly not limited to the sterilization of instruments, supplies, and accessories alone or to the establishment of good dressing-changing routines in the clinic or in professional office practice. Equally important is an awareness of the need for reduction of pathogens in the general environment, and, of course, the responsible surgeon is ever-alert to the need for preventing cross infection among circulating personnel, reducing microbes in room air, and eliminating human error and carelessness that tends to break down the chain of asepsis.

Currently physical technology continues to remain preferable to chemical methods for the sterilization of armamentarium and supplies. Moist heat is still the most reliable and least expensive means for destroying undesirable microbes. There are other, less effective, physical methods than steam, such as filtration, irradiation, and ultrasonics, but these are generally employed where the application of saturated steam is not feasible.

In the field of sterilization some hard facts important for the student of surgery to understand should be quickly established. For one thing, the rhetoric used must not be confusing or compromising. So, it is hereby agreed that sterilization shall mean the total destruction of microbial and viral life. Terms that are often related to sterilization, such as sanitation, antisepsis, and disinfection, must be clearly recognized as representing conditions *less than sterile* that thereby fail to meet the total requirements of sterility. As a basic principle of asepsis, there can be only one form of sterilization, the complete destruction of pathogens.

Textbook rhetoric permits the use of some commonly accepted suffixes such as ''cide'' and ''stat'', to name only two. These suggest a varying effect on the life cycle of microbes. For instance, a bactericide destroys bacteria but a bacteriostat only inhibits its growth. Similarly, a virucide kills virus, a fungistat slows the growth of fungus, and so on. Spore-forming pathogens provide the ultimate test for efficacy of sterilization practices, and, in this regard, saturated steam has proved to be the most practical, the most economical, and the most currently effective sporicide.

Principles of sterilization

The basic fundamentals of sterilization procedures will be briefly discussed to ensure that requirements of undergraduate education are fulfilled. The fact remains that today one rarely sees a boiling-water sterilizer or a dry-heat oven in operation on a ward or in the clinic. Presterilized, single-use disposables have largely eliminated the need for this equipment. Also, gas sterilization such as with ethylene oxide is being used on a progressively limited basis. Nevertheless, these are tried and proved techniques that have prevailed over the years and will continue to remain reliable until supplanted by better methods in the progressive evolution of medical technology.

Autoclaving. Autoclaving is the preferred method of sterilization and the most reasonably certain to destroy resistant spore-formers and fungus. It provides moist heat in the form of saturated steam under pressure. This combination of moisture and heat provides the bacteria-destroying power currently most effective against all forms of microorganisms. Instruments and materials for sterilizing in the autoclave are usually enclosed in muslin wrappers as surgical packs. Muslin for this purpose is purchased most economically in bolt lots and cut to desired size. It is used in double thickness, and each surgical pack is marked as to contents and date of sterilization.

Paper is now apparently supplanting muslin for wrapping surgical packs. Several manufacturers are producing various types of paper wrappers. These papers have clothlike handling properties and present several advantages over muslin. They are less porous than muslin and thereby are less likely to be penetrated by dust and microorganisms. However, they are sufficiently porous to permit required steam penetration under pressure. Crepe papers are currently in favor; they have some degree of elasticity and can be reused several times. Sterility under adequate paper wrapping appears to be effective for periods of 2 to 4 weeks' shelf life. This compares favorably with muslin-wrapped surgical packs.

Autoclaving time will vary directly with the size of the surgical pack. The smaller packs used for oral surgery usually require 30 minutes at 121° C under 1.40 kg^2 of pressure. Various sterilization indicators can be inserted into a pack to provide evidence that adequate steam penetration has been effected. Rubber gloves are more fragile than linens and most instruments. They are sterilized effectively after 15 minutes under 1.05 kg^2 of pressure at 121° C.

Boiling-water sterilization. Ordinarily boiling-water sterilizers do not reach a temperature level above 100° C. Some of the heat-resistant bacterial spores may survive this temperature for prolonged periods of time. On the other hand, steam under 1.05 to 1.40 kg^2 of pressure will attain a temperature of 121° C, and most authorities concur that no living thing can survive 10 to 15 minutes' direct exposure to such saturated steam at that temperature. If boiling-water sterilization must be used, it is recommended that chemical means be employed to elevate the boiling point of water and thereby increase its bactericidal efficiency. A 2% solution of sodium carbonate will serve this purpose. Sixty milliliters of sodium carbonate per gallon of distilled water will make a 2% solution. This alkalinized distilled water reduces the required sterilization time and the oxygen content of the water as well, thereby reducing the corrosive action on the instruments.

Dry-heat sterilization. Sterilization in dry-heat ovens at elevated temperatures for long periods of time is widely used in dentistry and oral surgery. This technique provides a means for sterilizing instruments, powders, oils (petrolatums), bone wax, and other items that do not lend themselves to sterilization by means of boiling water or steam under pressure. Dry heat will not attack glass and will not cause rusting. Furthermore, the ovens have additional uses in dentistry, such as baking out and curing plastic pontics and other applications. The general design of the ovens permits a heating range between 100° and 200° C. Overnight sterilization in excess of

6 hours at 121° C is widely employed. Adequate sterilization of small loads is attained at 170° C for 1 hour. Manufacturers of dry-heat sterilizers provide detailed instructions for their effective use. The major disadvantage of dry-heat sterilization obviously is the long periods of time required to ensure bactericidal results.

Cold sterilization. None of the chemicals used for cold sterilization satisfactorily meets all of the requirements for true sterilization. Alcohol is expensive; it evaporates readily and also rusts instruments. The widely used benzalkonium chloride, 1:1,000 solution, requires an antirust additive (sodium nitrate) and long periods of immersion (18 hours). The more recently introduced cold-sterilizing chemicals employ hexachlorophene compounds as the active base. These chemicals claim adequate sterilization of heat-sensitive instruments in 3 hours. Fundamentally, most of the cold sterilizing media that may be safely used probably kill vegetative bacteria, but there is doubt of their effectiveness against spores and fungus.

Gas sterilization. The limitations of chemical solution sterilization techniques have made is necessary to exploit other methods for sterilizing the heat-sensitive or water-sensitive armamentarium. One of these methods employs a gas, ethylene oxide, which has proved to be bactericidal when used in accordance with controlled environmental conditions of temperature and humidity as well as an adequate concentration of the gas for a prescribed period of sterilizing exposure. Ethylene oxide sterilizers are currently manufactured in varied sizes from the small portable table model (chamber measuring about 7.5 cm in diameter), to the large, built-in, stationary apparatus found in many hospitals. Smaller chambers use gas that is provided from convenient metal cartridges. The large, built-in sterilizers are hooked up to multi-liter tanks.

The relatively high cost of using ethylene oxide sterilizers frequently results in their being used only once or twice per day, more often for overnight sterilization of a capacity load. A hermetically sealed apparatus is necessary to economically ensure the retention of the expensive gas at its most effective concentration for a prolonged period of time ranging from 2 to 12 hours. Since ethylene oxide is highly diffusible, it requires a containing apparatus of precise manufacturing detail.

Under arid conditions, desiccated microorganisms are known to resist the bactericidal effectiveness of ethylene oxide. Therefore the relative humidity within the sterilizing chamber should be controlled at an optimum of 40% to 50%. Also the efficiency of the gas sterilizer is reduced directly by temperature drops below 22° C.

In general, gas sterilization as currently employed in ethylene oxide techniques does indeed fill a necessary void in presently available sterilization practices, but its shortcomings dictate the urgent need for better and less expensive methods.

Sterilization of supplies on industry-wide level

Our expanding population and the successful practice of geriatrics have greatly increased the demand for more medical services. Although the construction of hospitals to meet this demand has been slow, and the training of medical personnel has been even slower, it is encouraging to observe the notable achievements of the pharmaceutical and hospital industry in the mass production of medical supplies. One major achievement concerns the development and profession-wide acceptance of sterile disposable (single use) items. There are now so many disposable products in daily use that space precludes their individual discussion. Another achievement involves automation in manufacture, processing, sterilization, and packaging on an industrial scale. It is the *sterilization* of disposables and other mass-produced medical supplies that shall be discussed.

Modern manufacturing methods for medical supplies and their marketing have pointed out the shortcomings of former sterilization practices when applied to this industry. Although formerly heat, steam, gas, and bactericidal solutions were the only widely accepted means for sterilization, these methods could not be adapted to current mass production and marketing techniques. Many supplies, containers, illustrations, and enclosed printed matter could not withstand these sterilization procedures. The hermetic sealing of products and packages was impossible, since asepsis was dependent on permeation by heat, steam, gas, or bactericidal solutions. Heat-sensitive and water-sensitive equipment and supplies required special handling that was inadaptable to mass-production practices.

Recently a radical change has been instituted in sterilization procedures for manufactured and packaged medical supplies. The change has been expensive but effective. Its success in industry has focused the attention of the professions on some of the rather archaic sterilization techniques. Briefly, the improved sterilization techniques employ ionizing radiation. The pharmaceutical and hospital industries are credited with developing, at considerable expense, a successful radiation sterilization technology. The military establishment of the federal government has also played a major role with its studies of irradiation sterilization of foodstuffs for preservation purposes. Both groups have contributed knowledge and standardization of irradiation techniques to the degree that now permits the safe and efficient use of gamma rays and accelerated beta rays on the wide scale employed in food and drug technology. The manufacturer is now able to package the product in a variety of containers that could not be used with previous sterilization methods. Directions, legends, illustrations, and heat-sensitive and water-sensitive materials can be included and yet meet the professions' requirements of sterilization. As a matter of fact, in much of the industry the contents are packaged for final shipment before they are run through an irradiation building on a conveyor-belt system for the efficient sterilization of the entire shipping container and its contents.

Radiation sources. Ionizing radiation for sterilization as currently practiced is available from two sources: (1) machines of low energy but high output (electron accelerators) and (2) radioisotopes. The machines convert the electron output in a manner somewhat comparable to the output of an x-ray machine but with a higher potential of several kilowatts beyond x-ray output. Of the isotopes, cobalt-60 and cesium-137 emit the highly penetrating gamma rays. At the present time, isotopes are more widely used. However, electron accelerators (machines) have a number of advantages, and it is expected that they will ultimately supplant radioisotopes for these purposes.

Insight into current sterilization practices strongly suggests the need for improving the methods presently employed in the hospital and in the clinic. As previously indicated, the pharmaceutical industry is spending much time and money in furthering the use of radiation sources for sterilization of a wide array of products. Certainly irradiation is currently an expensive process. The capital investment and operating costs are beyond the scope of small institutions and private practice. But the overwhelming advantages of radiation sterilization dictate the continued exploitation of this field until it can be made available on a wide scale to the professions as well as to industry.

The presentation of this subject matter has been oversimplified. For this reason the discussions of Artandi[1] and Olander[5] are recommended for a more detailed and authoritative review of the technological aspects of radiation for sterilization.

General observations

1. Oils and grease are the major enemies of sterilization. Instruments exposed to oils should be wiped with a solvent and then

vigorously scrubbed in soap and water before being put through a sterilizing procedure.

2. When instruments are completely immersed in boiling water, they will not rust because dissolved oxygen is driven out of the solution by the heat and is no longer available for corrosion. However, if wet instruments are exposed to air for any considerable period of time, rusting will occur. After boiling-water sterilization, instruments should be dried with a sterile towel while they are still hot.

3. Instruments with movable joints will require much less oiling if sterilized by autoclave rather than by boiling. This is especially true if tap water is used in the sterilizer since such water has a high concentration of lime salts, which are deposited on the instruments in boiling.

4. Particular precautions must be exerted for the adequate sterilization of hypodermic needles and syringes. Injections with contaminated equipment may produce latent symptoms. With slow-incubating infections such as hepatitis, the infected patient may become jaundiced months after the injection. It is particularly recommended that hypodermic syringes and needles be sterilized preferably by autoclaving or by boiling water. Effectiveness of cold sterilization is always doubtful.

Currently almost all injectables are prepackaged as sterile, unit-dosing, single-use disposables. The closed-injection system is usually employed as a sterile, cartridge-needle unit. The injectable is accurately premeasured and identified as to contents, dosage, and expiration date. Since it is completely disposable after use, all risk of cross contamination is eliminated.

5. Instruments are best stored in autoclaved muslin or paper packs. If unused, these packs should be reautoclaved every 30 days unless there is a good reason for resterilization prior to that time.

6. Instrument packs should be organized in case pans so that the necessary instruments are included for routine procedures.

Instruments can be removed from the pack and arranged on a tray, such as a Mayo tray or a dental bracket table. To this arrangement can be added any additional instruments required to meet the needs of a special situation. An unscrubbed assistant should handle sterile instruments only with a sterile pick-up forceps that is kept constantly in a container of cold-sterilizing solution.

Comment

Currently notable achievements are being made in the better aseptic control of the entire hospital environment, including operating rooms, clinics, and supporting services. For example, successful efforts are being made to control the direction of flow, the temperature, and the purity of the air circulated through the surgical operatories. Filterable microorganisms are removed, and the temperature of the air is adjusted before it is permitted to flow at a measured rate in a predetermined direction. Furthermore, environmental technology has produced systems for air conditioning, heating, lighting, and ventilating many important patient-care centers of the hospital. This local environment is electronically monitored by means of computer (or minicomputer) control. Medical technology continues to strive for a goal of "germ-free" surfaces—and "germ-free" atmospheres—in surgical operating suites, acute-care units, and intensive-care centers. Progress in attaining these goals is slowed by the high cost of sophisticated equipment and the rapid obsolescence of this equipment occasioned by the accelerating rate of technological change.

Postoperative infection receives the constant vigilance of staff medical and nursing care. Dressings are changed, with strict adherence to aseptic principles. Resistant infections are identified and subjected to vigorous treatment when indicated, sometimes employing isolation of the patient or total bed rest or both. Infection committees composed of cognizant staff personnel are organized to ensure the proper care and disposition of unusual, acute, or persistent infections.

The central supply service must keep fully informed of the latest and best developments in the area of sterilization techniques so that there may be no doubt about the sterility of materials and equipment requested. Dietetics, food services, the many laboratories, and even the general overall housekeeping of the hospital environment require a thoughtful discipline and a constant surveillance in the maintenance of aseptic control.

METRIC SYSTEM CONVERSION

At this point it may be appropriate to recognize the national commitment to converting all mathematical data to metric terms. All pertinent measurements in the text will henceforth be written in metric terms. In the medical and dental professions this turnover from the United States' system to universal metrics will be easier than in other, unrelated areas because large, component parts, such as pharmacology, radiology, and pathology, have been using metric terms in their readings for a long time. Like pharmaceuticals, body fluids have also been measured in metric form. Nevertheless, the general conversion process may be slowed somewhat by the economic impracticability of replacing good-functioning, major pieces of equipment, such as steam gauges, pressure valves, and thermometers, just because they are not calibrated in metrics. However, cooperative manufacturers can speed the process of equipment conversion by providing recalibrated dials that can be pasted or otherwise inserted over now outdated dials.

In addition to metric changes, a better recording of time is also being effected and henceforth only the 24-hour clock will be universally employed. This change also requires only a new dial and not a new clock. During the conversion period, when everybody is trying to use Celsius in lieu of Fahrenheit and kilograms per square centimeter rather than pounds per square inch, the student may find some need for conversion calculations. The most important of the metric measurements will be concerned with weight, linear measurements, temperature, and time.

Simple conversion data

A. To change Fahrenheit to Celsius (centigrade)
Subtract 32 from Fahrenheit and multiply by $\frac{5}{9}$
Subtract 32 from Fahrenheit and divide by 1.8

B. To change Celsius to Fahrenheit
Multiply Celsius by $\frac{9}{5}$ and add 32
Multiply Celsius by 1.8 and add 32
Double the Celsius figure, subtract 10% of the total, and add 32

C. Linear comparisons
0.3937 inches	= 1 centimeter (cm)
1.0 inch	= 2.54 cm
1.0 foot	= 30.48 cm
39.37 inches	= 1.0 meter (m)
0.621 (or $\frac{5}{8}$) mile	= 1.0 kilometer (km)

To change kilometers to miles, multiply kilometers by 6 and divide by 10.

D. Weight comparisons
1.0 ounce	= 28.35 grams (gm)
1.0 pound	= 453.5 gm
2.2 pounds	= 1.0 kilogram (kg) or 1,000 gm

E. Volume comparisons
1.0 quart	= 0.9468 liters (l) (1.0 l = 1,000 cubic centimeters [cc] or 1,000 milliliters [ml])
1.056 quarts	= 1.0 liter
1.0 gallon	= 3.78 liter

OPERATING ROOM DECORUM

The work of Lister has proved conclusively the role played by bacteria in wound infection. It is now mandatory in all surgery, including oral surgery, that all intelligent, precautionary measures be taken to avoid the contamination of wounds.

Although the means for providing strictly aseptic mouth surgery are still unavailable, this is no reason for completely abandoning an aseptic routine. At the very least an aseptic routine for mouth surgery markedly eliminates some of the pathways of cross infection: the infection of the doctor from the patient, the infection of the patient from the doctor, or the infection of the patient from another patient through the doctor or through the contaminated armamentarium employed by the doctor. It has long been established that surgical wounds are contaminated chiefly from microorganisms harbored in the skin or mucous membranes that have been incised. Furthermore, the oral cavity is a normal breeding ground for a wide assortment of microorganisms. The noses, throats, and hands of the *operating team* are the next most common source of wound infection. Unsterile instruments and supplies follow in order of frequency. For the latter there is no excuse.

Complete asepsis in surgery may well be an ideal that is never fully attained. There may always be some doubt regarding the sterility of the skin or the mucous membranes to be incised. The air contamination of wounds is an omnipresent problem. But if wound infection in surgery is to be minimized, all logical precautions and preparations must be instituted. This should include the proper preparation of the operating team as well as the patient. Wherever surgery is done, in the hospital operating room or in the clinic, the surgeon wears a face mask of four-ply, fine-meshed gauze and a surgical helmet of linen or cloth such as the stockinette used under plaster casts. However, here as elsewhere throughout the hospital, paper is gaining favor over cloth for disposable face masks, headgear, and surgical gowns. The surgeon's hands are adequately scrubbed. Presently, highly detergent soaps containing hexachlorophene are commonly utilized in prescribed scrub techniques. Sterile gloves are employed for all surgery, and these, like sterile sheets, wraps, towels, and so on, serve bacteriologically to isolate the doctor from the patient.

Scrub technique

1. Street clothes are replaced with a scrub suit (Fig. 2-1, A). This consists of clean linen trousers and a short-sleeved blouse. In the operating room where static electricity may be a complicating problem, the surgical personnel wear appropriate conductive footwear. Each shoe has a sole and heel of conductive rubber or conductive leather or equivalent material. Such shoes have metal electrodes fabricated into the inner soles so that conductive contact is maintained with the stockinged foot.

2. It is necessary to stress that hair and hairy areas are extremely difficult to sterilize. This is the chief reason for preoperative shaving of surgical sites. Medical and paramedical personnel circulating throughout an operating room are an alarming source of infection. Along with many other precautions, the hair of these personnel must be adequately covered. Changing hair styles, such as fashionable long hair, flowing beards, and grandiose mustaches, have indeed compounded the problem of cross contamination in the operating room. Surgical helmets and face masks are becoming larger and less comfortable in the effort to adequately cover head and facial hair. One of these helmets is currently dubbed the "Lawrence of Arabia" helmet because it vaguely resembles the head and face wrappings that this legendary figure employed to protect himself against wind-blown sand. Such necessary full coverage of long hair and beards is most uncomfortable during prolonged and difficult procedures. Slits in these helmets must be cut for the ears when eyeglasses are to be worn or a stethoscope must be used.

In passing, a long-standing, unwritten rule can be repeated over and over again: "Sneezing and coughing are simply *not* permitted in the operating room."

3. The surgical scrubbing is carried out in the manner prescribed for major surgery. The hands and forearms are scrubbed to the elbows with brush and soap (or hexachlorophene detergents) and water according to prescribed plan. At many hospitals the recommended scrub technique is posted directly over the scrub sinks (Fig. 2-1, B). Two-minute scrubs between operations may be acceptable. However, numerous hospitals frown on any scrub technique

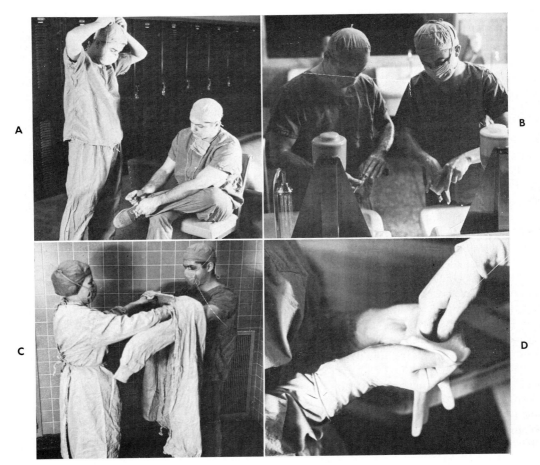

Fig. 2-1. A, Typical scrub suit attire. **B,** Scrub technique is in accordance with instructions usually posted over the scrub sink. **C,** The doctor is helped into the sterile gown by a scrubbed assistant. **D,** The doctor is helped into the gloves so that only the interior of the gloves is touched by the hand.

requiring less than 10 minutes. During the scrub, fingernails must be adequately cleansed. Sterile orangewood sticks are conveniently provided for this purpose. If nondetergent soap is used for the scrub, a longer scrub period is required, and a postscrub rinse with a low–surface tension antiseptic such as alcohol or Septisol is recommended.

4. The hands are dried in the operating room with a sterile hand towel. At this stage the hands are considered surgically clean but *not sterile*.

5. The surgeon is helped into the sterile

gown by a properly gowned and gloved surgical assistant (Fig. 2-1, *C*). A circulating assistant secures the gown ties at the surgeon's back. The surgeon's back as well as the gown below the level of the waist are considered *unsterile* (Fig. 2-1, *E*).

6. The surgeon is helped into the gloves in such a manner that *only the interior* of the gloves is touched by the hands (Fig. 2-1, *D*). The exterior and not the interior of the rubber glove is considered sterile.

Only a minimal amount of dusting agent is permitted in preparing the hands for the wearing of rubber gloves. Modified starch

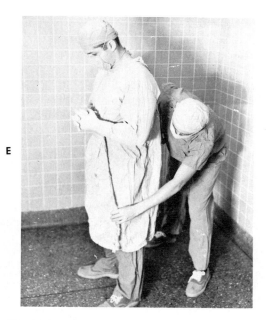

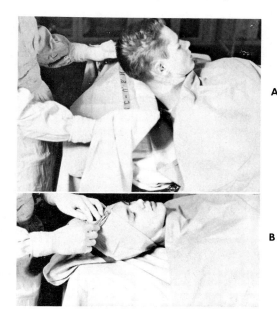

Fig. 2-1, cont'd. E, The entire back of the surgeon's gown and also that portion of the front of the gown below the level of the surgical table will be considered unsterile. (Official U. S. Navy photograph.)

Fig. 2-2. A, A drape and a hand towel are combined for wrapping the patient. Double hand towels may be similarly used. **B,** Towels and drapes are secured by clipping. (Official U. S. Navy photograph.)

powder has replaced talcum as the dusting agent of choice. However, sterile creams are being used for this purpose more than dusting agents. In the surgery of open wounds consideration must be given to the irritating, granuloma-producing propensity of foreign materials, such as talcum, starch, and creams, when used in excessive amounts and when inadvertently introduced into the wound.

Sterile isolation is provided only through the wearing of gloves. Sterile gloves are employed for the protection of the patient and the doctor. The dangers of cross infection make it imperative for the professional worker to wear gloves whenever the blood, tissue fluids, or saliva is contacted. Tuberculosis thrives in oral fluids. Serum hepatitis may be present in the blood of asymptomatic patients.

Isolation of patient from operating team

1. The site of incision is prepared. The operative field is cleansed by scrubbing with detergent soap, rinsing, and then painting with a suitable antiseptic.

2. The patient is further isolated from the doctor by means of sterile drapings of cloth or clothlike materials. The initial drape may be a single-thickness draw sheet measuring approximately 115 by 180 cm. A second drape called a front sheet, measuring about 115 by 175 cm, completes the major isolation (Fig. 2-2, *A*).

3. The patient's head is wrapped with a double-sheet technique, using a drape as the lower sheet and a hand towel as the upper sheet (Fig. 2-2, *A*).

4. Sterile drapings are secured with towel clips (Fig. 2-2, *B*). In some oral surgical problems requiring the manipulation of the patient's head from side to side, it is good practice to suture to the skin those sterile drapings outlining the periphery of the incision.

5. The anesthetist and his or her equipment are isolated from the operating team by a drape-covered screen.

6. Only that field above the level of the surgical table is considered sterile. Hands, equipment, and supplies lowered below the level of the surgical table are considered as having been contaminated.

7. Organization is such that once the surgeon has completed the scrub, put on sterile gloves, and draped the patient, it will be unnecessary to break scrub to obtain needed items.

8. It is important at this point to establish that a gown, drape, or covering is considered to be *contaminated when wet* unless the gown, drape, or covering is made of waterproof material or otherwise backed by a waterproof lining or sheathing.

Modifications of aseptic routine for office practice of oral surgery

One school of thought will insist that there can be no compromise with the aseptic measures employed in surgery. Another group may insist that a rigid aseptic technique is not practical in a busy office practice dealing with minor oral surgery in a large volume of patients. The fact remains that infection does not differentiate minor from major surgery, large numbers from small numbers of patients, or short operations from long operations.

It is generally believed that the reason for the relatively low incidence of oral infection after surgical procedures within the mouth can be traced directly to "man's acquired tolerance for his own microorganisms." No doubt these same organisms transmitted to another individual in cross infection are likely to result in virulent infection. In other words, man can tolerate his own organisms better than he can somebody else's. This fundamentally proper concept justifies the need for aseptic technique in surgical areas that defy complete bacterial sterilization, areas such as the mouth, the nasal and antral cavities, and the digestive and urinary tracts.

Despite the care that the operator may exert in preparing himself or herself, the instruments, the supplies, and the patient for oral surgery, the danger of cross infection is omnipresent. All reasonably intelligent efforts at limiting this danger of infection are the least that the patient should expect from the doctor.

Much of the operating room decorum employed for major surgery is within practical limits for oral surgical procedures. In the hospital operating room the level of the surgical table is the line of demarcation for asepsis. In the dental clinic the level of the armrests of the dental chair might be considered as a similar line of demarcation. Everything above the armrests should be subject to aseptic requirements.

The perioral facial skin should be as carefully prepared as the mucosa directly involved in surgery. This can be conveniently done by asking the patient to wash the face with detergent hexachlorophene provided in the washroom. Then a colorless, nonirritating antiseptic is applied to the perioral skin as well as to the mucosa. The patient's mouth is lavaged with a pleasant-tasting antiseptic solution, and the immediate area of the needle puncture or incision is painted with an antiseptic having staining qualities so that the area for surgery is clearly visualized as having been antiseptically prepared.

The patient's hair may be enclosed in a sterile wrapping such as that employing double hand towels.

Most patients are highly pleased with any extra effort that the doctor may choose to employ in assuring a safer operation (Figs. 2-3, *A* and *B*). Many patients prefer that the doctor's hands be gloved before they invade the mouth. In short-duration large-volume surgery, rubber gloves need *not* be changed for each patient. Instead the gloved hands may be scrubbed between patients, using a 2-minute scrub technique with detergent hexachlorophene soaps (Fig. 2-3, *C*). The difficulty with this method is that the rubber gloves, when washed and dried in this manner, become "tacky" and thereby somewhat difficult to use unless used wet.

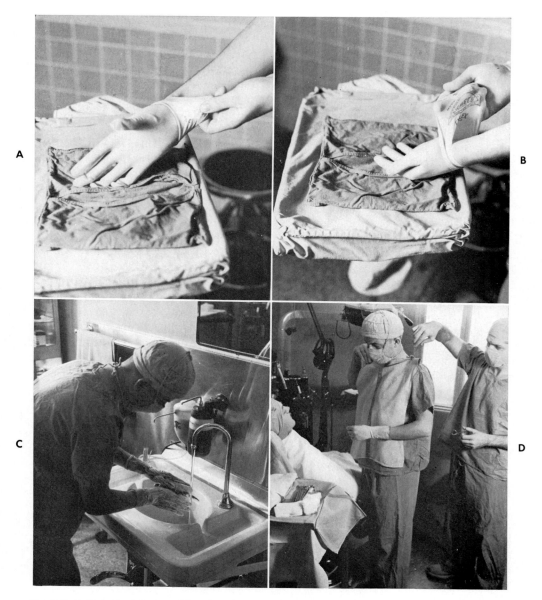

Fig. 2-3. A, Only the interior of the glove is touched by the bare hands. **B,** The sterile gloves may touch each other on their exterior surfaces. **C,** In large-volume, short-duration mouth surgery, it may be permissible to employ 2-minute scrub of the gloved hands between patients. This is in lieu of changing gloves for each patient. **D,** In office practice, a sterile hand towel is often used for isolating the surgeon's attire from the patient's draping. (Official U. S. Navy photograph.)

Surgical caps and masks need not be changed for each operation. The surgeon's gown can be isolated from the sterile sheets over the patient by clamping a sterile hand towel over that portion of the surgeon's gown contacting the patient's sterile coverings (Fig. 2-3, *D*). Uninformed patients and some doctors will oppose such recommendations concerning the need for sterile approach to so-called minor surgery in the mouth. But less than a hundred years ago there was similar opposition to the doctor who "fussed so much" washing his hands preparatory to surgery—and then proceeded to turn up the contaminated sleeves of his frock coat before reaching for the scalpel. In those days, "laudable pus" was erroneously accepted as a necessary sequel to surgery. There can be no justification whatsoever for permitting the "laudable pus" concept in oral surgery today.

Disposable (single-use) materials and equipment

Modern manufacturing, sterilizing, and packaging techniques are currently providing an ever-wider array of supplies conveniently packaged for single use and disposal thereafter. In many instances the increasing cost of labor in the multiple handling of reusable hospital supplies has resulted in making the use of disposables a more economical practice.

Paper and similar man-made fibers are replacing woven cloth for sheeting, drapes, toweling and similar supplies. Operating room gowns, scrub suits, lap sheets, stand covers, and surgical wrappings are now available in sterile, ready-to-use packages conveniently and economically disposable after single usage (Fig. 2-4). Seamless disposable latex gloves that can be placed on surgically scrubbed hands without the need of dusting powders or creams are now being used in many hospitals and clinics.

Hypodermic needles, syringes, and plastic collection tubes and containers for biological specimens are currently packaged as disposables. Intravenous techniques including those concerned with the collection and infusion of blood and administration of drug and fluid therapy are largely accomplished with disposable plastic supplies and equipment. Almost every department of the hospital or clinic concerned with dispensing professional care seems to be using more and more of the increasingly available disposables. Furthermore, improved packaging techniques have made disposables more reliable and more desirable. Sterility of the contents is better ensured by sequence wrapping and action folding. The package can be clearly marked in bold-faced type and color coded to facilitate differentiation or storage. The potential for single-use supplies seems limitless.

Of course, the more disposables used within an activity, the more an increased adequate storage area is required for supplies with such a rapid turnover.

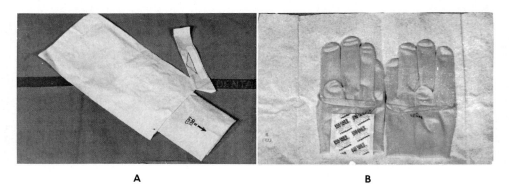

A   **B**

Fig. 2-4. A, Sterile, disposable latex surgeon's gloves are packaged in exterior and interior paper wrappings to permit usage under aseptic conditions. **B,** A packet of dusting powder or cream is included with the cuff-turned gloves enclosed in the sterile interior wrapping. Sterilization is by irradiation.

Some fundamental precautions with gaseous mixtures in operating rooms

The following anesthetic agents are considered combustible, and precautionary procedures must be employed in their administration: (1) cyclopropane, (2) divinyl ether (Vinethene), (3) ethyl ether, (4) ethyl chloride, and (5) ethylene. An explosion in an operating room is indeed a dramatic hazard, and unfortunately, like the automobile or airplane accident, it is classified as "something that happens to somebody else." As a regular operating room routine, the following precautionary measures are employed:

1. Modern operating rooms are built with conductive flooring. Operating room personnel and visitors must wear conductive footwear. Such shoes are usually made with conductive rubber or conductive leather soles and heels. They contain stainless steel conductors built into the inner sole so that frictional static electricity may be grounded and sparking avoided. Other floor-contacting devices are employed to ground equipment used in the vicinity of explosive, gaseous mixtures.

2. Wool, silk, and synthetic textures are known to produce electrical charge when subjected to friction. For this reason no woolen blankets and silk or nylon garments are permitted in the operating rooms.

3. Electrical equipment and anesthetic and other apparatus commonly used in the presence of combustible gases must be periodically examined to assure freedom from any defect that might emit spark in the presence of explosive mixtures.

4. Electrocautery, electrocoagulation, and other equipment employing open spark are of course not permitted in the vicinity of combustible gases.

Oxygen cylinders

Ordinarily oxygen is not considered an explosive agent, but it does support combustion, and thereby it may be considered as secondarily contributory to explosion. Some basic precautions must be taken with the care of oxygen cylinders[7]:

1. Fundamentally, oils, greases, and lubricants may be highly combustible with oxygen. Therefore their proximity to oxygen must be avoided. Regulators, gauges,

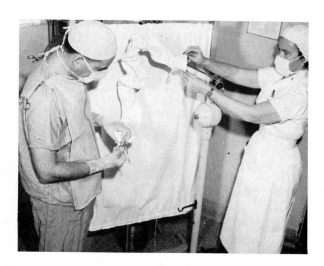

Fig. 2-5. The cable and extensions from the portable dental engine are covered with a sterile sleeve for operating room procedures. (Official U. S. Navy photograph.)

and other fittings on oxygen cylinders must not be lubricated when the cylinder contains the gas under pressure.

2. Oxygen cylinders must not be handled with oily hands or greasy gloves or rags.

3. Before applying fittings to the cylinder, clear the duct opening by allowing a momentary escape of gas.

4. Open the high-pressure valve on the cylinder *before* bringing the oxygen apparatus to the patient. Open this valve slowly and take common precautionary measures concerned with unexpected explosion.

5. Avoid covering the oxygen cylinder with gowns, linens, or other equipment that may serve to contain leaking gas.

6. Never use oxygen from a cylinder that does not have a pressure-reducing regulator.

7. Do not attempt to repair any attachments on a cylinder containing oxygen under pressure.

BASIC ORAL SURGERY
Incision

The efficient employment of a scalpel requires a basic knowledge of convenient fulcrum points already taught the dental surgeon during instruction in the use of motor-driven instruments within the mouth. The scalpel is gripped firmly but lightly in any one of several grasps. It should not be grasped too rigidly or in such a manner as to produce digital tremors and otherwise influence the unrestricted movement that is required in producing a clean, atraumatic incision or both.

Two scalpel grasps that are most commonly employed in oral surgery are illustrated in Fig. 2-6. The "pen grasp," in which the handle of the blade is engaged between the thumb and first two fingers, is favored for the delicate short strokes frequently required for intraoral surgery (Fig. 2-6, *A*).

Skin is more difficult to incise than mucosal tissue, and the steady pressure required for such cutting may be better obtained by grasping the scalpel in the "table-knife" manner illustrated in Fig. 2-6, *B*.

The choice between one scalpel grasp and another becomes a matter of individual preference. It is more important that an

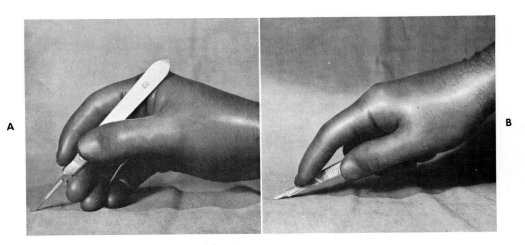

Fig. 2-6. A, The "pen grasp," commonly used in oral surgery, permits the grasping of the scalpel handle between the thumb and first two fingers. The third and fourth fingers provide a rest position (fulcrum) on a firm base from which short, deft, incising strokes may be safely instituted. **B,** The "table-knife" grasp permits the thumb and second finger to engage the scalpel handle, which is further supported in its upper end by the palm of the hand. The index finger rests on the dull edge of the blade and provides the necessary pressure for more vigorous incising.

atraumatic technique for incision and excision procedures be developed so that a sharp scalpel may be safely and efficiently employed. It is much safer to use a fulcrum point during surgical incision so that the scalpel may be braced by fingers resting on bone or tooth structure conveniently adjacent to the line of incision. A clear visualization of the area about to be incised is imperative.

Intraoral incisions involving the reflection of the mucoperiosteum for exposure of bone or dental structures are direct, straight-line, or curvilinear incisions taking the shortest distance through the tissues. However, where underlying bone may be remote from the site of the incision, such as when operating on the soft palate, tongue, cheeks, lips, and floor of the mouth, the incision is not necessarily direct. In these cases the incision is made only through the mucosa. Thereafter blunt dissection is combined with further sectioning, or scissors section, so that important anatomical structures are not needlessly sacrificed.

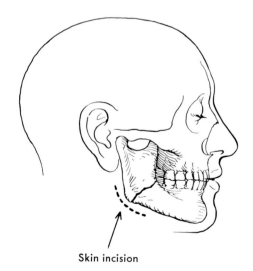

Skin incision

Fig. 2-7. Submandibular incision in natural shadow line of mandible. This approach is often employed for open surgical procedures on the body of the mandible.

Such dissection may be carried out with blunt instruments; the tissues layers are separated by actual tearing. Hemostatic forceps, rounded scissors, the handle end of a scalpel, or the gloved finger of the surgeon is commonly used for blunt dissection.

Cleavage dissection, in which the tissue layers are exposed by accurate snipping of the tissues with a sharp scissors or scalpel, produces less blind trauma than does blunt dissection. This, however, requires more detailed anatomical knowledge. The actual cutting is necessary only to expose a line of cleavage between tissue layers, permitting easy separation of the layers until another line of cleavage is exposed. The next tissue layer is then cut and dissected until another cleavage is encountered. Thus an orderly and atraumatic approach is made to the pathological area.

Skin surgery on the face carries the cosmetic requirement that the postoperative scar be minimal in size and so uncomplicated as to be esthetically acceptable. Whenever possible, these incisions are concealed in natural wrinkles, in the hairline, along the mucocutaneous junctions, or in shaded areas such as the nasolabial fold and the immediately submandibular-cervical zones (Fig. 2-7).

The skin of the face and neck is generously endowed with wrinkles and creases representing lines of tension and relaxation of the skin in its response to the action of the muscles of expression and mastication. The depth of the skin wrinkles varies with the age and weight of the patient and the placement of these creases is generally symmetrical. Planning the surgical scar for best esthetic results demands that the incision be placed into one of the creases of skin relaxation or, as a second choice, into an immediately parallel area. Furthermore, it is desirable that skin incisions be made along, not across, the grain of the skin. Incisions made in skin wrinkles will permit wide exposure of the operative field, since these are really cleavage lines of the superficial tissue planes. If incisions are made across these lines of tensions, sutures will be placed under maximum stress, and the possibility of unfavorable cicatricial formation will be enhanced.

Hair clipping, of course, is necessary when hairy areas are invaded. However, eyebrows are not shaved and eyelashes are not clipped.

Particular attention must be given to the prevention of wound infection because septic wounds may heal with irregular and extensive scarring. Depression contraction and hypertrophy along the line of incision produces unsatisfactory cosmetic results, which oftentimes require corrective surgery that might have been avoided if adequate early care had been thoughtfully administered. Incisions must be made with a sharp scalpel, perpendicular to the skin surface, and preferably in the natural skin creases. The capable surgeon is especially adept at the gentle handling of soft tissue. "Heavy-handed" retracting may result in the necrotizing of such injured tissue with subsequent healing by second intention and considerably more scarring than was necessary. In suturing a skin incision about the face, a slight eversion of the skin edges is preferred. This will compensate for anticipated swelling and permit the levelling out of the eversion without loss of the edge contact of the skin incision. It is simply a means for aborting a spreading of the line of incision.

Skin edges must not be sutured too tightly, and sutures should be removed on the third or fourth day to avoid suture scars. Halsted's basic teachings can well be repeated—the suture material should be no stronger than the tissue itself; a greater number of fine stitches is better than a few coarse ones; fine silk or cotton, Nos. 3-0, 4-0, and 5-0, is used to best advantage for skin incisions on the face. When it is necessary to support such fine skin suturing, this may be done by the following methods:

1. Deep, dermal tension sutures

2. Antitension elastic and adhesive bandaging across the suture line
3. Pressure bandaging
4. Subcuticular (intradermic) suturing with fine-gauge, stainless steel wire

Any history of keloid scar formation should be recorded in the patient's history, and both doctor and patient should be fully aware of the calculated risks assumed in this regard. The black race is thought to be most predisposed to keloid formation, but this problem is not limited by racial boundaries.

Comment. In terminating the discussion concerning the surgery of tissue injury and repair, the following thoughts prevail as basic requirements:

1. It is necessary to answer the question: "When are wounds left open?" Wounds should be left open in the following situations:

a. When the injury is the result of human bite and thereby contaminated by highly pathogenic organisms. Human bite wounds are never sutured.

b. When contamination appears certain or when infection with suppuration is already evident.

c. When there is so much loss of tissue substance as to preclude adequate primary approximation. In massive loss of tissue, such as the cheek or a lip, the oral mucosa of the defect can be sutured to the surrounding peripheral skin so that the circumference of the defect is maintained free of puckering and scarring while plastic surgery is pending.

2. Persistent complaint of pain in a sutured wound is most likely to be caused by skin sutures or retention sutures that are too tight. Usually after 3 or 4 days most sutures have fulfilled their greatest benefits and can be removed.

3. Contrary to common belief, an itching wound is certainly not indicative of normal healing. More likely, it suggests a hypersensitivity reaction to suture materials, bandages and dressing materials, topical medications, or other treatment materials.

4. Persistent suppuration in an otherwise healthy patient suggests a retained foreign body in or about a wound.

Suture materials

Currently in oral surgery there appears to be a preference for nonabsorbable suture materials for cutaneous, mucosal, and deeper layer approximations. However, absorbable suture materials are still widely used in subsurface closures. Of the absorbable sutures, catgut is commonly used. Actually catgut is a misnomer because the material is made from the serosa layer of sheep intestine. It is provided by manufacturers as plain and tanned (chromic) in a suitably wide range of sizes.

Of the nonabsorbable suture materials, black silk is widely used. It has an adequate tensile strength, produces minimal tissue reaction, and can be readily seen for convenient removal. No. 4-0 is popular in oral surgery. If purchased in spool lots, it is inexpensive. Ordinary cotton sewing thread, No. 40, quilting, has many of the advantages of silk and is even less expensive.

Atraumatic-type sutures of both absorbable and nonabsorbable materials are provided by various manufacturers in sealed ampules containing a cold sterilizing medium. The atraumatic feature comprises a fine, ½-circle or ⅜-circle needle, which is swaged on one end of the suture material.

Wire mesh

In oral surgery, wire mesh is sometimes used to fill in bony defects and to develop lost bony contours. Tantalum mesh is most satisfactory because it is best tolerated when buried in the tissues. However, it is expensive. Stainless steel mesh has been gaining popularity as a satisfactory, less expensive substitute for tantalum. Wire mesh is made of extremely thin wires about 0.008 cm in diameter. The mesh is woven with about 22 wires to the centimeter. This allows sufficient spacing to permit tissue to grow through the wire meshing. The mesh must be sutured with wire of the same material or with nonabsorbable silk or cotton to eliminate the possibility of galvanic current activity.

Dressings

The primary intent of dressings is to keep the surgical field free of infection. Second, dressings support the incision, protect it from trauma, and absorb drainage. Intraorally, dressings are not used for these purposes. Within the mouth they are utilized as drains or as vehicles for carrying medicaments and obtundents to the operative site. Sterile strip gauze, 1 to 2 cm wide, is preferred. This gauze may be plain or iodoform. The iodoform gauze has antiseptic qualities, but it also has a strong, persistent, medicinal odor. When used as a drain, strip gauze may be saturated in petrolatum to facilitate removal after its purpose has been served.

Dressing intraoral injuries. The propensity for thorough and rapid healing of oral mucosa is well-known. For this reason, minor injuries, such as bites, burns, and limited surgery, will heal in a clean mouth without treatment. Large lacerations and surgical flaps require adequate positioning and approximation by suturing or other splinting of the injured tissues. Denuded areas within the mouth are acutely painful until granulation and coverage has been effected in healing. During this short but painful period of healing, intraoral dressing may be beneficial. Such dressings find wide usage in postperiodontal surgery in which a denuded area is covered not only for the relief of postoperative pain but also to control desired gingival contour.

Many intraoral dressings combine a medicament with other substances that produce a cementlike set. The medication is usually an obtundent for the local relief of pain. The cement often comprises combinations of zinc oxide, powdered resins, and gums mixed with tannic acid. Topical varnishes that produce a protective film over denuded areas are also helpful in relieving pain and salvaging blood clots. Many topical varnishes are available for this purpose. Some employ ether and collodion; others use cellophane, Teflon, and the polycarboxylate, waterproof cements. In general, it is difficult to maintain any dressing comfortably within a wet mouth for any prolonged period. However, since oral epithelium regenerates so rapidly in an injured mouth, just a few hours of topical dressing may carry a patient through the most painful period and also provide protection for the continued healing of a granulating wound. A more detailed discussion of intraoral dressings ranging from adhesive foils to waterproof cements is readily available in any current periodontal textbook.

Dressing extraoral injuries. For extraoral wounds, gauze pads that are 5 by 5 cm and 10 by 10 cm squares are practical. Such gauze pads are maintained in position by adhesive or elastic bandage. Elastoplast bandage is a cotton elastic with adhesive on one side. Because it is elastic, it does not constrict, yet it provides the desirable gentle, even pressure required to firmly support a dressing and avoid incisional hernia. Pressure bandaging is frequently employed for dressing facial incisions. Pressure dressings are used chiefly to splint the soft tissues and minimize edema that might tear through sutures and reopen the incision. They also serve to eliminate dead space, control secondary capillary oozing, and abort hematoma. Pressure dressings consist essentially of bulky materials, such as fluffed gauze, mechanic's waste, sea sponges, and foam rubber. The bulky material is place directly over the sterile gauze pads covering a wound and is retained in position by an elastic bandage.

A few problems caused by compression bandaging should be pointed out so that they may be recognized and eliminated if possible. These dressings are constrictive by design and are painful when used over a progressively swelling area. They may be responsible for lymphatic and venous blockage and thereby increase rather than decrease the swelling for which they were used. Pressure bandages should be heavily padded to be effective. The bandaged areas should be carefully observed for stasis and swelling *beyond* the edges of the bandage. If this occurs, the bandage should be either eliminated or the compression released for short periods of time to relieve the stasis.

Compression bandaging, when intelligently employed, will promote good wound healing with excellent cosmetic results at the line of incision. When poorly employed, such dressings will not only retard healing but may also stimulate fibrosis through lymphatic and venous obstruction in areas somewhat remote from the site of actual wound healing.

OPERATIVE TECHNIQUE
General anatomy

It is not the purpose of this chapter to deal with the detailed anatomy in the oral surgery field. This information is readily and authoritatively available in many well-known sources. Fundamentally, the major facial vessels concerned in oral surgical exposures run a course that is (1) deep to the superficial muscles of expression (including the platysma but excluding the caninus and buccinator muscles) and (2) superficial to the muscles of mastication and, of course, the deeper facial bones. In a similarly general sense, the facial vein drains areas supplied by the facial artery and the posterior facial vein drains those deeper facial areas supplied by the terminal branches of the external carotid artery. The major sensory nerve to the face is the fifth cranial nerve. The major motor nerve to the face (other than to the muscles of mastication, which are supplied by the fifth cranial nerve) is the seventh cranial nerve. Surgical injury to the fifth cranial nerve may be considered of minor significance, since sequel to such injury most likely would be sensory paresthesia, with good chance for regeneration. However, surgical injury to the seventh cranial nerve and subsequent loss of function of the muscles of expression presents extreme cosmetic problems, without much hope for spontaneous and functional regeneration.

A thorough knowledge of the anatomical relations of the tissues that the surgeon is about to invade is of course mandatory. It is common practice among young surgeons of limited experience to perform the proposed surgery in cadaver dissection prior to the actual operation. Such procedure is good technique and is not to be misinterpreted as indicating deficiency.

Submandibular approach to the ascending ramus and body of the mandible

Most extraoral surgery requiring exposure of the mandible is done through a submandibular approach. The area about the angle of the mandible is considered more complex than are the more anterior zones, and this area will be discussed surgically.

The location of the incision must be given careful consideration to be sure that deeper anatomical structures are exposed to view in normal relationship. Positioning of the patient or rotating or extending his head may considerably alter the location of the incision as compared to its location when the patient is seated at rest. The incision in the submandibular approach should be made in one of the lines of skin tension, and it should be predetermined and marked either by superficial scratching with the back edge of a scalpel or by marking with an analine dye. The gonial angle of the mandible and the notch in the inferior border of the mandible (produced by the pulsating facial artery) should be marked as points of reference, the former indicating the posterior terminus of the operative field and the latter suggesting the location of the facial artery and the facial vein (Fig. 2-8). The incision is placed in the shadow line of the

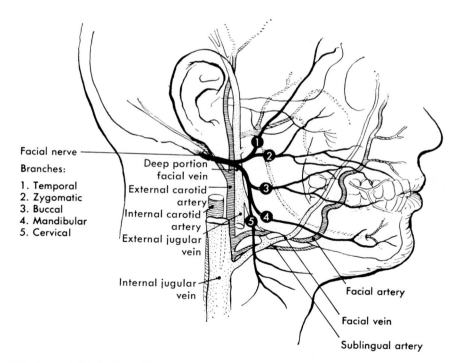

Facial nerve

Branches:

1. Temporal
2. Zygomatic
3. Buccal
4. Mandibular
5. Cervical

Deep portion facial vein

External carotid artery

Internal carotid artery

External jugular vein

Internal jugular vein

Facial artery

Facial vein

Sublingual artery

Fig. 2-8. General distribution of facial nerve, arterial blood supply to face, and venous return from face.

mandible about 2 cm below the inferior border of the mandible and curved in best cosmetic conformity with that bone. This distance below the mandible will avoid the cutting of the mandibular branch of the facial nerve. The total length of the incision may vary between 6 and 8 cm.

Crosshatching the line of incision. With the line of incision predetermined and marked, the patient's head is extended and turned as far as possible to one side. This is for the convenience and comfort of the operating team. A final, brief consultation is held with the anesthesiologist relative to the patient's readiness for immediate surgery. The line of incision, clearly marked, is then crosshatched by scratching vertical lines with the back edge of a scalpel, pendicular to the prospective line of incision. These vertical scratch lines should be about 1.5 cm apart and extend, so spaced, throughout the length of the incision. Such crosshatching serves only to ensure that subsequent skin closure is perfectly approximated, with the least possible scar.

The incision. The skin is stretched superiorly so that the marked line of incision rests on solid bone and thereby provides a firm base for a clean incision in one deft incising move. The depth of the incision should be vertical and completely through the skin. Cutting on the bias may result in widening of the ultimate scar. A Bard-Parker blade No. 10 or No. 15 is well suited to skin incisions in this area, but the choice of scalpel rests with the operator's individual preference. Some bleeding points may be anticipated at this subcutaneous level. If the bleeding is arterial, the vessel is clamped with a Halsted mosquito hemostatic forceps and ligated with either fine cotton (No. 3-0 or 4-0) or plain surgical gut (No. 3-0). A square knot is recommended for vessel ligation, and the free ends are cut short on the knot.

Deeper soft tissue dissection. With the skin and subcutaneous areolar tissue incised, they may be widely undermined by blunt dissection, using a 14 cm curved Mayo scissors, a hemostatic forceps, or the butt end of a knife handle. This will permit the insertion of retractors (such as a Kny-Scheerer trachea rake retractor) on each side of the incision to allow wide exposure and visualization of the underlying platysma muscle. A few points of interest relative to retraction technique might be developed now:

1. Good retraction includes gentle elevation as well as tractile force.

2. Good retraction should be reasonably firm and steady. Tissue is unnecessarily damaged and the operation time prolonged by the assistant who is persistently changing the position of the retractors.

3. When the operative technique so permits, the tractile force on the retractors should be periodically released without removing the retractors; thus circulation may be restored to the soft tissue flaps during that brief period.

4. Retraction must be continual and adequate during unexpected arterial hemorrhage until that immediate problem is solved.

With adequate exposure of the platysma muscle and its overlying and rather poorly defined superficial fascia, this muscle is now made ready for sectioning. It should be remembered that this muscle will later require suturing in closure by layers. At this time the muscle should be carefully dissected, elevated, and cleanly sectioned so that it can be conveniently found for later suturing. Immediately under the platysma muscle and along the border of the mandible, exploration should be provided for identification of the mandibular branch (ramus marginalis mandibulae) of the facial nerve. It is small and sometimes difficult to locate, especially if there has been surgical shredding of fascial tissue in the immediate field. It is often best found in the potential fascial space, just deep to the platysma and superficial to the anterior border of the masseter, or over the depressor anguli oris. Suspected segments of this nerve can be identified when stimulated with faradic current or by gentle clamping with a hemostatic forceps. The effect of such stimulation will be seen in noticeable contracture of the musculature at the corner of the mouth. The Bovie unit employing low current (noncoagulative) is frequently used in operating rooms to provide faradic current for such stimulation. Many surgeons consider that the most constant point of reference for convenient identification of the mandibular branch of the seventh cranial nerve is its relationship to the large, pulsating facial artery. The nerve is found lying directly over the facial artery as that vessel passes over the mandible. If the artery and vein are reflected superiorly from their location at the inferior border of the mandible, such retraction is certain to include and thereby salvage the more superficial mandibular branch of the seventh cranial nerve. This important nerve has considerable cosmetic and some functional significance, and it should not be inadvertently sacrificed.

The next step in orderly surgical approach concerns the identification and retraction of the facial artery and vein as they pass over the notching in the inferior border of the mandible just anterior to the angle. The parotideomasseteric fascia and other sheaths from the ascending deep cervical fasciae are first brought into surgical view. After adequate orientation by palpation of the inferomandibular notch, this fascia is separated by blunt dissection, permitting the large, pulsating facial artery to bulge into the created opening. The larger facial vein will be found slightly superficial and posterior to the artery but in close approximation. Both vessels are sacrificed if necessary. This is best done by first clamping each vessel and then ligating proximally and distally before sectioning. White cotton sutures, No. 2-0, are well chosen for this ligation. For smaller vessels, finer cotton sutures, Nos. 3-0 and 4-0, are used. Of course, other subcutaneous suture materials such as chromicized surgical gut and similar absorbable ligating sutures are equally acceptable for this purpose.

Glandular tissue will be observed in the dissection at this point. This is the submandibular gland (glandula submandibularis). Some difficulty may be encountered in separating the lower pole of the parotid gland from the submandibular gland. The stylomandibular ligament is often surgically viewed as a heavy fascial plane that serves to separate these glands. The glandular tissues should be separated by blunt dissection and carefully retracted. If incised, they may produce persistent hemorrhage that may be difficult to control. With the glandular tissue retracted, the facial vessels subsequently ligated and sectioned, and the seventh cranial nerve salvaged and protected in careful retraction, the remainder of the surgical exposure can proceed with greater speed and impunity. Other smaller vessels will be encountered, but these will be of no surgical significance, unless requiring ligation to preserve blood volume and maintain a dry surgical field. Surgery on the body of the mandible anterior to the facial artery and veins is seldom complicated by excessive bleeding. Minor and smaller bleeders will often coagulate under pressure tampons. Sometimes the clamping of such a minor bleeder with a hemostatic forceps for a few minutes will serve to enhance coagulation so that ligation is not required. However, when the hemostatic forceps is removed, the bleeding site must be carefully evaluated to establish that hemostasis is complete. If in doubt, ligate the bleeding point.

Minor variations of the soft tissue surgery described will be required to meet the demands of surgery in more anterior aspects of the lower face. If the body of the mandible is to be approached, the location of the incision is placed more anteriorly. The amount of exposure required determines the length of the incision. Usually 6 to 7 cm will be found adequate, but accessibility should not be sacrificed only to produce a slightly smaller scar. To do so may result in unnecessary trauma to adjacent soft tissue, postoperative swelling, poor healing, and ragged scarring. It is good technique to identify and retract or identify, ligate, and retract blood vessels overlying the operative field. It is *necessary technique* to identify and salvage nerve supply—especially *motor nerve* supply.

Soft tissue closure. As in all surgery, closure of the soft tissues in the submandibular approach to oral surgery is carried out in an orderly manner. The field is first scrutinized to assure that hemorrhage is controlled and ligated vessels are adequately secured. It is better that the time be taken to ensure these necessary precautions at this stage of surgery rather than that they be inadequately performed and the patient suffer postoperative hemorrhage on the ward in the middle of the night.

Closure of the soft tissues is then done in layers, with anatomical repositioning in proper relation. Periosteal tissues are difficult to suture. Fine surgical gut, No. 3-0 or 4-0, on a ⅜-circle, side-cutting needle is best used for this procedure. Whether the surgical gut is tanned (chromic) or plain is of small consequence. The chromic gut will resorb more slowly than will the plain, and this may be desirable in ligating large vessels and in suturing fascia. The cervical fascia is likewise closed. In operations on the ramus of the mandible in which the masseter muscle is detached and elevated, it is especially important that this muscle be well sutured at its origin in the vicinity of the angle of the mandible. This can be accomplished by suturing the lower end of the masseter muscle to the lower end of the medial pterygoid muscle (on the medial aspect of the mandible) at the angle of the mandible. The positions of these muscles may be slightly altered by this procedure, but no appreciable residual effect will be evident in their function.

It is important in closing by layers that approximation be reasonably accurate so that all dead space may be eliminated. Dead space is a harbor for a hematoma.

As the platysma is recognized and closed, assistants should hold skin hooks tautly at each end of the incision. In this manner, the longitudinal relation of this muscle is reestablished and smoother skin closure can be effected. Muscle closure at this superficial level can be established with No. 4-0 plain surgical gut (although silk or cotton may be acceptable) on a small ⅜-circle, round needle. To approximate skin with minimal scarring, it is wise to use first a subcuticular suture of plain surgical gut or stainless steel wire. If the wire is employed, it can be conveniently removed after the tenth day. The subcuticular approximation serves to relieve suture tension on the skin incision.

If subcuticular suture has not been employed, the skin wound may be closed with vertical mattress sutures. Interrupted sutures are preferable to continuous sutures, since approximation may be maintained even if one of the sutures should slip. The skin sutures should be of nonabsorbable material of extremely fine gauge (No. 4-0 or 5-0) on a ⅜-circle, cutting needle and spaced about 3 mm apart. The skin closure is initiated at each of the preoperatively marked crosshatchings to facilitate the exact repositioning of the skin.

It is considered good technique to slightly evert the line of skin incision in suture closure. Sutures must be removed on the fourth postoperative day to avoid suture scarring, and at that time there may be a tendency for some separation in the suture line. Everting the skin edges permits some subdermal contracture without separation in the line of incision. Irrespective of the care devoted to skin closure, unless careful attention has been paid to the closure by anatomical layers of all of the tissues, the cosmetic result may be unsatisfactory.

The skin incision line is first covered with a single-layer pad of sterile, lubricated gauze. The lubricant may be sterile petrolatum jelly. Over this is placed a 10 by 10 cm sterile gauze pad, and this is covered with a pressure dressing to limit postoperative edema. The dressing is part of the surgical procedure and is the responsibility of the surgeon. It is most important that all dressings, primary and reapplied, be sterile. The greatest complication to all wound healing is infection.

Surgical approach to the temporomandibular joint

Many of the so-called classic approaches to surgery of the temporomandibular joint mechanism have been complicated by the danger of surgical damage to the costmetically significant seventh cranial nerve.

Blair[2] used an incision resembling a reverse question mark or an inverted L, commencing in the temporal hairline and curving downward in close proximity to the anterior auricle (Fig. 2-9, *A*). Wakely[8] used a modification resembling a T incision with the horizontal bar of the T placed over the zygomatic arch. Lempert's[4] endaural approach to the middle ear suggested to numerous observers that, with some modifi-

cations, this basically could be employed as perhaps the safest surgical route to the glenoid fossae.

In 1951 Dingman and Moorman[3] reported such a new approach, which appeared to be initiated somewhat similarly to Lempert's second endaural incision. The major objective of this approach concerned sectioning the minor fibrous attachment of the lamina tragi at its superior aspect and reflecting this cartilage anteriorly and down over itself (Fig. 2-9, *B*). Rongetti[6] in 1954 reported another modification of the second stage of Lempert's endaural approach to the middle ear, which promised safe and direct invasion of the temporomandibular joint. However, for practical purposes Rongetti's approach is similar to Dingman's, differing chiefly in that Rongetti invades the external auditory meatus to a greater depth and does not extend his incision as far superiorly and inferiorly as does Dingman. Both are

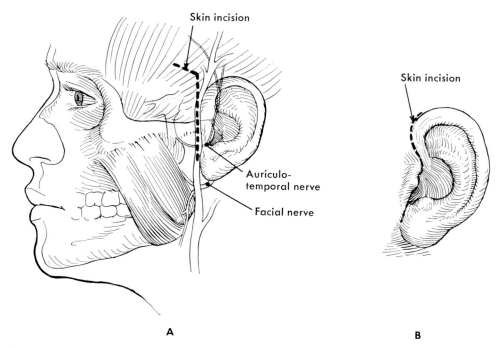

A

B

Fig. 2-9. A, Basic incision employed by Blair, Ivy, and others in surgical approach to the temporomandibular joint. **B,** Dingman's approach to the temporomandibular joint.

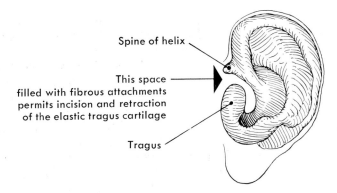

Fig. 2-10. Cartilaginous laminae of ear. The normally present space between the cartilaginous supports of the helix and the tragus allows for the convenient retraction of the tragus, anteriorly and inferiorly, for subsequent direct exposure into the temporomandibular joint.

endaural approaches, and both are designed to avoid injury to the facial nerve and to leave behind the least noticeable scar.

The endaural incision to expose the glenoid fossae has been used successfully for meniscectomy and condyloidectomy, but it is not necessarily limited to that surgery.

The hair in the temporal fossa is shaved, and the head is prepared and draped for sterile surgery. The incision is started in the skin crease immediately adjacent to the anterior helix. It is carried downward to the level of the tragus, at which point it passes in a gap to the deeper aspects of the external auditory meatus where it is cosmetically concealed. The gap is filled with a fibrous attachment for the lamina tragi, and no damage is done in this sectioning (Fig. 2-10). While in the auditory meatus, the incision remains in contact with the bony tympanic plate. As the incision leaves the external auditory meatus, it becomes just visible at the lower aspect of the tragus. It is not necessary to section the cartilage at this point since the cartilage has sufficient elasticity to permit adequate retraction without hazarding incision at this close proximity to the stylomastoid foramen (exit point for the facial nerve). In the upper aspects of this incision, the superficial temporal vessels and the auriculotemporal nerve may be encountered. These vessels are either re-

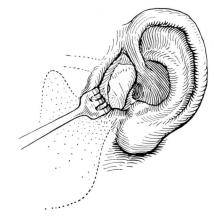

Fig. 2-11. This endaural incision permits the tragus to be incised at the fibrous bundle attachment at its superoanterior border so that it may be reflected anteroinferiorly, thereby exposing the articular ligamentous covering of the temporomandibular joint.

tracted or the artery and vein may be ligated and sectioned. The next landmark will be the temporalis fascia and then the exposed cartilage of the tragus. The fascia is sectioned with a scalpel or scissors, and the temporalis muscle is undermined with a periosteal elevator and raised from the root of the zygomatic arch. Some small portion of the upper pole of the parotid gland may be identified in this field. It is better to dissect and retract the glandular tissue since

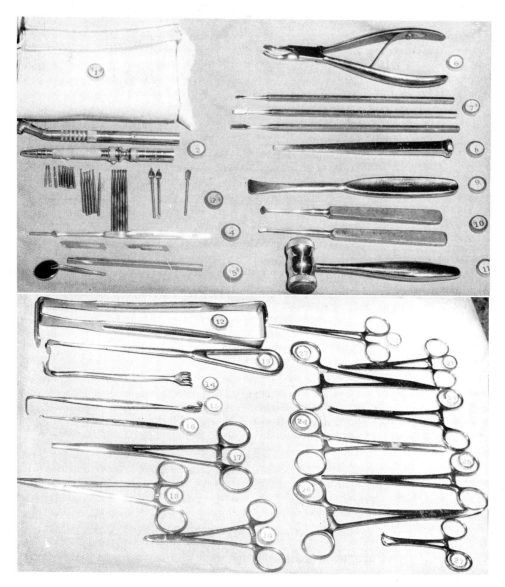

Fig. 2-12. *1,* Sterile sleeves for draping engine arms, cables, and extensions from portable dental engine. *2,* Straight and angle dental handpieces. *3,* Assorted burs—carbide preferred. *4,* Scalpel handle and blades Nos. 10 and 15. *5,* Mouth mirror and handle, plain. *6,* Bone rongeur No. 4. *7,* Osteotomes, Stout, assorted. *8,* Osteotome, single-bevel. *9,* Periosteotome, blunt, Lane, 19.5 cm. *10,* Curets, Molt, straight, Nos. 2 and 4. *11,* Mallet, metal. *12,* Retractor, set, general operating (Army-Navy). *13,* Retractor, vein, Cushing. *14,* Retractor, trachea, Hupp, 3-prong, blunt, 16 cm. *15,* Retractor, trachea, Kny-Scheering, 3-prong, blunt, 16 cm. *16,* Hook, skin, Dural-Adson. *17,* Forceps, straight, hemostatic, Rochester-Ochsner, 19 cm. *18,* Holder, needle, Mayo-Hegar, 17.5 cm. *19,* Holder, needle, Sterz-Brown, 14 cm. *20,* Forceps, hemostatic, straight, Halsted (mosquito), 12.5 cm. *21,* Forceps, hemostatic, curved, Halsted (mosquito), 12.5 cm. *22,* Holder, needle, Mayo-Hegar, 15 cm. *23,* Forceps, hemostatic, Kelly, curved, 14 cm. *24,* Forceps, tissue, straight, Allis, 15 cm. *25,* Forceps, hemostatic, straight, Rochester-Ochsner, 14 cm. *26,* Forceps, hemostatic, curved, Rochester-Pean, 15.5 cm. *27,* Forceps, towel, Backhaus, 8.3 cm.

Continued.

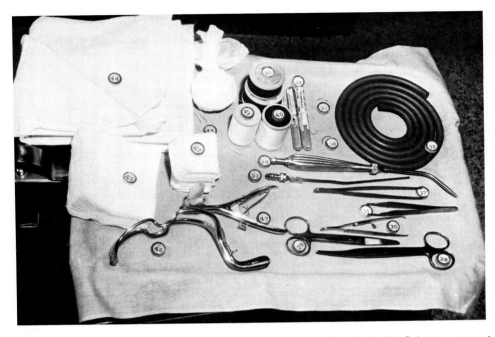

Fig. 2-12, cont'd. *28,* Scissors, general surgical, curved, Aufricht, 14 cm. *29,* Scissors, general surgical, straight, one point sharp, 14 cm. *30,* Forceps, fixation, straight, Graefe, 11.5 cm. *31,* Forceps, tissue, Brown-Adson, 11.5 cm. *32,* Forceps, dressing, straight, 13.2 cm. *33,* Suction tip, antrum. *34,* Suction tip, laryngeal. *35,* Rubber suction tubing. *36,* Needle, suture, ½-circle, taper, No. 12. *37,* Needle, suture, ⅜-circle, cutting, No. 20. *38,* Suture, surgical gut (plain and chromic), No. 3-0. *39,* Suture, silk, black, spools, Nos. 3-0, 4-0, and 5-0. *40,* Suture, cotton, white, No. 2-0. *41,* Suture, cotton, white, No. 3-0. *42,* Sponges, 5 by 5 cm. *43,* Sponges, 10 by 10 cm. *44,* Sterile drape, front sheet, 114 by 178 cm. *45,* Throat pack, with string attached. *46,* Mouth prop, Jennings. *47,* Mouth prop, Denhardt. (Official U. S. Navy photograph.)

incising may produce troublesome bleeding. Mandibular excursions at this point will clearly demonstrate the condyle enclosed in a rather loose articular capsule. Further exposure may be effected by blunt dissection. Any further incising at this stage is best made directly over the condylar head or along the inferior margin of the zygomatic arch (Fig. 2-11).

No surgical danger is anticipated deep to the temporalis fascia and lateral to the condyle. There may be some retraction paralysis of some of the branches of the facial nerve, since the area of exposure is small although adequate. This will be a temporary paralysis.

If further surgery deep to the neck of the condyle is required, this must be done with diligent respect for the maxillary artery, the middle meningeal artery, and the auriculotemporal nerve. Invasion of the pterygoid plexus of veins will result in persistent hemorrhagic seepage, but this is controlled by pressure tampons or Gelfoam strips saturated with a hemostatic. All gauze sponges used in this area should be tied on one end with long black suture silk to facilitate convenient removal.

The endaural approach to the temporomandibular joint, as for meniscectomy or condyloidectomy, is thought by many to be the most direct and perhaps the safest approach to a difficult area. The chief objections to it may be a limited range of exposure of the joint mechanism and the possibility of secondary infection of aural cartilage. However, these are small objections. Any surgical approach to this area that promises to eliminate the danger of damage to the facial nerve and provides a cosmetically acceptable postoperative scar is to be desired.

The Lempert operation for otosclerosis forms the basis for this modified approach to the temporomandibular joint by way of the external auditory meatus.

ARMAMENTARIUM

Some of the more frequently used instruments and supplies for oral surgery are illustrated and identified in Fig. 2-12. These are normally set up in sterile packs or case pans for routine use in oral surgical problems. To these routine setups the surgeon will add the special armamentarium required for a particular surgical problem.

REFERENCES

1. Artandi, C.: Production experiences with radiation sterilization, Bull. Parenter. Drug Assoc. **18:**2, 1964.
2. Blair, V. P.: Consideration of contour as well as function in operations for organic ankylosis of lower jaw, Surg. Gynecol. Obstet. **46:**167, 1928.
3. Dingman, R. O., and Moorman, W. C.: Meniscectomy in treatment of lesions of temporomandibular joint, J. Oral Surg. **9:**214, 1951.
4. Lempert, J.: Improvement of hearing in cases of otosclerosis: new, one stage surgical technic, Arch. Otolaryngol. **28:**42, 1938.
5. Olander, J. W.: New facilities and equipment for radiation sterilization, Bull. Parenter. Drug Assoc. **17:**14, 1963.
6. Rongetti, J. R.: Meniscectomy: new approach to temporomandibular joint, Arch. Otolaryngol. **60:**566, 1954.
7. Safe practice for hospital operating rooms, Booklet No. NFPA-56, July, 1956, National Fire Protective Association, 60 Batterymarch St., Boston, Mass.
8. Wakely, C. P. G.: Surgery of temporomandibular joint, Surgery **5:**697, 939.

CHAPTER 3

Introduction to exodontics

Gustav O. Kruger

GENERAL PRINCIPLES

A careful technique based on knowledge and skill is the most important factor in successful exodontics. Living tissue must be treated with gentleness. Rough handling, ragged or incomplete incision, excessive retraction of flaps, or uneven suturing, even though not painful to the anesthetized patient, will result in tissue damage or necrosis, which in turn provides an excellent medium for bacterial growth. Healing that could have taken place by primary intention must granulate from the bottom of the wound after necrotic tissue is phagocytized. This causes pain, excessive swelling, and possibly deformity. Gentle handling and instrumentation with a sharp, well cared for armamentarium are rewarded with a better tissue response.

Psychology

Science of behavior. The reaction with which different people respond to the same stimulus varies considerably. Individuals react to pain according to their basic make-up, which may range from stoicism to extreme sensitivity. An occasional patient who does not want an anesthetic may sit through an extraction with few outward signs of pain. Another patient with profound local anesthesia may jump when a forceps is placed on the tooth. The stoic patient is able to disregard a certain amount of the pain felt. A story is told of one Christian Science patient who refused an anesthetic of any kind. She telephoned her practitioner and left the telephone off the hook, even though it was across the room and therefore the reading was unintelligible to the patient in the chair. The patient did not move or make outward sign of discomfort during the extraction, although tears streamed down her cheeks.

The psychological effect of the placebo has been studied many times. A double-blind study to compare the sedative effects of a therapeutic agent with those of a bland pill of similar size and color was so conducted that neither the operator nor the patient knew which pill contained the active agent. Patients were told that a sedative or analgesic agent would be administered; they did not know that there was an equal possibility that a sugar pill might be administered. At the end of the experiment, after the reactions of all patients had been recorded, the code was opened, and the completed record cards were marked with the ingredients. In numerous such studies involving may ills and various drugs, no less than 35% of patients experienced relief using the placebo. The point was made that real pain was relieved in these patients, not merely imagined pain, indicating that physiological and psychological processes can be modified by psychological attitudes. In another double-blind experiment an injection of either a normal saline or a local anesthetic solution was given in the oral tissues of dental students. A significant number of students injected with saline had complete objective and subjective signs of anesthesia.

Circumstances have much to do with pain perception. Soldiers in the stress of warfare have been subjected to major injuries that were unfelt and unknown to them until the immediate objective was won. Children sometimes will react with fear to the white coat worn by the practitioner, and consequently some pedodontists wear street clothes in the office.[1]

The pain threshold varies significantly in individuals. What is major pain to one person at one time may be minor pain to another person. The introduction of a hypodermic needle into the vein of the arm may be barely felt by one individual, although it may be felt as excruciating pain by another.

Emotional control in the presence of pain varies considerably. Patients with the same threshold of pain can range from the individual who overreacts, such as the child who has no inhibitions, to the patient who will give no outward sign of pain.[4]

The anxious patient. Fear can be related to any one of several factors:

1. Fear of fear itself. Rembered fear from a painful childhood incident that has been relegated to the subconscious mind or even tales of painful experiences told by someone else can condition the patient to fear the fear he associates with the procedure. This is mainly an introverted reaction, although extraneous factors, such as long-remembered odors, colors, and situations, may stir latent memories.[3]

2. The operation. Any normal individual has some degree of concern about an impending operation. General surgeons say that the patient who approaches major surgery with no concern at all does not have the same chance of survival as the patient who has stimulated his adrenal cortices to some extent. Everyone has stresses in life, but the size of the factor required to stress an individual and his response to that stress vary. It is the concern of the dentist and his entire staff to reduce this normal fear to its absolute minimum. Every successful practitioner induces in patients confidence that ameliorates natural fear. The patient should be prepared psychologically before any operation is performed, and in many cases the preparation is done by thoughtful considerations by the staff and practitioner even without words. Most dentists will not extract teeth for the patient who grips the arms of the chair until white knuckles show, preferring to prepare him psychologically and by premedication for a more relaxed, subsequent appointment.

3. Esthetics. The menopausal matron whose children are married, whose husband, at the peak of his career, is busy and inattentive, and who has lost her girlhood beauty thinks beyond the full maxillary extractions for which she is sitting. This last insult to her beauty has been likened to a subconscious castration. She is fearful she is losing the power in society that beauty once gave her, and this is the last straw in that process. This fear can be aggravated by mental instability associated with the menopause. The wise dentist proceeds slowly in recommending such extractions, showing all the pathological reasons for removal of the teeth and allowing the patient herself to first express the conclusion that all teeth should be removed. Her first statement to this effect seems to prepare her better from a psychological standpoint. Of course, the practitioner in doing this occasionally encounters the matter-of-fact matron who says, "Come, come, young man, what are you saying? What is your diagnosis?"

It must be remembered that the pain the anxious patient experiences is really felt by that patient, even though in some psychosomatic illnesses no objective organic basis for the pain can be found.

Evaluation and preparation. The general psychological makeup of the patient should be evaluated before treatment is undertaken. His self-confidence, self-reliance, general attitude, and demeanor give clues to his later reactions. The neurotic patient has a nervous instability that must be taken into consideration when premedication and management are planned. The big policeman who swaggers in saying that he is afraid of nothing often is the first to go into syncope when the forceps appear. The banker's wife whose position has made her immune to physical and mental insult may react vocally on extraction even in the presence of adequate anesthesia; firmness by the operator at the moment, followed after the operation by kind words of commendation on her excellent behavior, with no mention of the unpleasantness, will make a firm friend. Age, race, health, physical considerations, and even vocation present variables that must be considered in evaluating the patient.

In verbal presentation of the exodontia problem, the patient should be told what to expect. Possible complications and postoperative problems can be identified without describing every catastrophic detail. The patient may have occasion to verify these experiences later and thereupon will have more confidence in the dentist who anticipated them. Terminology is important. For example, when considerable alveoloplasty is anticipated, the patient is told that the parts will be smoothed to create a better base for the denture in anticipation of natural resorption. The gory details are best left unsaid. During the operative procedure the patient is forewarned of noise made by instruments such as the chisel or rongeur.

Psychological office management. The office and its personnel should be geared to the instillation of confidence in the patient from the moment he arrives. Nothing defeats this objective as much as ignoring the patient in a bustling, impersonal office. As one of their primary functions the office personnel should show concern for the patient.

Another irritation in the office is extraneous noise. One practitioner had a quiet office in which the entire wall facing the chair was replaced by two pieces of plate glass extending from floor to ceiling, which formed a tropical fish tank. This was most restful to the patient.

Instruments should never be exposed to view. Odors suggestive of medication should be eliminated as much as possible. Adequate premedication is given if necessary. A towel head wrap can be placed over the patient's eyes if considerable instrumentation will be done.

The operator should exhibit sympathetic actions: gentleness and tranquility. He or she should be calm and self-reliant to inspire confidence. The terminology should be arranged so that if a new needle is desired he or she will call for a "point." The entire office should be devoted to eliminating psychological problems in patients and to ensuring them only minimum mental discomfort while in the office.

Psychiatric aspects. Neurotic patients need dental extractions just as much as normal patients do, but there are several differences to be observed in their management. First, the neurotic patient often has tensions that make management difficult. Second, the neurotic or slightly neurotic patient can exhibit bizarre postoperative reactions such as prolonged symptoms of local anesthesia, unnatural or prolonged wound pain, and other hysteria-like phenomena. The patient may return for months and then start legal action. Third, the neurotic patient will insist on prescribing operations for himself that will, in his mind, cure him miraculously of his troubles. He may complain of a vague pain in the maxilla for which no organic basis can be found and insist that the second molar be extracted. Complete examination will show a healthy tooth. After visiting several dentists he will find one who will extract the tooth. Immediately the pain will disappear, vindicating the patient's diagnosis and making this dentist the best one he has ever known. Unfortunately, within months the patient will return, complaining of the same pain and demanding that the second premolar be removed or, if all teeth on that side have been removed, that the maxilla be opened surgically to remove "bad bone." Once the initial nonpathological tooth is removed, it is almost impossible to convince the patient that this type of treatment will do no good and that psychiatric evaluation and treatment are necessary. If the dentist feels that the patient may take umbrage at such recommendation, he can always refer him to a neurologist for evaluation of the neurological pathways.

Anesthesia

Whether the operation is performed with the patient under local or under general anesthesia depends on many factors, including the custom, training, and equipment of the dentist, the wishes and physical status of the patient, the presence of an acute periodontitis or pulpitis that may make local anesthesia difficult, the presence of infection in the surrounding tissues, and the extent of the procedure.

Some operators use local anesthesia for every type of procedure, with major block anesthesia and premedication to manage the difficult cases. Others use general anesthesia for everything.

Premedication. Premedication with local anesthesia for extraction is helpful, especially if the operation is expected to involve complicated procedures.[5] Premedication must be tailored for each individual. It can vary from a barbiturate or ataraxic drug taken by mouth at home or in the waiting room to an intramuscular injection of a synthetic narcotic or an intravenous injection of a barbiturate given when the patient is in the chair.

Intravenous premedication is an art as well as a science. Techniques have been developed that range from a single intravenous injection to a continuous injection using a combination of drugs to provide se-

dation throughout a longer procedure. These techniques provide sedation and amnesia, but they do not create an unconscious patient with all the additional factors that need to be monitored such as respiration, blood pressure, and airway.

One widely employed technique involves the intravenous injection of diazepam in amounts of 20 mg or less before the local anesthetic is administered. The drug is injected into the median basilic vein or preferably into the hand vein. The latter is preferred because it is safer (the vein is never mistaken for the artery in the hand), although it is perhaps more painful. The drug is injected at the rate of 5 mg per minute, and injection is discontinued when the eyelids droop. Local anesthetic is injected into the oral tissues immediately after the needle is removed from the hand.

A better technique, however, seems to be the injection of the intravenous ataraxic immediately before the surgical procedure is started. In this procedure local anesthesia is administered without premedication, using a careful technique preceded by a topical anesthetic that has remained against the site of injection for 3 minutes. The patient is allowed to sit in the quiet operatory until profound anesthesia has occurred. Intravenous premedication given just before surgery changes his mental attitude at the most important time. Rarely is more than 10 mg necessary if given at this juncture.

Inhalation analgesia with nitrous oxide-oxygen is an important recent advance in sedation techniques.

Examination of the patient

The more experience a dentist has in exodontics the more aware he or she is of the complications that may occur and the more thorough is the examination. The dentist becomes adept at sizing up the patient and the area of the mouth involved. Legal considerations require that the examination be recorded. For the beginner the examination should be stylized and recorded in some detail. Examination is divided into several portions.

History is divided basically into the chief complaint, present illness, past history, and family history (see Chapters 1 and 27). To intelligently assess the problem an adequate knowledge must be obtained of both the background of the patient and of the present complaint. No problem is so simple that it cannot cause serious injury or death under the wrong circumstances. However, under apparently normal circumstances in which no diagnostic problem needs to be fathomed, the practitioner asks a few leading questions rather than attempting to write a complete, hospital-type history. The patient is asked if he has had major operations or illnesses, when he last was examined by his physician, if there were positive findings, and what drugs he is taking now. He is asked whether he has allergies or a history of rheumatic fever, how many pillows he sleeps on, and if he has difficulty climbing steps. Most offices used a rather sophisticated medical history form that obtains a good history of past and current systemic and oral problems. The form is completed by the patient in the waiting room and is followed by further questioning by the doctor to clarify positive findings.

Clinical examination consists of visual evaluation (color, swelling, and condition of tooth and surrounding structures), palpation and percussion, instrumentation, and vitality tests. The tooth in question is examined closely. In addition, adjacent teeth and surrounding structures are examined carefully for problems that may be pertinent. The overhanging margin of the restoration on the next tooth that will fracture on extraction, osteoradionecrosis in the underlying jaw, or a fractured jaw under the loose tooth in a patient who has come from a barroom fight should not be overlooked. A clinical survey of the general health status of the fully clothed patient in the dental chair also is a necessary art in the successful dental practice.

Radiographic examination is necessary, both preoperatively and postoperatively. Many conditions that could not be diagnosed otherwise are thus revealed, such as the curved root, the large cyst, a new abscess, or carious exposure of the pulp on an adjacent tooth that was not present on radiographs made several years earlier. The man whose jaw was fractured in the fight will sue when he becomes sober, claiming the jaw was fractured during the extraction, unless a preoperative radiographic record exists. A postoperative radiograph is equally important for clinical evaluation as well as for record purposes. It might be necessary to prove that a fracture received by the patient convalescing in a nightclub was not sustained during the extraction. With better radiographic procedures and protection, there is negligible radiation associated with these radiographs. However, children and pregnant women often are not given postoperative radiographs after uncomplicated procedures.

Blood pressure determination in the dental office has provided a service to the dentist in making him or her aware of the patient's hypertension and to the patient who often is not aware of his hypertension.

Laboratory tests are necessary adjuncts to diagnosis and management. Some tests, such as urinalysis, can be done in a well-equipped office, but most tests are done in a laboratory. Tests for bleeding are not done accurately in the office. If such tests are indicated, they should be done in a laboratory, in the hospital, or in the physician's office. Although such tests are expensive and time-consuming, there should be no hesitancy in ordering them if they are indicated.

Screening tests for diabetes and hemoglobin level are available from commercial firms in the form of treated paper strips. A service is performed if every dental patient is screened yearly, particularly if he does not obtain a yearly physical examination, since unknown cases of diabetes and anemia are thereby discovered in the dental office and referred to the physician for treatment.

INDICATIONS AND CONTRAINDICATIONS FOR EXTRACTION
Indications

Any tooth that is not useful in the total dental mechanism is considered for removal.

1. Pulp pathologic conditions, either acute or chronic, in a tooth that is not amenable to endodontic therapy condemns the tooth. A tooth that is not restorable by dental procedures can be considered in this category, even if a pulp pathologic condition is not demonstrable.

2. Periodontal disease, acute or chronic, that is not amenable to treatment may be cause for extraction.

3. Traumatic effects on the tooth or alveolus sometimes are beyond repair. Many teeth in the line of jaw fracture are removed to treat the fractured bone.

4. Impacted or supernumerary teeth often do not take their place in the line of occlusion.

5. Orthodontic consideration may require the removal of fully erupted teeth, erupting teeth, and overretained deciduous teeth. Malposed teeth and third molar teeth that have lost their antagonists can be included.

6. Devitalized teeth, radiographically negative, have been removed as a last resort at the request of the physician because of the possibility that they are foci of infection, although this concept is considered extremely questionable today, mainly because neither the dentist nor the physician can diagnose accurately whether such infection is present.

7. Prosthetic considerations may require the removal of one or many teeth for design or stability of the prosthesis.

8. Esthetic considerations at times transcend purely functional factors.

9. There may be a pathologic condition in surrounding bone that involves the tooth, or treatment of the pathologic condition may require removal of the tooth. Examples are cysts, osteomyelitis, tumors, and bone necrosis.

10. Teeth "in line of fire" of planned therapeutic radiation to a nearby area are removed so that a supervening osteoradionecrosis of the bone will not be complicated by radiation caries or by necrosing pulps and their sequelae.

Contraindications

Few conditions are absolute contraindications for extraction of teeth. Teeth have been removed in the presence of all types of complications because of necessity. In these situations much more preparation of the patient is necessary to prevent serious damage or death or to obtain healing of the local wound. For example, the injection of a local anesthetic, let alone the extraction of a tooth, can cause instant death in a patient in an addisonian crisis. Surgical intervention of any kind, including exodontics, may activate systemic or local disease. Therefore, a list of relative contraindications is given. In some instances these conditions become absolute contraindications.

Local contraindications. Local contraindications are associated mainly with infection and, to a lesser extent, with malignant disease.

1. Acute infection with an uncontrolled cellulitis must be controlled so that it does not spread further. The patient may exhibit a toxemia, which brings complicating systemic factors into consideration. The tooth that caused the infection is of secondary importance at the moment; however, to better control the infection, the tooth is removed as soon as such removal does not endanger the life of the patient. Before antibiotics became available the tooth was never removed until the infection had become localized, the pus was drained, and the infection had subsided to a chronic state. This sequence of events took much longer than the present method of removing the tooth as soon as an adequate blood level of a specific antibiotic had brought systemic factors under control.

2. Acute pericoronitis is managed more conservatively than other local infections

because of the mixed bacteriologic flora found in the area, the fact that the third molar area has more direct access to the deep fascial planes of the neck, and the fact that removal of this tooth is a complicated procedure involving ossisection.

3. Acute infectious stomatitis is a labile, debilitating, and painful disease, which is complicated by intercurrent exodontics.

4. Malignant disease disturbed by the extraction of a tooth embedded in the growth will react with exacerbated growth and nonhealing of the local wound.

5. Irradiated jaws may develop an acute radio-osteomyelitis after extraction because of a lack of blood supply. The condition is severely painful and may terminate fatally.

Systemic contraindications. Any systemic disease or malfunction can complicate or be complicated by an extraction. These conditions are too numerous to list. Some of the more frequently encountered relative contraindications are as follows:

1. Uncontrolled diabetes mellitus is characterized by infection of the wound and absence of normal healing.

2. Cardiac disease, such as coronary artery disease, hypertension, and cardiac decompensation, can complicate exodontia. Management may require the help of a physician. Usually a postinfarction patient is not subjected to oral surgery within 6 months of his infarction.[2]

3. Blood dyscrasias include simple as well as more serious anemias, hemorrhagic diseases such as hemophilia, and the leukemias. Preparation for extraction varies considerably with underlying factors.

4. Debilitating diseases of any kind make patients poor risks for further traumatic insults.

5. Addison's disease or any steroid deficiency is extremely dangerous. The patient who has been treated for any disease with steroid therapy, even though the disease is conquered and the patient has not taken steroids for a year, may not have sufficient adrenal cortex secretion to withstand the stress of an extraction without taking additional steroids.

6. Fever of unexplained origin is rarely cured and often is worsened by extraction. One possibility is an undiagnosed subacute bacterial endocarditis, a condition that would be complicated considerably by an extraction.

7. Nephritis requiring treatment can create a formidable problem in preparing the patient for exodontics.

8. Pregnancy without complications presents no great problem. Precautions should be taken to guard against low oxygen tension in general anesthesia or in extreme fright. Obstetricians hold varied opinions regarding the timing of extractions, but they usually prefer that necessary extractions be done in the second trimester. Menstruation is not a contraindication, although elective exodontia is not done during the period because of less nervous stability and greater tendency toward hemorrhage of all tissues.

9. Senility is a relative contraindication that requires greater care in overcoming a poor physiologic response to surgery and a prolonged negative nitrogen balance.

10. Psychoses and neuroses reflect a nervous instability that complicates exodontics.

THE OFFICE AND EQUIPMENT

The chief difference between the office devoted solely to oral surgery and the one designed for general practice is the lack of fixed equipment around the chair in the former. In the exodontist's office the space on the left of the chair, usually occupied by the dental unit and cuspidor, is left vacant so that the assistant can stand there. The patient either expectorates into a sterilized stainless steel basin that is held in the lap or held by the nurse, or a suction machine is used. If suction is used, it is more powerful than that produced by the average dental unit and often is central suction produced by a large compressor located in another room or area. If bone burs are used, a high-speed handpiece attached to an engine or

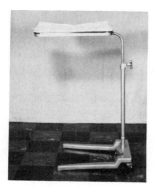

Fig. 3-1. Mayo stand holding covered instrument tray.

more often to a source of compressed gas is employed. A general anesthesia machine is brought near the chair after the patient is seated. Instead of a bracket table in front of the patient where its contents are in view, a Mayo stand is placed behind the chair (Fig. 3-1).

Little change is necessary to adapt the general office for exodontics, provided that several basic considerations are included in the design. The cuspidor on the unit can be pushed back so that the assistant can work on the side of the patient opposite the operator. A good light on the unit will suffice for exodontics. If suction on the unit is inadequate and central suction is not available in the building, a mobile suction machine can be purchased. A Mayo stand should be available behind the chair so that the bracket table is not used. The sink need not be larger than the conventional size, but it should have knee controls. No sink in a dental office should have hand controls. Foot pedals are difficult to clean under, and elbow controls sometimes get in the way.

Adequate storage space should be available for the sterile armamentarium, either out of sight in the room or in a nearby area. A place should be provided in the room for a sterile canister of sponges.

A radiographic viewbox should be placed in a prominent position facing the operator. This can be placed on the wall opposite the operator and to the left of the assistant. The room should contain an x-ray machine so that the patient does not have to move for postoperative or intercurrent radiographs.

ARMAMENTARIUM

The more experience the exodontist acquires and the greater volume of work he or she sees, the simpler and more standardized the armamentarium becomes. Because the practitioner does not wish to lose time picking up several instruments, because it costs more money to add another forceps to the complete sets, and because each additional instrument must be handled many times by the office personnel, he or she learns to do more with each instrument. Some practitioners boast that they can work with only two forceps. Although this philosophy seems foolhardy, since modern forceps are carefully designed to fit the anatomy of the various teeth, it nevertheless proves the ultimate in the "back pocket" philosophy.

Many practitioners have substituted universal forceps for paired (right and left) forceps. Another saving is the elimination of many, if not all, special forceps. Naturally, wide variation is found in individual likes and dislikes as well as in various techniques that call for specialized instruments. The beginner is well advised to start out with a basic armamentarium and to become thoroughly familiar with its use for at least a year before considering new or additional instruments.

An armamentarium that has proved satisfactory and complete over the years is as follows:

Forceps (Fig. 3-2)
    Standard forceps No. 1 for maxillary central and lateral incisors, canines, and premolars in some instances
    Standard forceps No. 65 for maxillary root tips
    Standard forceps No. 10S for maxillary molars
    Ash forceps, Mead No. 1, for mandibular teeth
    Standard forceps No. 16, cowhorn, for mandibular molars

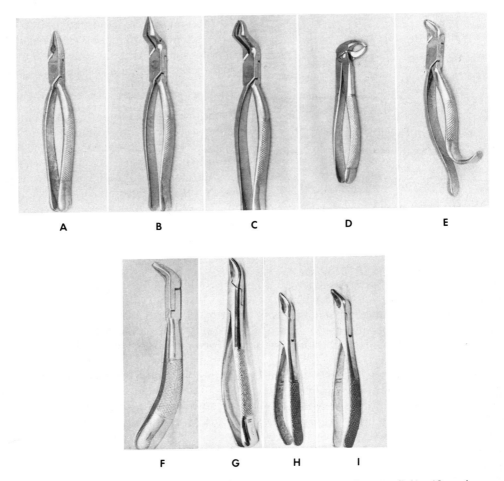

Fig. 3-2. Extraction forceps. **A,** No. 1. **B,** No. 65. **C,** No. 10S. **D,** Mead forceps. **E,** No. 16 cowhorn. **F,** No. 151. **G,** No. 150. **H,** Children's maxillary forceps. **I,** Children's mandibular forceps.

(Standard forceps No. 150 for maxillary premolars and standard forceps No. 151 for mandibular premolars can be added to these basic five forceps if desired. In addition, a maxillary and a mandibular child's forceps are desirable.)

Exolevers (Fig. 3-3)

Winter exolevers 14R and 14L, "long Winter exolevers," designed primarily for removing deep-seated mandibular molar roots

Winter exolevers 11R and 11L, "short Winter exolever," designed for elevation of tooth roots near the rim of the alveolus

Straight-shank No. 34, "shoehorn exolever," designed for elevating roots as well as entire teeth

Krogh exolever, Krogh 12B, designed for removal of third molar impactions

Root exolevers Nos. 1, and 3, Hu-Friedy, for removal of fractured root apices

Many designs are made, which vary in delicateness. The beginner needs a fairly stout instrument to minimize breakage, but sharp, delicate instruments are better. They are made in sets of three: right, left, and straight.

(Potts exolevers R and L can be added for deciduous root tips.)

Surgical instruments (Fig. 3-4)

Bard-Parker handle No. 3; No. 15 blade used most frequently

Rongeur No. 4, universal, for cutting bone

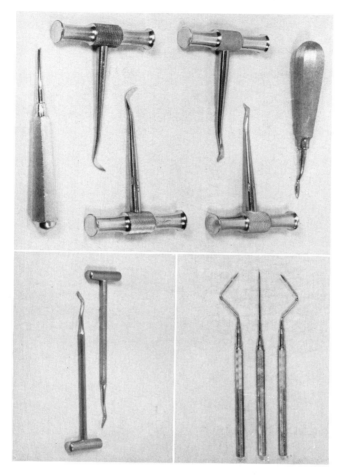

Fig. 3-3. Exolevers. Top row, left to right: straight-shank; long Winter (right and left); short Winter (right and left); Krogh spearpoint. Bottom row, left to right: Potts elevators (right and left); root exolevers.

Bone file No. 10

Chisel, Gardner No. 52, and Mallet, standard No. 1, if chisel technique is used

High-speed handpiece and burs if the bur technique is used

Retractors, Austin

Curets, Molt No. 2 for universal use, including breaking periodontal attachment before exodontia; Molt Nos. 5 and 6, same size, angled to right and to left; Molt No. 4 for periosteal elevator and for removal of large cysts

Needle holder, Mayo-Hegar 15-cm (A needle holder should be 15 cm long; a delicate hemostat is not adequate.)

Needles, ½-circle, cutting edge

Suture material, silk No. 3-0

Scissors, tissue

Scissors, suture

Hemostats, small curved

Allis forceps for grasping tissue

Single-tooth forceps, Adson 11-cm, for delicate grasp of tissue

College pliers

"Russian forceps," V. Mueller Co., 15-cm, for grasping teeth

Several general observations can be made about purchasing equipment. Stainless steel equipment is more costly initially, but it holds up better. It is mandatory that two

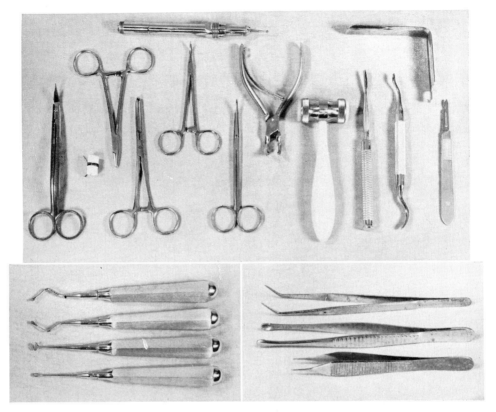

Fig. 3-4. Surgical instruments. Top row, left to right: suture scissors; suture and needle around cotton roll; needle holder; Allis forceps; hemostat; high-speed drill; tissue scissors; rongeurs; mallet; chisel; bone file; retractor; scalpel. Bottom row, left: Molt curets; right: Adson forceps (bottom), Russian forceps, college pliers.

complete sets of instruments be bought, although an office devoted to exodontics will have many sets. If an instrument is dropped or otherwise contaminated, time is too precious to await resterilization, even with high-speed autoclaving. If the bur technique for bone removal is employed, special care must be given by the operator and by all office personnel to provide a sterile handpiece for each procedure. Perhaps the greatest argument in favor of the chisel technique is that a sterile chisel is always available, whereas the general practitioner in a hurry might be tempted to employ the usual handpiece for what is considered to be just a small bone or tooth cut in the wound. Some of the worst infections in patients admitted to the dental service of a general hospital in the South Pacific in World War II were the result of exodontics complicated by handpiece infection.

Sterilization and care of instruments

The best way to sterilize instruments is by autoclaving. Sharp instruments such as chisels and scalpels can be sterilized by the hot oil sterilizer. Cold solutions are used for storing sterilized instruments or for primary sterilization if many hours of undisturbed time can be given. The autoclave is used for sterilization of gauze sponges, cotton applicators, and linen.

Storage of the sterilized instruments is a problem. In the office devoted to exodontia

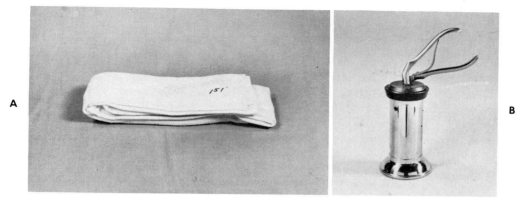

Fig. 3-5. A, Forceps in sterile towel. Note forceps number written on towel before autoclaving. **B,** Pick-up forceps.

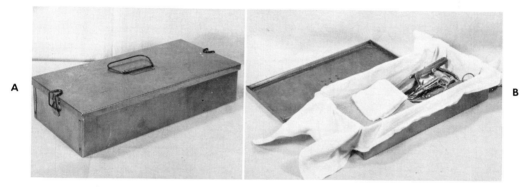

Fig. 3-6. A, Stainless steel box as removed from autoclave. **B,** Box opened, showing folded towels, gauze sponges, and accessory surgical instruments.

a sterile table can be set up each day. This is not feasible in a general practice. Here each forceps should be wrapped in a linen towel large enough to fit the Mayo stand, and towel and forceps should be sterilized together. A pencil mark on the outside of the pack before sterilization will identify the instrument (Fig. 3-5, A). Another technique employs a paper autoclave bag for each instrument. A complete tray of sterile accessory instruments covered with a towel should be available for more extensive surgery. The instruments can be sterilized on the tray if there is space to store the complete trays (which is the ideal way), or the instruments can be placed in a stainless steel box, which is more convenient to store

and fits the smaller autoclave (Fig. 3-6). In the latter case a sterile pick-up forceps (Fig. 3-5, B) is used to arrange the instruments on the Mayo tray, which has been covered with a sterile towel. Sharp instruments are placed in the autoclaved box or on the tray after they have been sterilized by other methods.

Instruments should be scrubbed with a brush and soap before being sterilized to remove blood and debris that would harden during the process. Hospitals do this with ultrasonic equipment. The hinge of forceps should be free swinging at all times. The patient lacks confidence in the operator who uses two hands to pull the handles of a frozen forceps apart just before an extraction. Rust has no place in the dental office.

The working points of all instruments should be sharp. Forceps with dull tips can be returned to the factory for refurbishing. A chisel that has been on a tray should be scrubbed and placed on the dentist's desk for inspection. If the chisel has been used, it should be sharpened on a stone so that it will cut hair. Scalpel blades and needles should be changed frequently if disposable items are not used.

REFERENCES

1. Baldwin, D. C.: An investigation of psychological and behavioral responses to dental extraction in children, J. Dent. Res. **45:**1637, 1966.
2. Glasser, S. P.: The problems of patients with cardiovascular disease undergoing dental treatment, J. Am. Dent. Assoc. **94:**1158, 1977.
3. Kruger, G. O., and Reynolds, D. C.: Maxillofacial pain. In McCarthy, F. M., editor: Emergencies in dental practice, Philadelphia, 1967, W. B. Saunders Co., p. 123.
4. McKenzie, R. E., Szmyd, L., and Hartman, B. O.: A study of selected personality factors in oral surgery patients, J. Am. Dent. Assoc. **74:**763, 1967.
5. Shannon, I. L., Isbell, G. M., and Hester, W. R.: Stress in dental patients. IV. Effect of local anesthetic administration on serum free 17-hydroxycorticosteroid patterns, J. Oral Surg. **21:**50, 1963.

CHAPTER 4

Forceps extraction

Gustav O. Kruger

After the history, radiographs, and examination have been completed, the exodontic procedure is discussed with the patient, and the operator makes notes concerning the planning of the procedure, including premedication if indicated. The anxious patient who will be accompanied to the office can start premedication the night before the procedure or one-half hour before arriving at the office. Other patients can be premedicated in the office while waiting in the reception room. Medications by mouth or by intramuscular or intravenous routes vary in depth of effect and time of onset according to the agent and the amount used.

ANESTHESIA

The armamentarium should be in place, covered with a sterile towel, when the patient enters the operatory. The patient is seated, and the chair is adjusted to the proper position for the administration of the anesthetic. A paper napkin is placed on the patient, and he is given one-third cup of mouthwash in a paper cup to rinse his mouth. The local anesthetic is administered. The operating light is turned off, and the patient is allowed to read or is engaged in conversation for a minimum of 3 to 10 minutes, depending on the tooth or teeth to be extracted. The operator should use at least a full minute of this time to study intently the radiograph of the tooth involved and its surrounding structures for anatomical and pathological variations from normal.

POSITION OF PATIENT

The chair usually has to be repositioned to be satisfactory for exodontics. For mandibular extractions it should be as low as possible. For maxillary extractions the upper jaw of the patient should be at the height of the operator's shoulder. These positions allow the upper arm to hang loosely from the shoulder girdle and obviate the fatigue associated with holding the shoulders in an unnaturally high position during the course of a day. The low positions allow the operator to bring the back and leg muscles into the operation to assist the arm. The chair can be tipped backward slightly for maxillary extractions. The present day contour chair has the patient in a semirecumbent position, which is ideal for oral surgery.

PREPARATION AND DRAPING

The operating light is turned on, the operator and the assistant scrub, and a sterile towel is placed over the paper napkin as the dentist admonishes the patient not to touch it. Since the towel is sterile,

49

gauze sponges or instruments can be placed on it. If a complicated exodontic procedure is planned or if the patient manifests anxiety, another sterile towel is placed over the eyes from behind the head and fastened with a sterile pin or towel clamp over the forehead. The operator and assistant may place sterile towels over their uniforms, fastening them with sterile towel clamps. The exposed portion of the patient's face is wiped with sponges dipped in benzalkonium chloride, 1:10,000 solution.

A 7.6 by 7.6 cm gauze sponge is placed in the mouth so as to isolate the operative field. The sponge allows the field to be dried, it keeps the tongue out of the way, it absorbs saliva and blood, it prevents teeth and fragments from slipping into the posterior pharynx, and it keeps the patient from leaning over the bowl to spit, which wastes time. If a continuous suction technique is chosen, the gauze sponge may or may not be used.

POSITION OF LEFT HAND

The fingers of the left hand serve primarily to retract the soft tissues and to provide the operator with sensory stimuli for the detection of expansion of the alveolar plate and root movement under the plate. It is for these reasons that one finger is always placed on the labial or buccal alveolar plate overlying the tooth and another finger retracts the lip or tongue. A third finger or the thumb helps guide the forceps into place on the tooth and protects teeth in the opposite jaw from accidental contact with the back of the forceps if the tooth loosens suddenly. In mandibular extractions, equal and opposite torquing force must be provided by the left hand to counteract the forces placed on the mandible by the extracting forceps in the right hand so that temporomandibular joint pain and injury do not occur. Each extraction and each type of forceps require different left-hand positions to accommodate the positions of the right hand, which holds the forceps.

FORCEPS EXTRACTION

A sharp No. 2 Molt curet is used to check the anesthesia. Then it is slid around the free gingival cuff to sever the gingival attachment of each tooth to be extracted in that quadrant. No force should be employed since this will alarm the patient.

The forceps are brought from the Mayo stand behind the patient, shielded from his view as much as possible, and guided into the mouth with the help of a finger or thumb of the left hand. The palatal or lingual beak is placed first, followed by the buccal or labial beak. The long axis of the forceps must be placed parallel with the long axis of the tooth. Failure to accomplish this is the most common cause of fractured teeth. (Use of the wrong anatomical forceps, such as a molar forceps on a premolar, is another common cause for fracture.) Pressure is placed toward the apex of the tooth to "set" the forceps at the cementoenamel junction.

Enough pressure is placed on the handles to hold the forceps on the tooth without slipping, but uncommon force may shatter a weak tooth. The forceps should be held near the ends of the handles to obtain the maximum mechanical advantage. No greater delicacy of touch is obtained by holding the forceps midway up the handles. In furniture factories, when an apprentice holds the hammer halfway up the handle, an old foreman takes it from him and cuts off the portion he was not using. This is a lesson he learns early, and he can hardly wait until evening to purchase a new balanced handle.

Each tooth requires a separate series of movements for extraction, which are described in the accompanying photographs and diagrams (Figs. 4-1 to 4-8).

POSTEXTRACTION PROCEDURE

After the extraction, all loose bone spicules and portions of tooth, restoration, or calculus are removed from the socket as well as from the buccal and lingual gutters and the tongue. If pathological tissue is

Text continued on p. 61.

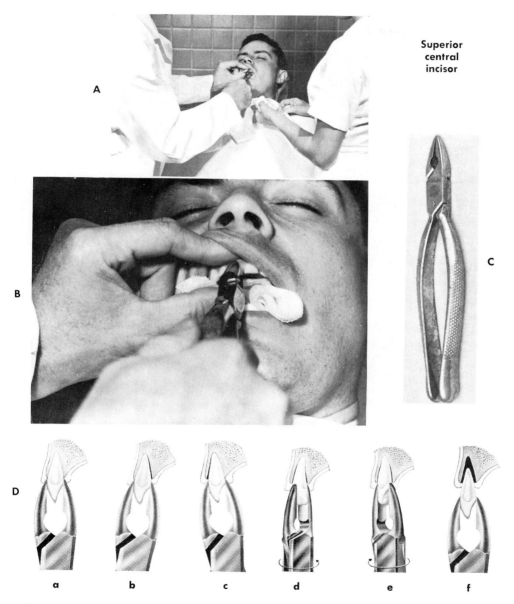

Superior central incisor

Fig. 4-1. A, Positions of patient, operator, and assistant. **B,** Fingers of left hand retracting tissues. **C,** Forceps No. 1. **D,** Extraction movements: *a,* forceps applied; *b,* first movement to labial side; *c,* movement to palatal side; *d,* rotatory movement from labial to distal side; *e,* reversed rotatory movement from labial to mesial side; *f,* downward movement in line with original position of tooth. (**D** from Winter, G. B.: Exodontia, St. Louis, 1913, American Medical Book Co.)

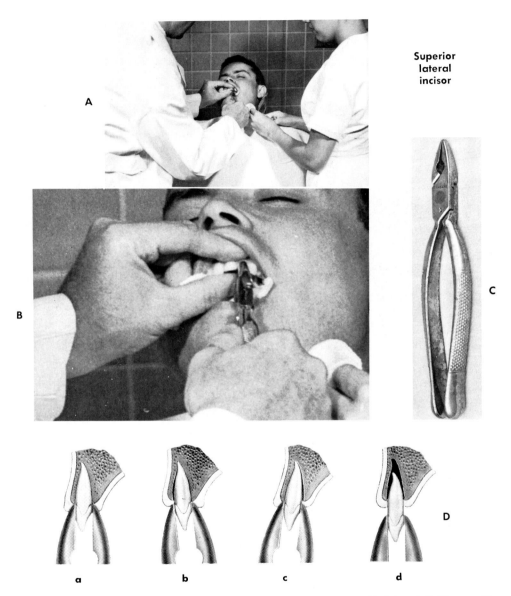

Superior
lateral
incisor

Fig. 4-2. A, Positions of patient, operator, and assistant. **B,** Fingers of left hand. **C,** Forceps No. 1. **D,** Extraction movements: *a,* forceps applied at anatomical neck; *b,* first movement to palatal side; *c,* movement to labial side; *d,* downward movement in line with original position of tooth. (**D** from Winter, G. B., Exodontia, St. Louis, 1913, American Medical Book Co.)

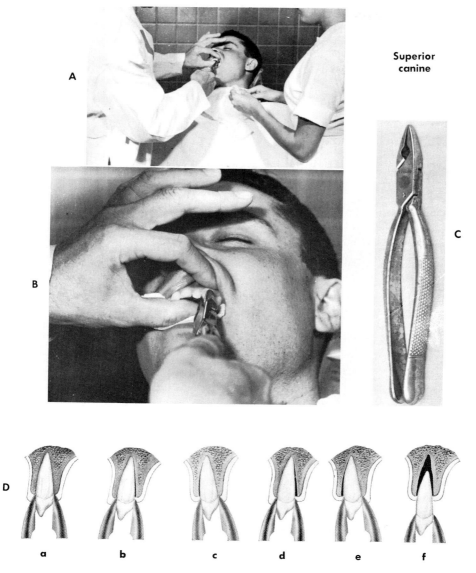

Superior canine

Fig. 4-3. A, Positions of patient, operator, and assistant. Note the straight line made by tooth, forceps, and lower arm while upper arm hangs from shoulder girdle. **B,** Positions of fingers of left hand. **C,** Forceps No. 1. **D,** Extraction movements: *a,* forceps applied at anatomical neck; *b,* first movement to labial side; *c,* movement to palatal side; *d* and *e,* labial and palatal movements more forcibly repeated; *f,* downward movement in line with original position of tooth. (**D** from Winter, G. B.: Exodontia, St. Louis, 1913, American Medical Book Co.)

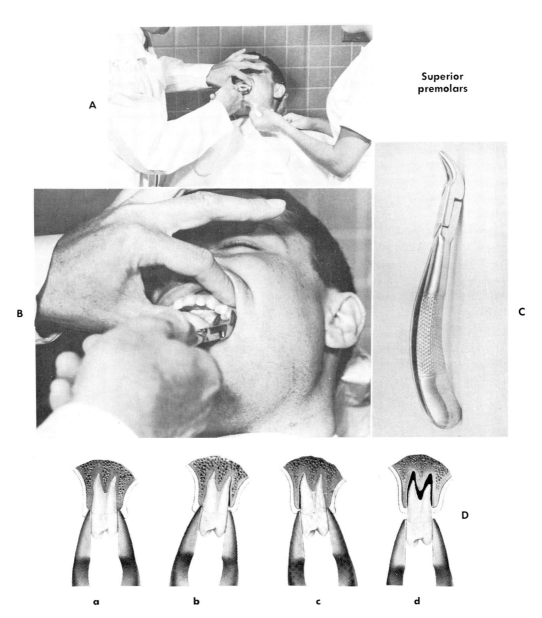

Superior premolars

Fig. 4-4. A, Positions of patient, operator, and assistant. **B,** Positions of fingers of left hand. **C,** Forceps No. 150 (No. 1 can be substituted). **D,** Extraction movements: *a,* forceps applied to anatomical neck; *b,* first movement to buccal side; *c,* movement to palatal side; *d,* downward movement in line with original position of tooth. (**D** from Winter, G. B.: Exodontia, St. Louis, 1913, American Medical Book Co.)

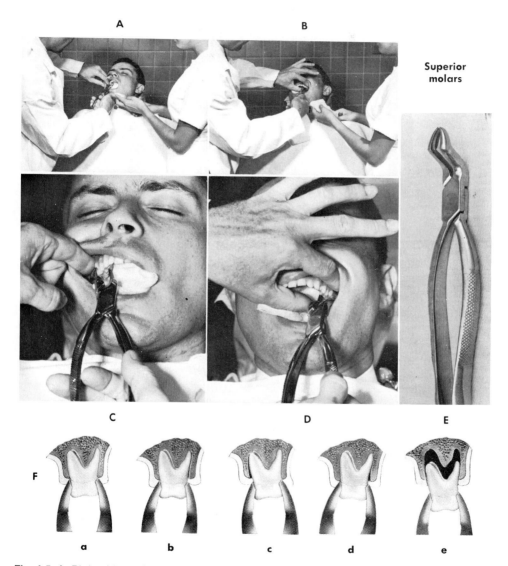

**Superior
molars**

Fig. 4-5. A, Right side positions. **B,** Left side positions. **C,** Retraction of tissues and palpation of buccal plate with radial side of forefinger, right side. **D,** Retraction of tissues, left side. **E,** Forceps No. 10S. **F,** Extraction movements: *a,* forceps applied at anatomical neck; *b,* first movement to buccal side; *c,* movement downward and to palatal side (do not thread lingual root back into socket; the downward and palatal movement may be stopped when the tooth is in its original buccopalatal position, but lower, rather than in palatoversion); *d,* buccal movement repeated more forcibly; *e,* downward movement in line with original position of tooth. (**F** from Winter, G. B.: Exodontia, St. Louis, 1913, American Medical Book Co.)

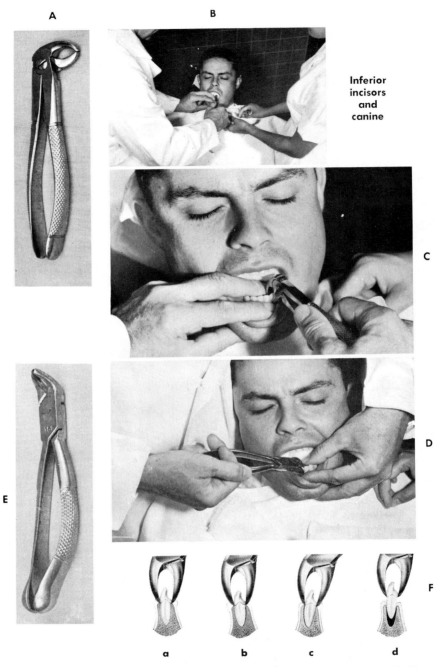

Inferior incisors and canine

Fig. 4-6. A, Mead forceps. **B,** Relative positions of patient, operator, and assistant. **C,** Fingers of left hand retract tongue and lip, while thumb supports jaw. **D,** Reverse position employed with forceps No. 151. **E,** Forceps No. 151. Either this forceps or Mead forceps may be used. **F,** Extraction movements: *a,* forceps placed at anatomical neck; *b,* first movement to labial side; *c,* movement to lingual side; *d,* upward movement in line with original position of tooth. (**F** from Winter, G. B.: Exodontia, St. Louis, 1913, American Medical Book Co.)

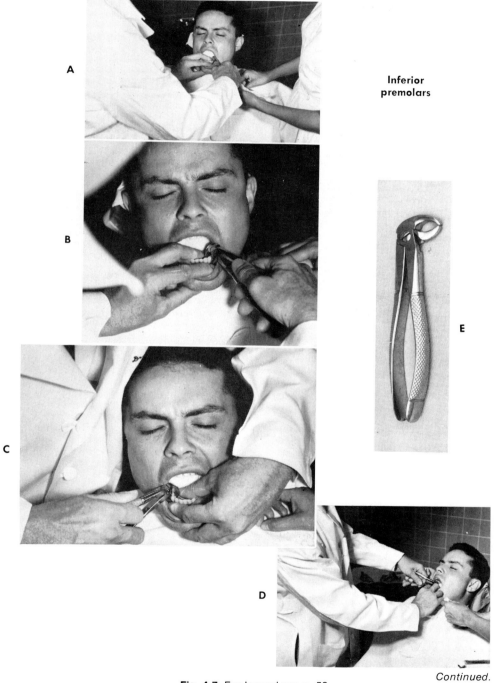

**Inferior
premolars**

Fig. 4-7. For legend see p. 58.

Continued.

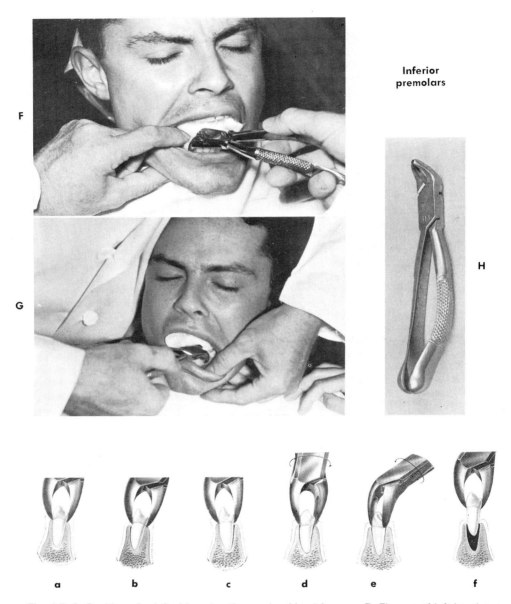

Inferior premolars

Fig. 4-7. A, Positions for left side extractions using Mead forceps. **B,** Fingers of left hand supporting jaw. **C,** Positions for right side extractions. **D,** Alternate position for right side extractions using Mead forceps in left hand. **E,** Mead forceps. **F,** Positions employed for right side extractions using forceps No. 151. **G,** Positions employed for left side extractions using forceps No. 151. **H,** Forceps No. 151. **I,** Extraction movements: *a,* forceps placed at anatomical neck; *b,* first movement to lingual side; *c,* movement to buccal side; *d,* rotatory movement from the mesial to the buccal side; *e,* reversed rotatory movement; *f,* upward movement in line with original position of tooth. (**I** from Winter, G. B.: Exodontia, St. Louis, 1913, American Medical Book Co.)

Inferior molars

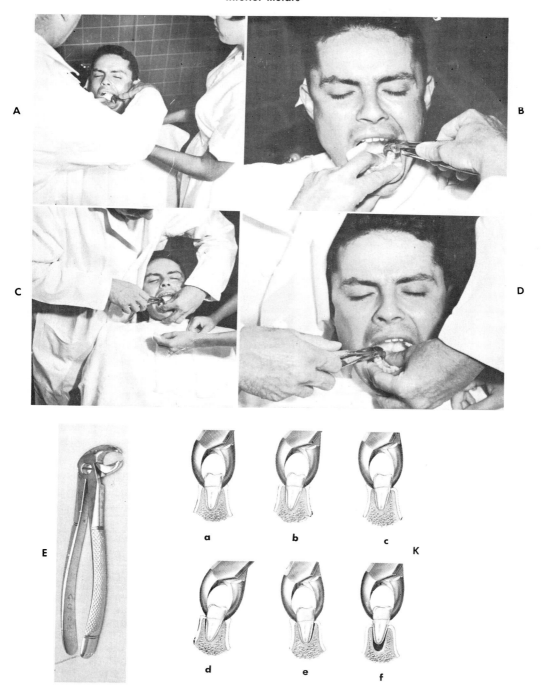

Fig. 4-8. For legend see p. 60.

Inferior molars

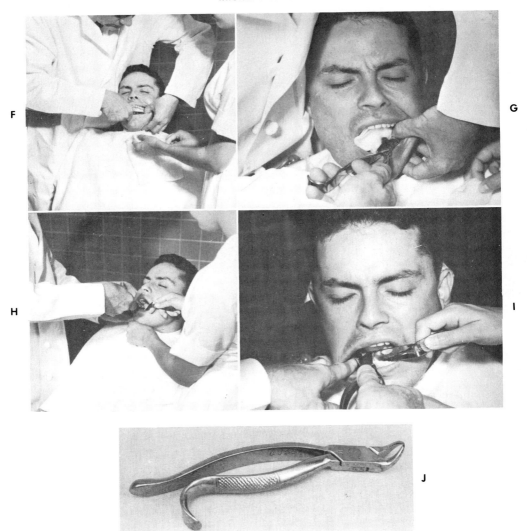

Fig. 4-8. A, Positions for extractions on left side using Mead forceps. **B,** Note positions of left hand. **C,** Positions for extractions on right side using Mead forceps. **D,** The thumb retracts the tongue, the forefinger retracts the lip, and the third finger supports the jaw. **E,** Mead forceps. **F,** Positions for extractions on left side using cowhorn forceps. **G,** Thumb is placed on occlusal surface of next posterior tooth or on ridge of mandible. **H,** Positions for extractions on right side using cowhorn forceps. **I,** Forefinger is placed on ridge of mandible. **J,** Forceps No. 16 (cowhorn). **K,** Extraction movements: *a,* forceps in position; *b,* first movement to lingual side; *c,* movement to buccal side; *d* and *e,* movements to lingual and buccal sides more forcibly repeated; *f,* upward movement in line with original position of tooth. With the cowhorn forceps the beaks are set into the bifurcation by squeezing the handles while moving them up and down. When the two beaks are in place, movements to the lingual and buccal sides are started. (**K** from Winter, G. B.: Exodontia, St. Louis, 1913, American Medical Book Co.)

present in the apical region, it is removed carefully with a small curet. The granulation tissue "velvet" is removed or broken up, but the bone is not scraped. This is *not* done in the maxillary incisor area because the veins here have no valves; consequently, infected material and thrombi may ascend into the cranial cavity to form a cavernous sinus thrombosis. If a recent radiograph does not show apical radiolucency, it is wise not to put a curet into any socket, since this will only inoculate the socket with organisms and debris from the free gingival margin if the original curet is used.

The socket must be compressed by the fingers to reestablish the normal width present before the plate was surgically expanded. In the case of multiple extractions, the sockets can be overcompressed by one third, which will eliminate the need for alveoloplasty in many borderline cases. Sutures usually are not necessary unless the papillae have been incised.

The socket is covered with a 7.6 by 7.6 cm gauze sponge that has been folded into quarters and moistened slightly at its center with cold water. This is done to prevent hemorrhage from the socket from penetrating the gauze at that point, which would be torn away from the remainder of the clot when the gauze is removed, resulting in new bleeding. The side of the gauze placed over the wound is not touched by the operator for aseptic reasons. When the covering sponge is in place, the sponge originally placed over the tongue is removed. Saliva and debris are kept out of the socket by this method. The patient is asked to bite down on the sponge for 5 minutes.

After that time has elapsed, a postoperative radiograph is made for legal as well as professional reasons and another moistened sterile sponge is placed, to be retained until the patient arrives home. Few cases of postoperative hemorrhage will occur if this procedure is followed. A printed instruction sheet is given to the patient, together with a prescription if pain is anticipated.

Analgesic drugs should be started as soon as the patient returns home, well before the local anesthetic effect disappears. An appointment for postoperative examination is given.

NUMBER OF TEETH TO BE EXTRACTED

Many variables exist in the health and fitness of the patient in addition to the condition of his teeth and their surrounding structures. The planned procedure may involve complicated extractions and alveoloplasty, which may take a considerable length of time and result in a loss of blood of up to 500 ml. In the uncomplicated case the remaining posterior teeth in the maxilla and mandible on one side can be removed in one visit. If an immediate denture will not be made, occasionally the mandibular canine will be removed too, so that an infiltration anesthetic can be given to remove the incisors later.

Further surgery is done no earlier than 1 week afterward, at which time swelling and discomfort have disappeared, and the white cell count has returned to normal. The posterior teeth on the opposite side are removed 1 week later. The anterior teeth are removed after another week, or whenever the posterior wounds have healed well.

ORDER OF EXTRACTION

The order of extraction is important. Since anesthesia becomes effective in the maxilla earlier, the maxillary teeth are extracted first (with the exception of impacted teeth). Also, debris such as enamel or amalgam fragments cannot be lost in open mandibular sockets. The most posterior teeth are removed first for better vision, since hemorrhage collects in the posterior region. In a mouth containing teeth that are difficult to extract, the first molar and canine teeth are extracted after their adjacent teeth are removed so that better purchase can be made on the tooth and so that advantage can be taken of earlier plate expansion resulting from adjacent extractions. These two teeth are encased in the so-called bony pillars of the face. Accordingly, the third molar, second molar, second premolar, first molar, first premolar, lateral incisor, and canine would be extracted in that order in difficult cases.

If a tooth or a root should break, it is best to stop and recover the root before proceeding to the next extraction. Consequently, the adjacent socket does not produce hemorrhage that obscures the field, and the location of the root is not lost. If there is a good possibility that adjacent teeth may break or if an alveoloplasty will be necessary, the operator may continue with the extractions, making careful note of the location of the root, and then design the surgical flap to accommodate the problem or problems that need attention.

REFERENCE

1. Rounds, F. W., and Rounds, C. E.: Principles and technique of exodontia, ed. 2, St. Louis, 1962, The C. V. Mosby Co.

CHAPTER 5

Complicated exodontics

Gustav O. Kruger

ALVEOLOPLASTY

Alveoloplasty or alveolectomy is the surgical removal of a portion of the alveolar process. When multiple extractions are performed, the contours of the alveolar ridge should be considered in the light of future prosthetic needs. The ideal ridge is U shaped. Natural resorption will contour the ridges, occasionally unevenly, but a longer period of time is required, and the patient may experience discomfort until the sharp bony edges underlying the sensitive periosteum round off. Judgment is required to determine whether alveoloplasty is necessary and how extensively it should be done.

Conservation of the maximum amount of bone consistent with a good ridge is the goal. Although the ridge that is extensively contoured by surgery is beautiful, with end-to-end mucosal closure over the sockets, the procedure is worthless if severe resorption of the remaining bone makes denture wearing impossible after a few years. On the other hand, laziness on the operator's part in smoothing obvious sharp edges, protuberances, and excessive undercuts that cause discomfort and an unsatisfactory denture base cannot be equated with conservatism.

Several years ago at a meeting of oral surgeons, discussion revealed that everyone had become more conservative in alveoloplasty procedures. The participants reported seeing greater numbers of elderly edentulous patients whose life-span had increased and in whom no alveolar bone remained. Finally, an elderly oral surgeon in the back of the room said, "I am a diabetic. As you know, diabetics experience rapid and extensive bone resorption. When my son removed all my teeth he said, 'Dad, I am going to remove only the teeth and not one sharp ridge or piece of bone because we have to save every bit of bone we can.' Gentlemen, I suffered the agony of the damned until the sharp edges rounded off. On the basis of my personal experience, I make sure that the bone is smooth, even if I have to remove a little bone in a patient who is expected to undergo extensive resorption."

The most conservative procedure is compression of the alveolar walls by finger and thumb pressure. Extraction usually expands the labial or buccal cortex. Pressure will restore the walls to their former position. Overcompression by heavy pressure can reduce the width of the sockets by one third.

If there is a question in the operator's mind about the amount of natural resorption that will take place, a better judgment is possible 3 weeks after the extractions are accomplished. Most of the initial resorption will be completed in 3 weeks. At that time an extensive alveoloplasty may still be necessary, but more frequently the operator will find that only a few small areas require contouring.

Simple alveoloplasty. After multiple extractions the buccal alveolar plates and interseptal bone are examined for protuberances and sharp edges. If alveoloplasty is necessary, incisions are made across the interseptal crests. The mucoperiosteum is raised carefully from the bone with a No. 4 Molt curet or a periosteal elevator. Diffi-

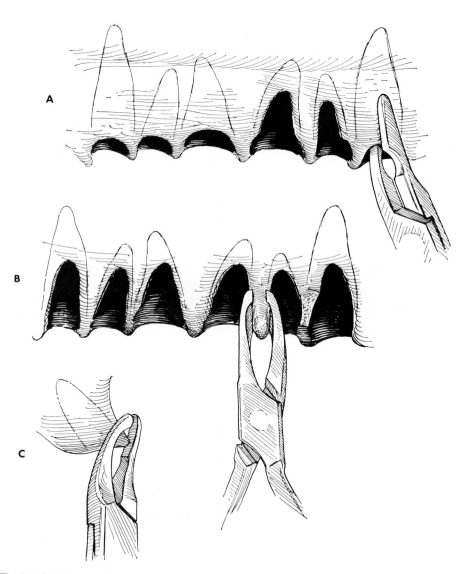

Fig. 5-1. Simple alveoloplasty. **A,** Rongeur removing labial plate. **B,** Removal of interseptal tip. **C,** Side view of interseptal tip removal.

culty is experienced in starting the flap at the edge of the bone because periosteum is attached at the ends of bones, but caution must be exercised in not raising the flap higher than two thirds of the way up the empty socket. To raise it further would strip the lightly attached mucobuccal fold, with the consequence of serious loss of space for denture flange height.

The flap is retracted gently and an edge of a gauze sponge placed between bone and flap. A universal rongeur is placed sideways halfway up the empty sockets, and the buccal or labial alveolar plate is resected to a uniform height in all sockets (Fig. 5-1, *A*). The rongeur now is placed at a 45-degree angle over the interseptal crest, one beak in each socket, and the labial or buccal interseptal tip is removed (Fig. 5-1, *B* and *C*). This procedure is accomplished on all interseptal crests. Bone bleeders are controlled by rotating a small curet in the bleeding point. A file lightly pulled in one direction over all cuts will smooth the bone. Loose particles are removed, the gauze is removed so that the flap resumes its place on the bone, and a finger is rubbed over the mucosal surface to examine the smoothness of the alveolus.

The buccal plate should be contoured to approximately the same height as the palatal plate to form a broad, flat ridge. Excessive undercuts in the upper posterior and lower anterior segments should be given particular attention. Excessive soft tissue and chronic granulation tissue are removed from the buccal and palatal flaps, which are then sutured over the interseptal areas but not over the open sockets. Interrupted or continuous sutures are placed without tension.

Radical alveoloplasty. At times radical contouring of the alveolar ridge is indicated because of extremely prominent undercuts or, in some instances, a marked discrepancy in horizontal relation of maxillary and mandibular ridges caused by marked overjet. Such patients may require complete removal of the labial plate to achieve satisfactory prosthetic replacement (Fig. 5-2).

In such cases a mucoperiosteal flap is raised prior to extraction. Extraction of the teeth can be facilitated by first removing the labial bone overlying the roots of the teeth (Fig. 5-3, *A* and *B*). This bone removal will also ensure preservation of interradicular bone. After removal of the teeth the remaining bone is trimmed and contoured to the desired labial and occlusal height with the chisel or rongeur and file (Fig. 5-3, *C*). Excessive tissue is trimmed

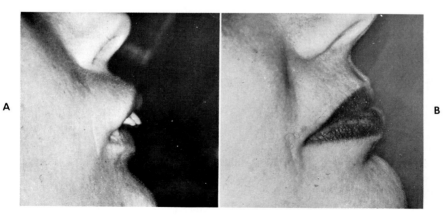

Fig. 5-2. Radical alveoloplasty. **A,** Preoperative overjet that was an esthetic and functional deformity. **B,** Postoperative result with denture in place.

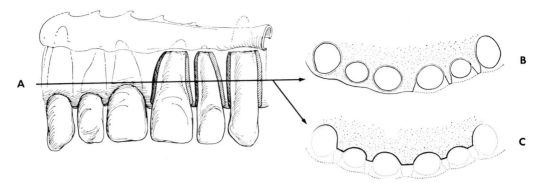

Fig. 5-3. Radical alveoloplasty. **A,** Mucoperiosteal flap raised and labial bone overlying teeth removed. **B,** Cross section showing removal of labial bone to encompass greatest width of tooth. **C,** Teeth removed and septa contoured back to palatal plate.

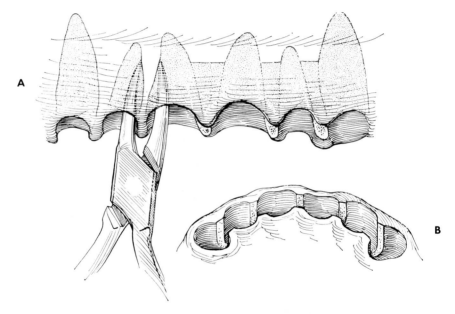

Fig. 5-4. Interradicular alveoloplasty. **A,** Narrow-beaked rongeur removes septa without raising a flap or destroying labial plate. **B,** The weakened labial plate is collapsed to the palatal plate by thumb pressure.

from the labial and palatal flaps, which are approximated with interrupted or continuous sutures over the septa.

In closing such a flap it may be necessary to remove a wedge of tissue in the premolar areas to allow for the decreased outer cir-

cumference of the labial bone. Care must be taken with this larger flap to preserve as much attachment at the height of the mucobuccal fold as possible, or else an excessively long flap is encountered at closure. If the flap is not supported by an immediate denture and the excess tissue is resected, the height of the mucobuccal fold will be diminished drastically.

Interradicular alveoloplasty. In this procedure interradicular bone is sacrificed rather than labial plate. The teeth are extracted. No attempt is made to raise a mucoperiosteal flap over the bone to be collapsed. Interradicular bone is removed with a narrow-beaked rongeur (one beak in each socket) to a height halfway up the sockets (Fig. 5-4). A notch is cut by rongeur or chisel in the labial plate in each premolar area to allow for the greater circumference of the labial plate to fit into its new position. The bone is collapsed to the desired contour by thumb pressure.

Less resorption and less postoperative pain are associated with this procedure since periosteum is not stripped from bone and does not rest on roughened bone.

SURGICAL FLAP

A surgical flap is a soft tissue flap that is incised and retracted so that underlying bone can be removed to expose teeth, roots, and pathological tissue. Extractions and root removal procedures accomplished through the intact alveolus are called closed procedures. Operations requiring a surgical flap are called open procedures.

Basically, the indication for the surgical flap is inability to remove the structure or tissue without traumatizing the surrounding tissues. If a closed procedure fails, adequate visualization and access are obtained by means of an open procedure. A root remnant that cannot be recovered by ordinary means is removed by making a surgical flap. A large tooth that is encased in dense bone and will not move with forceps pressure is dissected out under a surgical flap, making forceps delivery possible. However, there are indications for making a surgical flap without first attempting a closed procedure. For example, if there is a reasonable possibility that the crown of a tooth will fracture because it is

weakened by extensive caries or large restorations or if the crown is not present, a surgical flap should be considered. Some operators routinely prepare all devitalized teeth because the crown and root are friable after endodontic procedures. If the roots of a tooth are widely divergent, curved, or enlarged by hypercementosis, a flap may be prepared. If the overlying bone structure is enlarged or especially dense, or if the periodontal membrane is atrophic or absent (ankylosis), surgery is indicated. A large area of pathological tissue that cannot be removed through the narrow socket may be removed by way of a surgical flap.

Principles. Healing should take place without complication if basic surgical principles are followed. The incision should be designed so that the blood supply of the flap is adequate. If the free end of the flap is wide and the base containing the blood supply is narrow, nutrition to the flap may be inadequate. The flap should contain all the structures overlying bone, including mucosa, submucosa, and periosteum, with special care given to include the periosteum in the flap. The flap should be sufficiently large that adequate vision and space for removal of bone are present without damaging the soft tissue edges. The incision should always be made over bone that will not be removed, so that the sutured incisions are supported by bone. Incisions made in tissues that harbor uncontrolled infection may cause rapid spread of the infection.

Types. The two basic types of intraoral surgical flaps are the envelope flap and the flap that has a vertical component on the buccal or labial surface. The envelope flap is made by incising the tissues around the necks of several teeth anterior and posterior to the area and spreading the resultant labial or buccal flap away from the bone. This flap is used in removing impacted teeth more than in other extractions. The vertical flap employs a vertical incision extending from the mucobuccal fold to a horizontal gingival incision around the necks of the teeth. Less tissue is raised, and the free gingival fibers of adjacent teeth are not incised. Some operators prefer one type, some the other.

Surgical procedure. Incision with a No. 15 blade is made around the buccal or labial gingival cuff surrounding the tooth posterior to the one to be operated on, around the tooth itself, and then angled upward toward the mucobuccal fold away from the tooth to be removed (Fig. 5-5, *A*).

Elevation of the mucoperiosteal flap is started in the vertical component where the periosteal attachment is not tight, and the periosteal elevator is worked toward the gingival cuff incisions as well as backward. The thin periosteum overlying the bone must be included in the flap. The flap is raised. The edge of the elevator is inserted 2 mm under the attached anterior tissue midway between cuff and fold for later entrance of the suture needle.

The flap is held up from the incisal plane

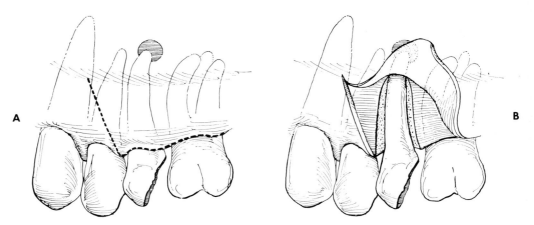

Fig. 5-5. Surgical flap. **A,** Incision. **B,** Retraction of flap and removal of labial bone to greatest width of tooth. Note that the edge of the flap, which will be sutured, will be supported by undissected bone.

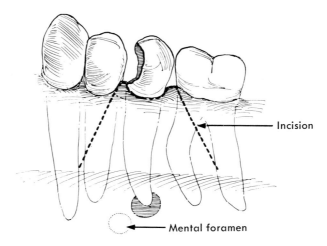

Fig. 5-6. Inverted incision for mandibular flap in the premolar-molar area.

with the periosteal elevator, or a piece of gauze is placed under the flap to retract it away from the field of operation with a finger. Retraction should be gentle to prevent damage and edema. The flap should remain retracted without relaxation of the retracting force until the operation is completed.

Bone removal may be accomplished by chisel, bur, or rongeur, the last being used to start ossisection if an empty socket is present. In dissection of a tooth, cuts parallel to the long axis of the tooth are made in the labial or buccal plate on the mesial and distal sides of the root. After removal of the buccal plate, further bone cuts are made on the two sides of the wound until the greatest width of the root is exposed. Care must be taken to avoid roots of the adjacent teeth (Fig. 5-5, *B*).

The tooth is removed with forceps or elevators. Pathological tissue at the apex is removed with curets. Edges of the bony incision are smoothed with a file or small curet. All debris and small spicules are removed. The flap is returned to position. A suture is placed through the edge of the free flap about halfway between cuff and fold and sutured to an opposite point in the fixed tissue anterior to the incision. It is tied without tension. A suture to the lingual tissues is not necessary. A folded, moist gauze sponge is placed over the socket to prevent bleeding.

Variations in basic flap design are necessary in special areas. In the mandibular premolar area a distal vertical incision is added so that the mental foramen structures can be protected (Fig. 5-6). The mandibular molar area benefits from a similar flap for better dissection of the distal root. The double flap is more difficult to suture.

ROOT REMOVAL

The removal of a freshly fractured root is attempted by the closed method, (that is, without a surgical flap) if there is likelihood of success. Many skilled operators

boast that they can remove all such roots through the intact socket. However, it is best to prepare a surgical flap if the technique is not successful within 4 or 5 minutes. Otherwise, a half hour can be wasted, the soft and bony tissues can be traumatized, and the flap has to be made anyway.

Closed procedures. A tooth fractured at its anatomical neck often can be grasped by an anatomical or a root forceps and delivered. An alveolar purchase may be obtained by loosening the buccal or labial gingival cuff with a small, sharp curet. The buccal beak of the forceps is then placed under the tissues on the buccal plate (Fig. 5-7). Pressure on a sharp forceps will bite down on the root, and the root, with the cut alveolar plate attached, is delivered. Occasionally pressure will fracture the plate enough to loosen the tooth, and the forceps is returned to its normal position at the anatomical neck for a normal extraction,

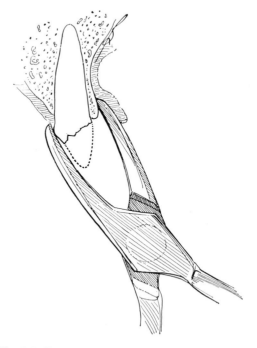

Fig. 5-7. Alveolar purchase. The labial tissues have been released, and the forceps beak is positioned on the labial alveolar plate.

without removing the alveolar plate. Alveolar purchase will not be successful if the buccal plate is excessively heavy or the palatal edge of the root cannot be grasped.

A straight-shank elevator is used to remove roots fractured just below the alveolar margin, especially in the maxilla. The instrument is held in a plane parallel to the long axis of the tooth and worked up along the palatal aspect of the root, with purchase placed on the palatal rim if necessary (Fig. 5-8, *A*) Another method of using the straight-shank elevator is to place it in the interdental area at a right angle to the long axis of the tooth, using a buccal approach. The root is elevated by using the interdental septum as a fulcrum (Fig. 5-8, *B*).

If the root is fractured more than halfway up the socket, root exolevers are used. These are delicate instruments that can break easily (Fig. 3-3). Pressure on the root tip itself may force the fragment into the antrum, the mandibular canal, or the soft tissues. A careful technique is necessary, the most important aspect of which is adequate vision. If bleeding obscures the field, pressure for several minutes on a piece of gauze held by an instrument in the socket, with or without 1:1,000 epinephrine, will allow the fragment to be seen. The light, positions of the patient and operator, retraction of tongue and cheek, and dryness must all be coordinated. Once the fragment is seen it often takes only a moment to remove it.

The object of the procedure is to place the instrument between the socket wall and the highest side of the fragment (that is, closest to the rim of the socket) and tip the fragment in the opposite direction. It can then be teased out. A clue to the inclination of the surface of the root can be obtained by observing the fracture in the tooth that has been removed. It is better to excavate slightly into the socket wall to obtain a good purchase than to risk placing apical pressure on the fragment.

Maxillary molar fragments, particularly those in the third molar area, are best visu-

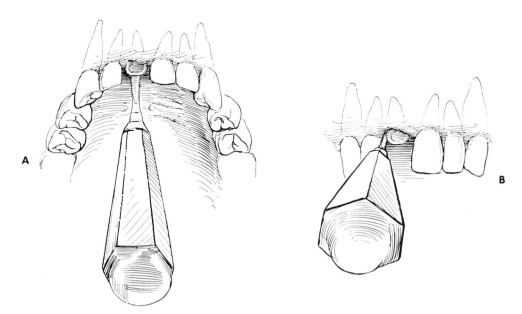

Fig. 5-8. Elevation of necrotic root remnant with straight-shank elevator. **A,** Palatal approach parallel with long axis of root. **B,** Labial-buccal approach at right angles to long axis of root.

alized and approached indirectly using a mirror. The operator stands behind the patient. Buccal roots may be curved, necessitating considerable teasing. Palatal roots of molars are large and are surrounded by unyielding socket walls. Because of their proximity to the antrum, no direct pressure is placed on the root. Space is gained between the socket wall and the root at the expense of the socket wall, and several sides are attacked before a curved root can be delivered.

Maxillary first premolar roots are small and thin. The buccal root can easily be pushed through the thin buccal wall so that it lies between periosteum and alveolar plate. A finger is placed over the buccal plate to prevent this occurrence or to feel the root if it does penetrate the plate. The palatal root is removed at the expense of the intervening septum between the roots.

Mandibular roots fractured at high level require separation of the roots if the crown is fractured below the alveolar rim and the two roots are still joined. Separation can be accomplished by chisel, bur, or elevator. The first root is removed with a short Winter elevator (No. 11); purchase is obtained between the two separated roots with the fulcrum on the second root (Fig. 5-9, *A*). An alternative method obtains purchase in the interdental area (Fig. 5-9, *B*). After the first removal the second root is removed with the same elevator by means of a high purchase in the interdental area, or, better, the long Winter elevator (No. 14) is placed in the depth of the empty socket (Fig. 5-10). With care that the heel of the elevator does not damage the adjacent tooth, the point of the elevator engages the septum and removes it with a turn. The elevator again is placed in the socket, engages the root, and delivers it. The latter method is used to remove all roots in the mandibular molar area.

Mandibular roots in the anterior and premolar areas are removed with root exolevers.

Open procedures. When unyielding

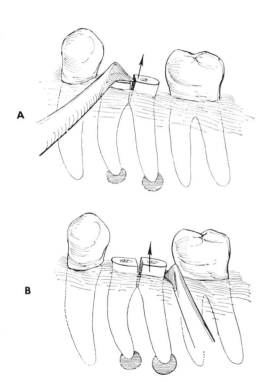

Fig. 5-9. Elevation of mandibular root with short Winter elevator. **A,** Fulcrum placed on shorter root by heel of elevator. **B,** Alternate procedure—fulcrum placed in interdental area.

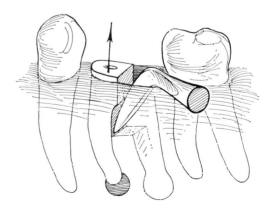

Fig. 5-10. Elevation of single mandibular root through adjacent empty socket with long Winter elevator. The alveolar septum was removed with the first turn; the root now is engaged.

socket walls, curved root tips, inaccessibility, or inadequate visibility preclude removal of roots by closed procedures, a surgical flap should be made before much time is wasted. The standard flap procedure is employed for buccal roots. Labial or buccal bone can be removed with a rongeur, although a chisel or bur is equally rapid. The root tip will come into view soon after the alveolar plate is removed.

An apicoectomy-type semilunar incision is advocated by some people for small buccal or labial root tips (Fig. 12-4). This procedure conserves considerable alveolar plate, but orientation is more difficult, and two areas—the wound and the socket—have be watched for delivery of the root.

Palatal roots in the maxillary premolar and molar areas are approached through the septum. The standard surgical flap is made, enough buccal bone is removed for access, and the septum is removed with cutting instruments. Since the antrum often extends low in the septal area of molars, deep cutting is hazardous. Palatal roots are not located close to palatal roots of adjacent teeth; therefore, bone can be removed mesial or distal to the root.

If a palatal root of a molar tooth suddenly disappears upward, the patient is directed to blow forcibly with the nostrils pinched together. If the root does not come down immediately, it is in the antrum. A Caldwell-Luc procedure is indicated (see Chapter 15). Occasionally a small root tip becomes wedged between the antrum membrane and the bone so that it will not be found lying within the antrum membrane.

The maxillary molar occasionally is fractured horizontally through the pulp chamber high enough so that forceps purchase is impossible, and still the roots are not separated. In this situation a surgical flap is raised, bone over the buccal surface is removed, and the buccal roots are separated with a bur, chisel, or elevator. The buccal root that has split free is removed with an elevator. If the other buccal root is still attached to the palatal root, an attempt is made to remove the combined structure. If this is not possible, the two roots are separated and removed individually.

Incidentally, if an intact maxillary molar tooth cannot be removed by a closed procedure because of an excessively rhomboidal shaped crown or other reasons related to the roots and surrounding structures, it must be removed surgically. After a surgical flap is raised, the two buccal roots are cut off from the crown above the bifurcation with a bur or chisel. The crown and its palatal root are removed with a forceps, followed by individual elevation of the buccal roots.

Surgical flap procedures can be complicated by bleeding in the mandibular incisor areas. In the premolar and molar areas the procedure becomes more formidable because of the presence of the mental foramen and heavy buccal bone strengthened by the external oblique ridge.

Residual roots. Residual roots that have been present in the jaws for some time are considered to be infected. Occasionally they appear on the radiograph circumscribed by a cemental line and a periodontal line. This signifies that healing has taken place, and a judgment must be made whether or not to remove them. Most dentists do not construct dentures over a residual root, and many physicians require that all residual roots be removed in the presence of specific types of systemic diseases. Each situation requires individual evaluation.

Of equal concern is the differentiation on the radiograph between osteosclerosis and root remnant. The oral surgery staff of a dental school made individual judgments for each such diagnostic problem during a school year, followed by surgical removal and histological diagnosis.[1] The staff was wrong in one third of the cases. Osteosclerosis does not have to be removed if proper diagnosis can be made. If it forms in a socket or between two nutrient canals, it is difficult to differentiate from a root.

Exact localization of the root is necessary, particularly in a completely edentulous area. If there are no anatomical landmarks, a suture needle is placed in the anesthetized tissues in the region of the root, and a radiograph is made to compare the location of the root to the needle. An occlusal view is helpful to ascertain the buccolingual position. The root may not lie within the bone at all, although it is superimposed over bone on the radiograph. The occlusal view will demonstrate the true position, and surgical search can be made between the bone and the periosteum on the buccal or the lingual side, whichever is indicated.

When the location of the residual root has been determined in the bone, a buccal mucoperiosteal flap is raised, usually by an incision over the crest of the ridge with a small anterior vertical incision. A window in the buccal cortex is made (1 chisel-width square), or a series of bur holes is made. After this portion of the plate is removed, exploration of the spongiosa is made with a sharp curet. If the root cannot be found or cannot be delivered through the small window, the window is enlarged in the proper directions. The wound is closed with sutures.

ELEVATOR PRINCIPLES

Two main forces are employed to raise an object from base level with the help of a fulcrum. Depending on the location of the fulcrum in relation to the object to be raised, a push or a pull force will dislodge the object upward (Fig. 5-11). In placement of a thin, flat elevator between the second molar and the third molar (in situations wherein the third molar cannot be grasped by forceps), the fulcrum can be established at the bottom edge of the elevator where it contacts septal bone so that the top edge of the elevator does the lifting or it can be established near the top edge of the elevator so that the bottom edge of the elevator does the lifting.

Consider the second situation first. When the bottom edge of an elevator is used to contact the object to be removed (the third molar), the top edge and back of the elevator form a fulcrum at the place of contact on the second molar (Fig. 5-12, *B*). The third molar is scooped out when sufficient space has been obtained by distal movement of the third molar. However, great force is placed on the second molar.

The first situation establishes the fulcrum in the proper place. When the top edge of the elevator is used to contact the third molar, the fulcrum is placed on the bottom edge of the elevator, which rests on the septum (Fig. 5-12, *A*). The top edge is leaned backward to obtain purchase on the anatomical neck of the third molar. The elevator does not exert force on the second molar at all. By means of an up-and-down "can opener" motion on the handle of the spearpoint elevator, the third molar is dislodged nearly straight upward so that the

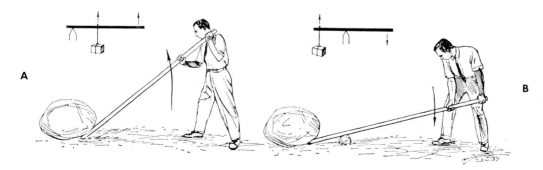

Fig. 5-11. A, Lifting an object with a pull force on an elevator. **B,** Lifting an object with a push force by changing the fulcrum location.

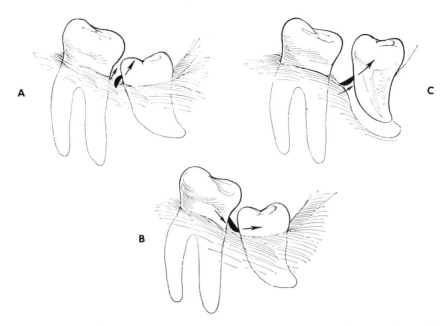

Fig. 5-12. Third molar elevation. **A,** Fulcrum established on septum by bottom edge of elevator while top edge engages tooth for straight upward movement. **B,** Fulcrum established near top edge of elevator, with bottom edge engaging tooth for "scooping" removal. Vector of forces moves tooth backward as much as upward and places more pressure on second molar. **C,** Proper use of "scooping" motion, when tooth has been raised partially in socket.

anterior ramus of the mandible does not interfere with the pathway of exit of the tooth. This is the recommended technique.

As the tooth rides upward it also rides backward to some extent so that continued contact of the elevator with the anatomical neck may be lost. If the tooth cannot be removed entirely with this technique, the fulcrum is shifted when the tooth is halfway out of the socket, and the bottom edge of the elevator scoops underneath the crown to complete the elevation (Fig. 5-12, *C*). This is the proper application of the second example. By this time there will be sufficient space between the teeth so that the top edge of the elevator can make contact with the septum as it is rotated and not with the second molar.

The straight-shank elevator (No. 34) is used in two ways (Fig. 5-8). It is placed parallel to the long axis of roots between the socket wall and the root and worked toward the apex. When purchase is obtained, the strongest portion of the alveolar socket may be used for a fulcrum if additional leverage is necessary. The older method is to place the elevator between the root and the adjacent tooth at right angles to the long axis of the root and to rotate it slightly. This motion should sever the pericemental attachments and deliver the root. The latter method is used sometimes to loosen teeth before forceps delivery is attempted, but because of discomfort associated with periodontal membrane pressure, it is used more commonly under general anesthesia.

The long Winter elevators (Nos. 14R and 14L) were designed for the removal of mandibular molar roots. They are never used elsewhere, with the possible exception of a special technique for elevating mandibular and maxillary third molar impactions. A crossbar elevator can develop tremendous pressure, and mandibles have been fractured with it.

The elevator is placed in the empty socket of the tooth being extracted, with the tip facing the root to be removed in the adjacent socket. The shank and handle are located on the buccal side. The interradicular septum is engaged near the apex of the socket, care being taken that the point does not invade the mandibular canal. The back of the instrument should ride buccal to the next tooth because contact with this tooth may damage it. A rotatory motion will cut through and deliver the septum. The elevator is placed is similar position, this time engaging the fractured root, and a rotatory motion will deliver the root (Fig. 5-10).

The No. 14 elevator is used to deliver a partially mobilized mandibular third molar impaction by engaging it in the area of bifurcation on the buccal side and elevating it upward, using the buccal plate as a fulcrum.

The short Winter elevators (Nos. 11R and 11L) are used for many purposes. Because the root surface must be engaged in each instance, these elevators (in common with all elevators) must be resharpened frequently. The No. 11 elevator is used to elevate molar roots that have been fractured near the alveolar rim (Fig. 5-9). Many situations that prevent forceps application on whole teeth are amendable to the use of this elevator. For example, a mandibular first premolar is crowded lingually so that the buccal beak of the forceps cannot gain access between the canine and the second premolar. In the example given, the anatomical neck of the tooth is engaged on the mesial side and loosened or delivered by use of the lingual alveolar rim as a fulcrum.

REFERENCE

1. McCarthy, F. M.: Osteosclerosis: a roentgenographic differential diagnosis of residual root tip and osteosclerosis, J. Am. Dent. Assoc. **55**:344, 1957.

CHAPTER 6

Impacted teeth*

Gustav O. Kruger

Anthropologists state that the constantly increasing cerebration of man enlarges his brain case at the expense of his jaws. The prepituitary line that sloped forward from receded forehead to protruded jaw in prehuman forms has become almost vertical in modern man as the number of teeth has decreased. A softer and more refined diet that requires less chewing enhances this trend, making a powerful masticatory apparatus unnecessary. Greater numbers of people have impacted teeth for this as well as other reasons. Eventually all third molars will be lost to man, followed eons later by the impaction and subsequent loss of the lateral incisors.

All teeth that do not assume their proper position and function in the arch should be considered for removal. There are exceptions to this general statement, but they are rare. For example, the youth who must lose all of his teeth for full dentures should not lose the unerupted maxillary third molars, since the eruption of these teeth will help to form the tuberosity. The denture can be made over the unerupted teeth if the patient is made cognizant of the situation so that the teeth can be removed later when they appear beneath the mucosa.

In the older individual, discretion may be the better part of valor. A tooth that has not erupted for 50 years is sometimes ankylosed, often has an atrophied periodontal membrane separating tooth and bone, and is always encased in inelastic, heavily mineralized bone. Unerupted teeth can and should be removed to ensure success for the denture, but in an occasional instance, removal may not be feasible.

PRELIMINARY CONSIDERATIONS

Presence of infection. Infection in the form of a pericoronitis should be treated before surgery. An acute pericoronitis around a mandibular third molar usually responds to the extraction of the maxillary third molar if the latter is impinging on the infected mandibular tissues. Probing with a sterile silver probe under the flap on the buccal side for the release of pus, subsequent irrigation, and antibiotic therapy may aid in treatment. Occasionally a tissue or high-level impaction can be removed as soon as a satisfactory antibiotic level has been established. If surgical complications arise, the fractured root can be allowed to remain undisturbed for a few days before removal. The removal of the crown will allow the pericoronitis to subside.

---

*Extensive portions of this chapter are quoted directly from Kruger, G. O.: Management of impactions, Dent. Clin. North Am., p. 707, Nov., 1959.

When no infection exists, oral or parenteral antibiotic therapy is unnecessary.

Premedication and preparation of patient. Premedication is helpful when impacted teeth are removed under local anesthesia. Orally an average dose for an outpatient is 0.1 Gm pentobarbital sodium. However, 1 to 2 ml of pentobarbital sodium can be given intravenously. The patient remains ambulatory but requires someone to accompany him home. Many other drugs or combinations of drugs can be given intravenously or intramuscularly. One of the most popular regimens today consists of diazepam titrated intravenously in dosages from 3 to 20 mg to achieve Verrill's sign. This may be supplemented with meperidine (Demerol) or nitrous oxide-oxygen.

Music, quiet surroundings, and interesting talk by the operator help to establish a favorable atmosphere. General anesthesia is preferred by many patients and operators.

Preparation of the patient starts with a mouthwash of any suitable antiseptic agent to reduce the intraoral bacterial count.

Draping. Drapes in the form of sterile towels will provide a sterile field as well as cover the eyes, thereby reducing psychological trauma. A sterile towel is placed under the patient's head, brought forward over the nose and eyes, and fastened by a sterile towel clip or safety pin (Fig. 6-1). Exposed portions of the face and chin are washed with an antiseptic solution. A sterile towel is placed over the patient's chest. Another sterile towel can be clipped over the chest of the operator. Sterile gloves may be worn. This draping, incidentally, does not represent too much attention to detail, since the incidence of dry socket is reduced considerably by its use.

Chair position. The chair position should be low enough that the operator's right elbow is opposite the patient's right shoulder.

Sponges. A curtain sponge is placed to isolate the field of operation if the chisel technique is used. A 7.6 by 7.6 cm exo-

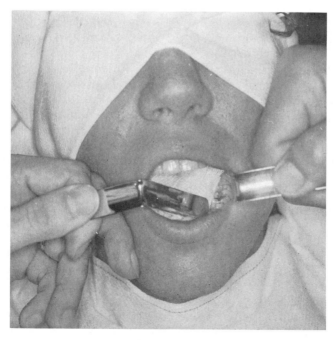

Fig. 6-1. Sterile drapes and retractors are in position. Note isolation of field with sterile gauze sponges. (From Kruger, G. O.: Dent. Clin. North Am., p. 707, Nov., 1959.)

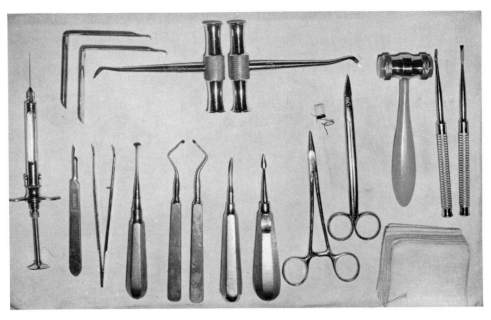

Fig. 6-2. Armamentarium: syringe, scalpel, thumb forceps, Molt curet No. 4, Molt curets Nos. 5 and 6, elevator No. 34, Krogh spearpoint elevator, needle holder, suture, scissors, mallet, Gardner No. 52 chisels, Winter elevators Nos. 14R and 14L, and Austin retractors. (From Kruger, G. O.: Dent. Clin. North Am., p. 707, Nov., 1959.)

dontic gauze sponge is placed with one corner near the mandibular incisors and another corner under the tongue on the side of the operation. The sponge keeps saliva from the field and fragments and blood from the throat and eliminates time loss associated with expectoration. The heavy, stringy, "sympathetic" type of saliva often encountered in surgery patients is difficult to remove from the mouth. By changing the sponge if it becomes wet, expectoration is eliminated and time is saved.

Retractors. The assistant should be trained to hold the retractor in the right hand. The edge of the gauze on the lingual side is held under the tip of the retractor, which in turn is held against the lingual plate when the practitioner is operating on the patient's right side. The tongue is not held toward the midline. When operating on the patient's left side, the tip of the retractor is held under the mucoperiosteal flap against bone. Heavy pulling on the flap by the as-

sistant will cause excessive postoperative lymphedema. Sponging and malleting can be accomplished by the left hand. If suction is used, another assistant is helpful.

Armamentarium. The armamentarium is illustrated in Fig. 6-2. The chisels are resharpened after each use, and they are changed frequently during the course of an operation. Many operators prefer to use burs.[3,4] Attention must be given to the sterility of the handpiece and burs if this technique is used.

Principle of removal of mandibular impacted teeth. The underlying principle in the removal of mandibular impacted teeth is a sectioning technique. Bone is removed to expose the crown. The tooth is split with a fresh sharp chisel so that a good portion of the crown is separated from the tooth. When this portion is removed, space is obtained so that the remainder of the tooth can be elevated into the defect. Before this technique was developed, space for eleva-

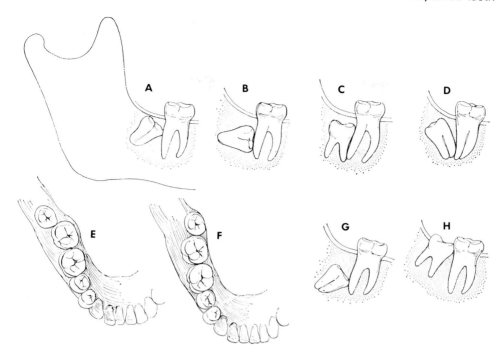

Fig. 6-3. Classification of mandibular impacted teeth. **A,** Mesioangular; **B,** horizontal; **C,** vertical; **D,** distoangular; **E,** buccoversion; **F,** linguoversion; **G,** low-level; **H,** high-level.

tion was obtained by more extensive bone removal and consequently more trauma.

Classification of mandibular impacted teeth. The classification of mandibular impacted teeth may be stated simply as (1) mesioangular, (2) horizontal, (3) vertical, and (4) distoangular. In addition, the tooth may be displaced to the buccal or to the lingual. Furthermore, it may be located at a high occlusal level (near the ridge surface) or a low occlusal level. (See Fig. 6-3.)

A tooth in any basic class is more easily removed if it is displaced to a buccal position and more difficult to remove if it is situated near the lingual plate or even directly behind the second molar. A tooth at a high occlusal level is easier to remove. A tooth may be prevented from erupting by the presence of bone (bone block), by the presence of an adjacent tooth (tooth block), or by both.

Preoperative evaluation. Careful preoperative evaluation will permit adequate planning for the subsequent surgery. The radiograph should be studied carefully to localize the impaction and to determine the shape, number, and inclination of the roots. Frequently, a root will be directed toward or away from the observer rather than mesially or distally. Small roots often are superimposed and can be missed in the radiographic diagnosis. The relationship of the tooth to the mandibular canal should be noted so that the patient may be warned of a possible postoperative paresthesia. The presence of a large restoration, particularly an old amalgam filling, on the second molar should be cause for warning the patient that the operator is aware of the situation and will attempt to save the restoration from inadvertent damage during the surgery.

MANDIBULAR MESIOANGULAR IMPACTION

A typical mesioangular impaction, low level, with bone and tooth block is illustrated in Fig. 6-4. Prior to removal of the impaction, the patient and the field of operation have been prepared adequately as described previously and a local anesthetic has been administered.

A curtaining sponge is placed in the mouth to isolate the operative site. Another sponge is used to dry exposed oral mucous membranes. Pressure over the area with a small Molt curet (No. 5) combined with positive statement rather than negative questions will ascertain the depth of anesthesia.

An incision is made into the tissues distal to the second molar with the scalpel. It is important to palpate the tissues before incision to keep the incision over bone. The vertical ramus of the mandible flares outward, and therefore a straight distal incision might extend into tissues medial to the mandible that contain important anatomical structures. A safe rule to follow is to place the incision back of the buccal cusp of the second molar, following the underlying bone, which may flare laterally (Fig. 6-4, A).

The second arm of the incision is made vertically from the first incision at its junction with the distobuccal cusp, extending downward and forward to the buccal tissues over the mesial root of the second molar.

Variations in flap design include the technique of detaching the buccal free gingival fibers around all the teeth forward to include the first molar and separating the large

flap buccally (Fig. 6-5). It is claimed that this flap is easier to suture, that it is less painful in the postoperative period, and that there is less distortion in healing. Another variation is the placing of the slanting vertical incision mesial to the second molar rather than mesial to the third molar.

The mucoperiosteal flap is raised carefully with a sharp No. 4 Molt curet, starting in the vertical incision where the periosteum is not attached to bone. The instrument is worked posteriorly and toward the alveolar ridge. When the operative site is widely exposed, a suitable retractor is placed under the flap and held against bone.

Ossisection is started in a vertical fashion parallel to and just back of the distal root of the second molar (Fig. 6-4, B). The bone incision should be one, two, or three chisel widths long, depending on the depth necessary to get under the enamel crown of the impacted tooth as determined on the preoperative radiograph. The chisel then is turned to face posteriorly, placed in the bottom of the first cut, and directed slightly toward the alveolar crest. Most of the buccal plate will be removed in one piece, which is desirable.

Further horizontal cuts are made as necessary to expose the crown (Fig. 6-4, C). In a wide mandible with a heavy cortical plate, the impacted tooth can be exposed further by angling one edge of the chisel toward the tooth in making a horizontal cut to create a

Fig. 6-4. Removal of impacted mandibular third molar, mesioangular position. **A,** Incision is made back of the buccal cusp of the second molar and then into the buccal tissues. **B,** Ossisection. The two check points that must permit entrance of the curet before ossisection is complete are marked with asterisks. **C,** Horizontal ossisection. **D,** "Ditching" to save height of buccal cortical plate. **E,** Sectioning of distal cusp. **F,** Position of elevator under cemento-enamel junction on mesial surface. **F₁,** Diagram represents the action of the top edge of the instrument in elevating the posterior object. Note that the bottom edge of the instrument rests on the ground surface and not on the anterior object. This is the recommended technique. **F₂,** "Scooping" with the instrument forces the posterior object backward rather than upward. Note that the opposite edge of the instrument now rests on the anterior object and tends to force it forward. **G,** The tooth is moved upward and backward as far as the distal rim of bone will allow. **H,** Further straight upward movement is accomplished with the No. 14 elevator if the tooth cannot be removed in an arc with the spearpoint elevator. **I,** Suture placed. (From Kruger, G. O.: Dent. Clin. North Am., p. 707, Nov., 1959.)

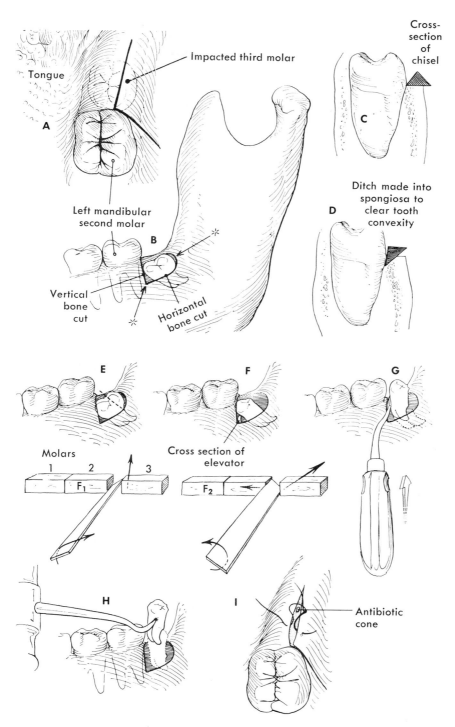

Tongue

Impacted third molar

Cross-
section
of
chisel

C

A

Left mandibular
second molar

Ditch made into
spongiosa to
clear tooth
D   convexity

B

Vertical
bone
cut

Horizontal
bone cut

E

F

G

Molars

Cross section of
elevator

1   2 F_1 3

F_2

H

I

Antibiotic
cone

Fig. 6-4. For legend see opposite page.

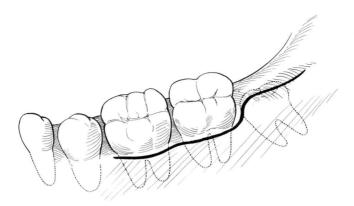

Fig. 6-5. Envelope flap.

"ditch" in the spongiosa between the tooth and the cortical plate (Fig. 6-4, *D*).

Two points are checked with the small curet. The bone over the distal or top surface of the impaction should be removed so that the crown can be removed after splitting. The bone at the junction of the vertical and horizontal cuts should be removed sufficiently to allow the curet to enter the spongiosa under the impacted crown. If either of these two check points is unsatisfactory, further bone is removed.

The tooth then is sectioned (Fig. 6-4, *E*). A new chisel is placed in the buccal groove, directed distally toward the distal anatomical neck of the tooth (not lingually, which may fracture the lingual cortical plate), and struck sharply. This blow should be a glancing blow with no "follow-through." The tooth will often split on the first attempt. The sectioned distal portion of the crown is lifted from the wound.

A binangled spearpoint elevator such as the Krogh elevator is placed under the crown, and upward motion is made (Fig. 6-4, *F*). The upper edge of this elevator is the portion of the instrument that lifts the tooth. To obtain a better purchase on the tooth, the leading (upper) edge is turned slightly distalward toward the tooth. The handle of the instrument is moved in a straight vertical plane (Fig. 6-4, *G*). It is not rotated at this time.

When the tooth moves, it will be forced to move in an arc. When it has moved upward and distally to the point where the instrument can no longer maintain contact with it, the instrument is rotated so that the inferior edge completes the tooth removal. Earlier rotation sometimes will fracture the root and may endanger the second molar.

Often the tooth will move upward far enough to clear the second molar, but it will not rotate distally. It is now in a vertical position, separated from the second molar far enough to lose the mechanical advantage of the elevator placed between the teeth. A long Winter elevator (No. 14) placed in the root bifurcation, with the buccal cortical plate utilized as a fulcrum, will elevate this tooth out of the wound (Fig. 6-4, *H*).

Bone fragments are lifted from the wound with a small curet. Particular attention is given to chips that lodge under the flap buccal to the second molar. The soft tissue remnants in the socket (for example, granulation tissue, eruption follicle) are removed carefully by means of sharp or blunt dissection. Heavy curettage is avoided in the depths of the wound where the inferior alveolar nerve and vessels lie. Edges of the

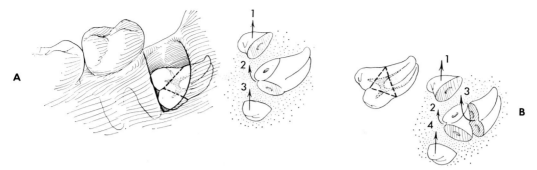

Fig. 6-6. A, Horizontal impaction. The superior (distal) cusp is sectioned, and the inferior (mesial) cusp is sectioned. The superior crown fragment is removed first, followed by the bulk of the tooth. The inferior crown fragment is removed last. **B,** Horizontal impaction (variation). If insufficient room is present for removal of the bulk of the tooth, a split is made near the anatomical neck of the tooth. (From Kruger, G. O.: Dent. Clin. North Am., p. 707, Nov., 1959.)

bony wound are smoothed with the curet. A small fragment of a sulfonamide tablet is placed in the wound if preoperative questioning indicated no sensitivity to the drug, or a Gelfoam wedge that has been soaked previously in an antibiotic solution and allowed to dry without losing its sterility is used by some oral surgeons.

A suture is placed over the socket from lingual to buccal (Fig. 6-4, *I*). This violates a surgical rule to suture the free flap to the fixed flap, but it seems to be simpler here because the retractor is not removed from the wound until the needle is recovered in the depth of the wound. A ½-inch round cutting needle and No. 3-0 silk is used, although No. 3-0 catgut does not have to be removed.[4] One suture is usually sufficient. The vertical cut is almost never closed. No drain is placed. A gauze sponge is placed over the area.

MANDIBULAR HORIZONTAL IMPACTION

The horizontal impaction situated at a low occlusal level requires a deep vertical bone cut, often extending almost to the level of the second molar apex (Fig. 6-6, *A*). The horizontal cuts should be sufficient to expose the anatomical neck of the tooth. The classic description of the removal of

this tooth includes a split at the anatomical neck to divide the crown from the root. This can be accomplished with a sharp chisel. However, the bur is especially efficient for this procedure, provided that a sterile bur and handpiece are available.

An alternate method involves placing the chisel in the buccal groove, directing it backward and upward and as little lingually as the access allows. The distal portion of the crown can be split off and removed. The chisel then is placed at the same site directed backward and downward. This will split the mesial (lower) portion of the crown, which cannot be removed at this time. If the angles of the sections have been wide enough, there may be enough clearance to remove the impaction, provided that sufficient bone over the crest of the ridge has been removed. Attention is directed to this area now. If all the ossisection is accomplished before the sectioning is attempted, the tooth may be loosened slightly, and a tooth loose in its bed is difficult to split. The sectioning is accomplished as soon as access to the crown is obtained, even though the parts cannot be removed, and then further ossisection is accomplished.

A further split in a near vertical (downward) direction can be made at this time

(Fig. 6-6, *B*). The exposed dentin surface can be split more easily than enamel, and, if the pulpal chamber is exposed, it is even easier to obtain a split.

The various superficial tooth fragments are removed. If the vertical bone cut has been made deep enough for elevator access and sufficient alveolar crest bone has been removed, the root portion can be removed with the No. 14 elevator, with or without further root sectioning. Heavy pressure should not be used. Further tooth sectioning or ossisection should be carried out until the impaction can be removed with relative ease. The mesial portion of the crown is removed last. Primary closure is effected after careful debridement.

MANDIBULAR VERTICAL IMPACTION

The removal of the vertical impaction is one of the more difficult operations because of the difficulty in placing an instrument between the second molar and the closely adjacent impacted third molar. This space is too small for adequate bone removal.

The area is exposed to view under a large mucoperiosteal flap. A long, vertical bone cut is made to expose at least the anatomical neck of the impaction. Bone is removed well behind (distal to) the impaction and

over its occlusal surface as well. A long, almost vertical split is obtained from the buccal groove through the distal portion of the tooth below the anatomical neck (Fig. 6-7). This portion is removed. A thin spearpoint elevator is forced between the teeth if possible, and the tooth is elevated. If access is not possible, a No. 14 elevator can engage the area of bifurcation on the buccal side, and force straight upward can be exerted.

MANDIBULAR DISTOANGULAR IMPACTION

The distoangular impaction is difficult to remove because its bulk lies in the vertical ramus. The crown of the impaction is situated away from the second molar, affording no mechanical advantage to the elevator.

A generous mucoperiosteal flap is raised, and the usual vertical and horizontal bone cuts are made. The tooth is sectioned in a vertical direction (Fig. 6-8, *A*). Depending on the curvature of the roots, the mesial bulk of the tooth first is moved upward by the spearpoint elevator placed on the mesial side of the tooth or by the No. 14 elevator placed in the area of bifurcation. At times the distal sectioned crown portion may be dissected out of the bone first. The tooth

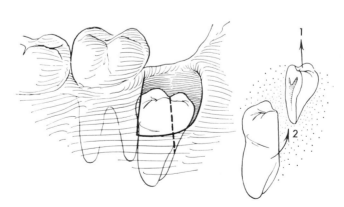

Fig. 6-7. Vertical impaction. A long split is obtained. The distal cusp is removed first, followed by elevation of the tooth. (From Kruger, G. O.: Dent. Clin. North Am., p. 707, Nov., 1959.)

then is rotated distally into the space created. It is often helpful to section the crown from the root in the distoangular impaction, remove the crown, split the root if feasible, and remove the separate root portions (Fig. 6-8, *B*).

• • •

Several points of caution in the operations for the removal of mandibular impactions should be noted. Force applied with elevators should always be controlled force, and it should be minimal. Greater than normal force is necessary in a few special situations, especially in forcing an elevator between two closely placed teeth. Some operators use more force than others. However, it is best to obtain multiple sections of the tooth and to clearly remove the bone blocks before attempting to elevate the tooth. A good many properly prepared impactions, even at low level, can be removed with a small curet rather than a heavy elevator.

Bone that has become traumatized exces-sively should be removed with a sharp chisel or bur after the tooth has been removed.

BUR TECHNIQUE

The high-speed surgical drill is employed extensively for the removal of impacted teeth and root tips. The technique has several advantages.

The first advantage is of special significance when dealing with the unsedated patient. The placement of the handpiece in the patient's mouth is a familiar experience, common to everyone who has occupied the dental chair, as contrasted to the use of the chisel and mallet.

The second advantage is that the physical blows and pressures associated with the chisel and mallet technique are eliminated.

The third advantage is that since the surgical handpiece technique eliminates the need for an assistant to do the malleting, fewer personnel are required in the operatory.

The fourth advantage is related to the

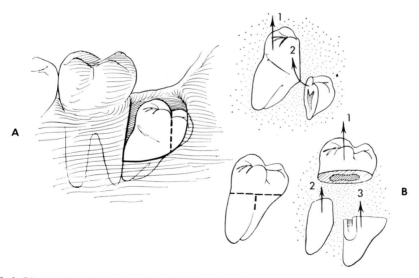

Fig. 6-8. A, Distoangular impaction. The distal cusp is split off. The tooth is elevated first, and then the sectioned distal cusp is removed. **B,** Distoangular impaction (variation). The tooth is sectioned at the anatomical neck. The crown is removed, and the roots are divided and removed separately. (From Kruger, G. O.: Dent. Clin. North Am., p. 707, Nov., 1959.)

need to irrigate the surgical field in order to reduce heat caused by the bur. This creates a continuously washed surgical field in which to work.

The fifth advantage is that the operator has the ability to trench around the impaction in a delicate and controlled fashion in order to remove osseous tissue so that an instrument purchase can be obtained. This feature of the bur technique is particularly useful for the recovery of mandibular molar root tips lying close to the mandibular canal and maxillary root tips lying close to the maxillary sinus. This eliminates apically directed forces such as occur in the case of an elevator purchase under or next to the impacted fragment. The instrument purchase can be enhanced when a notch is made with the bur on the remaining portion of the tooth, allowing an elevator to engage it more fully.

Early attempts to develop an effective technique for the removal of impacted teeth resulted in the establishment of two fundamental techniques. The first technique involved removal of the intact tooth after sufficient bone had been removed, and the second technique involved sectioning of the tooth so that less bone would have to be removed for its delivery. Present day techniques employ various combinations of these two fundamental procedures. The introduction of the air turbine drill, with rotating speeds in excess of 300,000 rpm, has brought about a marked increase in the use of the high-speed bur for the removal of impacted teeth.

Before description of the methods used to remove impacted teeth by the bur technique is begun, it must be emphasized that it is imperative that only an autoclavable handpiece and bur be used. The communication of the surgical site with the fascial spaces increases the possibility of serious complications resulting from instrumentation with less than sterile techniques. The use of the standard handpiece employed by the general practitioner for tooth preparation is absolutely contraindicated for the removal of impacted teeth.

Furthermore, irrigation of the surgical wound during and after the procedure cannot be emphasized enough. Copious amounts of coolant spray are crucial in minimizing osseous necrosis caused by heat generated by the bur. Irrigation serves also to cleanse the crypt and areas beneath the flap of bony debris, tooth fragments, and blood.

Techniques that combine certain advantages of the chisel and the bur methods and eliminate some of the disadvantages of both are finding increased acceptance. The flap design, reflection, and retraction for bur removal of impacted teeth is the same as for their removal by chisel.

The basic points of the high-speed bur-chisel technique are:

1. Dense bone is removed with a high-speed bur. The chisel is used to re-

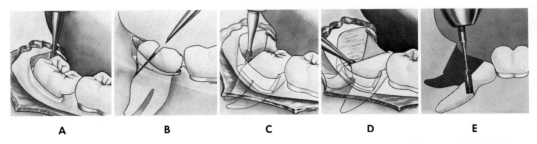

    A   **B**   **C**   **D**   **E**

Fig. 6-9. Bur technique. **A,** Removal of bone around crown. **B,** Sectioning of crown with chisel. **C,** Further ossisection to level of bifurcation. **D,** Sectioning of distal root. **E,** Sectioning of mesial root. (Courtesy Szmyd, L.: Dent. Clin. North Am., April 1971.)

move thin layers of relatively soft bone that commonly are encountered in the removal of maxillary third molars.

2. The use of a chisel in tooth division is usually limited to a single split along natural cleavage lines. Additional sectioning is carried out with a high-speed bur, usually in dentin.

3. Dense bone adjacent to the crown, which is to be sectioned with the chisel, frequently is removed not only to provide a path of delivery but also to aid in splitting the tooth.

MANDIBULAR THIRD MOLAR

Elevation of the mandibular third molar impaction usually is impeded by one or more of the following factors: (1) overlying bone, (2) anterior border of the ascending ramus, (3) adjacent second molar, and (4) unfavorable root formation. Proximity to the inferior alveolar nerve, thin lingual plate, lack of visibility, restricted access, and abnormal bone formation, as well as other surgical and anatomical problems, may be encountered.

Vertical impaction

Bone removal is begun at the mesiobuccal line angle of the third molar. The initial bone cut is made vertically down to expose the height of convexity of the third molar. The bur is passed distally at this depth to the distobuccal line angle and then lingually around the distal surface of the tooth (Fig. 6-9, A). This frequently results in a fragment of bone that can be flicked away and removed from the surgical site. A mallet and chisel are then employed to section the distal third from the crown (Fig. 6-9, B). Usually this is sufficient preparation to enable elevation of the tooth. Surgical experience and judgment will determine whether additional sectioning or bone removal is necessary. If the vertical impaction is not easily delivered at this juncture, the high-speed bur is used to increase the depth of ossisection to the level of the bifurcation

(Fig. 6-9, C). Starting at the bifurcation a deep groove is cut into the distal root of the impaction (Fig. 6-9, D). Separation of the coronal segment from the distal root is completed with an exolever. The coronal segment and mesial root are removed as a single element prior to elevation of the distal root.

Mesioangular impaction

Ossisection is carried out in a manner similar to that for the vertical impaction to widen the pericoronal space and eliminate the bone overlying the height of contour. The depth of ossisection is increased to the level of the bifurcation and the chisel employed to section the distal half of the crown of the third molar or to section vertically through its bifurcation if indicated. The distal crown segment, or distal crown segment and attached root, are then removed as a single element. In those cases in which the mesial portion is tightly wedged under the second molar, the bur can be used to cut a deep groove in the mesial root beginning in the pulp chamber so an exolever can split crown from root. They are then removed as separate units (Fig. 6-9, E).

Horizontal impaction

The anatomical neck of the tooth is exposed by bur technique as previously described, reducing the height of the buccal plate to the buccal groove of the tooth. A chisel is employed to section the distal third of the crown and expose the pulp chamber (Fig. 6-10, A). The high-speed bur is employed to expose the labial surface of the clinical crown without further reduction of the height of the buccal plate by "ditching."

As is demonstrated in Fig. 6-10, B, starting in the exposed pulp chamber, a T-shaped groove is cut with a high-speed bur. Two large segments of the clinical crown are split and removed as separate units. Two deep grooves are cut with the bur to facilitate separation of mesial root from distal root. Alternate techniques include bur division of the crown at the cervix and re-

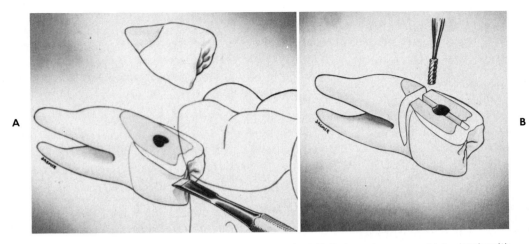

Fig. 6-10. Horizontal impaction. **A,** Initial split with chisel. **B,** T-shaped groove cut into dentin with bur. (Courtesy Szmyd, L.: Dent. Clin. North Am., April 1971.)

moval of the sectioned elements as separate entities.

Distoangular impaction

Variations of the surgical techniques previously described for mandibular third molar impactions are utilized for distoangular impactions. The vertical ramus presents a formidable obstruction to delivery of this type of impaction. Following bur removal of buccal bone to expose the tooth's height of contour, the bur is used to remove distobuccal bone. The distal portion of the tooth is then sectioned or the tooth divided through its bifurcation. Alternate approaches include bur division of the tooth in half or section of the crown from the roots followed by division of mesial root from distal root and removal of the separate elements.

MAXILLARY MESIOANGULAR IMPACTION

The maxillary impacted tooth usually is removed at the same sitting as the mandibular tooth on that side. An anesthetic is administered concomitantly with the mandibular anesthetic. The curtain sponge is replaced quickly with a dry gauze sponge. The buccal fold is dried, and the operator holds the buccal retractor.

Incision is made over the crest of the ridge, extending from the tuberosity to the second molar, and a vertical component is slanted upward and forward to end over the mesiobucal root of the second molar (Fig. 6-11, A). The mucoperiosteal flap is raised with a No. 4 Molt curet.

In the chisel technique, a new chisel is placed for a vertical cut parallel to the distal root of the second molar (Fig. 6-11, B). Light malleting will afford penetration into the soft spongiosa, and the enamel crown often is felt soon after entrance. The light cortical plate is raised slightly over the buccal aspect of the tooth, or, in a heavy impaction, it should be removed altogether. In the bur technique, bone is removed rapidly around the impacted tooth. A small curet is used to ascertain if access exists between the second molar and the impacted third molar. In some cases it does not exist. Further bone removal between the two teeth is almost impossible, and considerable controlled elevator pressure is necessary to force the point of the instrument into the interdental space. Distal bone should be removed in such an instance.

The tooth is removed with a spearpoint elevator, a No. 34 elevator, or a No. 14 elevator (Fig. 6-11, C). The point of the

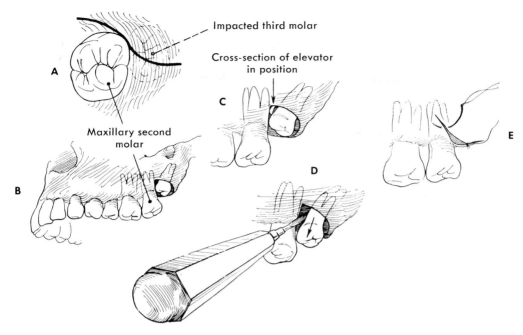

Fig. 6-11. Removal of impacted maxillary third molar, mesioangular position. **A,** Incision over alveolar crest extended to buccal tissues. **B,** Bone removal. Particular attention is given to access between the second and impacted third molars. **C,** Position of elevator at cemento-enamel junction. **D,** The handle of the elevator is moved up and down. **E,** Suture closure. (Modified from Kruger, G. O.: Dent. Clin. North Am., p. 707, Nov., 1959.)

elevator is forced between the teeth into the area of ossisection, and a straight downward and buccal force is applied (Fig. 6-11, *D*). The point and the inferior edge of the elevator make contact with the anatomical neck of the tooth and elevate it downward with these vantage points. Care is exercised in turning the elevator distally (backward), since to do so increases the possibility of fracturing the tuberosity.

The area is debrided for extraneous soft and hard tissue material, and bone edges are smoothed with the curet. A suture is placed across the crest incision, and another is placed across the vertical incision (Fig. 6-11, *E*).

The curtain sponge is removed. Another sponge, slightly moistened in water, is placed over the wound (mostly to the buccal), and the patient is directed to bite down on it with pressure. A few minutes later postoperative radiographs are made, and another sponge is placed between the jaws to remain until the patient has returned home. An ice bag to be placed on the face is ordered, on 10 minutes and off 10 minutes, for the remainder of the day. A therapeutic level of an analgesic drug is established, with the administration of the first dose on arrival home, before the effect of the local anesthetic has disappeared.

MAXILLARY VERTICAL IMPACTION

The maxillary vertical impaction, particularly if the crown rests close to the anatomical neck of the second molar, permits no access between the teeth for ossisection or for purchase by an instrument.

A vertical bone cut is made parallel to the mesial edge of the impacted tooth. The thin bone overlying the buccal surface of the tooth is removed carefully or sometimes

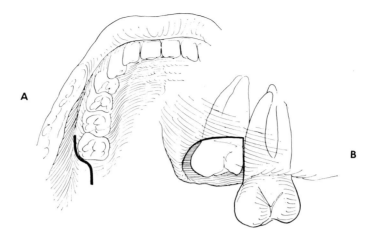

Fig. 6-12. A, Vertical impaction, incision. **B,** Bone removal. (Modified from Kruger, G. O.: Dent. Clin. North Am., p. 707, Nov., 1959.)

separated from the tooth and bent 1 to 2 mm buccally. The chisel or bur is introduced carefully back of the distal surface to create space for backward movement (Fig. 6-12).

A thin-bladed instrument of any kind described previously is introduced between the teeth. Since the removal of bone has not been possible in this space, considerable force is necessary. As soon as the instrument can be pushed into this space, the tooth can be removed easily. Occasionally it will move downward so rapidly that it may be swallowed or aspirated if a suitable gauze curtain does not cover the oropharynx.

If the instrument cannot be introduced into the space and considerable bone surrounding the tooth has been removed, a driving chisel can be placed on the buccal surface of the enamel in a vertical direction and gently tapped downward. If a bur is available, a hole is drilled into the buccal surface of the impaction to allow purchase by a sharp elevator to move the tooth downward and backward.

MAXILLARY DISTOANGULAR IMPACTION

The distoangular impaction, a rare situation, requires a larger surgical flap and ex-

tensive removal of surrounding bone. A midcrest incision is made, extending from the second molar to the tuberosity curvature, and vertical extensions to the buccal and lingual are made distal to the second molar. This flap exposes the entire bony tuberosity (Fig. 6-13, A).

A vertical bone incision is made distal to the second molar to the area of the apex. Buccal and alveolar crest bone is removed. The area distal to the impaction is carefully exposed with a chisel, mainly by hand pressure, or by bur (Fig. 6-13, B).

The tooth is elevated from a purchase on the mesial side as near to the apex as access will allow. The tooth can be pushed into the antrum or into the tissues back of the tuberosity. A second instrument (No. 5 Molt curet) occasionally is placed simultaneously on the distal surface to guide the tooth downward. Several alternate methods can be used. If the tooth is in severe distoangular position, a No. 14 elevator may be used on the distal (superior) crown surface to bring the tooth downward and forward. At times the tooth should be dissected extensively and removed with forceps. Gelfoam may be used to fill an extensive defect, and the wound should be closed tightly with multiple interrupted sutures.

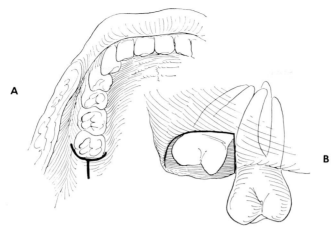

Fig. 6-13. **A,** Distoangular impaction, modified incision of soft tissues. **B,** Bone removal. (From Kruger, G. O.: Dent. Clin. North Am., p. 707, Nov., 1959.)

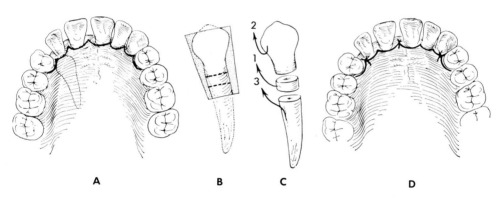

Fig. 6-14. **A,** Canine impaction, palatal position. Soft tissue flap design. **B,** Sectioning of tooth. **C,** Note that the middle section is removed first. **D,** Closure of flap. (Modified from Kruger, G. O.: Dent. Clin. North Am., p. 707, Nov., 1959.)

MAXILLARY CANINE IMPACTION

Impactions of the maxillary canine are classified as labial, palatal, and intermediate. Localization is important, since the surgical techniques for removal of the three types vary so much that they are almost unrelated operations. Intraoral radiographs can be read to determine the form of the tooth as well as its location (Clark's rule, buccal object rule). The true occlusal view made with an intraoral cassette and extraoral views often are necessary. Clinical pal-pation on the labial side is not reliable, since the bulge felt may be either the impacted tooth or the labially displaced root of the incisor or premolar.

Palatal canine position. The palatal position is the most frequent situation. Incision is made in the palatal interdental spaces, beginning with the space between the premolars on the one side and around the palatal free gingival fibers and interdental spaces to the premolar area on the other side (Fig. 6-14, *A*). The heavy mucoperiosteal flap is stripped from the bone with the No. 4 Molt curet. The contents of the incisive foramen are divided by scalpel where they enter the flap.

If bone is removed with the chisel, removal is started with a small rectangle back of the incisor that appears nearest to the impaction on the radiograph (unless an obvious protuberance locates the tooth). The rectangle is one chisel width in size initially, and it is enlarged as soon as the enamel crown is located. Care must be taken in dissecting anteriorly in the region of the incisors, and a 1 to 2 mm margin of bone around their sockets should be maintained. When one half to two thirds of the tooth is exposed, a split is made at the anatomical neck. If the crown is near the incisors so that its tip lies in an undercut, a second split is immediately made 3 mm toward the apex from the first cut (Fig. 6-14, *B*). The small piece is removed, the crown is backed into the space created and removed and the root is teased out with a No. 34 elevator or a Molt curet (Fig. 6-14, *C*).

Maxillary canine impactions are especially amenable to removal by the bur technique. A wiping motion is used until a portion of the impacted tooth is encountered. Further ossisection is made by creating grooves in the bone adjacent to the tooth until the tooth is exposed. The bur is excellent for sectioning the tooth, especially since the width of the bur creates space for maneuvering the parts.

Bone chips and debris are removed, edges of the bony wound are smoothed with a curet, and the wound is closed by means of three or four sutures through the interdental spaces, tying on the labial aspect (Fig. 6-14, *D*). Pressure on a large wad of gauze over the palate for 15 minutes helps to prevent formation of a gross hematoma. To support the palatal flap against bone, a preformed clear acrylic palatal splint is useful. A stab incision and rubber drain through the palatal mucosa is used by some operators to prevent formation of a dependent hematoma.

Labial canine position. After the impaction has been localized, a large semilunar incision is made extending from the labial frenum to the premolar area, with the curvature pointing toward the gingival margin (Fig. 6-15, *A*). Labial bone is removed in the usual fashion until the tooth is located; it may be high on the facial surface of the maxilla. Sufficient dissection is accomplished until the tooth can be elevated with suitable instruments.

Intermediate canine position. The usual position for an intermediate impaction is

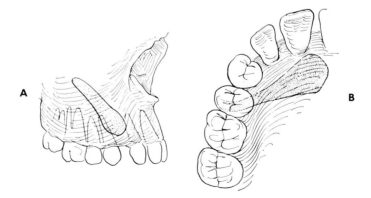

Fig. 6-15. A, Canine impaction, labial position. **B,** Canine impaction, intermediate position. (Modified from Kruger, G. O.: Dent. Clin. North Am., p. 707, Nov., 1959.)

the crown on the palate and the root lying over the apices of the premolar teeth near the buccal cortex (Fig. 6-15, *B*). Even if the condition is not diagnosed preoperatively, it should be suspected when difficulty arises in the removal of the root portion of any palatally placed canine.

The palatal exposure is made in the usual manner, and the crown is removed. A separate buccal flap is made in the region suggested by the radiographic and clinical findings, usually above and between the premolars on the same side. Careful bone removal will uncover the root end of the impaction, which can be pushed from the buccal opening into the palatal wound. The two operative sites are closed.

SUPERNUMERARY TOOTH IMPACTION

Although supernumerary teeth may be found impacted in any area of the alveolar ridges, the most common ones occur in the maxillary anterior region. They may occur singly between the central incisors (mesiodens), or they may be double (mesiodentes).

Under ordinary circumstances, removal of mesiodentes is not scheduled until the apices of the permanent incisors have closed, since then there is less danger of damaging the growing mesenchymal portion of the permanent teeth. Sometimes the permanent incisors will not erupt because of interference by the supernumerary teeth. The operation is complicated by the diffi-

culty in locating, identifying, and removing the supernumerary tooth without damaging the permanent tooth (Fig. 6-16, *A*).

Supernumerary anterior maxillary teeth usually are removed by a palatal approach. When radiographs are inconclusive in establishing the location of the supernumerary teeth anterior or posterior to the normal teeth, a palatal approach is made, since few are located in an anterior position.

The technique for removal is similar to that used for removal of the palatally impacted canine. An incision is made around the necks of the teeth on the palate from first premolar to first premolar, and a palatal flap is raised (Fig. 6-16, *B*). If no identifying protuberances are found on the bone surface, ossisection is started behind the central incisor, back of the incisive foramen. A collar of bone is left around the central incisor. Dissection is carried upward and backward until enamel is encountered. If the permanent central incisors have not erupted, the tooth encountered must be differentiated from the unerupted permanent central incisor by its anatomy. Sufficient bone is removed to deliver the tooth. When bilateral impactions occur, the second tooth often will be less difficult to find because of the experience gained in locating the first one. The wound is treated and closed in the usual manner.

Impacted mandibular supernumerary premolars are difficult to remove because of the presence of compact bone and vital

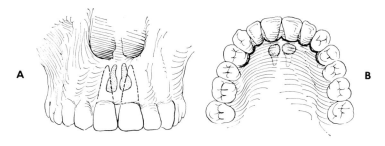

Fig. 6-16. Supernumerary teeth. **A,** Location anterior or posterior to central incisors can be difficult to determine. **B,** Incision around necks of teeth for palatally located mesiodentes. (Modified from Kruger, G. O.: Dent. Clin. North Am., p. 707, Nov., 1959.)

structures such as the contents of the mental foramen on the buccal side and salivary gland and neurovascular structures on the lingual side. Occlusal radiographs will locate the tooth as being on the buccal side or on the lingual side or midway beween the plates (the last is most frequent).

A double flap is made on the buccal side, consisting of two vertical components some distance apart joined by an incision around the necks of the teeth. Unless the tooth has erupted through the lingual plate, it is difficult and hazardous to make a lingual approach. Buccal bone over the tooth to be removed is removed through a square window until it is dissected out. If instrumentation is difficult because of narrow access between the erupted teeth, a thin instrument, such as a broken Molt curet, can be placed between the teeth to engage the impacted premolar and tapped with a mallet. A bur hole on the surface of the impaction will enhance purchase and prevent slip-page. If the supernumerary tooth is not fully formed, it is easier to remove (with a curet) than if it is completely formed. After removal, antibiotic-containing Gelfoam is placed in the wound and all borders of the incision are approximated with sutures.

Molar supernumerary teeth are managed much like an impacted third molar, since the supernumerary tooth occurs at the end of the molar series.

REFERENCES
1. Lilly, G. E., Salem, J. E., Armstrong, J. H., and Cutcher, S. L.: Reaction of oral tissues to suture materials, Oral Surg. **28**:432, 1969.
2. Szymd, L.: Combined chisel–air turbine technic for impacted mandibular third molar surgery, J. Oral Surg. **21**:114, 1963.
3. Szymd, L., and Hester, W. R.: Crevicular depth of the second molar in impacted third molar surgery, J. Oral Surg. **21**:185, 1963.
4. Szymd, L., Shannon, I. L., Schuessler, C. F., and McCall, C. M.: Air turbine in impacted third molar surgery, J. Oral. Surg. **21**:36, 1963.

CHAPTER 7

Special considerations in exodontics

Donald C. Reynolds

REMOVAL OF TEETH FOR CHILDREN

The management of a child who must undergo dental extractions is based on (1) age and maturity, (2) past medical dental experiences that might influence behavior, (3) physical status, and (4) the length of time and amount of manipulation necessary to accomplish the surgery.

The age and maturity of the child often determine the type of anesthesia best suited for the intended procedure. Children below the age of reason generally are best managed under general anesthesia, since a slight amount of discomfort is always associated with the administration of a local anesthetic. During the extraction the child will experience pressures and noises associated with the necessary instrumentation. If these phenomena cannot be explained to the child, he will become anxious and rebellious. For these reasons general anesthesia is often used for the very young patient.

Good rapport must be established between the dentist and the pediatric patient. The dentist should be friendly but firm. Short, simple explanations of the sensations the child will experience should be made. At the time of needle insertion he is told that he will feel a little "stick," and during in-

jection of the solution he is told that he will feel pressure. Forces that the child will experience during the extraction can be demonstrated by pushing gently but firmly on his shoulders. The child is told that he will feel the pushing in the area of surgery, just as he has felt it on his shoulders. It should be pointed out that pushing is the only sensation that will be felt. At no time should the word "pain" be mentioned.

The child should be verbally reprimanded for unwarranted actions. During and at the end of the procedure he should be praised for his cooperation. Speaking to the child in a friendly, understanding manner throughout the procedure will greatly enhance the efficacy of "verbal anesthesia."

Scheduling the pediatric patient in the morning is desirable. At this time he is less likely to be tired and difficult to manage. Delays should be eliminated as much as possible between the time the child enters the office and the initiation of treatment. Delays allow only for the development of apprehension. Premedication with a sedative is indicated if the child appears apprehensive. Such premedication will be helpful with the administration of a local as well as a general anesthetic. A sedative is indicated also if a lengthy procedure such as removal of supernumerary teeth is planned. A child will tend to become restless and unmanageable during prolonged procedures.

At no time should the child be allowed to see the instruments necessary for anesthesia and surgery. A Mayo stand is placed behind the chair and the instruments brought to the mouth from behind and below to keep them out of the child's visual field. Small syringes and extraction forceps are available that can be more easily hidden, but they are by no means necessary for the successful management of the pediatric patient. One example regarding the advisability of keeping instruments out of the child's view involves a youngster who became hysterical at the sight of a suture needle after having sat quietly throughout multiple extractions. On questioning the patient it was discovered that during the previous year the child had lacerated his scalp, which required suturing. The child associated the needle with the pain experienced during the suturing of his scalp and related it to the current operation.

In general, the removal of deciduous teeth is not difficult; it is facilitated by the elasticity of young bone and the resorption of the root structure. Children's upper and lower forceps can be used for the removal of all deciduous teeth (Fig. 7-1). These for-

ceps have the basic design of the universal upper and lower forceps (Nos. 150 and 151). If children's forceps are not available, deciduous teeth can be removed with the forceps used for the removal of their succedaneous analogues. However, the "cowhorn" (No. 16) forceps is not used for the extraction of lower deciduous molars because the sharp beaks of this forceps could cause damage to the unerupted premolar teeth.

The maxillary and mandibular six anterior teeth are removed by luxation to the labial side, followed by mesial rotation, and then pressure in the direction of removal. Because of the lingual position of the erupting permanent incisor teeth, little can be gained by placing lingual pressure on these teeth. The maxillary and mandibular molars are luxated to the buccal and lingual areas and delivered to the mesial or lingual. Frequently, a mesial or distal path of exit is necessary because of the root formation.

Adequate radiographs are invaluable for the removal of any deciduous tooth. The presence and position of the permanent successor must be established as well as the status of the root formation of the deciduous tooth that is to be removed. Many times the resorption of the deciduous root is unequal, leaving a long, thin root portion. If a root is fractured during the extraction, it should be removed by the judicious use of

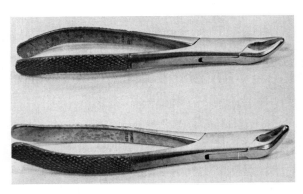

Fig. 7-1. Children's forceps.

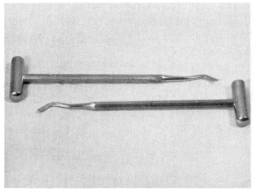

Fig. 7-2. Potts' elevators for removal of deciduous roots.

root exolevers or a small curet. The Potts elevators also are valuable here (Fig. 7-2). Care must be exercised not to injure the crown of the permanent tooth or its surrounding bony support. If the removal of the deciduous root tip jeopardizes the permanent tooth, it is better to leave the root tip intact. It will resorb or can be removed at a later date without jeopardy to the permanent tooth.

Occasionally the radiograph will demonstrate that the permanent premolar is wedged tightly between the bell-shaped roots of the deciduous tooth. This occurs most often in a deeply carious tooth of a young patient in which no deciduous root resorption has occurred. Care must be taken that the succedaneous tooth is not removed with the deciduous tooth because of the viselike grip of the roots. If the radiograph shows this condition, the deciduous crown should be sectioned into a mesial and a distal half before a forceps is placed on the tooth to remove the two portions separately. If at any time a permanent tooth is removed during the extraction of a deciduous tooth, it should be replaced in the alveolar bone with as little handling as possible and with the operator making sure that the buccal aspect of the tooth is placed on the buccal side of the alveolus.

SELECTION OF ANESTHESIA FOR EXODONTICS

The types of anesthesia available for exodontics are (1) regional or local anesthesia, (2) local anesthesia with heavy sedation or supplementation by light general anesthetic agents, and (3) general anesthesia induced intravenously or by inhalation.

Factors that determine choice of anesthesia are (1) age and physical status of the patient, (2) infection, (3) trismus, (4) emotional status of the patient, (5) nature and duration of the procedure, (6) allergies, (7) wishes of the patient, and (8) training and office equipment of the operator.

As stated previously, the very young patient is best managed under general anesthesia, usually of the inhalation type or in combination with small doses of intravenous barbiturates. The geriatric patient metabolizes barbiturates poorly and requires reduced dosages. Older patients are more likely to have systemic diseases that complicate the use of general anesthesia. The geriatric patient is often managed with local anesthesia, with judicious use of sedatives, when necessary, to relieve apprehension.

In the presence of infection, local anesthesia is not always profound. If local anesthesia is used, a nerve block is most effective and allows injection of the anesthetic solution in a noninfected area. Under no circumstances is a local anesthetic solution injected into or through an area of cellulitis. This serves only to spread the infection, with possible serious consequences. General anesthesia is often indicated in the presence of acute infection, except when the overall systemic condition of the patient precludes its use or the patient is in a toxic condition and dehydrated because of the infection. After the toxic manifestations have decreased and the patient is well hydrated, a general anesthetic may be given and the tooth removed. Before removal of any tooth during an acute infection, adequate blood levels of antibiotics should be obtained.

Trismus, the inability of the patient to open his mouth, may make the administration of a local anesthetic by the usual route difficult. Extraoral nerve blocks usually can be given. When the nerve block has alleviated the pain, the patient may be able to open the mouth so that the necessary extraction can be accomplished. Ethyl chloride sprayed on the skin overlying the muscles that are in spasm may enable the patient to open the mouth sufficiently to allow the surgeon to administer a local anesthetic and to perform the extraction. Care must be taken not to freeze the tissue with the ethyl chloride spray. General anesthesia, if deep enough to obtain muscle relaxation, is valuable when the trismus is caused by infection or trauma. When ankylosis of the temporomandibular joint is present, anesthesia can be accomplished by extraoral blocks or by performing a tracheostomy and administering a general anesthetic. If a general anesthetic is given to a patient with this condition, a tracheostomy is performed so that a patent airway can be maintained. Although adequate anesthesia can be obtained, this type of patient still presents many problems because of the inaccessibility of the teeth to be extracted.

The emotional status of the patient may determine the selection of anesthesia. Some people have a phobia regarding injections within the mouth. Because of the recent advances in general anesthesia, it is comparable in safety to local anesthesia. For this reason patients of this type are better managed under general anesthesia.

If the apprehensive patient must be treated under local anesthesia, sedation is necessary. The patient should receive a sedative at bedtime the night before surgery and again 1 hour prior to surgery. Intravenous sedation can be given at the time of surgery to augment sedatives already administered. Any patient who receives a sedative should be accompanied by a responsible adult. The surgeon is responsible for the patient while the latter is under the influence of the drug. Under no circumstances should a sedated patient be allowed to drive an automobile.

The nature of the procedure and the duration of time necessary to accomplish the exodontic procedure can govern the choice of anesthetic agent. In general, procedures requiring more than 30 minutes are better managed under local anesthesia with premedication or by admitting the patient to a hospital where adequate recovery facilities are available. With prolonged general anesthesia, a prolonged recovery time is necessary.

All patients should be questioned with regard to drug allergies. Patients having a possible history of allergy to local anesthetics should be questioned as to the type of reaction experienced and referred to an allergist for evaluation. Patients who have a history of allergic reaction to procaine often are not allergic to lidocaine because of the different chemical configuration of the drug. Although lidocaine has a low incidence of allergic reactions, reactions to this drug have been reported. Infrequently, adverse reactions to barbiturates are found. Most of these are not true allergic reactions but are failures of the patients to respond to the drug in the normal fashion. Nausea, vomiting, or changes in the psyche are common reactions. In any office in which drugs are administered, an emergency tray should be immediately available with the proper drugs necessary for treatment of allergic reactions. The treatment of these reactions will be described later in this chapter.

REMOVAL OF TEETH UNDER GENERAL ANESTHESIA

Organization and teamwork are essential when using general anesthesia. An efficient team is composed of three or four members: the surgeon, the anesthetist, the assistant, whose duty is to use the suction apparatus and retract tissues, and sometimes an instrument nurse whose duty is to pass instruments or wield the mallet if a chisel technique is used. Every member of the team must know the technique and anticipate the needs of the surgeon and the patient. Unnecessary acts should be avoided. Each motion should be smooth and purposeful.

All instruments that may be needed for a procedure should be available so that a member of the team does not have to break scrub to get an instrument. The instruments should be on a tray and always grouped in the same fashion, with the most frequently used instruments in the most accessible position.

For general anesthesia the patient may be supine or in a sitting position. Each position has its advantages.

The general anesthetics most frequently

used are inhalation alone, barbiturates alone, barbiturates with oxygen and nitrous oxide, and barbiturates with oxygen and nitrous oxide in combination with a more potent agent such as halothane (Fluothane). In addition, a local anesthetic is sometimes administered for vasoconstriction and to decrease the amount of barbiturate used in lengthy procedures.

A mouth prop is inserted immediately prior to induction of the anesthesia. Two types of mouth props are used—either a solid rubber bite block or a ratchet-type prop. If the latter is used, it is inserted in a closed position, and the patient is instructed to close on the mouth prop to hold it in position. After induction the mouth prop is adjusted to the degree of opening desired.

Immediately after induction a mouth pack is positioned. The pack is placed in such manner as to hold the tongue and soft tissues of the floor of the mouth anteriorly to maintain an airway. Care must be taken not to place the pack so far posteriorly that the oropharynx is stimulated. When an inhalation anesthesia is used, an airtight pack is more important so that anesthesia may be maintained by use of a nasal mask. Extra sponges may be added over the pack to absorb secretions and blood. With general anesthesia, more bleeding is experienced because of the lack of vasoconstrictive agents.

The surgical team should be ready to work as soon as the patient is anesthetized. One should not lose 2 or 3 precious minutes by not being prepared. The mouth prop is opened immediately and the mouth pack placed. The tooth is extracted and the socket compressed and covered with a gauze sponge. The mouth pack is removed and the mouth suctioned. The mouth prop is closed but left in place until the patient responds. The patient is transferred to a mobile chair or table and moved to a recovery room where he is watched carefully by an attendant.

During longer procedures a gauze sponge is placed over the mouth pack and changed as necessary. The assistant retracts and suctions in the most dependent portion of the mouth, not necessarily in a socket. A careful, efficient, unhurried technique is developed. Efficiency comes from precise instrumentation with few instrument changes. One should accomplish all that is to be done with a given instrument before the instrument is exchanged for another (for example, curet around all teeth that are to be extracted before picking up forceps). In multiple extractions the maxillary teeth are removed in one quadrant first, and the necessary alveoloplasty there is finished and sutured. A gauze sponge is then placed over this wound to help control hemorrhage. The mandibular teeth are removed in the opposing quadrant. After completion of surgery in this area, a new gauze sponge is placed over the wound before the mouth prop is shifted so that extractions can be done in the two remaining quadrants. Frequently, when a series of teeth are being extracted, as each posterior tooth is removed, the socket is covered with a sponge to help control hemorrhage while the next anterior tooth is removed.

A powerful suction apparatus is necessary. The greatest hazard when operating under general anesthesia comes from allowing blood, secretions, and debris to collect within the mouth. If these materials are allowed to descend, the larynx can be irritated and a laryngospasm caused, a lung abscess can be formed, or nausea and vomiting may follow entrance of these materials into the stomach. The average suction available in a dental unit is inadequate. Two types of suction tips should be available. A tonsillar suction tip is best adapted for handling a large volume of fluid efficiently, but it is too bulky to allow for suctioning within a socket. A neurosurgical suction tip will enter a small area. It is helpful to have two suction tips on the table in case debris clogs one of the tips.

The art of exodontics is never one of force. This is particularly true when operating on a patient under general anesthesia. Because of the loss of subjective symptoms in the patient, it becomes easy for the novice to apply great force with an exolever or to retract soft tissue carelessly. Meticulous surgery when using general anesthesia is important so that the postoperative healing will not be a painful experience for the patient.

REMOVAL OF TEETH IN THE HOSPITAL

Hospitalization of patients for exodontic procedures should always be considered when medical management of the patient may be a problem or the postoperative course may necessitate special care.

Before a patient is admitted to a hospital, arrangements must be made with the admitting office so that a bed will be available. The operating room secretary is also called so that an operating room can be reserved for the procedure.

The dental staff of the hospital is obligated to observe the basic rules of the hospital and the American Hospital Association. Although it is not the object of this text to outline hospital procedure, some basic rules should be noted. A patient who will undergo general anesthesia must have a physical examination, which includes a history. All patients admitted to a hospital for more than 24 hours should have routine laboratory tests. These usually consist of a hematocrit (HCT), a white blood cell count (WBC), a differential white count, and a urinalysis. A chest radiograph and serological tests may be required by some hospitals. Patients older than 45 years of age often are examined by an electrocardiogram (ECG) if general anesthesia is to be used. The dentist must write the necessary orders and an admission note, which includes the reason for the admission and the contemplated procedure. A dental history and oral examination should also be included in the dentist's note.

The dentist should check with the operating room personnel to be sure that all instruments necessary for the procedure will be available. In many hospitals the dentist must provide certain instruments.

In the operating room, sterile precautions are employed. The surgeon is expected to scrub and to wear a cap, gown, mask, and gloves.

The area around the patient's mouth should be prepared with an antiseptic solution to remove surface contaminants. If a single extraction or a minor procedure is to be performed, the simple placement of sterile towels to isolate the mouth is all the draping necessary. For multiple extractions or more extensive procedures, sterile sheets should be added so that the entire patient is covered to guard against contamination.

On completion of surgery a description of the operative procedure is dictated so that it may be added to the patient's chart. This note should include the following: date; names of the patient, surgeon, assistant, and anesthetist; type of anesthesia and agents used; surgical procedure and how it was accomplished; any complications (such as extensive hemorrhage); and condition of the patient at completion of surgery.

New orders are written, since preoperative orders are usually cancelled by the operating room procedure. Orders suggested by the consulting physician have to be rewritten to be given. Routine postoperative orders include patient's ambulatory status (bed rest until recovered, then up and about), hot or cold applications for swelling, antibiotics if needed for infections, diet, and an order for an analgesic and a hypnotic, if needed. Daily progress notes are entered by the dentist.

At the time of the patient's discharge from the hospital, a discharge summary of one paragraph is written, including reason for admission, surgical procedure, postsurgical course, and condition on discharge.

MANAGEMENT OF ACUTELY INFECTED TEETH

With the advent of antibiotics, the management of acutely infected teeth has changed. In the past it was necessary to treat the patient palliatively until the infection could be localized and drained and the tooth extracted. Today this sometimes long delay can be avoided by use of antibiotics. If the cause of the infection (that is, the tooth) can be removed, the resolution of the infection will be accelerated. The abscess formation may not have reached the stage at which tissue is broken down and pus formed. Antibiotics may control the acute infectious process, preventing pus formation. In any event, a blood level of antibiotics should be established as soon as possible. Once this blood level is established, the tooth should be removed if a surgical extraction is not deemed necessary. If a difficult extraction is anticipated, the patient should be placed on antibiotics until such time as a surgical flap can be raised and bone be removed without spreading the infection into surrounding tissues. The patient should remain on antibiotics after removal of an acutely infected tooth for 3 days after all evidence of the infection has disappeared.

COMPLICATIONS OF EXODONTICS

Complications arise from errors in judgment, misuse of instruments, exertion of extreme force, and failure to obtain proper visualization prior to acting. The old adage "To do good, you must see good" is apropos to exodontics, and one might add "Do well what you see."

Because of the anatomy of the maxillary antrum and its proximity to the maxillary premolar and molar roots, the antrum should always be considered when extracting teeth in this area.

Methods to remove maxillary roots are described in the section on root removal (Chapter 5).

Extreme force applied to upper molars can result in removal of the molar tooth along with the entire maxillary alveolar process and the floor of the antrum. The first, second, and third molars, along with the tuberosity, have been removed in one segment because of improper use of force in the maxilla. If during an extraction the surgeon feels large segments of bone moving with the tooth when pressure is applied, the forceps should be set aside and a flap raised. If judicious removal of part of the alveolar bone allows the tooth to be removed, then the remaining bone, which is attached to the periosteum, may be retained, and it will heal. This will minimize the bony defect. If the bone cannot be removed from the tooth, the mucosa should be incised and reflected so that the mucosa will not tear as the tooth and bone are removed. A laceration is much more difficult to repair than a well-planned incision.

Large antral perforations resulting from exodontics should be closed at the time of the extraction. The bone in the area should be smoothed with a rongeur or bone file. The mucoperiosteal flap is returned to position, and a watertight closure should be accomplished without putting undue pressure on the flap. If this cannot be done, the flap should be freed by means of an incision extending vertically into the mucobuccal fold and the mucosa of the flap undermined to allow it to advance over the defect.

When the antrum is entered during exodontics, the patient should be made aware of the situation and asked to not blow the nose and also to refrain if possible from coughing or sneezing. Antibiotics and vasoconstrictive nose drops are prescribed to guard against infection of the sinus and to allow for emptying of the fluid that will collect within the sinus.

Occasionally, buccal roots of premolars and molars are pushed laterally through the wall of the maxilla and lie above the attachment of the buccinator muscle. When the operator uses root exolevers in this area, a finger of the left hand should be held against the buccal plate so that he or she can be aware of any movement of the root in this direction. If the root is dislodged into these tissues, a small incision is made in the mucosa inferior to the root tip and the root tip is removed with a small hemostat or similar instrument.

The infratemporal space lies directly posterior and superior to the tuberosity of the maxilla. Within this space lie many important neurovascular structures. In the elevation of third molars or third molar root tips and in the removal of supernumerary molars, care must be taken not to dislodge them posteriorly. If an object is to be removed from the infratemporal space, adequate visualization and careful dissection are necessary. The incision should include the entire tuberosity and extend posteriorly to the anterior pillar of the fauces. Blind dissection and groping for objects in this area can be complicated by massive hemorrhage or nerve damage.

In the third molar region of the mandible, the lingual surface of the mandible curves laterally, close to the apices of this tooth. Therefore it is not difficult to dislodge a root tip inferiorly into this space when the lingual plate is fractured. When a root tip is displaced in this area, a finger should be placed inferior to the root tip (in the mouth) to stabilize the tip against the lingual plate of the mandible. Access to this area is gained by making a mucoperiosteal flap on the lingual side of the mandible and extending anteriorly enough that the tissues can be retracted lingually for good vision.

Recovery of a root tip in the mandibular canal is principally a problem of access and vision. Usually it is difficult to remove bone overlying the canal from within the depths of the wound, which is usually the third molar socket. Access may be gained by removal of bone from the buccal plate and by careful removal of bone that overlies the canal. If one of the vascular components of the canal has been injured, it may be necessary to pack the socket with gauze, allowing 10 minutes for control of the hemorrhage. If hemorrhage cannot be controlled in this manner, the injured vessel should be severed completely and allowed to retract into the canal. At this time the socket is again packed, and hemorrhage control is usually accomplished.

POSTEXODONTIC COMPLICATIONS

Postoperative hemorrhage is the most common complication after exodontics. If the patient calls from home to report that hemorrhage has started again, he should be advised first to clear the mouth of any blood clots with a gauze sponge and then rinse the mouth with warm salt water. All excessive blood clots should be removed from the vicinity of the socket, but the clot in the socket should not be removed. The patient is instructed to bite firmly on a sterile gauze sponge that has been folded so that pressure is exerted on the area of surgery. If a sterile gauze sponge is not available, the patient may use a tea bag that has been placed in cold water to soften the tea leaves. The patient is advised to bite (not chew) on the pad or tea bag for 20 minutes. If bleeding persists at the end of this period, the patient should be seen by the dentist.

In cases of persistent hemorrhage, gauze sponges and hemostatic agents such as Gelfoam, topical thrombin, and oxidized cellulose may be helpful for the local control of hemorrhage in addition to an adequate armamentarium.

The patient is seated and a local anesthetic administered. The clot that has formed within the socket is removed. Next, the area of hemorrhage is located. If the hemorrhage is coming from a bone bleeder within the socket, the dull side of a curet is used to burnish the bone in the area of hemorrhage. If generalized bone bleeding is present, the socket is packed with a hemostatic agent such as Gelfoam soaked in thrombin, and a purse-string suture is applied to hold the hemostatic agent in place. The patient is asked to bite on a moist gauze sponge. If the hemorrhage is from the surrounding soft tissue, a tension suture is placed to apply pressure to the area (see Chapter 13).

In patients with advanced periodontal disease, postoperative bleeding will occur if granulation tissue is allowed to remain after removal of the affected teeth. At the time of surgery a few minutes spent removing the granulation tissue and suturing the alveolar mucosa will assure good hemorrhage control.

Infection can occur as a postoperative complication. Treatment of such infection is managed by using the principles outlined in Chapter 11.

Dry socket (localized osteitis) is one of the most perplexing postoperative complications. The etiology of the dry socket is unknown, but the following factors increase the incidence of this painful post-extraction sequela: trauma, infection, decreased vascular supply of the surrounding bone, and general systemic condition.

This condition rarely occurs when minimal traumatic methods are employed during difficult or simple extractions. Meticulous debridement of all extraction wounds should be done routinely. The etiology may be related to factors that impede or prevent adequate nourishment from reaching the newly formed blood clot within the alveolus. Patients with dense osteosclerotic bone or with teeth that have osteosclerotic alveolar walls because of chronic infection are predisposed to dry sockets.

Dry socket most commonly develops on the third or fourth postoperative day and is characterized by severe, continuous pain and necrotic odor. Clinically the condition may be described as an alveolus in which the primary blood clot has become necrotic and remains within the alveolus as a septic foreign body until it is removed by irrigation. This usually occurs a few days after extraction, leaving the alveolar walls divested of their protective covering. The denuded bone is accompanied by severe pain, which can be controlled only by local application of potent analgesics and oral or parenteral use of analgesics or narcotics.

To treat a septic alveolus properly, one must understand the physiology of bone repair. If the loss of the primary blood clot results from a sclerotic condition of the alveolar walls and the absence of nutrient vessels, then the resulting denuded bone surface must be viewed as any other denuded bone surface and the dentist must rely on nature's methods of bone repair for ultimate recovery and not employ any other methods that would disturb the healing process.

A septic alveolus is a denuded bone surface. Nature abhors denuded bone and responds to repair it. Behind this denuded and traumatized surface an immediate mechanism is set up to physiologically correct the defect. All denuded bone becomes necrotic and must be removed before it can be replaced by normal bone. During this period the contiguous region behind the alveolus is defended against invasion of pyogenic organisms within the septic alveolus, provided nothing is done to break through or violate this wall until the repair mechanism is ready to replace the nonvital structure. This process usually takes 2 to 3 weeks, depending on the regenerative capacity of the individual.

With the completion of this cycle, the nonvital alveolar wall is sequestrated molecularly or en masse, and immediately behind it is a defensive and regenerative layer of juvenile connective tissue that ultimately fills the void and undergoes osseous replacement. During this period, treatment should be directed only to maintenance of wound hygiene, with employment of antiseptic, analgesic dressings within the alveolus of sufficient potency to keep the patient comfortable. Nature must do the repairing. Curettage is contraindicated and will not only delay physiological healing and repair but may also permit invasion of infection into and beyond the area of defense immediately behind the denuded alveolus.

Prevention, of course, is the best treatment. To this end, atraumatic surgery, avoidance of contamination, and maintenance of a good level of general health are important.

When a dry socket does develop, treatment should be palliative. The socket is gently irrigated with warm normal saline solution to remove all debris. After the socket has been carefully dried, it is lightly dressed with 1/4-inch plain gauze saturated with an obtundent paste, such as equal parts of thymol iodide powder and benzocaine crystals dissolved in eugenol. The dressing may be changed as necessary until pain has subsided and granulation tissue has covered the walls of the socket.

EMERGENCIES IN THE DENTAL OFFICE

The number of emergencies that arise in a dental office is inversely proportional to the preventive measures taken by the dentist. A good medical history, carefully evaluated, may be the best insurance against office emergencies. Although dental emergencies are rare, the dentist and staff must be prepared to manage those that do arise. A well-organized plan of treatment should be worked out and rehearsed to cope with these situations. Emergency drills, just like fire drills, may save lives. Emergency situations can be of a minor or a major nature, but, in all instances, if improper care is given the outcome can be disastrous.

The dental office should be equipped with oxygen that can be applied under positive pressure. An emergency tray containing all the necessary drugs should be readily available and checked from time to time to ensure completeness. Drugs should never be taken from an emergency tray for routine use.

Syncope (fainting) is probably the most common emergency and is usually associated with the administration of a local anesthetic. The etiology is cerebral hypoxia, resulting from the disturbance of the normal mechanism of blood pressure control. Dilation of the splanchnic vessels causes a fall in blood pressure with a decrease in cerebral blood flow. The initiation

of this reaction is of a psychic nature and should not be interpreted as a reaction to the drug administered. Symptoms include pallor, dizziness, light-headedness, clammy skin, nausea, and sometimes complete loss of consciousness. The treatment consists of placing the patient in a supine position, with the head lower than the rest of the body. An airway is maintained, and oxygen should be administered. Mild respiratory stimulants such as spirits of ammonia can be used, but analeptics and other more potent agents are generally not used unless specifically indicated. Prevention of syncope can be accomplished by considering the psychic constitution of the patient. Measures should be taken to allay apprehension.

Toxic reactions to local anesthetics are characterized by an initial excitatory phase followed by marked depression. The patient may become talkative and anxious. Nausea and vomiting may occur. If the drug is given intravenously, the initial excitatory phase may be brief, terminating in convulsions followed by marked depression. (When administering a drug intravenously, always aspirate before injecting.) If any signs of reaction to the drug are noted during an injection, the needle should be withdrawn immediately.

Most reactions to local anesthesia are of a minor nature and can be treated palliatively. If convulsions occur and become increasingly intense, a short-acting barbiturate or diazepam should be given intravenously to control the convulsion. Oxygen should then be given to ensure adequate oxygenation. When the stimulatory phase is mild or of short duration, no sedative is given but oxygen is administered, and steps are taken to maintain adequate circulation.

In cases of severe central nervous system stimulation or depression or cardiovascular collapse, the dentist should initiate treatment but call for additional professional help. The calling of other professional personnel does not indicate inadequacy on the part of the dentist but instead shows good judgment.

To avoid allergic reactions to medication,

the dentist should complete an adequate history and evaluation before using the drug.

Allergic reactions to drugs can vary from delayed reactions that are more annoying than dangerous to anaphylactoid reactions that are severe and often lead to the death of the patient. Most drugs at one time or another have been associated with allergic reactions. Penicillin, sulfonamides, and other antibiotics are the most common drugs the dentist may use that are associated with allergic reactions.

Delayed or less severe reactions may be characterized by swelling at the site of injection, angioneurotic edema, pruritus, and urticaria. Treatment consists of antihistamines and palliative care.

Anaphylactoid reactions develop quickly. The patient becomes extremely apprehensive, intensive itching occurs, and asthmatic breathing develops. Urticaria may develop rapidly; the blood pressure falls, and the pulse becomes weak or absent. The patient may lapse into an unconscious state with or without convulsions. Death may occur within a few minutes or several hours later.

Treatment of an anaphylactoid reaction consists of the immediate application of a tourniquet above the site of injection if possible.

Because of the vasopressor, bronchodilator, and antihistaminic effects of epinephrine, it is the drug of choice in reactions of this type. The dosage in the adult will range from 0.3 to 1 mg (0.3 to 1 ml of a 1:1,000 solution) subcutaneously or intramuscularly. In all severe systemic reactions, a cannulated vein allows for rapid use of drugs and fluid management. If possible, an intravenous route should be started and maintained. The intravenous route allows for titration or fractional doses of epinephrine, although the total dosage is approximately the same. Oxygen under pressure should be given with assisted respiration. Antihistamines, such as diphenhydramine, 50 mg, are given intravenously or intramuscularly. Corticosteroids such as hydrocortisone (Solu-Cortef), 100 mg intravenously or intramuscularly, are usually recommended for their peripheral vascular effect.

Professional aid should be called as soon as possible to consult in the further treatment of the patient. If symptoms continue, consider readministration of epinephrine or antihistamine. If the blood pressure is low, consider the use of a vasopressor drug such as phenylephrine, 1 to 5 mg intramuscularly.

During exodontics, teeth are sometimes inadvertently displaced into the oropharynx, larynx, trachea, and esophagus. Teeth in these positions can present serious problems that could be avoided by simple precautions. A gauze screen should always be placed to block off the oropharynx from the mouth. This is true whether the exodontic procedure is performed under general or under local anesthesia.

Teeth displaced into the oropharynx present no problem, provided they can be retrieved before they descend into the deeper structures. When a tooth is displaced in the oropharynx while the patient is under local anesthesia, the patient is instructed to hold perfectly still and not swallow or take a breath until the tooth can be retrieved. If this occurs under general anesthesia, everything stops until the tooth is retrieved. The assistant should be cautioned not to move the retractor or suction tip because any movement may cause the loss of the tooth into the larynx or esophagus.

When a tooth is displaced in the posterior portion of the mouth, the natural reflex of the patient is to cough or swallow. In the majority of cases the patient will swallow, carrying the tooth into the esophagus. Regardless of the patient's reactions, radiographs should be taken to determine the exact location of the tooth. If the tooth is found to be in the gastrointestinal tract, a high bulk diet should be prescribed, and the patient should contact the dentist if any gastrointestinal symptoms occur. Usually the tooth will be passed without incident.

In coughing, the patient can either cough up the foreign body or it will be lodged in the larynx or aspirated into the tracheo-bronchial tree. The abdominal thrust procedure should be used to dislodge large objects from this area. In the case of teeth in the larynx, a laryngeal spasm may occur, blocking the exchange of air. The tooth may be removed by means of a laryngoscope and a Magill forceps. If the tooth cannot be removed quickly, an airway must be established. This can be accomplished by a cricothyroidotomy through the triangularly shaped cricothyroid membrane and into the trachea. The cricothyroid membrane is located between the thyroid cartilage (Adam's apple), which is the largest of the tracheal cartilages, and the cricoid cartilage, which is the next inferior tracheal cartilage. Oxygen then should be given through the established airway until the tooth is removed and the laryngeal spasm is broken.

Teeth that are aspirated into the tracheo-bronchial tree present a serious problem. The removal of teeth in this position can be accomplished only by someone trained in methods of bronchoscopy. The patient may cough continuously, and cyanosis may occur. Oxygen should be given until the patient can be transferred to an area where a radiograph of the chest and direct bronchoscopy can be accomplished. The aspiration of teeth and other debris during dental operations has been associated with a high incidence of lung abscesses.

Under all circumstances a radiograph of the chest and possibly of the abdomen must be taken to establish the exact location of any tooth that is displaced.

REFERENCES

1. Auster, K. F.: Systemic anaphylaxis in man, J.A.M.A. **192**:116, 1965.
2. Calhoun, N. R.: Dry socket and other postoperative complications, Dent.Clin. North Am. **15**:337, 1971.
3. Erickson, R. I., Waite, D. E., and Wilkinson, R. H.: A study of dry socket, J. Oral Surg. **13**:1046, 1960.
4. McCarthy, F. M.: Emergencies in dental practice, ed. 2, Philadelphia, 1972, W. B. Saunders Co., pp. 239-250.
5. Norman, J. E., and Cannon, P. D.: Fractures of the maxillary tuberosity, Oral Surg. **24**:459, 1967.
6. Thoma, K. H.: Oral surgery, ed. 5, St. Louis, 1969, The C. V. Mosby Co.

CHAPTER 8

Preprosthetic surgery

Louis H. Guernsey

In a *Time* magazine essay,[46] it was noted that 20 million people in America are older than 65 years of age and that the aged have grown to represent approximately 10% of the total population. Actuaries have emphasized that the American life-span can be expected to increase as a result of public health measures, research, and the high quality of medical care that are the earmarks of our nation. Already the United States population of persons older than 75 years of age is increasing at two and one-half times the rate of the general population. This large, superaged citizenry, living in an era of social consciousness in which health and health care are believed to be rights that are to be guaranteed and even underwritten by government, will certainly create a colossal prosthetic restorative problem.

Prosthodontics aims to restore the functional and esthetic portions of the gnathological system that have been lost or are congenitally absent. Since a denture can be no better than its foundation of basilar bone with its proper tissue cover, it is axiomatic that every effort should be made by the dentist to prepare, improve, preserve, and reconstruct the jaws for prolonged denture wearing.

Many dentures that are worn with discomfort, annoyance, and embarrassment could be made comfortably functional if surgical alterations were accomplished to improve denture wearing.

EDENTULOUS RIDGE CRITERIA

Goodsell[24] outlined the criteria for prosthesis in an ideal edentulous mouth. Following are the criteria of an ideal edentulous ridge:

1. Adequate bony support for dentures
2. Bone covered by adequate soft tissue
3. No undercuts or overhanging protuberances
4. No sharp ridges
5. Adequate buccal and lingual sulci
6. No scar bands to prevent normal seating of a denture at its periphery
7. No muscle fibers or frenums to mobilize the periphery of the prosthesis
8. Satisfactory relationship of the maxillary and mandibular alveolar ridges
9. No soft tissue folds, redundancies, or hypertrophies of the ridges or in the sulci
10. Freedom from neoplastic disease

CORRECTIVE SURGICAL PROCEDURES

A large number of oral surgical procedures have been advocated to achieve the previously listed prerequisites. Recently a great amount of emphasis has been placed on ridge extension procedures. However, little attention has been given to surgical attempts to alter, improve, or replace faulty ridge-covering tissues with a functioning masticatory mucosa or skin. The principles of oral plastic surgery— gentle handling of tissues, preservation of blood supply, and prevention of infection—are particularly applicable to this type of surgery.[32]

Corrective procedures necessary to prepare the edentulous ridge for prosthesis can be divided into two basic groups with respect to time of surgery: *initial preparations* and *secondary preparations. Initial preparations* of the edentulous ridge occur at the time of tooth extraction or at the time of the first denture insertion. This group can be further subdivided into preparations to correct soft tissue and hard tissue deformities. Soft tissue preparation includes procedures to eliminate frena, scars, and high muscle attachments and to resurface the basilar bone with a new tissue covering; hard tissue preparation includes procedures for alveoloplasty, tori removal, and sharp ridge removal, which includes lingual shelf reduction. Correction for combined soft and hard deformities includes procedures for tuberosity alteration and reduction. These procedures are mostly supportive in nature.

Secondary preparations of the ridge occur after a period of protracted denture wearing during which excessive atrophy, scarring, or injury have caused a marked change in the basilar bone and its covering tissues, thus negating successful denture wearing. This group can also be further subdivided into soft tissue and hard tissue preparation. This preparation includes elimination of epulis fissuratum and scars, correction of reactive inflammatory papillary hyperplasia of the palate, ridge extension, and ridge augmentation in the maxilla and mandible. Special attention will be given to ridge extension and ridge augmentation procedures.

Initial preparations
Soft tissue deformities and corrective procedures

Soft tissue preparation of the edentulous ridge involves correction of soft tissue deformities. Deformities such as high muscle attachments and frena can occur normally, but they are usually found when excessive atrophy has decreased alveolar height. Scars can be residuals of previous periodontic, endodontic, or trauma surgery.

Correction is begun by transverse incision across and a supraperiosteal dissection of the attachment, followed by downward displacement and suturing of the muscle to the periosteum with No. 3-0 Dexon (polyglycolic sutures) in the new position. Additional stabilization is obtained by overextending the denture periphery with dental compound and guttaform or zinc oxide impression paste to support the attachment in this new position. Obwegeser[44] states that if there are three or more high muscle attachments or frena, consideration should be given to submucosal vestibulo-

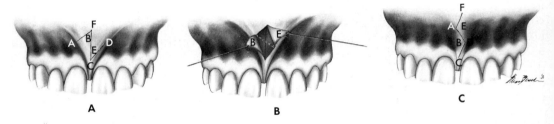

Fig. 8-1. Z-plasty. **A,** Tight frenum outline for Z-plasty technique. **B,** Angular flaps *B* and *E* raised. **C,** Flaps transposed into their new positions.

plasty in the maxilla or to vestibuloplasty with skin graft in the mandible.

Other useful corrective methods include Z-plasty, V-Y–plasty for lengthening tissue, Y-V–plasty for shortening tissue, and cross-diamond excision of frena (Fig. 8-1).

Hard tissue deformities and corrective procedures

Alveoloplasty. With alveoloplasty only the protuberances that prevent insertion of the denture or retard healing are removed.

Conservatism should be the paramount guide. Minimal raising of attached gingiva is accomplished (whether labially, lingually, or palatally) so that a minimum of the underlying bone is exposed. Wide retraction of tissues increases bony resorption and obliterates sulci.

In single tooth extraction with early loss of adjacent teeth, the collar of bone around the tooth must be reduced at the time of extraction (Fig. 8-2). Labial, lingual, and palatal sharp edges should be reduced to provide a U-shaped ridge. Bone should not be sacrificed for primary tissue closure.

During the procedure, inflamed or excessive interdental and interradicular tissue should be trimmed and removed. Copious irrigation with normal saline and final palpation and inspection should accompany the procedure to assure removal of debris and to ascertain smoothness of the bony base. Suturing with No. 3-0 silk or Dexon should be done across the interseptal bone while the assistant supports the sulcus superiorly with a retractor (Fig. 8-3).

Radical alveolectomy has a minimal role in special preparations of the mouth for specific conditions (Fig. 8-4). Correction of severe overbite and overjet can best be obtained by extensive labial removal of the buccal and interseptal bone or by interseptal alveolectomy.

Radical alveoloplasty is performed in patients with oral cancer who are to undergo radiation therapy as a part of the preoperative therapy for their cancer. In these patients periodontally involved, devitalized, and extensively restored teeth and teeth that are going to be in the direct path of the radiation are removed. Radical alveoloplasty of bone is accomplished at surgery to contour the bone to the level achieved by subsequent normal healing and atrophy. It has been noted that interseptal and alveolar bone that has been irradiated will not remodel itself, which may preclude forever the wearing of a denture, since decubitus ulcers, which expose a nonrecontoured ridge, can predispose the ridge to radio-osteomyelitis of the jaws.

Torus removal. Tori have no pathological significance, but occasionally they are misdiagnosed as tumors, thereby alarming patients. Tori that are impinged on by a prosthesis are sources of painful chronic irritation that can invite infection or denture failure or both or even become an etiological factor in oral malignancy.

MAXILLARY TORI. Maxillary tori should be studied by a true lateral radiograph to rule out the possibility of pneumatization of the tori. Removal of such tori could lead to an iatrogenic oral-nasal opening (traumatic cleft palate).

Indications for removal include a large, lobulated torus with a thin mucoperiosteal cover extending posteriorly to the vibrating line of the palate that prevents seating of the denture over the mass and prevents posterior seal at the fovea palatini.

The technique for removal of the torus is as follows (Fig. 8-5): The maxillary torus should not be excised en masse to prevent entry into the nose but should be subdivided into segments by a bur. The segments are then removed with an osteotome, and protuberences are finished down smooth with a bone file or a Hall Surgairtome under a constant stream of coolant. The flap is trimmed and loosely sutured.

The palate should be covered to prevent hematoma formation and to support the flap and is best covered by a palatal splint fastened to the teeth by clasps or by ligation with stainless steel wire. The splint remains in place for 48 hours at which time it is

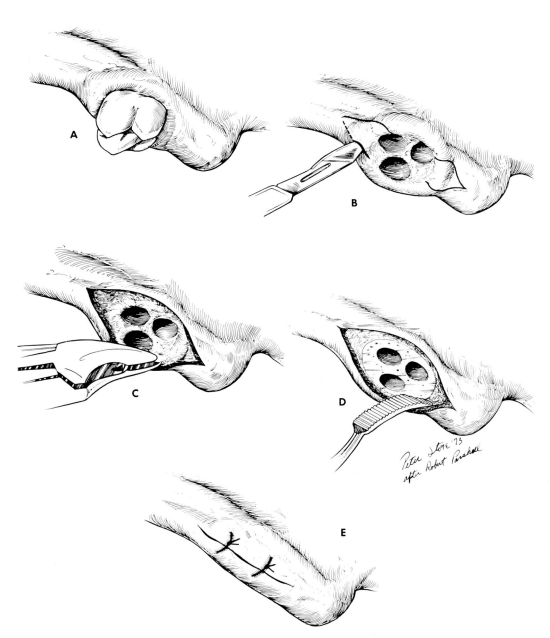

Fig. 8-2. Single tooth alveoloplasty. **A,** Isolated tooth with high alveolar bone. **B,** After tooth removal, wedge-shaped portions of gingiva are removed from mesial and distal borders of the socket. The mucoperiosteum is reflected buccally and lingually. **C,** Bony reduction with rongeur. **D,** Smoothing with bone file. **E,** Final suturing.

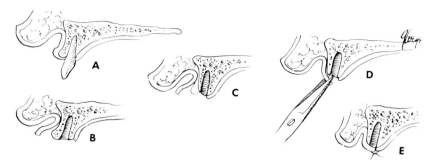

Fig. 8-3. Simple alveoloplasty. **A,** Cross section showing moderate undercut at labial alveolar crest. **B,** Extent of flap retraction should be limited to height of undercut only. **C,** Conservative bone removal. **D,** Excess tissue trimmed from labial flaps. **E,** Sutured flap.

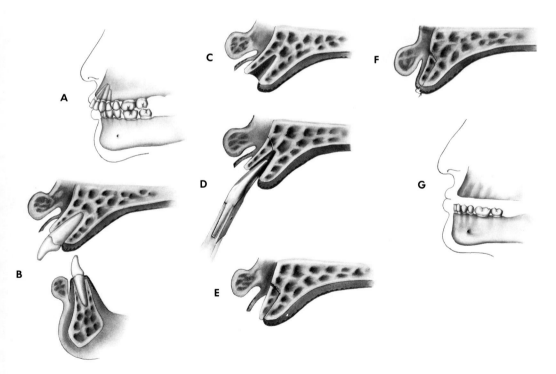

Fig. 8-4. Radical interseptal alveoloplasty. **A,** Cross section showing marked maxillary overjet. **B,** Wider flap retraction than for single alveoloplasty. **C,** Tooth extraction. **D,** Rongeuring of interseptal bone. **E,** Down fracture of buccal alveolar bone. **F,** Flap sutured. **G,** Cross section showing improved intermaxillary relation.

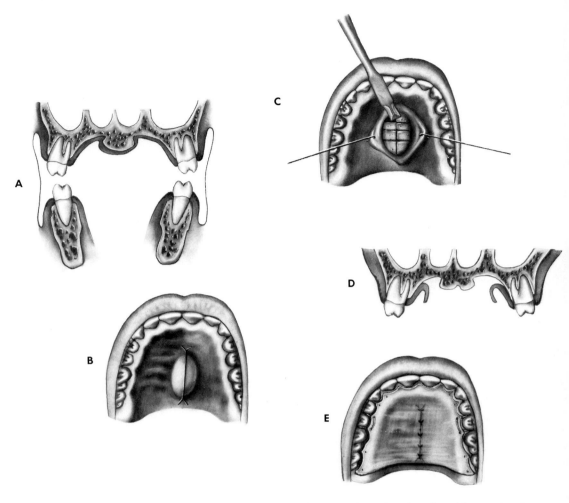

Fig. 8-5. Technique of maxillary torus removal. **A,** Cross section of oral cavity with prominent torus palatinus. **B,** Incision line. **C,** Divided segments of torus being removed with chisel. **D,** Lateral grooving of mass at its base (optional). **E,** Suturing completed with clear acrylic palatal splint wired in place.

removed to clean and inspect the wound. It is then worn as a bandage over the operative site until healing is satisfactory. The splint is removed, however, after each meal for cleansing and oral hygiene measures.

MANDIBULAR TORI. Mandibular tori occur primarily in the area lingual to the bicuspids. They are usually bulbar, can be single or multiple, and occasionally coalesce to form a thick lingual exostosis extending

from the cuspid posteriorly to the second molar.

The removal technique of mandibular tori is illustrated in Fig. 8-6. Placement of the incision over the crest of the edentulous ridge or around the necks of the teeth is important to afford proper closure. The incision should be long enough to encompass the entire torus and then extended beyond this to avoid tearing of the usually thin flap. Only the full thickness of the muco-

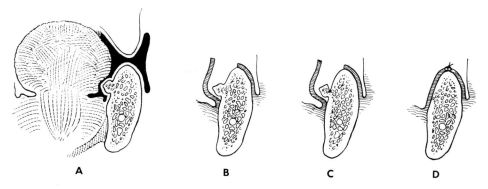

Fig. 8-6. Mandibular torus removal technique. **A,** Cross section of mandibular torus. **B,** Lingual periosteum reflected, exposing torus but leaving lateral periosteum attached. **C,** Superior grooving on torus. **D,** Incision sutured. (From Goodsell, J. O., and King, D. R.: Abnormalities of the mouth. In Kruger, G. O., editor: Textbook of oral surgery, ed. 3, St. Louis, 1968, The C. V. Mosby Co.)

periosteum on the lingual side is reflected. The labial tissues are not freed, providing a stable labial tissue for closure and preventing loss of sulcus depth.

A trough is cut by bur in the exposed torus to develop a plane from which the torus should split. A single-beveled osteotome with the bevel directed away from the cortex is placed in the cut, and the torus is split off by a sharp blow with a mallet. Bony smoothing is accomplished with a bone file or, if space permits, a rotating bone bur or both. The area is irrigated with normal saline. Closure is accomplished with interrupted No. 3-0 silk or Dexon sutures, and a clear acrylic splint is placed lingual to the teeth to prevent hematoma formation. Splint care is the same as for maxillary tori.

Sharp ridge removal. Sharp, sawlike edentulous ridges are a common cause of denture discomfort. The ridge is usually obscured by movable redundant tissue overlying the crest. Heavy finger palpation or underexposed x-ray films or both will reveal the sharp excrescences.

Removal is initiated by placing the incision through periosteum labially to the crest of the flabby ridge and reflecting the mucoperiosteum minimally to preserve the vestibule (Fig. 8-7). Bony trim is accomplished with rongeur, files, or surgical burs and involves only the sharp spines and knifelike bone. A maximum of 1 or 2 mm need be removed, since resorption during healing accounts for further loss. The flabby excess tissue is resected and sent to the pathologist. Closure is done with No. 3-0 silk or Dexon sutures. Additional tissue support is afforded by relining the patient's denture with periodontal pack or soft acrylic.

SHELF REDUCTION. Shelf reduction involves the sharp mandibular lingual shelf that houses the third molar and the mylohyoid ridge, which, although normal anatomy, becomes relatively more pronounced with extreme atrophy of an edentulous mandible (Fig. 8-8). Increasingly prosthodontists are extending the flanges of mandibular dentures lingually to increase stability and decrease lateral stresses. This requires the elimination of the naturally occurring undercut in the lingual shelf area. Significant ridge extension in this area can also be obtained by using techniques suggested by Trauner,[60] Obwegeser,[41] and Caldwell.[10]

The reduction of the shelf is predicated on the fact that mandibular bone contains

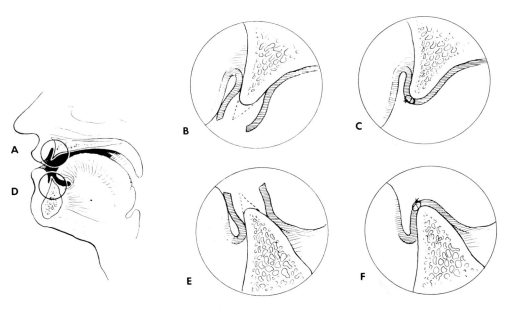

Fig. 8-7. Method for reduction of sharp edentulous ridges. **A** and **D,** Sharp edentulous ridges. **B** and **E,** Extent of bone trimming and amount of periosteal reflection. **C** and **F,** Utilization of palatal or lingual flaps to cover bony ridges. (From Goodsell, J. O., and King, D. R.: Abnormalities of the mouth. In Kruger, G. O., editor: Textbook of oral surgery, ed. 3, St. Louis, 1968, The C. V. Mosby Co.)

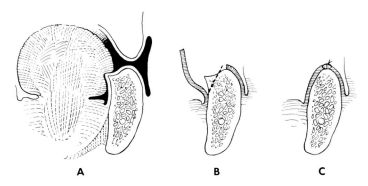

Fig. 8-8. Sharp mylohyoid ridge reduction technique. **A,** Sharp mylohyoid ridge. **B,** Reflection of lingual flap and extent of bone removed. **C,** Lingual flap repositioned and sutured. (From Goodsell, J. O., and King, D. R.: Abnormalities of the mouth. In Kruger, G. O., editor: Textbook of oral surgery, ed. 3, St. Louis, 1968, The C. V. Mosby Co.)

a grain similar to wood and that the grain direction is known.[61] This permits the surgeon to split bone off predictably for removal of the shelf (Fig. 8-9).

The procedure for shelf reduction is as follows. A special bite block with a self-retaining tongue retractor is used. Incision is made through the periosteum from the ridge crest laterally and superiorly onto the external oblique ridge. The periosteum is first detached buccally; a No. 4 Molt curet is then inserted into the lingual space under

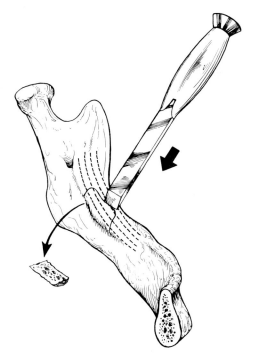

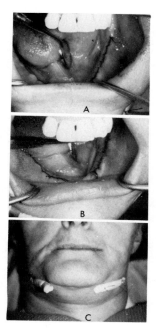

Fig. 8-9. Grain of mandible and chisel placement to split off the sharp lingual shelf. (Adapted from Guernsey, L. H.: Dent. Clin. North Am. **15**:459, 1971.)

Fig. 8-10. Catheter in floor of mouth. **A,** Lingual shelf reduction. **B,** French catheter placed in floor of mouth. **C,** Catheters sutured to poultice on skin.

the retromolar pad. At this point, care is exercised to not damage the lingual nerve. The lingual shelf is widely exposed by stripping the periosteum anteriorly. The lingual nerve and Wharton's duct are protected with a Lane retractor.

The shelf is chiseled free by placing a 1 cm, single-beveled osteotome parallel to the anterior border of the ascending ramus and driving the chisel downward and lingual to split off the bone shelf (Fig. 8-9). Significant bleeding can be encountered as the mylohyoid muscle is detached from the bone. Further trimming and smoothing is done with a bone bur or file to eliminate sharp spicules in the pterygomandibular space.

The wound is irrigated copiously with saline, followed by a loose closure of the tissues using No. 3-0 silk or Dexon. Down-

ward repositioning of the tissue can be maintained by placing a rubber No. 14 French catheter in the floor of the mouth and passing over it a No. 2-0 Tevdek suture that has been passed through to the skin with an awl. The sutures emerging on the skin are tied over a cotton roll or buttons and allowed to remain in position for 5 days (Fig. 8-10).

Pain on swallowing and edema of the floor of the mouth are the expected postoperative sequelae. This expected edema poses no significant threat to the airway. In more extensive procedures, edema can be controlled about the floor of the mouth and medial aspect of the mandible by using preoperative, interoperative, and postoperative dexamethasone (Decadron).[26]

MYLOHYOID MUSCLE RELEASE. As noted previously, mylohyoid muscle release is commonly a part of lingual shelf reduction since the posterior portion of the insertion of the muscle extends distally to the lingual shelf. Mylohyoid muscle release per se is indicated as part of preprosthetic surgery in two instances: (1) when the mandible is atrophic and the floor of the mouth tissues protrude above the crest of the ridge and (2) as surgical preparation for the insertion of the mandibular bone plate prosthetic fastener system. The surgical technique for the muscle release procedure will be detailed later in this chapter under floor of the mouth lowering with skin graft vestibuloplasty.

Combined soft and hard tissue deformities and corrective procedures

Tuberosities. Enlarged tuberosities of the maxilla can accompany submucosal fibrous

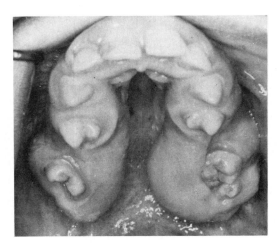

Fig. 8-11. Excessive fibrous tissue in maxillary arch.

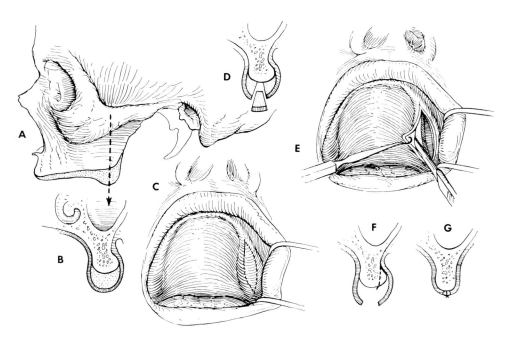

Fig. 8-12. Maxillary tuberosity reduction. **A** and **B,** Lateral and cross-sectional views of enlarged tuberosities. **C,** Elliptical incisions from tuberosity to bicuspid area. **D,** Cross section with area between elliptical incisions removed. Dotted area represents fibrous tissue to be removed. **E,** Removal of fibrous tissue by undermining buccal and palatal flaps. **F,** Removal of bony undercut. **G,** Closure of wound. (From Goodsell, J. O., and King, D. R.: Abnormalities of the mouth. In Kruger, G. O., editor: Textbook of oral surgery, ed. 3, St. Louis, 1968, The C. V. Mosby Co.)

hyperplasia or be the result of true bony enlargements that interfere with denture seating because of excessive undercut or impingement on the intermaxillary space (Fig. 8-11). Correction is accomplished by wedge resection of the fibrotic tissue down to bone over the crest portion of the ridge, followed by submucous resection of this tissue from beneath both the buccal and palatal flaps. In this palatal undermining, care should be taken to avoid the palatine artery (Fig. 8-12). Excess or undercut areas in bone are removed with rongeurs or surgical burs, irrigated, and smoothed with files. When the desired bony base contour is achieved, excess tissues are trimmed to afford closure without tension. Closure is made with No. 3-0 silk sutures left in place for 5 days.

TUBEROSITY REDUCTION, LATERAL APPROACH. A modification of tuberosity reduction using a lateral rather than crest-of-the-ridge

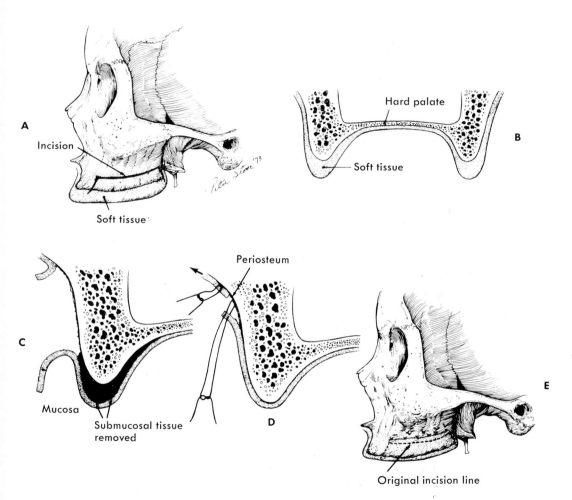

Fig. 8-13. Maxillary tuberosity reduction, lateral approach. **A,** Outline of main incision and two relaxing incisions on lateral aspect of the alveolus. **B,** Outline of flap to be raised. **C,** Submucosal connective tissue and bony undercut removed. **D,** Submucosal dissection and apical flap repositioning to deepen the sulcus. **E,** Final flap suture.

incision has been designed to conserve the limited amount of keratinizing mucosa overlying a narrow tuberosity,[20] thus saving it for local advancement vestibuloplasty at the end of the operation (Fig. 8-13). An incision to bone is made on the lateral side of the maxillary ridge from the tuberosity anteriorly but inferiorly enough to pass below the malar buttress. A relaxing incision is extended down onto the crest of the ridge anteriorly and posteriorly as needed to obtain tissue relaxation. The thickened fibrotic tissue overlying the bony tuberosity is elevated with periosteal retractors, and a submucosal excision of the fibrotic tissue is accomplished. The sulcus is extended superiorly from the height of the lateral incision by submucosal dissection

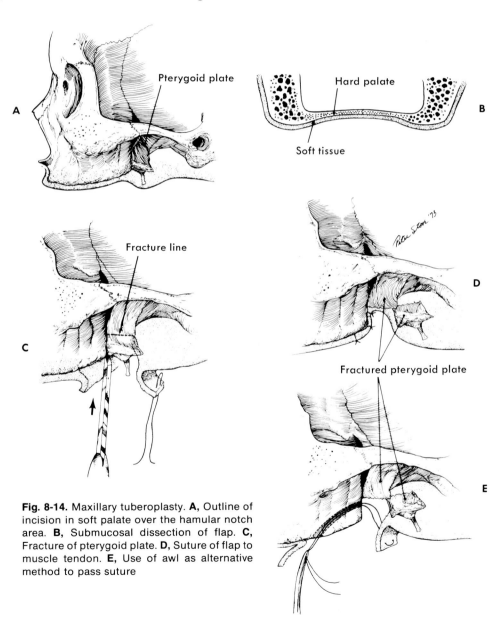

Fig. 8-14. Maxillary tuberoplasty. **A,** Outline of incision in soft palate over the hamular notch area. **B,** Submucosal dissection of flap. **C,** Fracture of pterygoid plate. **D,** Suture of flap to muscle tendon. **E,** Use of awl as alternative method to pass suture

as needed to deepen the sulcus. The palatally based keratinizing mucosa flap can now be advanced to cover the bone and line the new sulcus where it is sutured to periosteum with No. 3-0 Dexon. A maxillary denture splint with extended periphery is immediately introduced to stabilize the tissue in the new position.

TUBEROPLASTY. This procedure, advocated by Obwegeser,[44] is specifically designed to increase the depth between the hamular notch and the distal aspect of the maxilla. It is particularly useful for creating a space in a flat maxilla when extreme atrophy has caused complete loss of the tuberosity for the denture flange to rest on (Fig. 8-14).

This is usually a general anesthesia, operating room procedure, since hemorrhage from the pterygoid venous plexus can be significant. The operative technique is as follows. The area is infiltrated with 2% lidocaine with a 1:100,000 solution of epinephrine for hemostasis. An incision is made over the hamular notch, and the mucosa of the soft palate is undermined and mobilized. The tissue overlying the hamular notch is dissected down to the bone with curved scissors. A 1 cm osteotome is introduced into the area until it encounters bone; then it is driven into the bone, fracturing the pterygoid plate loose to a depth of approximately 1 cm. Bleeding is usually profuse at this time and can be controlled by saturating a 1-inch selvage gauze with a 1:50,000 epinephrine solution and packing it, under pressure, into the wound. Once hemostasis is obtained, the undermined mucosa is sutured at the depth of the tuberosity with a fishhook needle and No. 3-0 chromic gut or No. 3-0 Dexon to the remnants of the pterygoid muscle. The exposed bone of the distal aspect of the maxilla can be covered by secondary epithelization or, if desired, by a split-thickness skin graft. Should difficulty be encountered with the suturing method just described, an awl carrying a No. 3-0 Dexon suture can be passed through the sinus, exiting at the level of the posterior

tuberoplasty. This will afford an excellent means for pulling the tissue downward into the newly created space. Healing continues for at least 1 week before a temporary denture can be worn.

Secondary preparations

Epulis fissuratum and corrective procedures. Soft tissue trapped between an ill-fitting denture flange and the underlying bone will lead to tissue fibrosis and scarring of the sulcus, which is known as epulis fissuratum. Traumatic occlusion of natural teeth opposing an artificial denture is also a cause. Severe scarring of the sulci is also seen in acute trauma injuries incurred in auto accidents and gunshot and mortar fragment avulsive injuries.

Correction of epulis fissuratum is accomplished by excising the fold, if small, or by sharp submucosal dissection to develop a flap and then by sharp submucosal excision of the scarred tissues. The flap is sutured to the periosteum so as not to lose vestibular height (Fig. 8-15).

In severe scarring or avulsive wound cases or both, the method just described frequently fails because of extensive contracture relapse, which further decreases the vestibule height. In these cases the epulis is excised, the vestibule is extended supraperiosteally, and a free mucosal palatal graft is placed in a manner similar to that described for ridge extension procedures. If a small graft is placed, it can be protected and stabilized with isobutyl cyanoacrylate or a special denture splint to protect the graft site (Fig. 8-16).

Reactive inflammatory papillary hyperplasia of the palate. Reactive inflammatory papillary hyperplasia of the palate is commonly associated with prolonged wearing of an ill-fitting, maxillary, full or partial denture or with relining or remaking the denture over a preexisting papillomatosis, which perpetuates the condition (Fig. 8-17). Day and night wearing of a denture and poor or ill-timed oral hygiene measures (such as allowing food to remain for long

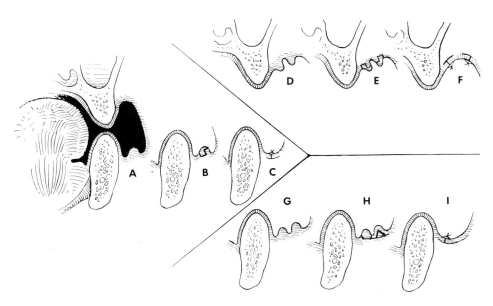

Fig. 8-15. Outline of technique to eliminate epulis fissuratum. **A,** Single fold in buccal sulcus. **B,** Edges undermined and section to be discarded outlined. **C,** Wound sutured. **D,** Two folds in sulcus. **E,** Tissue to be excised is outlined. Removal of both these folds in one piece without saving any of the inner fold membrane would result in serious loss of sulcus depth. **F,** Sutures applied. **G,** Alternate method of removing double fold. **H,** Medial fold is excised, and mucosa is dissected from second fold. Fibrous tissue that underlies lateral fold is carefully dissected away and discarded. **I,** Flap slid across denuded area and sutured in place. Patient's old denture with attached surgical cement periphery is now inserted as previously described. (From Goodsell, J. O., and King, D. R.: Abnormalities of the mouth. In Kruger, G. O.: editor: Textbook of oral surgery, ed. 3, St. Louis, 1968, The C. V. Mosby Co.)

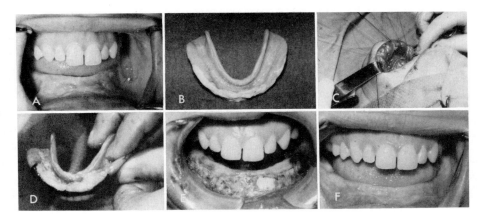

Fig. 8-16. Epulis fissuratum corrected by mucosa graft. **A,** Preoperative epulis fissuratum. **B,** Rough self-relined denture that caused condition. **C,** Excision of epulis and vestibuloplasty. **D,** Palatal mucosa fastened to relined denture with dermatone cement. **E,** Graft 1 week postsurgery. **F,** Healed graft 6 months later.

periods in the denture), are important contributing causes. The condition is recognized as reddened, nodular, or papillary excrescences arising from the palatal mucosa. It is occasionally found over the ridge and in labial or buccal sulci.[25]

Removal can best be accomplished with the patient under sedation or nitrous oxide–oxygen analgesia and local anesthesia, using a fully rectified electrosurgery unit and a loop electrode (Fig. 8-18). Depth of removal is to the submucosa. The proper depth is determined by the absence of the "wheatfield-in-the-wind" effect when the tissues are subjected to a stream of compressed air. The yellow-gray color of the submucosa is a useful guide to adequate depth of removal. Penetration of the periosteum must be avoided to prevent a bony slough, resulting in delayed healing. A biopsy of the affected tissue is performed toward the end of the procedure, and the

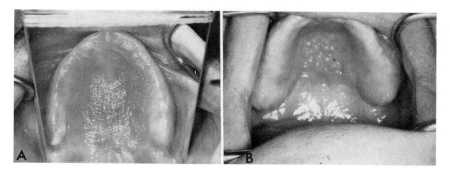

Fig. 8-17. Reactive inflammatory papillary hyperplasia of palate. **A,** Diffuse type. **B,** Nodular or polypoid type. (From Guernsey, L. H.: Oral Surg. **20:**814, 1965.)

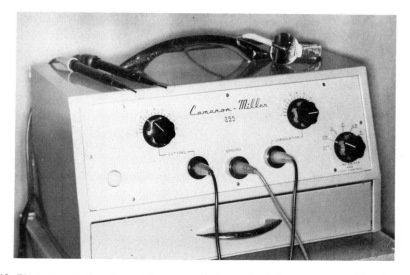

Fig. 8-18. Electrosurgical unit used for removal of reactive inflammatory papillary hyperplasia.

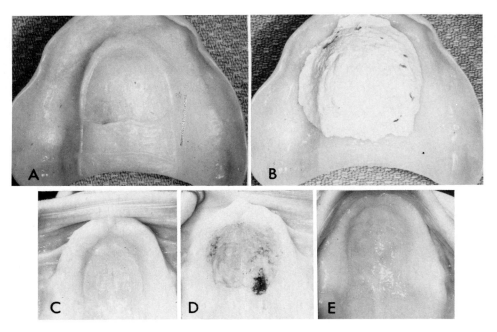

Fig. 8-19. Photographic summary of operative technique. **A,** Marked relief chamber in denture. **B,** Zinc bacitracin periodontal pack before insertion after surgery. **C,** Preoperative reactive hyperplasia. **D,** Appearance after electrosurgery. Darkened areas are sites of biopsy and bleeders, which have been cauterized. **E,** Healed case. (From Guernsey, L. H.: Oral Surg. **20:**814, 1965.)

tissue is sent to the pathologist to confirm the diagnosis (see Fig. 8-19).

A palatal splint lined with special periodontal pack[3] is used to minimize postoperative bleeding and pain. The splint is allowed to remain in place (except for oral irrigations for hygiene purposes) to allow for a good start of granulation to occur. The dressing is changed weekly under a topical anesthetic to allow for healing by granulation and secondary epithelization.

Postoperatively, pain lasting for 1 week can be severe. A narcotic analgesic is prescribed. Hemorrhage can occur for 5 to 7 days postoperatively when eschars soften and break loose during eating or oral hygiene measures. This is controlled by pressure on the splint, a sponge saturated in sodium hypochlorite solution, or anesthetizing the palate adjacent to the bleeding site to achieve vessel pressure and vaso-

constrictor effect. Between 3 and 5 weeks is required for healing prior to the new denture construction period.

RIDGE EXTENSION PROCEDURES

The goal of ridge extension is to uncover existing basal bone of the jaws surgically by repositioning the overlying mucosa, muscle attachments, and muscle to a lowered position in the mandible or to a superior position in the maxilla. The resultant advantage is that a larger denture flange can be accommodated, thus contributing to greater denture stability and retention.

Not all cases of maxillary or mandibular basal bone atrophy can be surgically treated by sulcus extension. There must be adequate alveolar bone with sufficient height remaining to allow for repositioning of the mental nerves and the buccinator and mylohyoid muscles in the mandible. In the maxilla the anterior nasal spine, the

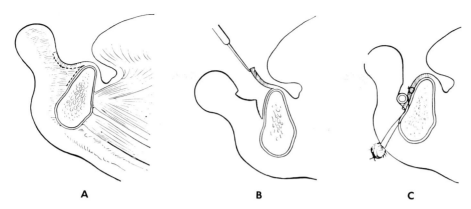

Fig. 8-20. Kazanjian's method. **A,** Incision is made through the mucosa of the inner surface of the lip. **B,** The mucosa is dissected back to a base on the crest of the alveolar ridge. The flap is held out of the way with an instrument while sulcus depth is obtained by supraperiosteal dissection. **C,** The mucosal flap is sutured to the periosteum. A rubber or polyethylene tube is held in place at the bottom of the new sulcus by circumferential sutures tied around cotton rolls. (Redrawn from Kruger, G. O.: J. Oral Surg. **16:**191, 1958.)

nasal cartilage, and the malar buttresses may interfere with repositioning the sulcus superiorly.

Conversely not all cases require a full skin or mucosa graft vestibuloplasty with floor of the mouth lowering. Many cases have success with a vestibular extension anterior to the mental foramina or a lingual procedure to reduce the genial tubercles or release the mylohyoid muscle posteriorly in the floor of the mouth, which may well solve the problem of lack of denture stability and retention.

Principles of plastic revision of tissues

Many basic and well-known procedures have been recommended to correct the many oral abnormalities encountered. However, the principles of plastic revision of tissue must be understood before these procedures are discussed. According to Ashley,[2] these principles are as follows:

1. Bare soft tissue should be covered surgically with epithelium to prevent subsequent contracture.

2. Whenever local tissue is not available to obtain the anticipated final result or to cover the defect without tension, distant tissue should be used.

3. In creating a new cavity, allowance should be made for contracture whenever the cavity is lined with remote grafted tissues or local flaps. Contracture is usually prevented by overcorrection of the cavity defect without tension on the lining tissues.

4. The greater the thickness of split-skin grafts, the lesser the tendency for contracture.

Review of the literature

Kruger[31] in an excellent review article in 1958 evaluated the Kanzanjian, Clark,[11] and Collett[12] vestibular extension techniques and the lingual approaches of Trauner[60] and Caldwell[10] (Figs. 8-20 to 8-23). He found that the main differences in techniques lie in the location of the incision, which was either over the crest of the ridge or in the lip and buccal mucosa, and in whether the periosteum was incised and retracted. The techniques of Clark and Kazanjian were more difficult to accomplish than Collett's full-thickness pushback of the mucoperiosteum, supported in its new position by an appropriately extended denture periphery. In comparing the techniques of Clark and Kazanjian, Kruger concluded that placement of the

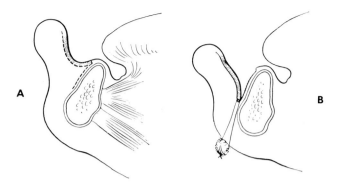

Fig. 8-21. Clark's technique. **A,** Incision is made slightly labial to the crest of the ridge. Sulcus depth is obtained by supraperiosteal dissection. The lip mucosa is undermined from the edge of the incision to the vermilion border. **B,** The mucosal flap is held over the wound by sutures placed to the skin surface. (From Kruger, G. O.: J. Oral Surg. **16:**191, 1958.)

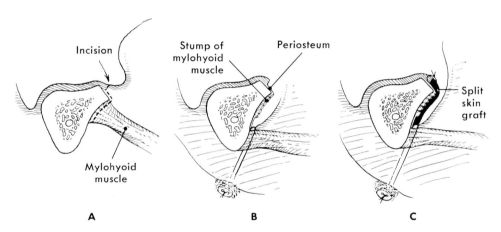

Fig. 8-22. Lingual mylohyoid muscle repositioning according to the technique of Trauner. **A,** Line of incision through mucosa and mylohyoid muscle. **B,** Anchorage of mylohyoid muscle to floor of mouth by means of external sutures. **C,** Surgical defect on mylohyoid stump may be covered with split graft or allowed to heal by granulation. (From Goodsell, J. O., and King, D. R.: Abnormalities of the of the mouth. In Kruger, G. O., editor: Textbook of oral surgery, ed. 3, St. Louis, 1968, The C. V. Mosby Co.)

incision made little difference in the result. There was in all cases an obliteration of the artificially created new sulcus by contracture from the bottom, which occurred early, usually before placement of the final denture. This was also confirmed in a study by Spengler and Hayward[57] who used these techniques on dogs.

The location of the surgical scar in the sulcus in the Kazanjian technique was considered helpful or detrimental to denture retention by various prosthodontists.

The following outline lists ridge extension procedures with appropriate references to publications containing detailed reviews. Only those operations that have given the best results will be described in more detail later in the chapter.

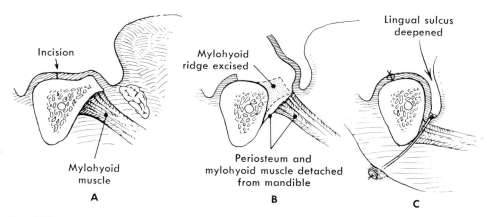

Fig. 8-23. Lingual mylohyoid muscle repositioning according to the technique of Caldwell. **A,** Line of incision. **B,** Periosteum and mylohyoid muscle detached from mandible. **C,** Suturing and anchorage to floor of mouth. (From Goodsell, J. O., and King, D. R.: Abnormalities of the mouth. In Kruger, G. O., editor: Textbook of oral surgery, ed. 3, St. Louis, 1968, The C. V. Mosby Co.)

I. Maxillary procedures
  A. Buccal approach
    1. Secondary epithelization vestibuloplasty
       a. Full thickness mucoperiosteum dissection—Collett[12]
       b. Submucosal dissection, periosteum intact—Szaba[59]
    2. Submucosal vestibuloplasty—Obwegeser,[42] Yrastorza[64]
    3. Ridge skin grafting vestibuloplasty—Weiser,[63] Schuchardt[51]
    4. Buccal sulcus skin grafting—Esser,[17] Gillies[21]
    5. Ridge mucosa grafting vestibuloplasty—Obwegeser,[45] Steinhauser,[58] Maloney and associates[36]
II. Mandibular procedures
  A. Buccal approach
    1. Submucosal dissection, periosteum intact
       a. Secondary epithelization vestibuloplasty
          (1) Incision in lip mucosa—Kazanjian[30]
          (2) Incision over crest of ridge—Clark[11]
       b. Ridge skin grafting vestibuloplasty—Obwegeser,[43] McIntosh and Obwegeser[38]
       c. Mucosa grafting vestibuloplasty—Propper,[47] Nabers,[39] Hall and

O'Steen,[28] Maloney and associates,[34] Shepherd and associates,[52] Guernsey[27]
    2. Full thickness mucoperiosteum dissection
       a. Incision in lip mucosa—Godwin[23]
       b. Incision on crest of ridge with mental nerve lowering and lingual frenotomy with genioglossus transplant—Cooley[14]
       c. Incision in lip mucosa and incision of periosteum over the crest of the ridge—Edlan[16]
       d. Ridge skin grafting and incision on crest of ridge, with genial tubercle removal and repositioning of genioglossus and geniohyoid muscles—Anderson[1]
  B. Lingual approach
    1. Submucosal dissection, periosteum intact
       a. Secondary epithelization
          (1) Lingual sulcus extension with resection of mylohyoid muscle and with or without lingual skin graft—Trauner[60]
          (2) Floor of mouth lowering—Trauner,[60] Obwegeser[43]
          (3) Sublingual ridge extension with free mucosa graft—Lewis[33]
    2. Full thickness mucoperiosteum dissection

a. Lingual sulcus extension with resection of mylohyoid ridge, mylohyoid muscle, and lingual flap cover of bone—Obwegeser[44]
b. Lingual ridge extension—Caldwell[10]
c. Lingual sulcus extension with free skin graft—Ashley[2]

C. Labiolingual approach
  1. Submucosal approach, periosteum intact
    a. Anterior buccal and sublingual sulcus extension with fenestration procedure—Baurmash[4]
    b. Ridge skin grafting vestibuloplasty combined with total lowering of floor of mouth—Obwegeser[43]

Recommended procedures
Maxillary procedures
SUBMUCOSAL VESTIBULOPLASTY

Indications. This procedure is indicated for patients with a small clinical ridge and healthy overlying mucosa and without excessive submucosal fibrosis, hyperplasia, or scarring. A useful test to determine whether there is sufficient mucosa to warrant sulcus extension is to push a mouth mirror superiorly into the labial sulcus. If the upper lip is significantly inverted or drawn superiorly, there is insufficient mucosa for this type of vestibuloplasty. Submucosal vestibuloplasty should be performed in the operating room using general anesthesia.

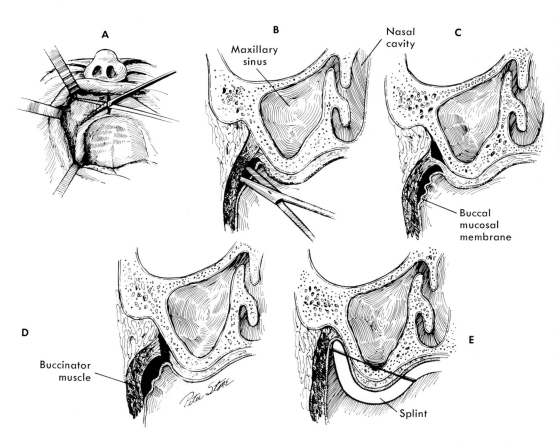

Fig. 8-24. Submucous vestibuloplasty. **A,** Vertical incision provides access for undermining the mucosa and severing the muscles from their attachment. **B,** Undermining of the mucous membrane. **C** and **D,** Supraperiosteal detachment of muscle. **E,** Retention of sulcus depth with acrylic splint. (Ends of the peralveolar wire should be tucked into a nearby hole.)

Technique. The submucosal soft tissues are distended with local anesthetic solution, using 1:100,000 epinephrine solution for hemostasis and to facilitate the dissection. A midline vertical incision is made from the nasal spine to the incisive papilla (Fig. 8-24). From this incision, dissection of the submucosa proceeds distally on either side (preferably with a Lincoln or small Metzenbaum scissors), separating the tissues inferiorly to the crest of the ridge and superiorly to restore good vestibular height. If the malar buttress cannot be negotiated blindly in this tunnel, another vertical incision can be made in the mucobuccal fold at the root of the zygoma, enabling the dissection to be completed posteriorly to the region of the tuberosity.

The next dissection frees the submucosal connective tissue from the periosteum. This is done by establishing a supraperiosteal plane and is best accomplished with curved scissors. The freed tissues now can either be repositioned superiorly to fill in a defect in the canine fossa or resected. The anterior nasal spine, if prominent or interfering with denture seating, is approached by the same vertical incision and is resected with an osteotome. The incisions are closed with No. 3-0 Dexon. The patient's denture periphery is extended with dental compound and guttaform to the new vestibular height. Excess blood is then drained from the tunnel to prevent hematoma formation. The splint is fixed to the maxilla with peralveolar wires or nylon sutures. The stent is removed in 1 week, at which time impressions are made for immediate relining of the denture.

SECONDARY EPITHELIZATION VESTIBULOPLASTY

Indications. According to McIntosh and Obwegeser,[38] secondary epithelization vestibuloplasty is the procedure of choice for patients with extensive scarring or epulis fissuratum in the sulcus or who have good quality mucosa cover available without sufficient height.

Secondary epithelization vestibuloplasty requires supraperiosteal dissection of the mucosa to form a flap (similar to a periodontal mucosal flap for push-back procedure) and superior repositioning by suturing the flap high onto the periosteum. The exposed periosteum is allowed to granulate and reepithelize without benefit of cover from a denture (Fig. 8-25).

Neidhardt[40] studied a large number of cases in which this technique was used and found that 50% of maxillary cases relapsed in three years. This relapse incidence can reach 80% to 95% for patients subjected to this surgery in the mandible and is the reason for using skin or mucosa grafts to hold the repositioned muscles in their new position to gain a more acceptable, less frequent, contracture relapse incidence of 20% to 30%.

Free mucosa grafts transplanted from one site in the oral cavity to another are not new. Many authors have advocated their use for specific surgical problems.* In my experience with patients suffering from war injuries to the maxilla, which result in extensive scarring and loss of substance, I have found that it is best to replace the lost tissue with like tissue whenever possible. Similarly Steinhauser[58] has pointed out that skin-grafting extension vestibuloplasty in the maxilla has been unsatisfactory for denture retention and has instead recommended free cheek mucosa grafts, which provide an autochthonous vestibular mucosa that enhances denture adhesion.

Maloney and associates recommend free split-thickness mucosa grafts from the cheeks for all types of preprosthetic and oral reconstructive soft tissue procedures. Their method of obtaining split-thickness donor tissue will also be described (see p. 129).[36]

Although I agree with Steinhauser, I have found that masticatory, stress-bearing mucosa similar to attached gingiva works better for me. This mucosa can readily be

---

*See references 6, 28, 33, 34, 36, 47, 52, and 58.

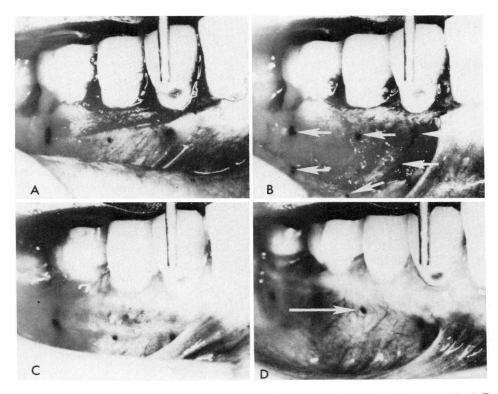

Fig. 8-25. Contracture relapse in apical flap repositioning. **A,** Gingivectomy accomplished. **B,** Supraperiosteal flap dissection and apical displacement. Note that the two sets of methylene blue dye markings are well apart. **C,** Healing at 3 weeks. Note that the two dye marks are coming closer together by contracture relapse. **D,** Healing at 6 weeks, with complete contracture relapse back to preoperative condition. (Courtesy Billy M. Pennel, D.D.S.)

procured from the covering of the hard palate. The palatal mucosa is an ideal tissue for stress bearing since it is keratinized, and therefore, it is the preferred transplant tissue to the maxilla when increased vestibular height is needed. With the new technique of fenestrating palatal mucosa grafts, small donor sources can be expanded to cover larger areas.

BUCCAL MUCOSA GRAFT VESTIBULOPLASTY

Technique. This is usually a general anesthesia operation in the hospital operating room, although a short-span, spot graft can certainly be an office procedure (Fig. 8-26).

Preparation of the recipient bed involves submucosal infiltration with 2% lidocaine and 1:100,000 epinephrine solution to distend the tissues, provide hemostasis, and facilitate the dissection. Incision is made through the mucosa at the junction of the attached and nonattached mucosa from malar buttress to malar buttress. A supraperiosteal flap is developed by sharp dissection. It is carried superiorly and laterally from the canine fossa to the region of the infraorbital nerve. Anteriorly at the midline, the dissection approaches the pyriform aperture without perforating the nasal mucosa. The anterior nasal spine, if prominent, is removed as outlined previously.

The margin of the freed flap is sutured superiorly to the periosteum with No. 4-0 Dexon so as to delineate the new vestibular

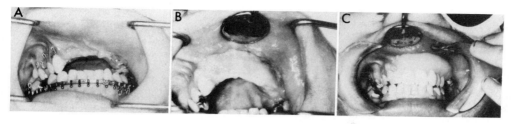

Fig. 8-26. Maxillary ridge extension to restore the vestibulum lost from a gunshot injury. **A,** Preoperative appearance of the scarred vestibulum. **B,** Healed mucosa graft 3 months after operation. **C,** Final prosthesis in place. Note the more than adequate flange for lip support. (From Guernsey, L. H.: Dent. Clin. North Am. **15:**459, 1971.)

height. This would normally complete the procedure for secondary epithelization vestibuloplasty, but the placing of a denture over this raw tissue tends to accelerate secondary granulation and contribute to relapse. As previously mentioned, to avoid relapse the operator can use mucosa grafts to secure the repositioned flap.

The procedure to obtain the donor mucosa graft is as follows: The size of the donor mucosa is measured on the recipient site, using sterilized tinfoil. The foil is adapted to the palate, which was previously injected with 2% lidocaine and 1:100,000 epinephrine for hemostasis. The outline of the graft is incised down to the submucosa but above the periosteum. The submucosa dissection is started by mobilizing an end of the graft with a scalpel and maintaining it under tension with a skin hook. Once the graft is well mobilized, mucosa removal proceeds rapidly, using periodontal knives and strabismus scissors. The graft is severed at its base and stored in a saline-moistened sponge.

Hemostasis of the vascular bed is the first consideration after removal of the donor mucosa, since the palate contains many vessels. This is accomplished by electrocautery and ties as indicated. A previously prepared palatal stent or denture with an extended periphery is tested for fit.

After the graft is tried and measured to cover the recipient bed particularly at the height of the extended sulcus, it is trimmed and then tacked to the periosteum with No. 6-0 Dermalon sutures when hemostasis has been meticulously achieved. This is the most delicate and time-consuming part of the operation. If the recipient bed has any tendency to ooze, horizontal mattress sutures are placed in the middle of the graft to hold it in place. The graft is further covered with an acrylic splint lined with dental compound and guttaform and is fastened to the maxilla with peralveolar wires or nylon suture. Areas of localized necrosis caused by excessive pressure on the graft occasionally occur with this method. Unless suitable relief can be afforded in the stent, I recommend suturing the graft and covering it with isobutyl cyanoacrylate.

The procedure for obtaining split-thickness cheek mucosa grafts is described by Maloney and associates.[34] A suitably bent Deaver retractor is secured to the patient's cheek with heavy silk sutures so that it can serve as a handle to evert and support the cheek while the graft is taken (Fig. 8-27). A Castroviejo Electro-Keratotome set at 0.3 mm thickness is used to obtain the donor split-thickness mucosa. Up to two specimens of mucosa (4.0 by 1.5 cm) can be obtained from each cheek. Additional pieces can also be taken from the extended lower lip mucosa. Since the thickness includes only the epithelium and tunica propria, the donor sites need little postoperative attention beyond a coating of

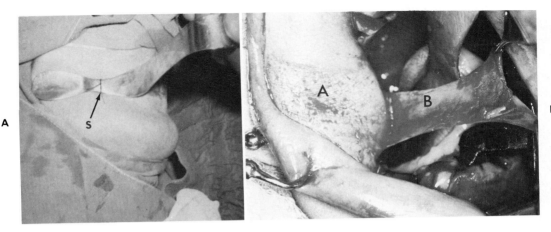

Fig. 8-27. A, Stainless steel retractor, bent at right angle, fixed to cheek with a through-and-through silk ligature *(s)*. **B,** Retractor rotated to evert buccal mucosa to provide access and support to graft. The split-thickness mucosal graft is being removed from buccal mucosa after application of the Castroviejo Electro-Keratotome. *A,* Donor bed; *B,* graft. (From Maloney, P. L. and others: J. Oral Surg. **30:**717, 1972. Copyright by the American Dental Association. Reprinted by permission.)

tincture of benzoin. The raw surfaces will reepithelize rapidly without scarring.

Postoperative care and sequelae. The splint remains undisturbed for 7 days, after which time it is removed to check on healing of the donor site and the viability of the graft. The mucosa will be covered with a white coagulum of desquamated cells that, when lavaged or wiped gently, will peel off to leave a bleeding granular surface. This is normal and is evidence of a viable graft. In less than 2 weeks the graft will assume the appearance of normal mucosa again. The patient wears the splint as a denture during the healing period. A soft wax impression is taken as soon as healing permits, and the splint is relined with acrylic as needed. It is important not to overextend but rather to underextend the periphery between 1 and 2 mm because this minimizes granulations, which are the cause of contracture relapse. An initial contracture of 20% to 30% occurs at the entire periphery of the vestibule during initial healing. Overcorrection is accomplished when possible for this reason. A final prosthesis can be made approximately 4 weeks after grafting.

Mandibular procedures
BUCCAL MUCOSA GRAFT VESTIBULOPLASTY

Buccal mucosa graft vestibuloplasty is the procedure of choice in avulsive or severely traumatized patients in whom the sulcus is entirely obliterated by scarring or by bone grafting reconstructive procedures. Small spot grafts can be accomplished in the office using local anesthesia.[49] However, since many patients with this problem require varying amounts of extensive dissection, the operation should be performed in the hospital operating room using general anesthesia.

Indications. This procedure is indicated for patients in whom there is a sulcus obliterated by high muscle attachments, extensive local scarring, extensive mandibular bone atrophy with the mental nerves emerging at the crest of the ridge, or extension of a normal sulcus from canine to canine resulting from premature tooth loss caused by periodontal disease.

Technique. The procedure is identical to that of the maxillary mucosa graft, except in the manner of treating the lingual sulcus, which will be discussed in detail in

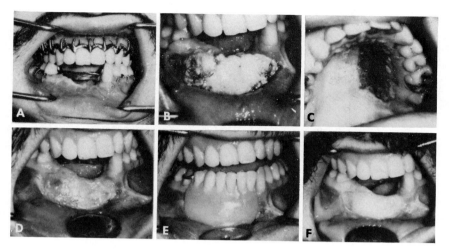

Fig. 8-28. Palatal mucosa graft to extend an inadequate anterior mandibular vestibulum. **A,** Preoperative condition as a result of mortar fragment injury. **B,** Graft 1 week postoperative, after removal of the splint. **C,** Palatal donor site granulations 1 week after operation. **D,** Graft healing at 2 weeks. **E,** Final dental prosthesis. **F,** Grafted mucosa appearance 8 months later. (From Guernsey, L. H.: Dent. Clin. North Am. **15:**459, 1971.)

the following section on buccal skin graft vestibuloplasty. The procedure parallels the method recommended by McIntosh and Obwegeser,[38] except that it is accomplished in a localized area (Fig. 8-28).

USE OF SPLINTS. A full palatal acrylic splint is used to cover the donor site in the palate. For the mandible, particularly for the partially edentulous one, an overextended splint relieved at the mental nerve is used. The splint is used to take a compound impression of the extended vestibule and is relieved to accommodate a guttaform liner. The graft is sutured in place as in the maxillary procedure, and the splint is inserted over the graft and immobilized with No. 2-0 Mersilene or Tevdek sutures circumferentially placed around the bone and the splint. This minimizes pressure necrosis of the graft, effected by too much pressure from circumferential wirings.

Postoperative care. Both splints are removed in 7 days, and the healing of the donor site and the viability of the graft are checked. If the palatal spint was lined with a periodontal dressing, it is changed weekly to allow for granulation to proceed unimpeded. The mandibular splint is now relined and extended 1 to 2 mm short of the periphery and is worn as a temporary denture. In mandibular cases, a watchful postoperative course is required to prevent pressure points and granulations that predispose to contracture relapse. Definitive denture construction can start in 3 to 4 weeks.

BUCCAL SKIN GRAFT VESTIBULOPLASTY WITH COMPLETE LOWERING OF THE FLOOR OF THE MOUTH

Although I prefer to use free mucosa transplant grafts in vestibuloplasty since mucosa has definite advantages over skin, enough palatal mucosa to cover the entire extended sulcus area cannot always be procured. As mentioned earlier, a system of extending donor mucosa and skin tissue is now available through fenestrating or meshing both skin and mucosa grafts using either a Padgett Graft Expander* or a Tanner Van Derput mesh-graft dermatome.† Grafts can be increased up to nine times the original

---

*Padgett Instrument Co., Division of Kansas City Assemblage Co., Kansas City, Mo.
†Zimmer USA, Warsaw, Ind.

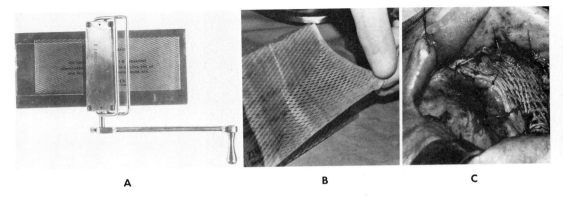

A　　　　　　　　　　　　　**B**　　　　　　　　　　　　　**C**

Fig. 8-29. A, Tanner Van Derput mesh-graft dermatome and plastic skin holder meshing the donor skin. **B,** Donor skin meshed to a 3:1 expansion. **C,** Skin graft in place and excellent adaptation afforded.

size, but the ratio of 3:1 is the most commonly used (Fig. 8-29). The advantages to mesh grafts, besides the obvious one of limited donor tissue coverage of a larger area, include a better adaptation of the fenestrated grafts to all types of recipient sites, seepage of fluids precluding formation of hematomas and dead space, shorter operating time, less hemorrhage, less discomfort, and shorter healing time of the donor site.

For patients needing extensive grafting, it is necessary to use skin from a nonhair-bearing area, such as the inner thigh, regions of the buttocks, and the lateral abdomen.

Indications. Indications for this procedure include an atrophic, but not pencil-thin, mandible, with high buccinator, frenum, and mylohyoid attachments covered by thin, movable, atrophic nonkeratinizing mucosa. In addition, the floor of the mouth bulges up to displace the lingual flange of the denture. The typical patient is one with a denture-sore mouth and a history of being unable to juggle or retain a full lower denture in a functional stress-bearing situation.

Case selection. With this surgery, more than with any other surgery discussed, thorough case selection and expected sequelae counseling is mandatory. The

sequelae of mental nerve hyperesthesia, paresthesia, or anesthesia coupled with the severe dysphagia and pain on swallowing that is associated with operations in the floor of the mouth must be thoroughly explained in advance. The need for a splint fastened to the lower jaw for 1 week must be understood. The donor site will require special care until the fine mesh gauze dressing falls off between 3 and 5 weeks after surgery and new skin covers the donor site.

Preoperative planning. After patient counseling and workup, complete radiographic study of the mandible is accomplished to ascertain the size and shape of the basal bone, position of the mental foramina, and presence or absence of sharp ridges. An overextended compound impression is used to pour a mandibular model, on which is made an overextended acrylic tray that is relieved in the mental nerve region and in which is embedded a U-shaped wire to be used as a handle during impression taking at surgery.

On the day before surgery the patient is typed and cross matched for two units of whole blood. The corticosteroid dexamethasone (Decadron), 4 mg intramuscularly, and procaine penicillin G, 600,000 units intramuscularly, are administered the evening before surgery and twice on the day of surgery. The dexamethasone is then

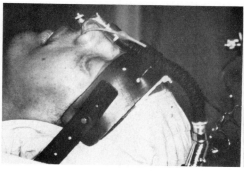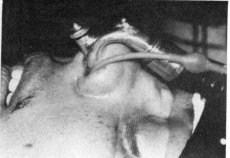

Fig. 8-30. Low silhouette, general anesthetic technique with extension tubing to the anesthesia machine, which permits the surgeon to operate on the floor of the mouth from a position at the head of the table.

decreased to 2 mg twice a day, then to 1 mg twice a day, then discontinued on the third postoperative day. This combination will materially decrease postoperative edema and the likelihood of postoperative infection, which could be a threat to the airway.

This is clearly a major operation and can only be done under general anesthesia in the operating room. It is greatly facilitated by a low-profile, endotracheal, general anesthesia technique that places the anesthetist at the level of the patient's thigh. This allows special head draping and the oral surgery team to stand around the head of the patient when operating in the floor of the mouth (Fig. 8-30).

Technique. The operation involves the following procedures.

DONOR SKIN PROCEDURE. The area of the lateral thigh is prepared and draped. A 4 by 10 cm split-thickness (0.18- to 0.25-inch) piece of skin is procured with a Brown or Padgett dermatome. The skin is stored until needed in a saline-moistened, fine mesh gauze.

More recently, because of the excellent adaptability of the donor skin, we have been fenestrating it at 3:1 expansion on a Tanner Van Derput mesh graft dermatome prior to storage (Fig. 8-31).

The donor site is immediately dressed with fine mesh gauze and covered with a temporary pressure dressing throughout the remainder of the operation. Postoperative care to the donor site is minimized if it is exposed to a dry heat lamp in the immediate postoperative period. This will result in a dry donor site, with eventual loss of the dressing in 2 to 3 weeks as re-epithelization occurs under the dressing.

FLOOR OF THE MOUTH PROCEDURE. Two percent lidocaine with 1:100,000 epinephrine is infiltrated immediately below the mucosa lingual to the mandible to balloon the tissue and provide vasoconstriction. A mucosal incision is made just medially to the crest of the ridge from retromolar pad to retromolar pad. The tongue is vigorously retracted laterally with a sponge stick to place the mylohyoid muscle on tension. This facilitates the dissection. By alternating sharp and blunt dissection, the muscle fibers can be made to bulge into the incision. A curved Kelly hemostat is threaded under the muscle, which is cut with scissors near the mandible without injury to the periosteum or the lingual nerve in the posterior portion of the incision. The remaining dissection from the lateral pharyngeal wall to the genioglossus attachment is done bluntly with the gloved finger. A similar dissection is performed on the other side at an angle to the symphysis area. In the

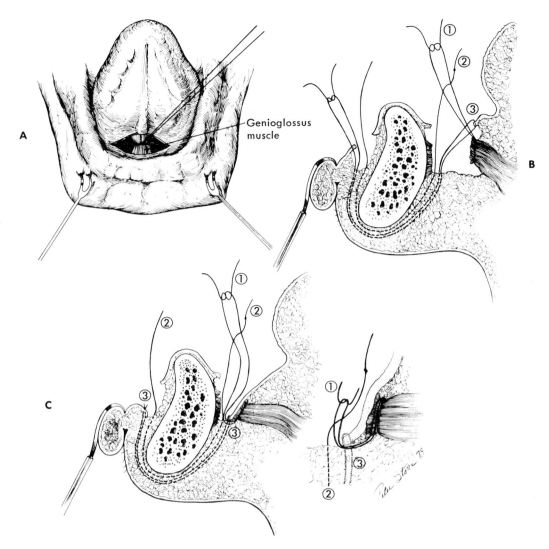

Fig. 8-31. Modification suggested by Anderson and co-workers[1] to reposition the genioglossus and geniohyoid muscles inferiorly while accomplishing the ridge skin grafting and full floor of the mouth lowering procedure. **A,** Retraction suture. **B,** Suture looped around genioglossus used to reposition the muscle attachment: *1,* retraction suture; *2,* circummandibular suture with knot; *3,* hammock suture for vestibuloplasty. **C,** Hammock suture tied to position mucosal margins. Retraction suture *(1)* is tied with knotted circummandibular suture *(2)* included. One arm of retraction suture is cut off; the other arm is tied to labial strand of circummandibular suture.

midline, the lateral and superior fibers of the genioglossus muscle are sectioned, but the inferior muscle bundle is left intact to support the tongue. Although Obwegeser[44] has cautioned against severing both the mylohyoid and the genioglossus-genio-hyoid muscles because of the resulting total loss of tongue control and swallowing difficulty, a modification suggested by Anderson and associates[1] (Fig. 8-32) has solved this problem when the genial tubercles are particularly high or large.

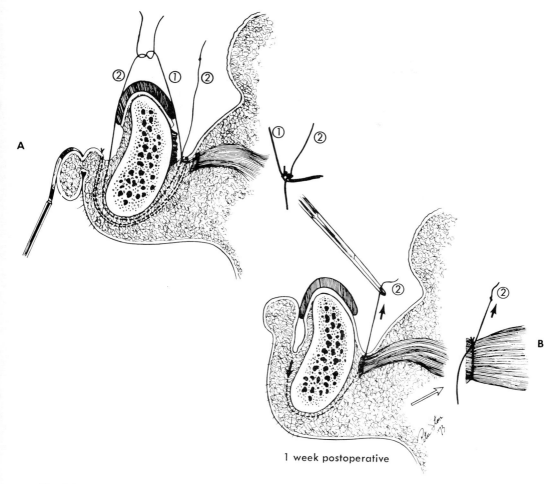

1 week postoperative

Fig. 8-32. A, Circummandibular suture being tied around stent. Note that the knot on strand *2* has been pulled inferiorly to reposition severed muscles. **B,** Later removal of circummandibular suture.

The periosteum over the tubercle is incised vertically, and the attached muscle insertions are identified. A No. 2-0 chromic gut suture is tied to the bundle to serve as a traction suture. The bundle is severed from the insertion. The tubercles are reduced by mallet and osteotome. The periosteum is closed with chromic sutures.

When the skin graft, which is glued to the splint, is later inserted, a midline circumferential, splint-holding No. 3-0 Tevdek suture is placed. The chromic traction suture is tied below a knot placed in the circumferential suture, thus permitting the

bundle to be displaced inferiorly, and then held there when the circumferential suture is tied over the splint.

RIDGE PREPARATION AND SKIN GRAFTING PROCEDURE. The *lateral* mandibular mucosa is infiltrated with lidocaine to distend this tissue and to provide hemostasis. A superficial mucosal incision is made from retromolar pad to retromolar pad just lateral to the crest of the ridge. Two lateral relaxing incisions are made posteriorly. Through these incisions a supraperiosteal flap is developed laterally and inferiorly, stopping short of the external oblique line. The mental nerve region dissection is meticulous to identify and dissect free these important nerves. If lowering is needed (which is determined by the presence of the foramen at the crest of the ridge) to eliminate undue nerve pressure that could be expected under the skin graft, then the nerve is retracted with a blunt nerve hook while the foramen is lowered and a trough is made in the bone with a No. 6 round bur.

The anterior sulcus between the mental foramina is dissected laterally and inferiorly enough to sever part but not all of the mentalis and caninus muscles. If these muscles are severed completely, the patient will have a flaccid-appearing lower lip.

The same procedure is carried out on the other lateral side of the mandible.

SPECIAL SUTURING TECHNIQUE. The freed mucosal edges obtained by means of the

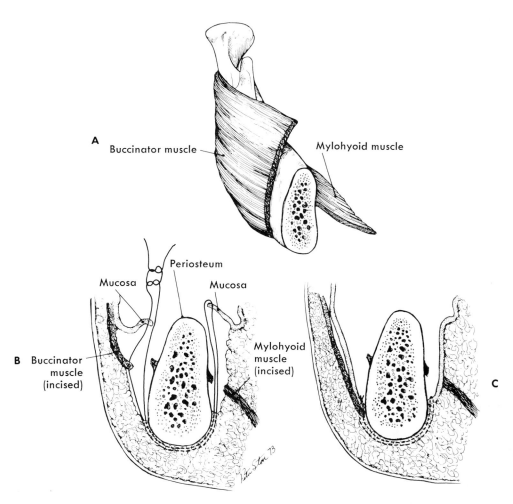

Fig. 8-33. Placement of special "hammock" sutures. **A,** Preoperative view. **B,** Schematic illustration of suture placement. **C,** Sutures tied, repositioning the floor of mouth inferiorly. (**B** and **C** adapted from Guernsey, L. H.: Dent. Clin. North Am. **15:**459, 1971.)

lingual and buccal flap dissections need to be repositioned and stabilized at their most inferior position. This is accomplished with eight carefully placed No. 2-0 Mersilene or Tevdek sutures in sling position under the mandible (Fig. 8-33). Eight sutures, four on each side of the midline with the first suture 1 cm from the midline, near the genioglossus bundle are passed through the lingual flap mucosa and are tagged with hemostats. Starting from lateral to the midline, an awl is passed from the submandibular skin into the floor of the mouth; both ends of the suture are threaded into the eye of the awl, which is withdrawn to the inferior border of the mandible, then passed buccally into the vestibule where one suture is removed from the awl's eye. The remaining strand is then passed through the mucosa of the buccal flap with the awl and removed from the eye of the awl, which is withdrawn. This completes placement of a single hammock suture. The suture is again tagged with a hemostat. Separate awls are used, and the remaining sutures are placed and tagged.

Suture tying is done over a No. 2-0 black silk pullout suture that has been placed loosely in the lingual sulcus and threaded under all the hammock sutures. This will facilitate their removal in 7 days. This step can be omitted if No. 2-0 Dexon resorbable sutures are used instead of No. 2-0 Mersilene or Tevdek. The hammock sutures are brought under tension by alternating the pull on each end of the suture. Buccal and lingual tissues are pulled downward under the mandible, thus deepening the buccal and lingual vestibules. Excess fibrous tissue, muscle attachments, and gingival scar tissue are now removed with scissors, with care taken not to perforate the periosteum.

IMPRESSION OF THE RECIPIENT SITE. The clear acrylic tray is filled with soft red dental compound, and an impression of the extended ridge is taken, keeping the lingual flange short, since no skin graft will be placed in this undercut area. The compound is relieved, trimmed, and flamed until the fit is satisfactory and is further refined by lining the impression with low-fusing guttaform. The impression is then painted with a skin adhesive, such as gum mastic or a compound containing one-half dermatome cement and one-half

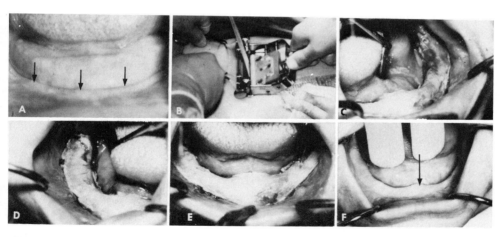

Fig. 8-34. Mandibular skin graft ridge extension and lowering of the floor of the mouth. **A,** Preoperative condition. **B,** Obtaining a split-thickness skin graft with Brown dermatome. **C to E,** Appearance of the skin graft 1 week after operation. **F,** Healed skin graft and extended labial and lingual vestibulum 2 months after operation. (From Guernsey, L. H.: Dent. Clin. North Am. **15:**459, 1971.)

ether, which is allowed to dry for at least 1 minute.

The skin is now placed in the splint (epithelial side against the adhesive) and is massaged into place with moistened cotton-tipped applicators. Excess skin is trimmed away at the periphery.

FINAL PREPARATION OF THE RECIPIENT BED. While the surgeon places the skin in the splint, an assistant obtains careful hemostasis of the bed by electrocautery of bleeders, pressure, and application of ice water. When hemostasis is satisfactory, the skin-containing splint is positioned over the recipient site and maintained with two circumferential No. 2-0 Mersilene or Tevdek sutures (one anterior and one posterior to the mental foramen) tied circumferentially over the splint. This completes the procedure except for a superficial dressing over the awl skin puncture wounds.

Postoperative course. The immediate postoperative edema and swelling are controlled by dexamethasone, ice packs to the area, and withholding oral feedings until swallowing is less painful. Clear liquid, oral alimentation is usually started in 24 hours, progressing to a full dental liquid diet of a high caloric and protein nature.

The splint is removed in 7 days to check for viability of the graft and to trim excess skin that has not taken. Immediate prosthetic care is provided by relining the old dentures and relieving the periphery, short of the new sulcus extension by at least 1 to 2 mm. These dentures can be worn as long as 3 months under close supervision to prevent pressure points or granulations or both from developing (Fig. 8-34). Final dentures can then be fabricated.

RIDGE AUGMENTATION PROCEDURES

Ridge augmentation procedures must be considered for cases in which atrophy or injury to the jaws has been such that, although maximum ridge extension by sulcoplasty has been accomplished, the ridge is still inadequate to allow for a functional denture. This area of preprosthetic surgery has received little attention from surgeons, possibly because there seemed to be no effective operation for ridge augmentation using a sterile extraoral method of insertion. Since penetration into the oral cavity during the procedure was deemed tantamount to failure, few surgeons or patients would undertake this risk for elective augmentation of the mandible. This method of treatment was not accepted until the advent of antibiotics and early reports in the literature of successful peroral bone grafting.[13,20]

Iliac bone crest and rib have traditionally been used to augment the jaws, but more recently, Boyne[8] has described a bone regeneration method that employs a Vitallium mesh tray containing hemopoietic bone marrow encased in a nylon reinforced Millipore filter. The filter appears to enhance osseous generation at the surgical site by exclusion of connective tissue cellular elements from the defect where osseous healing is desired. This method has been successful in loss-of-substance bone grafting, particularly in the symphyseal region, and now it is being clinically tested in patients as a means of ridge augmentation.

Oral surgeons are constantly seeking to improve existing augmentation procedures in order to minimize the shrinkage by resorption that occurs when grafted bone is placed into function under a prosthesis. Danielson and Nemarich[15] presumed that a subcortical insertion of the bone graft would have the advantage that the grafted tissue would be approximated on both sides by viable bone and used a Kazanjian modified flap. Farrell, Kent, and Guerra[18] have reported on a similar interpositional bone graft and vestibuloplasty for the atrophic edentulous maxilla. Sanders and Cox[50] advocated the use of inferior border rib grafting for augmentation of the atrophic mandible to minimize bone resorption and the delay in allowing a patient to return to denture wearing.

Lastly, Peterson and Slade[53] have described a body sagittal osteotomy to raise the lingual cortical portion of the atrophic mandible without detaching the lingual tissues for blood supply, fixing the ridge in the new position while augmenting it buccally with cancellous marrow from the ileum. They claim less shrinkage by resorption because the lingual cortical basilar bone has already undergone atrophy and an immediate extension of the vestibulum can be done over the cancellous marrow graft, thereby assuring early return to denture wearing.

Freeze-dried bone, aorta, and cartilage grafts have been used in dogs by Blackstone and Parker[7] to restore atrophic ridges. A large variety of alloplastic materials ranging from tantalum mesh to silicone plastics have been used to restore portions of the human body lost through atrophy, trauma, or radical surgical procedures.* In general, these materials, except autogenous bone, do not do well when placed under functional stress.

For ridge augmentation surgery, I prefer iliac crest. Although a notched rib can readily be contoured to the arc of the mandible, as much as 50% loss by shrinkage can be expected in this type of augmentation surgery. My experience with purely cancellous iliac graft and iliac cortical-cancellous sectional grafts introduced perorally, with appropriate immobilization of the graft, shows excellent healing even in the event of an occasional incision dehiscence. It is noteworthy that best results are obtained if the augmented mandible is not stressed by denture wearing or a vestibuloplasty procedure for 4 months after grafting. This allows time for an excellent layer of cortical bone to form at the graft site.

Technique. After injection of 2% lidocaine with 1:100,000 epinephrine for hemostasis, a crest of the ridge incision is made from retromolar pad to retromolar pad,

with care exercised not to incise the mental nerves if they emerge high on the crest. A full-thickness mucoperiosteal flap is reflected. The mental nerves are identified and dissected free as they enter the lip to minimize stress on these nerves during retraction. If pressure is going to be exerted on the nerve by the augmentation bone graft, the mental foramina are lowered as in the skin graft vestibuloplasty.

While the oral graft site is being prepared, another surgical team obtains an iliac inner-table, cortical-cancellous graft of the appropriate size.[22] The average adult can easily provide a 8 by 3 cm block graft and approximately 25 to 30 ml of cancellous marrow for further deposition at junctions of the segments of the graft.

After exposure of the mandible to the oral cavity, the mucoperiosteum is widely relieved on the buccal side. The mylohyoid muscle insertion is severed on the lingual site to free the tissue enough to close over the graft. Increased tissue relaxation can be accomplished by cutting the intact periosteal sling as low as possible near the inferior border of the mandible and by further submucosal dissection of the flap. A similar bone augmentation technique can be performed in the atrophic maxilla, with special care exercised during the undermining of tissue for closure to avoid entering the nasal cavity.

BONE GRAFT TECHNIQUE. The iliac crest block graft is sectioned into 1 to 1.5 cm wide pieces with an oscillating Stryker saw. These are tried for fit and contoured as needed, the cortex is thinned but not completely removed, and fenestrations are made in the mandibular cortex, with care taken not to penetrate into the neurovascular canal. The individual pieces are notched, scored, and bent if necessary, and fixed by a combined transosseous circumferential technique (Fig. 8-35). In a severely atrophied mandible, a circumferential wire can erode through the cortex, producing an iatrogenic fracture.

The fragments, usually three, are fixed

---

*See references 5, 9, 19, 29, and 48.

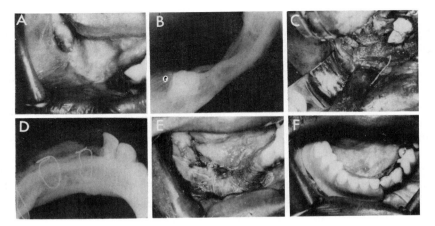

Fig. 8-35. Ridge augmentation with iliac crest bone graft. **A,** Preoperative condition, alveolar bone loss after gunshot injury. **B,** X-ray film of deficient alveolus. **C,** Bone graft wired in place by means of peroral approach with suture closure. **D,** X-ray film of augmentation on bone graft. **E,** Skin graft ridge extension vestibuloplasty appearance at 1 week. **F,** Final prosthesis.

to the host mandible. Cancellous marrow is packed into interstices beneath the graft around the butted joints to achieve good bone contact between graft and host bone, as well as to give a U-shaped form to the augmented ridge.

Closure is by continuous horizontal mattress sutures with No. 3-0 Dexon, with care taken not to close the tissues under any tension. Interrupted sutures reinforce the incision for watertight closure.

Because all floor-of-mouth procedures are prone to significant edema and swelling, patients are placed on the same corticosteroid and antibiotic regimen as those who undergo the skin graft vestibuloplasty.

Postoperative course. If meticulous tension free closure has been accomplished, the incision heals by first intention. In several war wound cases in which there was extensive scarring, the incision dehisced to expose small fragments of bone or wire. For exposed bone, good results can be obtained by allowing the exposed bony spicule to sequestrate or by removing it with a rongeur while irrigating the dehiscence with 9-aminoacridine and normal saline. For exposed wire, removal of the wire usually is necessary before irrigation,

and secondary granulation succeeds in covering the graft. In all cases, the patient is not ready for final prosthesis insertion until after 4 to 6 months has been allowed for healing and extension vestibuloplasty with either mucosa or skin graft.

MANDIBULAR STAPLE BONE PLATE FASTENER SYSTEM

Small,[54] in reviewing the efforts of early prosthodontists, dentists, implantologists, and oral surgeons to find a suitable metallic implant that could be placed in the jaws to replace lost teeth and act as abutments for either fixed or removable prostheses, came to the logical conclusion that the stress of function, the biological incompatibility of certain implants, the interface reaction between the tissues and the implant, the nature of the host tissue, and the host-invader relationship were responsible for the almost universal failure of dental implants.

He set for himself the task of finding a successful metallic implant device that would not have these difficulties and yet would be effective in retaining a full lower prosthesis.

He looked at the advantages of metal as

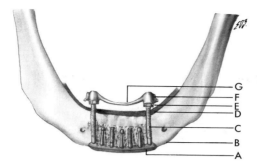

Fig. 8-36. Diagram of Tivanium mandibular staple bone plate illustrating, *A*, staple base and retentive pins; *B*, inferior border of mandible; *C*, transosseous pin; *D*, mucosal covering; *E*, locknut; *F*, coping; *G*, connecting bar.

an implant material, such as strength, resistance to fracture during intermittent loading, and ability to be fashioned into any desirable form. However, metals implanted into the body were well known as potential causes of corrosion, fatigue, and stress fracture. He reviewed the properties of pure metals and found them to be lacking either in strength, ductility, or hardness to perform well as implants. Alloys were the solution to these deficiencies. Starting with a pure metal such as titanium, various other metals were added to achieve the properties of resistance to corrosion through protection of the implant with an oxide layer; elimination of crevices, cracks, and areas of stress concentration; and lastly minimization of the amount and area of metal in contact with oral mucosa.

Those metals near the noble end of the periodic chart were best suited for implantation into the body since they were the least reactive to chloride ions and corrosion. In 1959 Zimmer USA was developing an alloy of titanium (6 ACHV) later to be named Tivanium in 1970. Extensive research was done on the new alloy for orthopedic implants, bone screws, Jewett nails, Schneider intramedullary nails, Steinman pins, and allied surgical instruments to be used in insertion procedures.[58]

Dr. Small asked Zimmer USA to fabricate the mandibular staple bone plate out of Tivanium since this alloy shaped into the design chosen for the seven-pin staple (Fig. 8-36) best and could fulfill the criteria for a desirable implant, that is, keep as much metal as possible away from the oral mucosa, make it possible to bury the retentive pins into cortical bone at the inferior border of the mandible, allow placement of the transosseous bone holes in between the mental foramina, and permit the joining of the intraoral fasteners to form a rigid metal frame (Fig. 8-36).

The principle of minimizing direct stress on the implant and distributing it over the entire ridge area seemed paramount to prevent stress. A Dalbo stress-breaking precision attachment was used to fasten the prosthesis in the mouth, providing for resistance to lateral and superior displacing forces while avoiding direct pressure on the transosseous pins of the implant.

The implants were thoroughly investigated in animals[56] and were given an extensive clinical trial. They were subjected to peer review with a rigid 5-year follow-up and were deemed worthy of continued clinical study and application.

I have followed with great interest Dr. Small's study[55] and success over an 8-year period and have reported on a case to illustrate the surgical and prosthetic techniques involved.[62] A case report will be used to illustrate the techniques involved.

Case report

The patient was a 62-year-old white man in good health. His chief complaint was inability to function satisfactorily with a mandibular complete denture. The patient had been completely edentulous for 10 years, having lost the mandibular anterior teeth last. Previous to these extractions he had worn successfully for 3 years a maxillary complete denture and a mandibular removable partial denture. The patient had a total of four maxillary dentures (all reasonably well tolerated) but only one mandibular com-

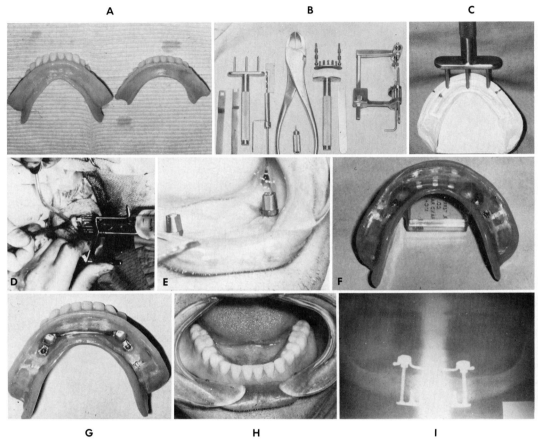

Fig. 8-37. Mandibular staple bone implant. **A,** Comparison of borders of new mandibular complete denture (left) and old denture (right). Surgical extensions were made in the retromylohyoid and anterior lingual areas. **B,** Instruments (left to right): tightening wrenches for the threaded fasteners and locknuts, transosseous pin marking guide, Allen wrench, twist drill and drill stop assembly with L-shaped depth gauge, pin cutter, beveling instrument, staple driver with plastic end, seven-pin staple, drill guide tightening wrench, and drill guide with stabilizing pins. **C,** Location of mental foramina transferred from template to mandibular cast. The lateral extensions of the instrument correspond to the distance between the transosteal pins of the implant. **D,** Pin guide in place on mandible. Transosseous and blind holes being drilled. **E,** Staple immediately after insertion into the mandible with metal fasteners and locknuts screwed down into place. **F,** Finished prosthesis. Note cobalt-chrome framework. **G,** Finished prosthesis illustrating relationships between the removable component (denture) and the fixed component (coping bar). **H,** Completed prosthesis exhibits excellent stability and retention. **I,** Radiograph taken 10 months postoperatively. (**A, C, F, G, H** and **I** from Weintraub, G. S., and Guernsey, L. H., Oral Surg. **43:**828, 1977.)

plete denture, which did not meet his functional and social needs. He expressed the opinion that it would be a waste of time and effort to undergo additional conventional mandibular complete denture therapy. The patient reported that he had tried all type of powders, pastes, and relining devices in order to function with the denture but that none was successful. He had read about the staple implant in a national magazine and was referred to me for consultation.

Oral examination revealed no apparent soft tissue pathosis. The maxillary edentulous ridge had favorable local and anatomic factors, offering a good prognosis. The mandibular edentulous ridge was moderately atrophied. Shallow vestibular depth was noted in the anterior lingual and labial segments. Severe bilateral undercuts of the mylohyoid ridges were present.

Radiographic examination revealed no osseous pathosis. There was sufficient bone height in the anterior segment of the mandible to accommodate the staple implant (a minimum of 9 mm is necessary).

The existing maxillary denture exhibited adequate retention and stability, although it was underextended labially, buccally, and posteriorly. The mandibular denture was grossly underextended. Its form appeared to be totally unrelated to the functional anatomy of the bordering tissues (Fig. 8-37, *A*).

The vertical dimension of the occlusion was insufficient. Centric relation and centric occlusion were not coincidental. New complete dentures were indicated.

A diagnosis of functional masticatory insufficiency caused by an atrophic mandible was determined.

Phases of therapy

Five distinct phases of therapy are involved in oral rehabilitation with the mandibular bone staple implant:

1. Conventional preprosthetic surgical preparation
2. Conventional complete dentures or correction of existing dentures. This procedure will permit a determination of the prognosis of the mandibular denture and will serve as a prototype for the ''implant prosthesis''
3. Hospitalization for surgery and implantation of the orthopedic appliance
4. Conversion of the existing mandibular denture for use as an interim postsurgical prosthesis

5. Construction of the definitive prosthesis

The patient's expectations of potential treatment results were judged reasonable and obtainable, and he was accepted for treatment.

Phase I. This important phase of treatment involved routine and special preprosthetic surgical procedures the objective of which was a more suitable bony base and tissue foundation for dentures. The definitive prosthesis was to be supported by the edentulous ridge and had to be maximally extended within the limitations presented by the patient's tissues and functional anatomy. Maximum extension minimized the amount of force delivered to any given area supporting the prosthesis. Reduction of the mylohyoid shelves and of the genioglossus-geniohyoid attachment was indicated and accomplished for this patient (Fig. 8-37, *A*) to provide maximum extension. Additional considerations in this phase of therapy included a tuberosity reduction, excision of hyperplastic tissue, tori reduction, alveoloplasty to reduce spinous ridges, and mucosa or skin grafts to provide suitable tissue cover.

Phase II. Properly extended maxillary and mandibular complete dentures were constructed. The vertical dimension of occlusion was restored. Routine postinsertion adjustments were made. This patient expressed definite criteria of function that he expected as a result of his treatment. It was recognized that conventional complete denture therapy could not meet his expectations and that the mandibular staple bone plate fastener system was indicated. The patient realized, however, that the new mandibular prosthesis would serve as the prototype for the definitive implant prosthesis. The basic differences were (1) an increase in stability and (2) positive resistance to vertical displacement.

Phase III. Specialized surgical instruments and armamentarium were needed for the insertion of the mandibular staple (Fig. 8-37, *B*). In preparation for the surgical procedure, a dual-purpose clear acrylic resin template was constructed on a cast of the patient's mandible. The locations of the mental foramina were scribed on the template and transferred to the cast (Fig. 8-37, *C*). The intraoral pin positions were marked medial to the foramina and in the center of the ridge, and two holes corresponding to the transosseous pin positions were drilled through the template. The template also could be used to position the drill guide accurately while seven parallel holes from the inferior border of the mandible, of which the two most lateral would be transosteal, were drilled.

The location of the incision was the crease line beneath the patient's chin. The mandibular bony symphysis was fully exposed, followed by insertion of the acrylic resin template intraorally. The drill guide and director rods were positioned and secured, and the seven holes were drilled with a low-speed, high-torque, air-driven bone drill (Fig. 8-37, *D*). The Tivanium implant was tapped into place, and the wound was closed in layers. Two metal fasteners machined to resemble premolar crown preparations were threaded on the intraoral pins and secured with locknuts 0.5 to 1 mm above the gingiva. The pins were cut off flush with the top of the fasteners (Fig. 8-37, *E*).

Postoperative swelling and morbidity were controlled by the use of preoperative, interoperative, and short-term postoperative anti-inflammatory corticosteroids (Decadron in 4 mg doses). Infection was minimized by the use of therapeutic levels of penicillin during hospitalization and a prophylactic dose of 250 mg of pencillin V per day for 1 year after the surgical procedure. A pressure dressing was placed for 48 hours. Postoperative discomfort was considerably less than that which follows third molar surgery.

Phase IV. After the patient was discharged from the hospital 2 to 3 days postoperatively, his existing mandibular denture was converted to an interim prosthesis. Holes corresponding to the intraoral position of the fasteners were placed through the denture, allowing generous clearance around the fasteners. The tissue surface of the prosthesis was relieved and subsequently relined with a soft tissue–conditioning material. This procedure provided the patient with a stabilized, well-retained, and functional interim prosthesis.

The soft lining served as a stress-breaking mechanism between the prosthesis and the implant. For this reason, as well as for maintenance of tissue health, the lining was changed as frequently as required during the time that the interim denture was in use, a period of approximately 90 days.

Phase V. During this period, cast gold copings were fabricated for the fasteners. The copings were joined to a 14-gauge round gold bar that was positioned 1.5 to 2 mm above the gingiva over the ridge crest. Eventually the coping bar

component was cemented to the fasteners, which, with the staple implant, completed the boxlike formation (Fig. 8-37, *G*). This rigid form was designed to allow a passive relationship to exist among the denture, the implant, and bone. Forces transmitted by the denture during function need to be distributed as broadly as posssble to the supporting ridge.

The coping-bar component was picked up in a final impression from which the master cast was constructed. Dalbo stress-breaking precision attachments were soldered to the distal aspect of both copings, with their counterparts welded to a cobalt-chrome meshwork that was to be embedded in the denture (Fig. 8-37, *F*).

The mandibular denture was constructed following accepted principles of conventional denture therapy. The prosthesis was processed and finished, with adequate relief between the copings and the denture (Fig. 8-37, *G*). This allowed slight movement of the denture supported by the mucoperiosteum while it was positively retained by the implant. Compressive forces transmitted by the denture to the implant had to be minimized. It is theorized that eventually such forces may exceed the physiologic tolerance of the bone, resulting in bone resorption and loosening or failure of implanted devices. The designer of the staple implant concedes that some resorption will occur in the presence of a complete denture, but this resorption should not exceed normal resorption with age and should not jeopardize the staple implant since the bulk of the metal is away from the surface tissues and the objective of the prosthesis design is to minimize compressive forces transmitted to the transosteal pins.

The coping-bar component was temporarily cemented to the fasteners, and the patient was allowed to wear the prosthesis for 2 weeks, during which time postinsertion adjustments were made. This was followed by permanent cementation of the copings.

The implant has been in place for more than 18 months, and the definitive prosthesis has been in use for 1 year (Fig. 8-37, *H* and *I*). The tissue response has been excellent. The patient is extremely well satisfied with the results and has commented that his ability to function with the prosthesis has far exceeded his expectations. In addition to immediate postoperative instructions, the patient has been provided with special home care instructions for the maintenance of the tissues around the transosseous pins and the cleansing of the denture. Patients must understand the importance of their role in maintaining tissue health and must establish a routine procedure for this.

CONCLUSION

The magnitude of sulcus extension and ridge augmentation procedures combined with the expected patient discomfort should not be used as excuses to deny patients the benefit of preprosthetic surgery. Patients who have been in pain or embarrassed by juggling an ill-fitting denture for years are most grateful when these conditions are corrected and successful denture wearing is restored.

The mandibular staple implant has application for the patient with severe mandibular atrophy with at least 9 mm of alveolar crest height and for the patient who has an absolute need for a stable and retentive prosthesis in order to lead a normal life, regardless of the degree of mandibular atrophy exhibited.

This preprosthetic surgical approach, however, calls for the utmost of surgical and prosthetic preplanning and cooperation, as well as meticulous attention to detail in all phases of treatment. When the principles of case selection and treatment outlined previously are followed, excellent results and patient satisfaction can be expected.

REFERENCES

1. Anderson, J. O., Benson, D., and Waite, D. E.: Intraoral skin grafts, an aid to alveolar ridge extension, J. Oral Surg. **27:**427, 1969.
2. Ashley, F. N., Schwartz, A. N., and Dryden, M. F.: A modified technic for creating a lower lingual sulcus, Plast. Reconstr. Surg. **22:**204, 1953.
3. Baer, P., Sumner, C., and Scigliano, J.: Studies on hydrogenated fat-zinc bacitracin periodontal dressing, J. Oral Surg. **13:**494, 1960.
4. Baurmash, H., Mandel, L., and Strelioff, M.: Mandibular sulcus extension—a new technic, preliminary report, J. Oral Surg. **20:**390, 1962.
5. Bellinger, D. H.: Preliminary report on the use of tantalum in maxillofacial and oral surgery, J. Oral Surg. **5:**108, 1947.
6. Bjorn, H.: Free transplantation of gingiva propria, Sveriges Tandlukarforbunck Tidung. **22:**684, 1963.
7. Blackstone, C. H., and Parker, M. L.: Rebuilding of resorbed alveolar ridge, J. Oral Surg. **14:**45, 1956.
8. Boyne, P. J.: Restoration of alveolar ridges by intramandibular transposition osseous grafting, J. Oral Surg. **26:**569, 1968.
9. Brown, J. B., Tryer, M. B., and Lu, M.: Polyvinyl and silicone compounds as subcutaneous prostheses, Arch. Surg. **68:**744, 1954.
10. Caldwell, J.: Lingual ridge extension, J. Oral Surg. **13:**287, 1955.
11. Clark, H. B., Jr.: Deepening the labial sulcus by mucosal flap advancement: report of a case, J. Oral Surg. **11:**165, 1953.
12. Collett, H. A.: Immediate maxillary ridge extension, Dent. Dig. **60:**104, 1954.
13. Converse, J. M.: Restoration of facial contour by bone grafts introduced through the oral cavity, Plast. Reconstr. Surg. **6:**295, 1950.
14. Cooley, D. O.: Method for deepening maxillary and mandibular sulci to correct deficient edentulous ridges, J. Oral Surg. **10:**279, 1952.
15. Danielson, P. A., and Nemarich, A. N.: Subcortical bone grafting for ridge augmentation, J. Oral Surg. **34:**887, 1976.
16. Edlan, A.: Combining a modified lingual plastic operation of the lower jaw with a vestibular plastic operation in the frontal region, Csek. Stom. **5:**202, 1954.
17. Esser, J. F.: Studies in plastic surgery of the face, Ann. Surg. **65:**297, 1917.
18. Farrell, C. D., Kent, J. N., and Guerra, L. R.: One-stage interpositional bone grafting and vestibuloplasty of the atrophic maxilla, J. Oral Surg. **34:**901, 1976.
19. Flohr, W.: Zur Implantation alloplastishes Materialen, Zahnaerztl. Prax. **4:**1, 1953.
20. Gerhard, R. C.: Personal communication, 1971.
21. Gillies, H. D.: Plastic surgery of the face, London, 1920, Oxford University Press.
22. Gillies, H. D., and Millard, D. R.: Principles and art of plastic surgery, Boston, 1957, Little, Brown & Co.
23. Godwin, J. G.: Submucous surgery for better denture service. Amer. Dent. Ass. **34:**678, 1947.
24. Goodsell, J. O.: Surgical aids to intraoral prosthesis, J. Oral Surg. **13:**8, 1955.
25. Guernsey, L. H.: Reactive inflammatory papillary hyperplasia of the palate, Oral Surg. **20:**814, 1965.
26. Guernsey, L. H.: Preprosthetic surgery, Dent. Clin. North Am. **15:**478, 1971.
27. Guernsey, L. H.: Free mucosal grafts in major reconstructive oral surgery, Proceeding of the International Oral Surgery Conference, Amsterdam, Copenhagen, Dec. 1972, Munksgaard, International Booksellers & Publishers Ltd.
28. Hall, H. D., and O'Steen, A.: Free grafts of palatal

mucosa in mandibular vestibuloplasty, J. Oral Surg. **28**:565, 1970.

29. Hecht, S. S.: Improving mandibular ridge form by means of surgery and drug implanation, J. Oral Surg. **3**:1096, 1950.
30. Kazanjian, V. H.: Surgery as an aid to more efficient service with prosthetic dentures, J. Am. Dent. Assoc. **22**:566, 1935.
31. Kruger, G. O.: Ridge extension: review of indications and technics, J. Oral Surg. **16**:191, 1958.
32. Lane, S. L.: Plastic procedures as applied to oral surgery, J. Oral Surg. **16**:489, 1958.
33. Lewis, E. T.: Surgical correction to the sublingual region, J. Am. Dent. Assoc. **67**:364, 1963.
34. Maloney, P. L., Doku, H. C., and Shepherd, N. S.: Mucosal grafting in oral reconstructive surgery, J. Oral Surg. **32**:705, 1974.
35. Maloney, P. L., Garland, S. D., Stanwich, L., Shepherd, N. S., and Doku, H. C.: Immediate vestibuloplasty with fenestrated and intact full thickness mucosal grafts, Oral Surg. **42**:543, 1976.
36. Maloney, P. L., Shepherd, N. S., and Doku, H. C.: Free buccal mucosal grafts for vestibuloplasty, J. Oral Surg. **30**:716, 1972.
37. Maloney, P. L., Shepherd, N. S., and Doku, H. C.: Immediate vestibuloplasty with free mucosa grafts, J. Oral Surg. **32**:343, 1974.
38. McIntosh, R. B., and Obwegeser, H.: Preprosthetic surgery: a scheme for its effective employment, J. Oral Surg. **27**:427, 1969.
39. Nabers, J. M.: Free gingival grafts, Periodontics **4**:243, 1966.
40. Neidhardt, A.: Die Mund Vorhofplastik mit sekundarer Epithelieserung an Oberkiefer: Entwicklung, Methodik, Ergebnisse, Inaugural dissertation, Zurich, Switzerland, 1963, Benzinger and Co. AG.
41. Obwegeser, H., cited in Trauner, R.: Alveoplasty with ridge extension on lingual side of the lower jaw to solve the problem of a lower dental prosthesis, J. Oral Surg. **5**:340, 1952.
42. Obwegeser, H.: Die submuköse Vestibulumplastik, Deutsch. Zahnaerztl. Z. **14**:629, 1959.
43. Obwegeser, H.: Die totale Mundbodenplastik, Schweiz. Monatsschr. Zahnheilkd. **73**:565, 1963.
44. Obwegeser, H.: Personal communication, 1968.
45. Obwegeser, H.: In Thoma, K. H.: Oral surgery, ed. 5, vol. 1., St. Louis, 1969, The C. V. Mosby Co., p. 445.
46. The old in the century of the young, Time, vol. 49, Aug. 3, 1970.
47. Propper, R. H.: Simplified ridge extension using free mucosal grafts, J. Oral Surg. **22**:469, 1964.
48. Rieger, H. G.: Tantalum as a replacement for bone in oral surgery, J. Oral Surg. **3**:727, 1950.
49. Sanders, B.: Palatal patch-grafts in post areas of subperiosteal implants, J. Oral Surg. **34**:995, 1976.
50. Sanders, B., and Cox, R.: Inferior-border rib grafting for augmentation of the atrophic edentulous mandible, J. Oral Surg. **34**:897, 1976.
51. Schuchardt, K.: Die Epidermis Transplantation bei der Mund Vorhofplastik, Deutsch. Zahnaerztl. Z. **7**:364, 1952.
52. Shepherd, N. S., Maloney, P. L., and Doku, H. C.: Expanded split thickness mucosal grafts, J. Oral Surg. **31**:687, 1973.
53. Slade, E.: Personal communication, July 1977.
54. Small, I. A.: Metal implants and the mandibular staple bone plate, J. Oral Surg. **33**:571, 1975.
55. Small, I. A.: Experiences with the mandibular staple bone plate, J. Oral Surg., in press.
56. Small, I. A. and Kobernick, S. D.: Implantation of threaded stainless steel pins in the dog mandible, J. Oral Surg. **27**:99, 1969.
57. Spengler, D. E., and Hayward, J. R.: The study of sulcus extension wound healing in dogs, J. Oral Surg. **22**:413, 1964.
58. Steinhauser, E. W.: Free transplantation of oral mucosa for improvement of denture retention, J. Oral Surg. **27**:955, 1969.
59. Szaba, Ganzer, and Rumpel, Cited in Obwegeser, H.: Surgical preparation of the maxilla for prosthesis, J. Oral Surg. **22**:127, 1964.
60. Trauner, R.: Alveoplasty with ridge extension on lingual side of the lower jaw to solve the problem of a lower dental prosthesis, J. Oral Surg. **5**:340, 1952.
61. Ward, T.: The split bone technique for removal of lower third molars, Br. Dent. J. **101**:297, 1956.
62. Weintraub, G. S., and Guernsey, L. H.: Mandibular staple bone plate implant and prosthesis, Oral Surg. **43**:827, 1977.
63. Weiser, R.: Ein Fall von Ankylose, verlust des Alveolarforsatzes und der Vestibulum oris in bereiche fast des ganzen Unterkiefers-Oester. Hungra Viertelfahrsschr. Zahnheilk. **34**:147, 1918.
64. Yrastorza, J. A.: Mandibular sulcus deepening: a modified technic, J. Am. Dent. Assoc. **67**:859, 1963.
65. The Zimmer Company: Tivanium a new orthopaedic alloy from Zimmer USA, Warsaw, Ind. 46580.

CHAPTER 9

Surgical bacteriology

S. Elmer Bear

INFECTION

An ever present problem in the field of oral surgery is infection. Under normal circumstances the oral cavity is never sterile, and, if it were not for certain intrinsic and extrinsic factors, the care of a dental patient would be immeasurably more difficult.

The intrinsic factors include the normal regional immunity of the host to the bacterial flora of the mouth, the natural slough or desquamative function of the adjacent epithelium, the abundant blood supply present in the oral cavity, and the immediate response of the leukocytes when bacteria invade the host. In addition, saliva has been found to have an inhibitory effect on some bacteria, particularly those foreign to the normal flora. The normal flora also acts as a barrier to invading microorganisms.

The extrinsic factors that may aid in the control of oral infections are many; the most notable are the observance of good surgical and aseptic techniques (discussed in detail in Chapter 2) and the use of antibiotics and chemotherapeutic agents. The philosophy behind the use of antibiotics and chemotherapeutic agents is similar, and although the terms are not technically interchangeable because of their deriva-

tion, the former term shall be used henceforth for the sake of brevity and simplicity. Other factors aid in the control of infection, but a review of the source and physiological response, both local and systemic, should be evaluated before specific therapy is discussed.

In any discussion of surgical bacteriology applicable to the oral cavity and its adjacent structures, one must be aware of the existence of innumerable microorganisms that are normal inhibitants of this region. The most common bacteria found in the mouth include the alpha and beta streptococci, nonhemolytic streptococci, *Staphylococcus aureus, Staphylococcus albus,* Vincent's spirochetes, and fusiform bacillus. Increasing numbers of antibiotic-resistant organisms have been noted in saliva, particularly those resistant to penicillin. The virulence and quantity of these bacteria are generally controlled in the oral cavity by the mild bactericidal effect of saliva and the deglutition of oral fluids into the stomach, where the pH level is sufficient to destroy the majority of the bacteria and digest the balance. These two factors are not always sufficient to abort an infectious process; therefore, those factors that contribute to an inflammatory reaction will be considered first.

Local factors

A mouth that is already chronically infected or contains large deposits of calculus and debris is a poor environment for a surgical procedure. Chronic irritation damages tissues to the point at which the normal resistance is markedly impaired, and the area is therefore more prone to infection. Invading bacteria will frequently destroy the protective reparative properties of the blood clot, preventing normal consolidation by the adjacent tissues. Operating in a mouth in which evidence of necrotic gingivitis is present is extremely hazardous. The gingival structures are necrotic, and a surgical procedure performed in this field places the general health of the patient in jeopardy, not only because of localized infection and pain in the field of operation but also because the fascial spaces of the head and neck may be readily invaded, and a general septicemia may result if the bacteria are of sufficient virulence.

Systemic condition of the patient

Numerous factors of a systemic nature play a role in the predisposition to infection. Diabetes mellitus is a classic illustration of a disease that, if uncontrolled, provides a poor environment in which to perform surgery. This is a disease of carbohydrate metabolism, characterized by hyperglycemia and glycosuria, and is directly related to insufficient insulin. A characteristic feature of diabetes is increased susceptibility to infection, and, once established in diabetics, infection can proceed rapidly. Under these conditions, insulin demand is increased enormously, leading to additional complications. The oral manifestations of the diabetic, such as dryness of the mouth, lingual edema, and periodontal disease, are well known but may not be demonstrable on clinical examination if the disease is partially controlled. Surgical intervention, however, may precipitate an infectious process because of the lowered local and systemic resistance. Impaired healing may also occur, making the patient more susceptible to infection.

Patients who give any indication of diabetes, either by history or by clinical examination, should be evaluated carefully. If the patient is under a physician's care and his condition is under control, surgery can be performed in the usual manner. If, on the other hand, some doubt exists about the diabetic status, treatment should be deferred until a physician has been consulted and a urinalysis and fasting blood sugar study completed.

It should be stressed that although surgery is sometimes more hazardous in the diabetic patient, the elimination of oral infections is most important. Surgery should be done as soon as practical, since the removal of an infectious process may aid in the control of the disease symptoms.

Blood dyscrasias

Several blood dyscrasias are predisposing factors of oral infection, the most notable of which are the leukemias. In acute leukemia and acute exacerbations of chronic leukemia, infections of the oral cavity are frequently seen and are difficult to treat. Surgical intervention in patients so afflicted is hazardous not only because of the excessive hemorrhages that frequently occur in these patients but also because of these patients' susceptibility to infection and poor healing qualities. The use of antibiotics is imperative if surgery must be done, and these drugs are often used to reduce the oral symptoms of the disease.

Agranulocytosis and the anemias cause a general lowering of the host's ability to resist infection, and serious consequences may result if the dyscrasia is marked. In agranulocytosis, spontaneous hemorrhages of the oral cavity are not unusual, and this condition may be accompanied by various ulcerations of the mucosa. The clinical picture of anemia in the oral cavity is exactly what one would expect to find in a situation in which either a decrease in the number of red cells or a decrease in the hemoglobin content of the cells is present. The lips and mucosa are pale in color and delicate in texture. The tongue is often smooth, glossy, and painful. This may be the first clue to the systemic problem and should never be ignored. The decreased number of leukocytes and the subnormal oxygen-bearing elements are the systemic manifestations and make the patient easily susceptible to infection.

Malnutrition

Malnutrition may result from the failure to ingest, assimilate, or utilize any or all substances essential for normal body metabolism. In some parts of the world, starvation may be the predominate cause of malnutrition, but in a modern society the most obvious causes are probably a poorly balanced diet, alcoholism, and old age.

Longevity, one of the accomplishments of modern science, has presented dentistry with many new problems, including denture construction on atrophied ridges, poor tissue tolerance to stress, and impaired healing. In the elderly patient and the alcoholic, the digestive tract may not have the ability to properly assimilate amino acids or other substances necessary to tissue repair. When this happens, the patient is more susceptible to infection and may require parenteral therapy with antibiotics and vitamins.

A thorough past history is important relative to tissue healing and other untoward sequelae resulting from prior surgery. Suspected impaired antibiotic function, from whatever cause, cannot be ignored and should be treated accordingly.

Miscellaneous systemic problems

Numerous other systemic diseases have some direct or indirect relationship to infections· of the oral cavity and adjacent tissues, either preoperatively or postoper-atively. Any debilitating disease or affliction of the host can cause impairment of healing and decreased body resistance to infection.

Liver diseases. In the field of oral surgery one normally is concerned with cirrhosis of the liver, hepatitis, and other liver diseases because of the impaired clotting mechanism. A sufficient degree of liver damage can cause considerable impairment of the healing process associated with the resultant anemia and poor metabolism. Any patient having the obvious clinical manifestations of jaundice should be carefully evaluated before surgery is attempted.

Renal diseases. The kidneys are responsible, in part, for the elimination of the nitrogenous waste of the body, in maintaining the normal fluid and electrolyte balance, and in maintaining the proper level of plasma protein. Any disease or abnormality of these organs may well complicate the progress of a patient undergoing a surgical procedure and may in fact cause the death of the patient if sufficient caution is not exercised. It is generally agreed that an abnormal immune response to the hemolytic streptococcus usually precedes glomerulonephritis. Although this disease entity usually gives a history of prior respiratory tract infection, the possible occurrence of hemolytic streptococcus in the oral cavity cannot be ignored by the dentist. A history of oral infections predisposing to nephritis, pyelitis, and other kidney diseases is not uncommon, and one must be careful about subjecting a patient with a history of kidney disease to reinfection. Patients with active renal disorders should definitely be protected with prophylactic antibiotics for two reasons. First, the renal function has been impaired by disease and any bloodborne infection, however transient, may produce serious consequences. Second, local resistance and healing properties of the tissues operated on have been reduced because of the increased uremia and other waste materials in the blood. Infection after surgery is not uncommon in patients so afflicted, and every supportive measure available must be instituted.

Cardiovascular diseases. All patients who have a history of cardiovascular disease should receive special attention at all times, but the treatment varies considerably, depending on the type of cardiac disease. In angina pectoris, coronary occlusion, hypertension, and congestive failure, the primary concern of the dentist is the control of pain and apprehension that may precipitate a relapse. A history of rheumatic fever, chorea, congenital heart disease, or cardiovascular surgery requires specific attention for an entirely different reason—infection. These cardiovascular problems are often aggravated by a transient bacteremia, however brief, and the literature is replete with cases showing the relationship of extractions and bacterial endocarditis. Alpha hemolytic streptococcus is the organism usually responsible for this cardiac complication. These organisms can be found almost routinely in a blood culture after an extraction or extensive periodontal therapy. Consequently, it is good medical and dental practice to protect patients with rheumatic or congenital heart disease by prophylactic measures.

The procedures that would fall within the scope of dental interest include root canal therapy, periodontal treatment regardless of its extensiveness, and, of course, all surgical procedures within the oral cavity. If uncertainty exists about the degree of gingival manipulation that may produce a transient bacteremia, then antibiotics should be administered. Although the exact dosage and duration of therapy are somewhat empirical, it is generally agreed that high concentrations are desirable before any dental procedure is undertaken.

The American Heart Association constantly reviews and evaluates the need for and modality of antibiotic therapy in patients with structural heart disease. The following discussion reflects some of their philosophies and recommendations in the administration of antibiotics.

Bacterial endocarditis remains one of the most serious complications of cardiac disease. Surgical procedures or instrumentation involving the upper respiratory tract, geniotourinary tract, or lower gastrointestinal tract may be associated with transitory bacteremia. Bacteria in the bloodstream may lodge on damaged or abnormal valves such as are found in rheumatic or congenital heart disease or on endocardium near congenital anatomic defects, causing bacterial endocarditis or endarteritis.

Prophylaxis is recommended in those situations most likely to be associated with bacteremia since bacterial endocarditis cannot occur without a preceding bacteremia. Antibiotic prophylaxis is recommended with *all* dental procedures (including routine professional cleaning) *that are likely to cause gingival bleeding.* Chemoprophylaxis for dental procedures in children should be managed in a manner similar to that used in adults.

In general, parenteral administration of antibiotics provides more predictable blood levels and is preferred when practical, especially for patients thought to be at high risk to develop bacterial endocarditis.

Since it is not possible to predict those patients with structural heart disease in whom this infection will occur nor the specific casual event, optimal prophylaxis requires proper consultation between the treating dentist and the patient's physician to determine whether the patient is a high risk and should be given parenteral prophylactic antibiotics or a relatively low risk and can be covered with oral prophylactic antibiotics. The determination as to the relative risk (high or low) should be made by the patient's physician, not the dentist. In cases where the patient's physician is not available for consultation the parenteral route is preferred.

Table 9-1 contains suggested regimens for

Table 9-1. Prophylaxis for dental procedures and surgical procedures of the upper respiratory tract*

	Most congenital heart disease[3]; valvular heart disease; idiopathic hypertrophic subaortic stenosis; mitral valve[4] prolapse syndrome with mitral insufficiency	Prosthetic heart valves[5]
All dental procedures that are likely to result in gingival bleeding[1,2]	Regimen A or B	Regimen B
Surgery or instrumentation of the respiratory tract	Regimen A or B	Regimen B

[1]Does not include shedding of deciduous teeth.
[2]Does not include simple adjustment of orthodontic appliances.
[3]E.g., ventricular septal defect, tetralogy of Fallot, aortic stenosis, pulmonic stenosis, complex cyanotic heart disease, patent ductus arteriosus or systemic to pulmonary artery shunts. Does *not* include uncomplicated secundum atrial septal defect.
[4]Although cases of infective endocarditis in patients with mitral valve prolapse syndrome have been documented, the incidence appears to be relatively low and the necessity for prophylaxis in all of these patients has not yet been established.
[5]Some patients with a prosthetic heart valve in whom a high level of oral health is being maintained may be offered oral antibiotic prophylaxis for routine dental procedures except the following: parenteral antibiotics are recommended for patients with prosthetic valves who require extensive dental procedures, especially extractions, or oral or gingival surgical procedures.
*From American Heart Association Committe Report: Prevention of bacterial endocarditis, Circulation **55**:139A-143A, 1977, by permission of the American Heart Association, Inc.

chemoprophylaxis for dental procedures or surgical procedures and instrumentation of the upper respiratory tract. The order of listing does not imply superiority of one regimen over another, although parenteral administration is favored when practical. The authorities favor the combined use of penicillin and streptomycin (Regimen B), or the use of vancomycin in the penicillin-allergic patient, in those patients felt to be at high risk (such as those with prosthetic heart valves).[2]

Regimen A—Penicillin
1. Parenteral—oral combined
   Adults: Aqueous crystalline penicillin G (1,000,000 units intramuscularly) mixed with procaine penicillin G (600,000 units intramuscularly). Give 30 minutes to 1 hour prior to procedure and then give penicillin V (formerly called phenoxymethyl penicillin) 500 mg orally every 6 hours for 8 doses.
   Children: Aqueous crystalline penicillin G (30,000 units/kg intramuscularly) mixed with procaine penicillin G (600,000 units intramuscularly). Timing of doses for chil-

dren is the same as for adults. For children less than 60 lbs., the dose of penicillin V is 250 mg orally every 6 hours for 8 doses.
2. Oral
   Adults: Penicillin V (2.0 gm orally 30 minutes to 1 hour prior to the procedure and then 500 mg orally every 6 hours for 8 doses.)
   Children: Penicillin V (2.0 gm orally 30 minutes to 1 hour prior to procedure and then 500 mg orally every 6 hours for 8 doses. For children less than 60 lbs. use 1.0 gm orally 30 minutes to 1 hour prior to the procedure and then 250 mg orally every 6 hours for 8 doses.)
   For patients allergic to penicillin use either vancomycin (see Regimen B) or use
   Adults: Erythromycin (1.0 gm orally 1½-2 hours prior to the procedure and then 500 mg orally every 6 hours for 8 doses).
   Children: Erythromycin, (20 mg/kg orally 1½-2 hours prior to the procedure and then 10 mg/kg every 6 hours for 8 doses.)

Regimen B—Penicillin plus streptomycin
   Adults: Aqueous crystalline penicillin G (1,000,000 units intramuscularly) mixed with procaine penicillin G (600,000 units

intramuscularly) plus streptomycin (1 gm intramuscularly). Give 30 minutes to 1 hour prior to the procedure; then penicillin V 500 mg orally every 6 hours for 8 doses.

Children: Aqueous crystalline penicillin G (30,000 units/kg intramuscularly) mixed with procaine penicillin G (600,000 units intramuscularly) plus streptomycin (20 mg/kg intramuscularly). Timing of doses for children is the same as for adults. For children less than 60 lbs the recommended oral dose of penicillin V is 250 mg every 6 hours for 8 doses.

For patients allergic to penicillin

Adults: Vancomycin (1 gm intravenously over 30 minutes to 1 hour). Start initial vancomycin infusion ½ to 1 hour prior to procedure; then erythromycin 500 mg orally every 6 hours for 8 doses.

Children: Vancomycin (20 mg/kg intravenously over 30 minutes to 1 hour). Timing of doses for children is the same as for adults. Erythromycin dose is 10 mg/kg every 6 hours for 8 doses.

Footnotes to Regimens

In unusual circumstances or in the case of delayed healing, it may be prudent to provide additional doses of antibiotics even though available data suggest that bacteria rarely persists longer than 15 minutes after the procedure. The physician or dentist may also choose to use the parenteral route of administration for all of the doses in selected situations.

Doses for children should not exceed recommendations for adults for a single dose or for a 24-hour period.

For vancomycin the total dose for children should not exceed 44 mg/kg/24 hours.

For those patients receiving continuous oral penicillin for secondary prevention of rheumatic fever, alpha hemolytic streptococci which are relatively resistant to penicillin are occasionally found in the oral cavity. While it is likely that the doses of penicillin recommended in Regimen A are sufficient to control these organisms, the physician or dentist may choose one of the suggestions in Regimen B or may choose oral erythromycin.[2]

Other indications for prophylactic antibiotics are:

1. Those patients who have had a documented previous episode of infective endocarditis, even in the absence of clinically detectable disease

2. Those patients with indwelling cardiac catheters, especially those that reside in one of the cardiac chambers

3. Those patients with indwelling transvenous cardiac pacemakers, even though at low risk; the dentist should consult the patient's physician, and they may choose to employ prophylactic antibiotics to cover dental and surgical procedures in these patients

4. Those patients on renal dialysis with implanted arteriovenous shunt appliances

5. Those patients with orthopedic joint replacements (such as total knee, total hip)

It is not possible to make recommendations for all possible clinical situations. Practitioners should exercise their clinical judgment in determining the duration and choice of antibiotic(s) when special circumstances apply. Consultation between the dentist and the patient's physician in these cases is stressed.

Since endocarditis may occur despite antibiotic prophylaxis, dentists and physicians should maintain a high index of suspicion in the interpretation of any unusual clinical events following the above procedures. Early diagnosis is important to reduce complications, sequelae, and mortality.

Physiology of infection

A frequent cause of acute inflammation in the oral cavity and its adjacent structures is the invasion of microorganisms. The response to infection of the host follows a relatively normal pattern. Accepting this premise, one can state that the physiological response to infection is inflammation. The nature of the inflammatory reaction is dependent in turn on the site, type, and virulence of the bacteria. In addition, the physical status of the host may determine the degree of inflammation, depending on the local and systemic factors that have already been discussed.

The response of the host to infection may be local and systemic. The local reaction is inflammation, which is defined by Moore as "the sum total of the changes in the tissues of the animal organism in response to an injurious agent, including the local reaction, and the repair of the injury. If the inflammatory reaction is adequate, it minimizes the effect of the injurious agent, destroys the injurious agent, and restores the part to as near normal structure and function as possible. If it is not adequate, there is extensive destruction of tissue, invasion of the body, and somatic death."[29] More briefly stated, one might say that inflammation is the reaction of the body to irritants, the most common of which are bacterial. The classic signs of inflammation are redness, swelling, heat, and pain. The degree and frequency of these signs vary considerably, depending on the virulence of the bacteria and their location. For example, in the oral cavity one might find a mild gingivitis, which is a minimal inflammatory reaction, and at the same time find a fulminating cellulitis of the neck caused by the same microorganisms. The different response is dependent in part on the location of the bacteria involved and may vary considerably if its environment is aerobic or anaerobic. In addition, the various body tissues respond differently to the same invading organism.

The signs and symptoms of inflammation can be explained when the tissue response to an irritant is understood. Initially a marked dilation of the vascular bed occurs, which is accompanied by a deceleration of the blood flow resulting from the greater volume of the vascular bed. The increased capillary volume is responsible for the cardinal signs of redness, swelling, and heat. As the rate of blood flow decreases, leukocytes begin to penetrate through the vessel walls into the surrounding tissues. This phenomenon is accompanied by an exuding of blood plasma through the walls,

producing an inflammatory edema. The escape of the blood plasma may be caused by the toxic reaction of the capillary walls to infection or to an increased osmotic pressure of the surrounding tissues. This tissue distention produces pressure against the neurogenic fibers and may actually cause the destruction of these fibers. This pressure phenomenon, along with the release of histamines from injured cells, plays a major role in the appearance of the fourth classical sign of inflammation—pain.

Varied types of inflammation are seen, depending on the tissue involved, the type of bacteria, and the resistance of the host. The most important are pyogenic, serous, catarrhal, fibrinous, hemorrhagic, and necrotizing inflammation.

The type of inflammation encountered most frequently in the field of oral surgery is pyogenic, meaning "pus forming." Most infections in this region, if allowed to progress without treatment, will eventually produce pus. The invasive bacteria or their toxins or both may produce several different clinical entities that will be discussed in detail in Chapter 11. They include lymphadenitis, cellulitis, abscess formation, phlegmon, and osteomyelitis. All may be either acute or chronic, and combinations of two or more of these clinical manifestions may be present. The pattern of infection is dependent on the numerous factors discussed previously, the length of time the infection has been present, and the mode of treatment.

Systemic effects of oral infection

In all infectious diseases except the most trivial, systemic manifestations of bacterial invasions are found. The reaction may be produced by the actual destructive ability of the bacteria, as in an abscess, or by its toxins, as in diphtheria. When bacteria are present in the blood, the condition is known as "bacteremia." Most authors use the term "septicemia" when the bacteria and their toxins are found in large numbers, suggesting actual growth while in the bloodstream. Transient bacteremias are usually seen after the removal of teeth or periodontal therapy. This is generally of little consequence except when a cardiac valve deformity exists or the resistance of the host is impaired or the organism is highly virulent.

Fever is perhaps the most outstanding symptom of a systemic infection and probably results from the action of the bacterial toxins on the heat-regulating mechanism of the brain. As one might suspect, fever may vary considerably from one individual to another, even though they may be afflicted with the same infectious process. The exact nature of temperature control is not clearly understood, but with sufficient fever, an accompanying reduction in blood volume is caused by a shift of blood fluids to the tissues and extravascular spaces. This phenomenon together with the loss of fluid caused by excessive perspiration leads to decreased urinary output (oliguria) and retention of chlorides. An increase in the nonprotein nitrogen, both in the blood and urine, results from an increased metabolism, which is also a consequence of fever. If the kidneys are functioning properly, this is not a serious problem, but if marked dehydration goes uncorrected, the patient may be in real difficulty because of the abnormal electrolyte balance and retention of nitrogenous waste products.

The elevated metabolism resulting from a fever also causes an increased pulse rate, cardiac output, and respiratory rate. These clinical symptoms of a fever are invaluable in determining the progress of the disease and the effectiveness of the therapy used. Any marked deviation of these manifestations from normal would require an alteration of the therapy and increased supportive care.

Focus of infection

The principle of focal infection has been a controversial issue for many years. The pendulum of opinion has swung in both directions many times since the turn of the century. The modern concept of focal infection was given strong support by Billings[5] and Rosenow[37] so that in the 1920s considerable importance was placed on this concept. Since that time many studies have been conducted to ascertain the validity of the earlier conclusions. Some have substantiated the principle of focal infection and some have not. Today the pendulum has gradually swung back to a more conservative concept. It is generally agreed that the principle of focal infection is valid and that a focus of infection should be eliminated when possible. However, the general consensus is that a minor focus is, as a rule, not capable of producing exacerbations of unrelated disease except in specific and occasional instances.

In the last half century, many teeth have been condemned on the block of focal infection. Today with the aid of roentgenograms, vitalometer tests, and better clinical judgment the dentist is able to defend his or her position in attempting to salvage a patient's dentition. A focus of infection may act as a depot from which bacteria or their products may be disseminated to other parts of the body, or it may act as a site in which bloodborne bacteria may localize, setting up an acute inflammatory reaction.

The concept of elective localization of microorganisms is not fully understood, but it explains in part why certain bacteria have an affinity for one or more specific tissues of the body. Undoubtedly some close chemical interplay takes place between bacteria and tissues. This would explain why most apical lesions do little damage elsewhere unless the body resistance is depressed or a specific area elsewhere has been damaged. An excellent illustration of this phenomenon is the effect of the alpha hemolytic streptococcus on a previously damaged mitral valve.

The practitioner must keep these possibilities in mind when making a decision concerning the preservation of a tooth or its supporting tissues. If a tooth is infected, the infection must be removed. Little controversy exists about this basic tenet of good dental practice. This does not necessarily mean the extraction of the tooth. One can and should do root canal therapy if indicated in relation to the remaining dentition, and, in addition, a root resection should be performed if the apical lesion cannot definitely be eliminated by more conservative means. A root resection ensures a complete seal of the accessory canals and also eliminates the area of infected cementum. If the question of focal infection arises, it seems reasonable to accept the principle of root resection as being more reliable regarding the elimination of a focus of infection.

Periodontal disease of varying degrees has been accepted as a frequent site of focal infection. This disease, except for caries, is perhaps the most common chronic infectious process in man. Clinical evaluation regarding the presence of pus and inflamed gingiva is perhaps more reliable in determining if the disease is infectious than are roentgenograms. The latter may show bone loss, which may be persistent over a period of years, although the surrounding tissues show no clinical evidence of infection. When the dentition is firm even in the presence of moderate bone loss and clinical evidence of infection is absent, conservatism is justified in considering the teeth as a possible focus of infection.

As mentioned previously, specific diseases have been shown to have a direct relationship to oral foci of infection. Acute infections of the eyes, heart, kidneys, and joints have on occasion shown a direct correlation to oral infection. Some forms of optic neuritis and iritis have been traced directly to a chronic periapical or periodontal lesion. In the past it was not unusual to remove a chronically infected tooth and find a sudden exacerbation of a chronic iritis. The bacterium causing the initial eye condition, being suddenly released into the bloodstream in relatively large quantities, may produce an acute condition. Today this clinical observation does not occur as frequently, since most patients with iritis are given some supportive therapy with antibiotics prior to extractions.

Arthritic patients as a group have in the past probably lost more teeth under the guise of focal infection than all other groups combined. Arthritis is a painful and debilitating disease, and everyone associated with the case makes every effort to leave no stone unturned in the hope of finding the etiological factor. Arthritis occurs in a number of different forms, dependent on various etiological factors. In infectious arthritis (such as gonococcal and pneumococcal) and in degenerative arthritis, the etiological factors are readily established. Thus no effort is made to establish an oral focus. In rheumatoid arthritis, however, the exact etiology is unknown, although it is thought to be infectious. For this reason the dentist invariably sees the patient to eliminate any possible focus of infection. This is not an unreasonable request, since the patient is in desperate need of assistance. Any active infectious process of the oral cavity should be eliminated. Teeth that have root canals and no apical involvement and areas of condensing osteitis should not be removed unless the dentist is convinced that infection is present or unless the physician insists and has examined the patient for all other possible foci of infection. In this way it is possible to aid the patient and yet protect him in the retention of his dentition.

Studies have been reported that attempt to explain one of the disturbing aspects of focal infection. Some infectious processes in specific areas of the body are definitely believed to result from a primary focus of infection yet do not respond favorably when the primary focus is removed. These studies have shown that the secondary focus has been present long enough and the damage is of sufficient magnitude to be irreversible. The secondary site then is no longer dependent on the primary focus. This would explain the absence of dramatic results in many cases where teeth are removed as a focus of infection. An illustration of this problem as it relates to dentistry is the presence of some long-standing apical infection, which might well be the primary focus for pyelitis, bacterial nephritis, or other infectious processes. Although the apical infection is eliminated, the secondary focus will not respond, since the process is no longer reversible.

ANTIBIOTICS
Historical background

The antagonism of microorganisms to each other and the ability of various bacteria and fungi to produce antibacterial substances have been known since the late nineteenth century. Prior to 1938 this phenomenon was a scientific curiosity, utilized only to separate various bacterial species from one another. Since that time, however, this well-known fact has all but revolutionized modern medicine. Fleming in 1928 reported the value of penicillin in the isolation of *Haemophilus influenzae*. It was not until 1940 that a group from Oxford was able to develop penicillin as a therapeutic agent. The investigation of Waksman and associates and Dubos and his group at about the same time led to the development of numerous other antibiotic agents suitable for clinical use. Some time earlier, in 1935, Domagk observed the therapeutic value of Prontosil in the treatment of mice with streptococcal septicemia. This was only the beginning of a new era in the treatment of infection. Countless lives have been saved by sulfanilamide and related sulfonamide drugs, although since 1944 the antibiotics have largely supplanted the sulfonamide drugs.

General considerations

The ideal antibiotic has not yet been found. If one is ever discovered, it would have to have numerous important attributes. (1) It should be antimicrobial and therapeutically effective in vivo in concentrations that would not injure the host. (2) It should be able to attack the pathogenic organisms regardless of their location within the host. (3) It should have con-

sistent therapeutic value. (4) It should not impair normal antibody or phagocytic activity. (5) It should not readily induce the development of resistant strains of microorganisms. (6) Its effectiveness should not be impaired in the presence of other therapeutic agents that might be administered concurrently. (7) It should be stable and easy to administer. (8) It should be inexpensive.

Before an antibiotic can be administered safely and effectively, certain factors require careful consideration.

Nature of the lesion

The nature of the lesion caused by microorganisms commonly found in the field of oral surgery may fall into one of three categories. The one encountered most often in general practice is wound contamination, as in a "dry socket." Although the clinical picture is not necessarily caused by infection, wound contamination is not uncommon when teeth have been removed in the presence of oral filth and chronic infection. The blood clot is delicate, and if bacterial enzymatic action occurs before vascularization from the side walls of the wound, the clot will be destroyed. The use of unsterile instruments and materials is likely to cause wound contamination, since the bacteria are foreign to the oral flora and thus normal local tissue resistance is absent.

Abscess formation is the second most common bacterial lesion related to the oral cavity. These lesions may be chronic or acute, depending on the virulence of the bacteria, resistance of the host, and location of the infectious process. Apical abscesses are generally chronic, since the microorganisms in this location are not particularly virulent, and the normal body responses are able to build up a protective reaction as seen in a granuloma. Only when the body resistance is lowered or the environment altered to favor bacterial growth do these lesions become acute.

The third type of bacterial lesion is the invasive type of infection, which spreads through the soft tissues and usually results from an acute episode of an apical abscess. Until evidence of purulent material appears, this clinical entity is known as a cellulitis. An inflammatory reaction occurs in response to the invading microorganism or its toxins or both. In the field of oral surgery it almost invariably involves the connective tissues and muscles adjacent to the mandible or maxilla or both, since the lesion generally results from a breakdown of the periosteum. Unless prompt measures are taken to control the infection, abscess formation with necrosis of tissue, lymphadenitis, and bacteremia will occur.

The effectiveness of antibiotic therapy has a direct bearing on the nature of the lesion. If a wound is contaminated and is on a surface where the antibiotic can be applied topically and maintained in sufficient quantity without producing senstivity to the drug, then topical administration may be the method of choice. However, in the majority of instances an infected oral wound cannot be treated topically, since the concentration of the drug is difficult to maintain because of saliva dilution. More important, however, is the fact that the oral mucosa is highly prone to produce a drug sensitivity in the host. For this reason alone the use of topical antibiotics is to be avoided and is contraindicated except in a few instances in which the more insoluble antibiotics may be beneficial. Before any type of antibiotic therapy is effective in wound contamination, it is usually necessary to debride the area of necrotic material. This will ensure a healthy wound periphery for healing and an adequate blood supply.

Extracellular microorganisms are most often responsible for acute infections, and unless an accumulation of pus has developed they can generally be destroyed by phagocytic cells and antibiotics. The absence of normal tissue structures in an abscess deprives the leukocytes of the surface on which they operate effectively, and when deprived of oxygen, as in the case of an abscess, leukocytes become nonmobile and lose their phagocytic properties. To be effective an antibiotic must come into direct contact with the infective agent. This is not possible in many abscesses since the only contact can come through the intact capillaries at the periphery of the lesion. The larger the abscess the less effective is the antibiotic. This fact alone illustrates the necessity for continued surgical intervention when fluctuant material is within a tissue space. It has become apparent in recent years that antibiotics are only adjunctive aids in the presence of pus and that the purulent material must be evacuated surgically.

A cellulitis, on the other hand, that has not undergone sufficient degenerative changes to produce pus may be amenable to antibiotic therapy alone. The rich blood supply, characteristic of early inflammation, provides optimal transport of the antibiotic to the involved tissues. In addition, the drug tends to accumulate in the infected area because of the increased vascular bed and permeability of the vessel walls. Antibiotic therapy, therefore, must be instituted promptly if surgery is to be avoided. Before therapy is discontinued it is advisable to remove the causative factor to eliminate the possibility of a relapse.

Sensitivity of microorganisms

An ever-increasing problem in the treatment of an infectious process is the response of the causative organisms to antibiotics. When the antibiotics were first introduced and as each new one was placed on the market, the manufacturer could generally predict, on the basis of laboratory data, which of the species and strains of bacteria would be sensitive. This is no longer the case. Although antibiotics are effective against certain bacterial groups, specific effectiveness is no longer the general rule. On the contrary, individual strains and species are showing wide variations in susceptibility to the same antibiotic. Making the treatment even more complex is the fact that initial susceptibility to an antibiotic

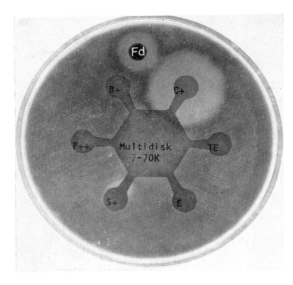

Fig. 9-1. Disk method for determining sensitivity of microorganisms to multiple antibiotics. The organism tested was inhibited by chloramphenicol and Furadantin, as shown by the lack of bacterial growth. The size of the clear area should not be taken as an indication of the relative degree of sensitivity. The center section is commercially prepared and contains a predetermined amount of drug on each segment, *C,* Chloramphenicol; *TE,* tetracycline; *E,* erythromycin; *S,* streptomycin; *P,* penicillin; *B,* bacitracin; *Fd,* Furadantin.

by a specific strain of bacteria may change during treatment.

It is difficult to explain why microorganisms change in their response to an antibiotic. Most investigators feel that bacteria actually undergo sufficient change to be considered mutations. Some, however, feel that an organism initially sensitive to one or more antibiotics gradually builds up a resistance and is no longer affected by the bacteriostatic or bactericidal property of the drug. The exact explanation is still controversial.

The resistance of microorganisms to antibiotics is a serious problem and promises to become even more difficult. For example, in numerous hospitals throughout the United States, strains of staphylococcus have been found that are resistant to all available antibiotics. Research installations are working overtime to produce new drugs that hopefully will be effective. Because of the numerous deaths caused by this strain, it has been necessary in some hospitals to close their operating suites for long periods of time.

One of the most effective means of determining the antibiotic sensitivity of the causative microorganism is to test it in the laboratory. It is first necessary to secure

Antibiotic sensitivity tests		
Organism: STAPH. AUREUS - COAG. +		
Inhibited by		
Penicillin ( )		Tetracycline ( )
Erythromycin ( )		Streptomycin ( )
Bacitracin ( )		Chlormycetin (✔)
No inhibition ( )		

Terramycin ( )	Neomycin ( )
Aureomycin ( )	Polymyxin B ( )

Fig. 9-2. Typical laboratory report sent by the bacteriologist after sensitivity test. This organism is a resistant strain of *Staphylococcus aureus* found in hospitals. A coagulase-positive test is presumptive laboratory evidence for pathogenicity of the genus *Staphylococcus.*

some of the purulent material. This is usually accomplished early in the treatment of oral surgery cases, since prompt incision and drainage of the abscess, as stated earlier, is generally indicated. An agar plate is inoculated with the freshly obtained material, and medicated disks, each containing a measured amount of antibiotics, are

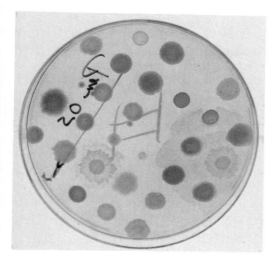

Fig. 9-3. Each disk contains various concentrations of penicillin, thus determining the degree of sensitivity more accurately.

spaced over the plate. If the microorganism is sensitive to the antibiotic, it will fail to grow around the medicated disk (Fig. 9-1). Resistant organisms will grow to the disk, and gradations of sensitivity or resistance may be present that can be evaluated by an experienced observer. If, however, the degree of susceptibility is important or if a mixed infection (more than one organism) is anticipated, other laboratory aids, such as the tube dilution method, are available.

It should be emphasized that although the laboratory procedures are important and should be used whenever possible, antibiotic therapy should not be delayed until results of the test are available. On the contrary, these drugs should be used and the antibiotic therapy altered if the laboratory studies warrant the change (Fig. 9-2).

For more sophisticated and sensitive determinations the agar-gel dilution method may be used for each antibiotic in which the concentration of the antibiotic tested is in micrograms per milliliter (Figs. 9-3 and 9-4).

Dosage and route of administration

When use of an antibiotic is contemplated, the dosage and route of administration are important considerations. The purpose of the therapy is to produce as

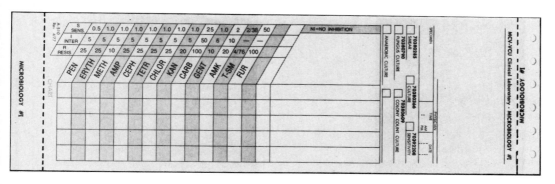

Fig. 9-4. In the agar-gel dilution method the results are interpreted in the following manner: S, Sensitive—no growth of the organism is found at the optimum concentration of the antibiotic. I, Intermediate—no growth of the organism is found at a much greater concentration. R, Resistant—very high concentrations of the antibiotic are required to ensure no growth of the organism. NI, No inhibition—there is growth of the organism regardless of the antibiotic exposure.

promptly as possible an optimum concentration of the drug at the site of infection and to maintain it at an effective level. The causative bacteria must, of course, be sensitive to the antibiotic used. Each antibiotic has its own characteristics regarding rate of absorption and excretion, which in turn are dependent on the mode of administration. For example, penicillin has a slower rate of absorption when administered orally as compared to parenteral injection, although some of the newer oral preparations have increased the rate of absorption considerably. The rate of absorption will also vary with the vehicle, whether oil or aqueous. In addition, penicillin combined chemically with a procaine radical has a much slower rate of absorption than potassium penicillin alone.

Dosage is also determined by the rate of inactivation and excretion of the drug used. When administered orally, several antibiotics are destroyed readily by the lower digestive tract, whereas some are absorbed very slowly and may be excreted before therapeutic value can be obtained. At one time it was thought that the maximum tolerated dose was the only limitation on the amount given a patient. This has been found to be an erroneous conception and can cause untoward side effects in the host. The premise that if a little does some good then a lot will do better does not apply in the use of antibiotics.

Antibiotics may be administered intramuscularly, intravenously, orally, or topically. With the exception of the latter method, the antibiotics reach the area of infection by way of the bloodstream. When placed intramuscularly, the site acts as a depot from which the drug is taken slowly into the bloodstream.

Intravenous administration produces a rapid, high level of concentration in the bloodstream, but the excretion rate is even more rapid. This method of administration is generally used when an acute fulminating disease must be treated with the utmost haste. To maintain an adequate level the intravenous method is often combined with one or more other routes of administration.

Originally the oral administration of some antibiotics was necessary, since this was the only route available other than the intravenous. This is no longer true, but this mode of administration has become popular with the doctor and the patient. It is painless and convenient and particularly valuable when children are concerned. Palatable oral suspensions are most advantageous in treating children. Several disadvantages occur with the oral route of administration, the most serious being the reliability of the patient. Therapy depends on the cooperation of the patient, who is likely to be lax and forgetful about maintaining the dosage at regular intervals for as long as it is necessary. Some clinicians have taken the attitude that if a patient is ill enough to warrant an antibiotic, they would rather administer the drug themselves, thereby having the assurance that the patient receives the drug and also the added opportunity of evaluating the patient's progress more often.

One of the most controversial subjects with respect to antibiotics is the topical use of these drugs. Perhaps the greatest hesitancy has arisen because serious complications have occurred with the use of the sulfonamide preparations in topical form. It has been well established that the topical use of the sulfonamides often induces allergic reactions in the host. This has caused severe complications, even death, and is definitely contraindicated except in specific and rare instances under strictly controlled conditions.

Antibiotics have caused similar allergic responses in the host and also tend to produce resistant strains of bacteria. In addition, in the oral cavity the topical use of some antibiotics leads to partial destruction of the normal oral flora, permitting the rapid overgrowth of some of the fungi. Normal antagonisms as well as normal symbiotic associations are eliminated, and a flora that is naturally resistant to the drug becomes predominant. Thrush, cheilitis, and the production of resistant strains that can cause superinfections may be the result of the indiscriminate use of topical antibiotics.

Some antibiotics cannot be given systemically without hazard to the host because of toxic reactions to the drug. On occasion it is most beneficial to use this group topically, particularly when the offending organism is resistant to the drugs normally employed. Fortunately these agents (bacitracin, tyrothricin, neomycin, polymyxin) are rather insoluble, which is a distinct advantage when used topically, and relatively nontoxic. They seldom produce allergic manifestations and only occasionally produce resistant strains.

The therapeutic value of these drugs in the field of dentistry is still questionable except in isolated instances. Maintaining sufficient concentration for therapeutic efficacy in the oral cavity is well nigh impossible because of the constant dilution by saliva. They can be used effectively in ointment form on the lips and soft tissues outside of the oral cavity, primarly as prophylactic agents. In the presence of a chronic osteomyelitis the topical antibiotics have been found most beneficial, particularly when one can be placed in a cavity of bone and maintained there in adequate concentration. Antiobiotics administered parenterally do not diffuse into infected bone in therapeutic concentrations as a result of a variety of factors, including impaired circulation and fibrous barriers. When this is the case, the practitioner must resort to any method left open to him. Parenteral therapy is indicated to prevent the spread of the infection, and topical administration is indicated in an effort to control and abort the infective process within bone.

Indiscriminate use of antibiotics

Undoubtedly the discovery of the antibiotics as therapeutic agents must be considered among the greatest advancements of medical science, but with their discovery came the unnecessary, indiscriminate, and dangerous use of these drugs. Antibiotics have their therapeutic limitations and on occasion can produce toxic results far more serious than the initial disease for which they may have been given. On the basis of present-day knowledge the practitioner must make a new appraisal of the situation and use these drugs in a more reasonable manner.

The two most hazardous sequelae of antibiotic therapy are the toxic reactions exhibited by the host and the increasing problem of drug resistance by numerous microorganisms. Bacterial resistance can occur in two basic forms—the naturally insensitive strains, which are present to some degree in all bacterial populations, and by far the most dangerous, resistant strains developed as a result of inadequate and indiscriminate use of antibiotics. Resistance to the drugs has been shown to develop when the bacteria are exposed to suboptimal concentrations. The practicing dentist must be made acutely aware of this problem since in some locales the habit of administering antibiotics in insufficient dosage has become common practice. After the removal of an impacted tooth, for example, the operator gives the patient a "shot" of penicillin as a prophylactic measure and then does not see the patient for subsequent antibiotic therapy. This procedure is to be condemned because it has little therapeutic value and can produce resistant strains of organisms that may cause the patient considerable damage.

Drug resistance is not dependent on inadequate dosage alone. Antibiotics administered therapeutically for protracted periods of time and producing excellent results for a specific organism may still cause alterations of other bacteria that can produce difficulty at a later date either for the host or by cross infection. As mentioned earlier, the problem of cross infection has become a serious one in hospitals throughout the country because of the production of resistant strains of staphylococcus. Rigid aseptic techniques must be adhered to in the dental office for this reason alone if for no other. Most of our population has received antibiotic therapy at one time or another and may be carriers of resistant strains of bacteria. It is imperative that those associated with the healing arts, as well as the lay public, be apprised of the ever-increasing problem of drug resistance, since the incidence is related in large measure to the indiscriminate use of antibiotics.

A toxic reaction of the host to antibiotic therapy is another complicating factor in the use of these drugs. It is more prevalent when the drugs are used indiscriminately and may be produced in two ways. First, a sensitivity or allergic response of the host to the drug may be produced, and second, the alteration of certain normal physiological activities of the host may be disturbed either by prolonged or massive dosage. The incidence of allergic responses to antibiotics is increasing primarily because of the repeated indiscriminate use of the drugs for trivial problems. As has already been pointed out, one of the best means of sensitizing a patient is by the use of topical preparations, particularly on the skin and oral mucosa. Erythemas, hives, and exfoliative dermatitis, are not uncommon and are occurring more frequently as the population becomes increasingly sensitive to the drugs. Having been forwarned by relatively minor reaction or by the patient's history, the practitioner should avoid the use of the offending drug or the results may be disastrous. Anaphylactoid reactions generally occur after the patient has had a minor reaction on a previous occasion. This reaction is characterized by the rapid onset of cyanosis, coughing, tonic spasm, a weak and thready pulse, and a marked drop in blood pressure. The incidence of serious and fatal results is increasing, and although more common after the use of penicillin, the problem cannot be ignored whenever any antibiotic is used.

Several antibiotics other than penicillin are capable of producing episodes of headaches, nausea, vomiting, and diarrhea.

Most often these reactions are mild and can be controlled with adjunctive therapy, but occasionally the symptoms become acute and difficult to treat. Vertigo, nerve damage, renal disorders, blood dyscrasias, and resistant secondary infections are but a few of the additional complications that may evolve from the use of antibiotics. The specific toxic reactions and contraindications of each drug will be discussed independently.

Masking of the true clinical entity is another complication of the indiscriminate use of antibiotics. When a patient has symptoms that suggest infection, treatment must not consist of antibiotic therapy alone. It is equally important to establish the diagnosis before treatment is instituted. For example, if a patient gives symptoms of infection in the maxillary arch, an acute sinusitis and even a malignancy of the maxillary sinus might be masked if antibiotics are given on the premise that an acute apical abscess is the causative factor. Once the drug has been administered it is conceivable that the acute symptoms may subside and lie dormant only to arise again at some later date with more serious consequences. Antibiotics administered in the presence of pus may also complicate the problem. Surgery is still the best means of treating a fluctuant infected area, and it should be borne in mind that antibiotic therapy is only adjunctive therapy. Failure to evacuate pus might well produce what is known as a "sterile abscess," and although dormant for awhile, it will be activated again with increased virulence.

Specific antibiotics

New antibiotics and modifications of old ones are being released frequently by various pharmaceutical houses. This is a natural by-product of active and competitive research and is to be encouraged. It is necessary if the increasing number of resistant strains and incidence of superinfections are to be combated. The antibiotics of today may be useless or outmoded tomorrow, although the ones that are to be discussed have stood the test of time reasonably well.

Recent laboratory investigations suggest that there may be some previously undetected anaerobic bacteria that may be causing some severe infections of dental origin. Until recently most cultures have been only for aerobic bacteria. The penicillin-resistant, anaerobic bacteria may require dentists to alter their choice of antibiotics. More research is in progress.

An effort has been made to discuss the antibiotics on a generic basis rather than by proprietary names.

Penicillin

Although the oldest antibiotic, penicillin is still the most widely used. Penicillin is a selective inhibitor of bacterial cell wall synthesis in multiplying bacteria because of its capacity to inhibit formation of the cross linkages in the mucopeptide lattice. The inhibiting of cell wall synthesis may not in itself be lethal, but under the osmotic conditions in body fluids, which are normally hypotonic in relation to the interior of the bacteria, lysis of the organisms results. Penicillin is effective against gram-positive streptococci and staphylococci, which are of particular interest to the oral surgeon. It is also effective against several gram-negative cocci, notably meningococci and gonococci, but most gram-negative rods are naturally resistant. In addition, most spirochetes are sensitive, making penicillin the drug of choice in syphilis. With the exception of those infections in which resistant organisms and some gram-negative organisms are present and those patients in which allergic responses occur, penicillin is still the desirable drug for the treatment of oral infections.

Preparation and dosage. Penicillin is available in numerous preparations for intramuscular, oral, and intravenous use and is combined with various chemical radicals and carrying agents to produce short or long effective doses.

INTRAMUSCULAR. Because of the recent increase in allergic reactions to penicillin, some clinicians have discontinued the use of intramuscular penicillin except when the patient is hospitalized. Treatment of allergic manifestations after intramuscular injection is more difficult than treatment of those reactions resulting from the oral route.

1. Procaine penicillin G is the preparation most frequently used today as a prophylactic and therapeutic drug. One milliliter contains 300,000 units, and the recommended dose is 600,000 units a day for moderately severe infections, with a reduction in dosage toward the end of treatment. When the patient requires hospitalization, it is practical and desirable to administer the drug every 12 hours.

2. Crystalline potassium penicillin G in aqueous suspension was one of the original preparations, but because of its rapid absorption, it is used in combination with procaine penicillin G, except in intravenous therapy. The combining of these two penicillin preparations (referred to as fortified) permits a rapid, high blood level (30 to 60 minutes) with a maintenance level. The usual dosage is 1 ml (300,000 units of procaine penicillin and 100,000 units of crystalline potassium penicillin) given every 12 or 24 hours, depending on the severity of the infection.

3. Benzathine penicillin G is a long-acting preparation that has found favor with those who feel the need for a prolonged blood level in their patient. The average dose is 300,000 to 600,000 units every 10 days. Like procaine penicillin it can be combined with aqueous penicillin, thus giving a high level for 24 hours and then sustaining a low blood level. Its most frequent use in oral surgery is as a prophylaxis against secondary infection or in treatment of a systemic condition such as rheumatic fever. It is not generally used in the treatment of acute infections and should not be used if the patient is sensitive to iodides.

4. More recently the semisynthetic derivatives methicillin, oxacillin, and nafcillin have become available. As noted previously, the indiscriminate use of antibiotics can produce resistant strains, and many in-

fections today are caused by resistant penicillinase-producing staphylococci These new semisynthetic penicillins may be used for this type of infection, in which resistant strains such as those of hospital-acquired infections are suspected. However, sensitivity of the bacterium should be determined by in vitro tests when possible.

Penicillinase-resistant drugs should be restricted to treatment of resistant staphylococcus infections, since extensive or indiscriminate use of these drugs may produce more resistant strains of bacteria.

The intramuscular dosage and frequency of administration for the new semisynthetic penicillins vary from 250 mg to 1.5 Gm every 4 to 6 hours, depending on the drug used, size and age of the patient, and severity of infection. Before the dosage is established, all pertinent factors should be evaluated and a review of the prescribed dosage studied.

ORAL. The more recent preparations of oral penicillin have an excellent absorption rate in the bloodstream. When one is assured of a cooperative patient, these preparations are effective even for serious infections. It should be emphasized that the oral penicillins should be taken when the stomach is empty, to minimize gastric retention, and preferably with an antacid.

1. Penicillin G, as an oral preparation, has been available for some time, but some hesitancy has prevailed about its use because the degree and rate of absorption are variable. In addition, one must depend on the patient to take the drug exactly as prescribed, since a high blood level is not sustained for any length of time. When used, the average dose is 250 mg (250,000 units) given four times a day. This is believed to be equal in effectiveness to one injection of 300,000 units intramuscularly.

2. Penicillin V (pheneticillin) is a more recent and popular development and is being used rather extensively for the oral administration of penicillin. This drug has been found to be reliable in its rate of absorption and effective blood level. It is also compatible with penicillin G, which may have been given during the acute phase of an infectious process. It is generally administered three or four times a day and is available either in tablets or capsules containing from 125 to 300 mg (200,000 to 500,000 units). Oral suspensions containing 125 mg. per teaspoonful are available for children.

3. As noted previously, a number of new semisynthetic penicillins are available. Those that are prepared for administration by the oral route are ampicillin, cloxacillin, nafcillin, and oxacillin. Here, too, the exact dosage depends on the age and size of the patient and severity of the infection. The dosage for these drugs will vary from 250 mg to 1 Gm every 4 to 6 hours. A careful evaluation of the problem is imperative.

TOPICAL. In the past, penicillin had been available in various topical forms, but because of the high incidence of sensitivities reported, the Food and Drug Administration no longer permits the sale of topical penicillin preparations.

Precautions. As noted previously the route of administration must be carefully considered before penicillin is prescribed. In addition, the following precautions must be prudently observed.

1. Penicillin should not be administered if the patient has a history of reaction, however mild, after previous use of the drug.

2. The administration of penicillin to patients with a history of allergy, such as hay fever, should be viewed with caution, since these individuals are more prone to sensitization.

3. Penicillin therapy should be discontinued at the first sign of allergic symptoms to the drug, including minor reactions such as itching and redness at the site of injection (Fig. 9-5).

4. When penicillin is administered intramuscularly, extreme care should be taken to avoid an accidental intravenous injection.

5. If used intramuscularly, it is preferable to administer penicillin in the deltoid or

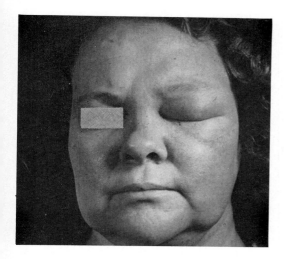

Fig. 9-5. Allergic response after the administration of penicillin.

triceps of the arm so that a tourniquet may be applied if the patient gives any indication of an anaphylactoid reaction.

Erythromycin

Erythromycin has a bacterial spectrum similar to that of penicillin, and because of its unequaled safety record it is used by many clinicians in preference to penicillin, particularly for oral infections. It is active against the gram-positive cocci and a few of the gram-negative rods. It has also been reported to be effective against some of the viruses, rickettsiae, and certain strains of the diphtheria bacilli. Like penicillin, it may be either bactericidal or bacteriostatic, depending on the concentration of the drug and the organisms involved. Strains of *Staphylococcus aureus* that are insensitive to penicillin may be susceptible to erythromycin. This drug has its chief usefulness in the management of infections produced by staphylococci or other penicillin-resistant gram-positive organisms.

Erythromycin is indicated for treatment of a large variety of infections caused by a wide spectrum of susceptible microorganisms. Indications include cases in which use of other antibiotics is limited by unde-

sirable or serious side effects. In cases in which organisms have become resistant to other antibiotics, particularly penicillin, erythromycin is often the drug of choice.

Side effects from the administration of erythromycin are rare. The oral administration may occasionally cause mild gastrointestinal disturbances, but the withdrawal of the drug is rarely necessary, since the symptoms disappear promptly.

Serious complications are extremely rare, but several proprietary preparations should be used cautiously when liver function is impaired.

Preparation and dosage. The usual mode of administration of erythromycin is orally, but it is available for intramuscular or intravenous use if the infection is of sufficient magnitude. It is supplied in enteric-coated tablets of 100 and 250 mg. The usual dosage for an adult is one or two tablets every 6 hours, depending on the severity of infection. Pediatric oral suspensions are available that contain 100 mg per teaspoonful (5 ml) and should be given every 4 to 6 hours.

The tetracyclines

The tetracyclines are a group of antibiotics that has been developed over the past several years, and although they differ slightly chemically, their pharmacological and therapeutic actions are essentially the same. The most notable of this group are chlortetracycline, oxytetracycline, and tetracycline. Although they are dispensed under numerous proprietary names, they will be discussed together.

The tetracyclines belong to the so-called broad-spectrum antibiotics because they are effective against many gram-positive and gram-negative bacteria. They are primarily bacteriostatic in their action and normally are effective against all pathogenic organisms arising from the oral cavity. They are also effective in the treatment of some rickettsiae infections. These drugs are of considerable importance in that many gram-positive organisms resistant to penicillin and some of the gram-negative organisms resistant to streptomycin are susceptible to the tetracyclines.

Like most antibiotics, these drugs produce resistant strains, but fortunately the susceptible organisms do not develop resistance rapidly, with the exception of certain gram-negative strains.

Preparation and dosage. The tetracyclines are generally administered orally, but intravenous preparations are available if desired. The standard oral regimen for the average acute infection is 0.25 to 0.5 Gm (250 to 500 mg) every 6 hours for a total daily dose of 1 to 2 Gm. For children this dosage is reduced to 100 mg every 6 hours. Most of the proprietary preparations are available in oral suspension in which 5 ml (1 teaspoonful) contains 100 mg of the antibiotic. This is a particularly effective mode of administration for children who are unable to tolerate a capsule. When the infection is of sufficient magnitude, the drug may be prescribed every 4 hours instead of every 6. Interestingly enough, increasing the antibiotic intake by increasing the dose is of little value, since the use of a dosage beyond the optimum amount fails to produce proportionately higher blood levels because of some limiting factor in the ability of the intestinal mucosa to absorb the antibiotics.

Intravenous preparations are available for those patients who require a rapid high blood level as a result of the severity of the infection. In instances in which the patient cannot take oral medications, this mode of administration is most acceptable. Unconsciousness, trismus produced by infection, and mechanical immobilization of the mandible are several instances that would warrant the use of the intravenous preparations. The dosage will vary from 500 to 1,000 mg administered with 5% glucose intravenous solution every 12 hours. Injecting these antibiotics in concentration should be done with some hesitancy because they can produce a thrombus within the vessel. Intramuscular and subcutaneous injections are not recommended, since they are painful and may cause tissue damage associated with their irritating action. Several new preparations have eliminated this problem.

Topical preparations have been withdrawn from the market by the Food and Drug Administration. In dentistry, topical preparations have been used in the past to treat various manifestations of periodontal disease and postextraction wounds. Some clinical evidence has supported their use, but systemic administration is undoubtedly more effective and less likely to produce resistant strains and host sensitivity.

Precautions. Signs that indicate discontinuance of the tetracyclines include the following:

1. Perhaps the most frequent untoward reaction of the host to the tetracyclines is the occurrence of nausea and diarrhea. Should the diarrhea continue unabated the drug must be discontinued immediately to avoid severe complications. Discontinuing the drug will usually permit the gastrointestinal flora to return to normal, thus aborting a possible fatal outcome.

2. Glossitis, stomatitis, and skin eruptions are not unusual after the administration of one of the tetracyclines, particularly when a topical preparation has been employed. The appearance of these relatively minor allergic manifestations warrants the prompt discontinuance of the drug—they may be a warning of more serious manifestations of drug sensitivity.

3. Prolonged use of the tetracyclines may permit the overgrowth of organisms that are not susceptible to the antibiotic. The overproduction of *Candida albicans,* for example, can produce symptoms that are painful and persistent. Oral discomfort and anal and vaginal itching are common manifestations of moniliasis and may be very difficult to treat. The drug should be discontinued promptly if these symptoms arise.

4. When an infectious organism fails to show any clinical sensitivity to one of the tetracyclines, it is most unlikely that it will respond to any in the group. Similarly, a patient with an allergic response to one is

likely to have the same response to any of the tetracyclines.

5. Of particular interest to dentists is that the tetracyclines are deposited in calcifying areas of bones and teeth and may cause a yellow to gray discoloration. The discoloration of the teeth was first noted by Schwachman and associates during assessment of long-term tetracycline therapy in children with fibrocystic disease. The phenomenon has been confirmed by many investigators since then, and long-term therapy with tetracycline in children is to be strongly discouraged because the cosmetic effect on the dentition can be severe.

Streptomycin

Streptomycin and dihydrostreptomycin are effective against a number of gram-positive and gram-negative organisms. These antibiotics interfere with bacterial protein synthesis, and it is postulated that this effect may account for their bactericidal activity. These drugs are ineffective in syphilis and in infections caused by clostridia, fungi, and rickettsiae. Because of their toxic side effects and the relative ease with which microorganisms become resistant, their general use for infections about the oral cavity is not recommended except as a last resort.

Preparation and dosage. Intramuscular injection of streptomycin (or dihydrostreptomycin) is the only effective means of administering the drug. Dosage ranges from 1 to 3 Gm daily in divided doses of 0.5 Gm.

Precautions. The following complications may accompany the use of these two drugs and must be watched for carefully. These drugs should be discontinued immediately if untoward symptoms appear.

1. The topical use of streptomycin is contraindicated because of the high degree of sensitization.

2. Both streptomycin and dihydrostreptomycin have been reported as producing vestibular and auditory damage even in small doses. Recovery of vestibular function may occur after the drug is withdrawn, but auditory damage may be irreversible.

3. Renal complications may occur after the use of these drugs, and when renal malfunction is present, the drug is contraindicated.

Chloramphenicol

Chloramphenicol is a broad-spectrum antibiotic and is effective against most pathogenic organisms associated with the oral cavity. In addition, the rickettsiae and some viruses respond to this drug. It is a specific therapeutic agent for typhoid fever. The spectrum is not unlike that of the tetracyclines, and chloramphenicol is bacteriostatic in its action. Its molecular weight is lower than that of the other broad-spectrum antibiotics, and thus it is capable of producing a rapid, high blood concentration, which is advantageous in severe infections. The drug's high diffusibility results in effective concentration in the cerebrospinal fluid. This attribute makes the drug particularly valuable in treatment of severe maxillary fractures complicated by cerebrospinal rhinorrhea. It is effective against many microorganisms that have developed a resistance to the older, more frequently used drugs. Chloramphenicol, like all antibiotics, produces resistant strains, and its indiscriminate use, particularly in minor infections, should be avoided, or its present advantage will probably be dissipated.

Preparation and dosage. The average adult daily dose of chloramphenicol is 1 to 2 Gm in divided dosage, either four times during the day or every 6 hours, depending on the necessity of a constant blood level. The drug is dispensed for oral administration in 50, 100, and 250 mg capsule form. For children an oral suspension is available that provides 125 mg per teaspoonful (5 ml).

For the average infectious process the oral administration is preferred, but when indicated, chloramphenicol may be administered intravenously or intramuscularly. The adult dose for intravenous administration is 0.5 to 1 Gm every 6 to 12 hours, either with a physiological sodium chloride solution or 5% dextrose in normal saline solution. This mode of administration should be discontinued as soon as the patient can take oral medication.

Chloramphenicol also may be administered intramuscularly in 1 Gm doses and because of its repository quality can be given only every 12 to 24 hours. This generally sustains an adequate blood level to combat most infections.

Precautions. Continuing and careful study of the patient who is taking this drug is necessary. Chloramphenicol should not be used when other and less potentially dangerous agents will be effective.

1. Chloramphenicol is a potent therapeutic agent, and certain blood dycrasias have been associated with its administration, although to a lesser degree of frequency than was originally thought when the drug was first introduced. Depression of the bone marrow may result in neutropenia, agranulocytosis, or, in extreme cases, aplastic anemia. Prolonged administration is to be avoided, and blood studies (complete blood count [CBC] and differential) should be made every 48 hours during treatment. It has been suggested that chloramphenicol not be administered longer than 10 days to an adult and 7 days to a child.

2. Like the tetracyclines, chloramphenicol is capable of producing nausea and diarrhea, but the latter complication occurs much less often since this antibiotic does not suppress the intestinal flora as readily. This is explained on the basis that it is absorbed more rapidly in the upper intestinal tract and does not reach the large bowel in any quantity.

3. Moniliasis, which occurs with the use of most of the antibiotics, may also result from prolonged or topical use of this drug.

Novobiocin

Novobiocin is an antibiotic that has been found to be effective in treating infections caused by both gram-positive and gram-negative bacteria. It has been effective against some strains of *Staphylococcus aureus* and is also used in infections caused by hemolytic streptococcus, *Diplococcus pneumoniae,* and *Proteus vulgaris*.

Preparation and dosage. The recommended dosage in adults is 500 mg every 12 hours or 250 mg every 6 hours, continued for at least 48 hours after the temperature has returned to normal and all evidence of infection has disappeared. In particularly severe infections it may be desirable to double the average dosage. The route of administration is orally in the form of capsules and a syrup for children. The syrup contains 125 mg per teaspoonful.

Precautions. Novobiocin is not recommended for treatment of any infection because of frequency of cholestatic jaundice, allergic reactions, gastrointestinal disturbance, neonatal hyperbilirubinemia, and fatal blood dyscrasias.

Lincomycin

Lincomycin has an antibacterial spectrum similar to that of erythromycin. In vitro it inhibits the growth of many gram-positive organisms, especially staphylococci, including penicillinase-producing staphylococci, pneumococci, and some streptococci. It appears to have little effect on enterococci, meningococci, and gonococci, and it is inactive against gram-negative bacilli.

Favorable responses have been reported from its use in cases of osteomyelitis. Lincomycin is useful in the treatment of infections caused by sensitive organisms when resistance to penicillin or erythromycin has developed or when these drugs cannot be used because the patient is allergic to them. The drug may be administered in combination therapy with other antimicrobial agents when indicated.

Preparation and dosage. Lincomycin is adequately absorbed either by the oral or intramuscular route. The oral dosage for adults is 500 mg given three or four times daily. The intramuscular dosage is 600 mg every 12 hours or more frequently in severe infections. Oral dosage for children is based on weight (15 to 30 mg per pound).

Precautions. Since lincomycin is a relatively new drug, patients must be observed carefully for the appearance of unforeseen reactions. Patients receiving treatment for longer than 1 or 2 weeks should have liver function tests.

1. Because of the lack of adequate clinical data, use of the drug is not indicated in those patients with preexisting kidney, liver, or metabolic diseases.

2. Evidence of moniliasis or monilial infection necessitates prompt discontinuance of the drug.

3. Minor gastrointestinal disturbances such as nausea, vomiting, abdominal cramps, and diarrhea have been reported.

Clindamycin

Clindamycin phosphate is produced from the same synthetic group as lincomycin. Although clindamycin phosphate is inactive in vitro, rapid in vivo hydrolysis converts the compound to the antibacterially active clindamycin, and orally it is more rapidly absorbed from the gastrointestinal tract than lincomycin. Recent studies seem to indicate that clindamycin is more potent than lincomycin.

It is believed that this drug is effective against *Staphylococcus aureus* and *S. epidermidis,* streptococci, and some anaerobic organisms such as the *bacteroides* species. Clindamycin is widely distributed in body fluids and tissues, including bone, and for this reason is found to be effective when treating chronic bone infections of dental origin such as osteomyelitis.

Preparation and dosage. Clindamycin may be administered intravenously, intramuscularly, or orally, with about the same effectiveness, except for severe infections. When administered parenterally the usual dosage is from 600 to 1,200 mg daily divided into two, three, or four equal doses. Oral administration is usually 150 mg every 6 hours but may be increased to 300 mg per dose without any untoward reactions.

Precautions. The following factors are to be considered for the safe use of clindamycin.

1. Clindamycin is contraindicated in those patients who may have exhibited a hypersensitivity to lincomycin.

2. During prolonged therapy, periodic liver and kidney function tests and blood counts should be performed because transient neutropenias and transient liver abnormalities have been noted.

3. Gastrointestinal symptoms, such as nausea and vomiting, occasionally occur with the oral administration of clindamycin.

Kanamycin

Kanamycin sulfate is the salt of an antibiotic derived from strains of *Streptomyces kanamycetius.* The antibacterial activity is similar to that of neomycin. It is active against many aerobic gram-positive and gram-negative bacteria. This drug is indicated for the treatment of serious infections caused by susceptible organisms. When osteomyelitis, bacteremias, and soft tissue have shown resistance to conventional antibiotics, kanamycin may be used if the causative bacteria have been shown to be sensitive by in vitro studies.

Preparation and dosage. Kanamycin may be administered by the intramuscular, intravenous, or oral route. The oral administration of the drug should be reserved for those patients with gastrointestinal problems, since the drug is poorly absorbed from the gastrointestinal tract and therefore not too effective in systemic problems. The intramuscular route is generally the route of choice, and the dosage is calculated not to exceed 0.7 mg per pound of body weight in two or three divided doses.

Precautions. As noted previously, kanamycin should be reserved for infections resistant to other antibiotics. Patients should be carefully evaluated during the administration of the drug and probably should be hospitalized.

1. The major toxic effect of parenterally administered kanamycin is its action on the

auditory portion of the eighth nerve. Excessive dosage seems to be a factor, and use of the drug should not be prolonged unnecessarily. Deafness may be partial or complete, and in most cases it has been irreversible.

2. Renal irritations frequently occur in those patients with prior kidney problems or in those patients who are not well hydrated.

Cephalosporins

The cephalosporins are bactericidal by inhibition of cell wall synthesis. They are not hydrolyzed by penicillinase, and there is little or no cross resistance with penicillins. They have a broader spectrum than penicillins but are less active against grampositive organisms. Resistance can develop by cephalosporinase production. In distribution, 55% to 65% of the drug is bound to plasma protein. From 70% to 80% is excreted unchanged in the urine.

Dosage types are as follows: cephalexin monohydrate (Keflex) is oral, cephaloridine (Loridine) is parenteral, and cephalothin (Keflin) is parenteral. the last two are nephrotoxic in high doses.

Toxicity is low compared to penicillins. Adverse effects include skin rashes and occasional allergic reactions and cross allergenicity to penicillins. In addition, gastrointestinal disturbance occurs occasionally with cephalexin monohydrates, and rare hepatic dysfunction occurs with cephaloridine and cephalothin.

Polymyxin B

Polymyxin B has its principal effect on gram-negative bacteria (except proteus species) and should be reserved for this group. It has been used primarily as a topical drug, but the incidence of gram-negative strains has forced clinicians to resort to polymyxin B for systemic use.

Topical polymyxin is usually nontoxic and nonsensitizing. It has been combined in complex preparations for use as troches and ointments.

Systemic administration must be carefully controlled, since the drug may induce nephrotoxic or neurological disturbances (dizziness, facial paralysis) or both. The problems are not pronounced when the recommended dosage range is not exceeded.

Preparation and dosage. The suggested route of administration is by intramuscular injection at intervals of 8 hours. The total daily dose is from 1.5 to 2.5 mg per kilogram of body weight. The maximum dosage must not exceed 200 mg.

Precautions. In those patients who exhibit any impairment of renal function, the use of polymyxin should be avoided. If the patient has normal renal function, the nephrotoxic effects of the drug may become evident on the fourth or fifth day of treatment, but these can generally be controlled if the recommended dosage is not exceeded. The same is true regarding the neurological disturbances.

It should be emphasized that polymyxin B must be reserved for those patients afflicted with an infection caused by organisms proved to be sensitive to the drug.

Local antibiotics

Antibiotics that are not normally used as systemic drugs because of their toxicity but have some benefits when used topically are referred to as local antibiotics. Used systemically they produce untoward complications and are therefore contraindicated except under dire circumstances. One common characteristic is their ability to be used topically with allergic reactions held to a minimum. These agents do have a place in dentistry, but it should be borne in mind that the concentrations employed are insufficient to control the infection and should be used as adjunctive therapy. These local antibiotics have been prepared commercially in various combinations and concentrations. Only a brief résumé of their specific characteristics seems indicated.

Bacitracin. Bacitracin is active against fusiform bacilli and some spirochetes and has a range similar to that of penicillin. Because of this relationship in activity it may be effective when employed with systemic penicillin in combating Vincent's infection. The effectiveness of bacitracin is not altered by serum, pus, or necrotic tissue. This characteristic makes it valuable in the treatment of osteomyelitis when the infected area can be approached directly and an adequate concentration maintained. To be effective the drug must be in contact with the pathogenic organisms.

Neomycin. Neomycin is bactericidal in vitro against both gram-negative and gram-positive organisms. Although occasionally administered parenterally, it has no general application because of the toxic effect on the kidneys and on the eighth nerve. Topically it is effective in skin infections and has been combined with other local antibiotics in the preparation of troches and ointments. The troches have been of value in controlling secondary local infection, particularly in those persons who are allergic to a number of the parenteral antibiotics.

Tyrothricin. Tyrothricin, like bacitracin, is particularly effective against the gram-positive organisms. It is made up principally of two active ingredients, gramicidin and tyrocidine. It is most effective when in direct contact with the offending microorganisms. Applied in compress form to open wounds it has been effective, and infected bone lesions have responded favorably when the drug, in solution, is carried directly to the injured part. The usual concentration is 0.01% to 0.05% in isotonic solution irrigated directly into the wound through a drain two or three times daily. Tyrothricin is also prepared in troche form, particularly to combat streptococcal oral infections.

SULFONAMIDES

As a group the sulfonamides have been replaced by the antibiotics primarily because of the dramatic effect of the newer agents and the toxicity of the older drug. Now, however, the antibiotics are producing resistant organisms that can be treated with the sulfonamides, and improvements have been made in these drugs that make them less toxic.

The primary toxic complication of the sulfonamides when they were first introduced was crystalluria, resulting in renal shutdown. Drug fever, dermatitis, and alterations in the blood-forming organs, with resultant hemolytic anemia, leukopenia,

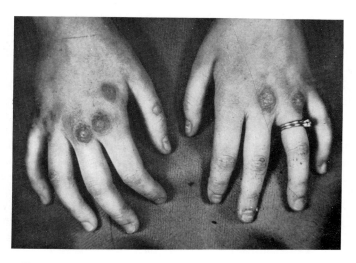

Fig. 9-6. Skin reaction after the adminstration of sulfadiazine.

and agranulocytosis, were additional complications (Fig. 9-6). Most of these complications have been eliminated or at least minimized by proper controls during administration and by the combination of three of the sulfonamides into one medication. The combination of sulfadiazine, sulfamerazine, and sulfamethazine into a triple sulfonamide preparation has reduced toxic reactions considerably. Sulfisoxazole and sulfadimetine are also well tolerated when properly administered and controlled.

Triple sulfonamides are prepared in 0.5 Gm tablets, and the dosage is generally 2 Gm initially to be followed by 1 Gm every 6 hours. Oral suspension for children is also available in concentrations of 0.5 Gm in each teaspoonful. Dosage for a child is usually one-half the adult dose. Most authorities recommend that an equal amount of sodium bicarbonate be given with each dose of the sulfonamides. This will reduce the incidence of urinary tract complications.

Precautions. The following factors are considered in the safe use of the drugs:

1. A history of previous sulfonamide sensitivity would normally contraindicate the further use of these drugs unless the exact sensitizing drug could be ascertained.

2. Daily supervision of the patient and constant observation for signs of toxicity are imperative in sulfonamide therapy.

3. High fluid intake is mandatory to avoid renal complications, and urinary output should be above 1,200 ml per day.

4. Measurement of sulfonamide blood concentrations is indicated in severe infections to maintain a sufficient therapeutic level.

5. CBC and urinalysis should be done every other day to ascertain any early toxic reaction.

6. Patients should be advised to avoid any unnecessary exposure to ultraviolet rays, since photosensitivity may result.

ADJUNCTIVE THERAPY

In the use of antibiotics the practitioner is often confronted with the necessity of using other drugs as supportive therapy or to combat the complications of the antibiotic. To discuss the relative merits and defects of each drug would be impossible but an awareness of what agents are available seems appropriate.

Vitamins

Vitamins are well established as an effective group of drugs in the treatment of dental problems; they have been useful in treating gingival disorders, cheilitis, and impaired healing. When antibiotics are used, vitamins are valuable in supplementing the dietary intake, particularly when the antibiotics are administered orally. Several of the broad-spectrum drugs cause a decrease in the intestinal flora, which may produce an avitaminosis. Numerous vitamins are dependent on the intestinal bacteria for their production, and, in the prolonged use of antibiotics, supportive vitamins should be administered. A therapeutic vitamin preparation that includes the B complex, ascorbic acid, and various minerals is usually adequate. A recent study indicated that tetracycline therapy is more effective and rapidly induced with minimum dosage when administered with ascorbic acid. The recommended dosage is 500 mg of ascorbic acid for every 250 mg of the tetracyclines.

Antihistamines

Allergic reactions to antibiotic therapy make it imperative to have some effective means of treating these untoward manifestations. The antihistamines are useful in treating urticaria, itching, allergic rhinitis, serum sickness, and angioneurotic edema. Penicillin is undoubtedly the antiobic that produces most of the local reactions, and should mild symptoms appear, antihistamine therapy is indicated to keep the reaction to a minimum. Prompt therapy will make the patient more comfortable and may prevent more serious complications.

Many antihistamines are available in the form of elixirs, tablets, and nasal sprays and in combinations with other drugs. Intravenous and intramuscular preparations are also available when a rapid high level is necessary. Most of these drugs currently available may produce drowsiness or vertigo in some patients. Less frequently encountered is nausea. The advantages, disadvantages, and dosage of each antihistamine are not within the scope of this text. A pharmacology reference provides an excellent source in the selection of the proper drug and dosage.

Cortisone, hydrocortisone, and epinephrine are used when the allergic manifestations become marked. Administered in suitable formulations and by the appropriate route, these drugs usually give dramatic relief. They should be used judiciously and in consultation with the patient's physician if the symptoms are severe or therapy is prolonged.

Penicillinase

An enzyme, penicillinase, has been introduced for the specific purpose of combating allergic reactions to penicillin. It catalyzes the hydrolysis of penicillin to penicilloic acid, which is nonallergenic. Whereas the antihistamines and steroids treat the effects of an allergic response to penicillin, this specific enzyme counteracts the cause of the reaction by neutralizing the penicillin itself.

The drug is administered intramuscularly as soon as signs and symptoms of a reaction appear. It may be repeated daily if needed and should be given intravenously in the presence of an anaphylactoid reaction to penicillin.

SEQUELAE

The use of antibiotics as a prophylaxis against possible infectious complications has become fairly common practice. It is now clear on the basis of recent studies that in most situations such prophylaxis is of no value and in many cases superinfections result. It appears that the unnecessary and prolonged use of antibiotics may induce, rather than prevent, infection. One recent assessment on a general surgical service showed that when antibiotics were used arbitrarily the incidence of infections in the group receiving systemic prophylactic antibiotics after clean surgery was three times higher than in the group receiving none.

These findings do not preclude the necessity of administering antibiotics in selected cases, giving them to the patient with rheumatic fever or severe facial injuries, but one should develop a cautious approach to the use of these drugs.

REFERENCES

1. American Dental Association: Accepted dental therapeutics, ed. 36, Chicago, 1977, The Association.
2. American Heart Association Committee Report: Prevention of bacterial endocarditis, Circulation **55:**139A-143A, 1977.
3. American Medical Association: Drug evaluations, Chicago, 1972, The Association.
4. Archard, H. O., and Roberts, W. C.: Bacterial endocarditis after dental procedures in patients with aortic valve prostheses, J. Am. Dent. Assoc. **72:**648, 1966.
5. Billings, F.: Chronic focal infections and their etiological relations to arthritis and nephritis, Arch. Intern. Med. **9:**484, 1912.
6. Burton, D. S., and Schurman, D. J.: Hematogenous infection in bilateral total hip arthroplasty, J. Bone Joint Surg. **57A:**1004, 1975.
7. The choice of antimicrobial drugs, vol. 18, no. 3, New Rochelle, N.Y., Jan. 1976, The Medical Letter, Inc.
8. Cruess, R. L., Beckel, W. S., and Van Kessler, K.L.C.: Infection in total hips secondary to a primary source elsewhere, Clin. Orthop. **106:**99, 1975.
9. D'Ambrosia, R. D., Shoji, H., and Heater, R.: Secondary infected total hip replacement by hematogenous spread, J. Bone Joint Surg. **58-A:**450, 1976.
10. Davis, W. M., Jr., and Balcom, J. H., III: Lincomycin studies of drug absorption and efficacy, Oral Surg. **27:**688, 1969.
11. Donoff, R. B., and Guralnick, W.: Shock due to odontogenic infection, J. Oral Surg. **35:**569, 1977.
12. Editorial: Prophylaxis of bacterial endocarditis. Faith, hope and charitable interpretations, Lancet **1:**519, 1976.
13. Edlich, R. F., Madden, J. E., Prusak, M., and others: Studies in the management of the contaminated wound; the therapeutic value of gentle scrubbing in prolonging the limited period of effec-

tiveness of antibiotics in contaminated wounds, Am. J. Surg. **121:**668, 1971.

14. Feder, M. J., Stratigos, G. T., and Marra, L. M.: Idiopathic submandibular and submental infections in children, J. Oral Surg. **29:**255, 1971.

15. Gabrielson, M. L., and Stroh, E.: Antibiotic efficacy in odontogenic infections, J. Oral Surg. **33:**607, 1975.

16. Goldberg, M. H.: Antibiotics and oral and oralcutaneous lacerations, J. Oral Surg. **23:**117, 1965.

17. Goodman, L. S., and Gilman, A.: The pharmacological basis of therapeutics, ed. 5, New York, 1975, The Macmillan Co.

18. Gould, L., and Sperber, R. J.: Prevention of subacute bacterial endocarditis associated with dental procedures, Am. Heart J. **71:**134, 1966.

19. Handbook of antimicrobial therapy, vol. 14, New Rochelle, N.Y., 1972, The Medical Letter, Inc.

20. Hooley, J. R., and Meyer, R.: Anaphylactic reaction to oral penicillin, Oral Surg. **22:**474, 1966.

21. Johnston, F. R. C.: An assessment of prophylactic antibiotics in general surgery, Surg. Gynecol. Obstet. **116:**1, 1963.

22. Khosla, V. M.: Current concepts in the treatment of acute and chronic osteomyelitis: review and report of four cases, J. Oral Surg. **28:**209, 1970.

23. King, G. C.: The case against antibiotic prophylaxis in major head and neck surgery, Laryngoscope **71:**647, 1961.

24. Kislak, J. W.: The treatment of endocarditis, Am. Heart J. **79:**713, 1970.

25. Kucers, A.: The use of antibiotics, Philadelphia, 1972, J. B. Lippincott Co.

26. Mehrhof, A. I., Jr.: Clindamycin: an evaluation of its role in dental patients, J. Oral Surg. **34:**811, 1976.

27. Meyer, R. D., and Finegold, S. M.: Anaerobic infections: diagnosis and treatment, South. Med. J. **69:**9, 1178, 1976.

28. Moellering, R. C., Jr., and Swartz, M. N.: The newer cephalosporins, N. Engl. J. Med. **291:**1, 24, 1976.

29. Moore, R. A.: A textbook of pathology, Philadelphia, 1948, W. B. Saunders Co.

30. Nakajima, T., and others: Surgical treatment of chronic osteomyelitis of the mandible resistant to intraarterial infusion of antibiotics, J. Oral Surg. **35:**823, 1977.

31. Parker, M. T., and Ball, L. C.: Streptococci and aerococci associated with systemic infection in man, J. Med. Microbiol. **9:**275, 1976.

32. Physician's desk reference, ed. 27, Oradell, N.J., 1973, Medical Economics Co.

33. Quayle, A. A.: Bacteroides infections in oral surgery, J. Oral Surg. **32:**91, 1974.

34. Report of Council on Dental Therapeutics: Prevention of bacterial endocarditis, J. Am. Dent. Assoc. **95:**600-605, 1977.

35. Reports of Council and Bureaus: Prevention of bacterial endocarditis, J. Am. Dent. Assoc. **95:** 600, 1977.

36. Robson, M. C.: A new look at diabetes mellitus and infection, Am. J. Surg. **120:**681, 1970.

37. Rosenow, E. C.: Studies on elective localization of focal infection with special reference to oral sepsis, J. Dent. Res. **1:**205, 1919.

38. Rosoff, C. B., and Fine, J.: Antibiotic therapy for major trauma, Surg. Clin. North Am. **46:**605, 1966.

39. Sabiston, C. B., Jr., Gold, W. A., and Grigsby, W. R.: Bacteriology of the acute oral abscess, 1972, Program and Abstracts of Papers, International Association for Dental Research, Fiftieth General Session, Abstract No. 737, p. 231.

40. Shapiro, S. L.: Ludwig's angina in the antibiotic age, Eye Ear Nose Throat Mon. **50:**229, 1971.

41. Shapiro, S. L.: Notes on some recent antibiotic literature, Eye Ear Nose Throat Mon. **50:**492, 1971.

42. Sprenkle, P. M., and others: Abscesses of the head and neck, Laryngoscope **84:**1142, 1974.

43. West, W. F., Kelly, P. J., and Martin, W. J.: Chronic osteomyelitis, J.A.M.A. **213:**1837, 1970.

44. Woods, R.: Antibiotic treatment of pyogenic infections of dental origin, Aust. Dent. J. **13:**151, 1968.

45. Zallen, R. D., and Strader, R. J.: The use of prophylactic antibiotics in extraoral procedures for mandibular prognathism, J. Oral Surg. **29:**178, 1971.

46. Zallen, R. T., and Curry, J. T.: A study of antibiotic usage in compound mandibular fractures, J. Oral Surg. **33:**431, 1975.

CHAPTER 10

Special infections and their surgical relationship

Edward R. Mopsik

When performing surgical procedures within the oral cavity, the surgeon must be aware that the tissue surfaces harbor microbiota. Although the microbial flora is complex, containing overtly pathogenic strains of microbes, natural body defense mechanisms allow the patient to successfully be healed of wounds in the oral cavity. But despite the patient's ability to withstand potentially harmful sequelae, the surgeon is still confronted with a varying incidence of infected lesions.

Since the microbial flora is so varied, diagnosis of infected wounds can be troublesome, particularly if the commonly used antibiotics having gram-positive activity fail to resolve the infection. Although it is stressed that culturing techniques be used to avoid these pitfalls, the isolation of the specific organism responsible for the infection from the vast array of microbes present within the tissues cannot always be accomplished. The specimen sent for laboratory analysis is usually contaminated, and standard laboratory analysis does not always consider the more exotic species, the potential pathogens as they are called. In addition, bacteria are not always responsible; fungi and viruses must be considered, as well as diseases of unknown etiology that can mimic the clinical appearance of the more common infections encountered. This chapter will be concerned with this diagnostic situation as well as the special care and considerations needed to manage these patients.

GRAM-NEGATIVE INFECTIONS

In the literature, authors have reported the presence of gram-negative organisms causing infections within the oral cavity. Enteric gram-negative rods are normally found within the intestinal tract of man. When they are present in the oral cavity, gram-negative organisms are considered to be a contaminant. The possibilities of dealing with this vast array of organisms should never be ignored, particularly when an infectious process does not seem to be responding quickly to penicillin or other antibiotics having predominantly gram-positive spectra. This is perhaps more significant in debilitated patients. Culturing techniques can identify these organisms, and a suitable antibiotic regimen can be chosen. Since many antibiotics having gram-negative activity possess nephrotoxic or ototoxic properties or both, their use must be well specified. In addition, adequate incision and drainage must not be overlooked. It is essential to avoid the development of endotoxin shock, which can be fatal. Only by early suspicion, quick and vigorous drug therapy, and adequate incision and drainage will this situation be avoided.

ANAEROBIC INFECTIONS

In anaerobic infections the clostridia, a group of anaerobic, gram-positive, spore-forming rods are the most dangerous. In particular, *Clostridium tetani,* the agent causing tetanus or lockjaw, and the clostridia causing gas gangrene are the most important pathogens contaminating wounds.

C. tetani are found in soil throughout the world. Spores infect the wound and develop into the bacilli, which produce a neurotoxin. This toxin causes the disease state of tetanus. Fortunately, only one antigenic type of toxin is involved, and an effective monovalent toxoid for prophylactic immunization has been developed. Since tetanus immunization is so widespread in this country, few cases are seen.

Because these organisms are anaerobic, thus having predilection to necrotic wounds, routine cleaning of wounds with resultant bleeding and oxygen perfusion suppresses their growth. This is particularly true within the mouth where tissues are highly vascularized. However, in traumatic injuries with penetration into deep tissue spaces, only adequate immunization can protect the patient. Should tetanus be suspected, massive doses of intravenous aqueous penicillin (10 million units per day), along with the administration of 3,000 to 6,000 units of human immune globulin, are indicated. Additional patient management involves airway assistance, bowel and bladder functions, and sedation of the patient to control seizures and convulsions.

The clostridia of gas gangrene are chiefly *Clostridium perfringens, C. novyi,* and *C. septicum.* Although the classic description of a crepitant, gas-filled wound is most frequently given, the condition may be manifested in different ways. Hence, like tetanus, gas gangrene should always be suspect in penetrating wounds and proper precautions taken. Whenever pain suddenly is felt around the site of soft tissue injury or the pain suddenly intensifies, gas gangrene should be suspected. Wide, radical surgical debridement with massive doses of intravenous penicillin and tetracyclines must be undertaken. Polyvalent antitoxin should also be administered. Hyperbaric oxygen techniques have been employed successfully, but this requires special facilities not readily available.

Bacteroides, a group of nonspore-forming, strictly anaerobic, gram-negative bacteria, have recently been implicated in oral infections as a result of better isolation techniques and renewed interest in anaerobic organisms. *Bacteroides* species are normal inhabitants of the respiratory, genital, and intestinal tracts. They are rarely involved alone in disease but are almost always associated with underlying debilitating disease or trauma impairing the host defense mechanisms. *B. fragilis* and *B. melaninogenicus* are found within the oral cavity and have been implicated as the cause of osteomyelitis of the mandible.

Bacteroides infections can only be identified by employing anaerobic culturing techniques. Treatment with penicillin and tetracycline gives only haphazard results, with resistant strains appearing. Chloramphenicol is considered an effective agent, but clindamycin has been shown to be effective and offers a safer alternative to chloramphenicol therapy. Metronidazole has been shown to be bactericidal in vitro.

FUNGAL INFECTIONS

The most commonly encountered fungal infection of the oral cavity is moniliasis, which is characterized by white, adherent patches on the oral mucosa. Pain, soreness, and disturbances in taste sensation are frequently noted. The etiological agent, *Candida albicans,* is normally present within the oral cavity. Monilial infections are caused by overgrowth of these organisms, which is a result of either debilitation of the patient or of chemotherapeutic agents affecting the balance of the oral flora. Most typical is the appearance of moniliasis after the use of broad-spectrum antibiotics such as the tetracyclines.

The diagnosis of moniliasis depends on the surgeon recognizing its clinical appearance as well as obtaining a specimen for culture and identification. A direct smear will reveal gram-positive, oval, budding yeasts and gram-positive, budding cells that are similar to hyphae. These fungi will grow on Sabouraud's glucose agar.

The treatment of oral monilial infections involves the use of nystatin suspension. These infections respond rapidly to the administration of 100,000 to 300,000 units nystatin held in the mouth for 3 minutes, then swallowed; this regimen is repeated three to four times daily. Recognizing the underlying causes of these infections is most important because monilial infections will return unless these causes are corrected.

Actinomycosis manifests itself as a chronic granulomatous lesion with fistula formation and pus production. Cervicofacial actinomycosis accounts for approximately 60% of all actinomyces infections. The remaining infections involve the abdominal and thoracic areas. The cause of actinomycosis is believed to be the endogenous spread of *Actinomyces israelii,* a gram-positive, nonacid-fast, nonmotile, filamentous organism found within the oral cavity. *A. bovis,* a closely related species, may also cause the disease. These two species are of interest for identification purposes only.

A history of trauma or one of tooth extraction is commonly found in patients with actinomycosis. The tongue is involved in roughly 4% of all forms of the disease. The tongue lesions must be distinguished from neoplasms, tuberculous lesions, syphilitic gummas, or other fungal lesions. Whenever a chronic infectious process occurs after tooth extraction and does not readily respond to the usual modes of treatment, actinomycosis should be suspected.

Diagnosis of this disease depends on the identification of the organisms from cultures taken from the pus of the draining lesions or from biopsy specimens of the lesions. The pathognomonic findings of sulfur granules can be obtained by placing one granule on a slide and crushing it under a cover slip. The typical appearance of the organism will be readily observed.

There are various opinions concerning the choice of antibiotics for treatment of this infection. Some practitioners recommend penicillin, and others recommend tetracyclines. Generally this infection requires massive doses of either antibiotic (a minimum of 3 to 4 million units penicillin or 500 mg tetracycline every 6 hours) over prolonged periods of time. The antibiotic must be continued weeks after clinical resolution of the disease. Surgical drainage of the abscess cavity must be accomplished and forms a vital part of the treatment plan.

Blastomycosis is a fungal infection of the skin and viscera. However, lesions have been reported within the oral cavity. Two types of infections are recognized: North American blastomycosis caused by *Blastomyces dermatitidis* and South American blastomycosis caused by *Paracoccidioides brasiliensis.* Most cases of North American blastomycosis are found in the southeastern United States and the Mississippi River Valley. Both forms produce firm, erythematous, ulcerative lesions, with massive regional lymphadenopathy.

Since clinical and epidemiological features are nonspecific, diagnosis depends on isolation and identification of the specific organism from these lesions. The accuracy of skin tests for blastomycosis is questionable.

Treatment of these infections depends on the use of amphotericin B along with surgical excision of the destroyed tissues. South American blastomycosis responds to sulfa drugs.

Histoplasmosis is a fungal infection that is caused by *Histoplasma capsulatum,* with cutaneous and pulmonary lesions. The pulmonary infection may lead to a more overwhelming systemic infection with resultant multiplication of the organisms within the reticuloendothelial cells and anemia, fever, hepatomegaly, splenomegaly, leukopenia, ulcerative lesions of the gastrointestinal tract, and adrenal necrosis. Oral manifestations of histoplasmosis involving the lips, tongue, nose, and larynx seem to occur mainly in adults and are seen in about one third of all fatal cases. Many cases of histoplasmosis go unnoticed with minimal consequences. It is only in the chronic localized forms of the condition that two main clinical types occur. One is pulmonary and resembles tuberculosis in all respects; the other is mucocutaneous, with ulcers of the mouth, tongue, pharynx, penis, and bladder. These ulcers are painful, granulomatous lesions, with associated regional lymphadenopathy.

Diagnosis of disseminated or chronic localized histoplasmosis can be made from cultures of blood, bone marrow, biopsied lesions, sputum, or exudate obtained from the ulcerated lesion. *H. capsulatum* will grow on Sabouraud's medium. Complement fixation tests and a histoplasmin skin test are available, with the latter resulting in a delayed hypersensitivity reaction similar to the tuberculin skin test. Unfortunately, false negatives are numerous. Histopathological examination of tissue lesions is another proved method of diagnosis for histoplasmosis.

Amphotericin B given intravenously in dosages of between 50 and 100 mg daily has been shown to be effective in treating most patients with histoplasmosis. Sulfadiazine has also been shown to be effective for some adult patients and can be given in conjunction with amphotericin B.

TUBERCULOSIS

Although oral lesions of tuberculosis are rare, these granulomatous ulcerations can easily be misdiagnosed as fungal infection, carcinoma, gumma, or chancre. These lesions are usually extremely painful, with a predilection for the tongue, although the cheeks, lips, and palate have also been reported as areas of involvement.

Mycobacterium tuberculosis, the infectious agent, is a rod-shaped bacterium that is rendered acid-fast when stained by the Ziehl-Neelsen technique. Another characteristic of the tuberculous lesion is the development of chronic granulomas with central areas of caseation necrosis. Within the center of this lesion are multinucleated giant cells containing the tubercle bacilli.

The diagnosis of oral tuberculous lesions is not easily achieved unless the Ziehl-Neelsen stain is employed. Ordinary histopathological study is inconclusive. Unless special culture methods are requested, these organisms will not grow using ordinary methods. When the diagnosis is made, however, it then becomes imperative to examine the chest for pulmonary lesions and the other organ systems for possible involvement.

In addition to the oral lesions just described, another form of tuberculosis, which is characterized by marked lymphadenopathy of the cervical nodes, may present itself to the dentist. This tuberculous involvement of the cervical lymph nodes is called scrofula and was frequently associated with drinking unpasteurized raw milk from tuberculous cows. The major salivary glands may also be involved, making a differential diagnosis between tuberculosis, mixed tumor, and malignancy difficult. Diagnosis is made by histopathological examination.

Treatment of choice for these tuberculous lesions is administration of isoniazid, streptomycin, and para-aminosalicylic acid (PAS). For the more seriously infected patients, isoniazid and PAS are used concurrently to prevent the appearance of resistant strains.

SYPHILIS

Despite improved methods for treating syphilis, every year the number of reported cases of infectious syphilis continues to rise at an alarming rate. In 1968, 75,000 cases were estimated in the United States. A complete discussion of syphilis is not suited for this text, but it is highly recommended that every dentist consult a standard reference text and familiarize himself or herself with this disease.

Briefly, syphilis is divided into the primary, secondary, and tertiary stages. The chancre is associated with the primary stage; the macular-papular skin rash and raised, grayish erosions of the mucosa (mucous patches) are associated with the secondary stage; the gumma, a chronic granulomatous lesion, is associated with the tertiary stage.

The chancre, which is an indurated solitary ulceration with dark encrustations, is generally found about the genitalia, although oral lesions of the gingiva, tongue, and pharynx have been reported. The painful mucosal erosions of the secondary stage, the mucous patches, are highly infectious and represent a potential source of infection to the dentist and the assistants. These lesions are commonly found on the tongue, lips, buccal mucosa, and pharynx. The gumma, which is a painless, granulomatous lesion that ulcerates and undergoes central necrosis, is commonly found within the tongue or on the palate. Perforations of the palate and nasal septum are associated with these lesions. The syphilitic interstitial glossitis associated with advanced leukoplakia is often considered a precancerous lesion and should be viewed with suspicion. It must be stressed that syphilis has often been called the "great mimic," and one's suspicion should always be aroused when confronted with unusual case presentations. For this reason as well as for public health measures, serological testing for syphilis is widely employed on a regular screening basis.

Diagnosis of syphilis relies on serological test, dark-field microscopic examination, and histopathological examination. Briefly, serological tests are negative during the first stage (when dark-field examination should be employed), positive during the second stage, and equivocal during the third stage. Of the serological tests, the most frequently employed is the Venereal Disease Research Laboratory (VDRL) slide test, which is a nontreponemal flocculation test. The Kolmer test, another nontreponemal test, relies on complement fixation. These tests are associated with false positive results but are useful during treatment because the titers observed parallel the infectious course.

Treponemal tests generally employed are the *Treponema pallidum* immobilization test (TPI) and the fluorescent treponemal antibody (FTA) test. These tests are generally more specific than the nontreponemal tests. The most specific treponemal test for diagnostic purposes seems to be the fluorescent treponemal antibody absorption (FTA-ABS) test. But this too is not without occasional false positive results, particularly for those patients with increased or abnormal globulins.

Treatment of syphilitic patients is a public health measure. Penicillin is still the first drug of choice; a single injection of 2.4 million units of benzathine penicillin is often curative. Another schedule recommends procaine penicillin, 600,000 units daily for 8 to 10 days. Other alternatives to penicillin include tetracycline, erythromycin, and cephaloridine.

ERYTHEMA MULTIFORME

Erythema multiforme is a vesicular, bullous lesion of unknown etiology. The sudden onset of large bullous lesions, which are relatively nonpainful but frequently are secondarily infected by the time they affect the oral mucous membranes, is typical of the disease. In addition, the extremities, the face, and the neck may be involved. Spontaneous remission occurs in 2 to 3 weeks after considerable discomfort, encrustation, and bleeding from these lesions. Commonly, erythema multiforme is associated with high temperature (102° to 105° F or 38.8° to 40.5° C) and joint pain. This disease is frequently associated with drug eruptions caused by drugs such as antisera, sulfonamides, quinine, and arsenicals.

Various entities of this disease have been described, helping to confuse the issue. The Stevens-Johnson syndrome occurs in the younger age group, with accompanying high fever, headache, and overwhelming stomatitis. Other mucous membranes may be involved, leading to conjunctivitis, urethritis, and balanitis. Arthralgia and myalgia are common. Behçet's syndrome involves erosive lesions of the eye, with oral and genital lesions. Reiter's syndrome includes acute arthritic manifestations along with the triad of conjunctivitis, oral lesions, and urethritis.

Treatment is symptomatic with no known cure. Oral hygiene, bland mouthwashes, antibiotics to control secondary infection, and systemic steroids when indicated for severe cases are the treatment measures usually employed.

HERPETIFORM LESIONS

Because so much has been written about oral herpes simplex and recurrent aphthous ulcers, they will be discussed briefly in this chapter. These recurrent mucosal and lip lesions are self-limiting and regress in 10 to 14 days. Although the etiological agent in herpes is known (the herpes simplex virus), speculation still exists concerning the etiological agent of recurrent aphthous ulcers.

Herpetic lesions frequently occur after upper respiratory illnesses, gastrointestinal upsets, and menstrual disorders. It is important to avoid steriod therapy whenever herpes simplex infection is suspected for fear of dissemination, particularly to the conjunctiva and central nervous system. Idoxuridine (IDU), although shown to be effective with herpes simplex keratitis, has been a disappointment in the treatment of herpes labialis.

Aphthous ulcers (canker sores) still remain an enigma to treat because of their obscure etiology. Social and economic factors, psychic tension, autoimmune mechanisms, and L-forms (pleuropneumonia-like organisms or PPLO, *Mycoplasma* organisms) have all been implicated. Since these are spontaneously regressing lesions, patient comfort is strived for during the acutely painful episodes. Various regimens of multivitamins, steroids, and topical tetracycline and repeated smallpox vaccinations have been suggested with varying claims of success. Generally the simplest palliative therapy is suggested, with care to control secondary infections if they should arise.

Clinical entities such as pemphigus, mucous membrane pemphigoid, periadenitis mucosa necrotica recurrens, herpes zoster, and herpangina are similar, regarding treatment modalities, to oral herpes simplex and aphthous ulcers. In herpes zoster the etiological agent is the varicella virus, and in herpangina it is the Coxsackie virus. Causes of the other clinical entities listed are unknown. In all cases these ulcerative lesions of the oral mucous membranes should be treated symptomatically in the simplest manner. Although the viral infections are self-limited and regress, the other entites may follow a chronic course. When this is the case, steroid therapy may be tried, usually being reserved for the most difficult cases. However, steroids do not always bring about resolution, although they may retard the course and progression of these ulcerative lesions.

REFERENCES

1. Burket, L. W.: Oral medicine, Philadelphia, 1965, J. B. Lippincott Co.
2. Davis, B. D., Dulbecco, R., Eisen, H. H., Ginsberg, H. S., and Wood, W. B.: Microbiology, New York, 1967, Hoeber Medical Division, Harper & Row.
3. Early care of acute soft tissue injuries, Committee on Trauma, American College of Surgeons, Philadelphia, 1965, W. B. Saunders Co.

4. Harrison, T. R., editor: Principles of internal medicine, New York, 1966, McGraw-Hill Book Co.
5. Jawetz, E., Melnick, J. L., and Adelberg, E. A.: Review of medical microbiology, Los Altos, Calif., 1964, Lange Medical Publication.
6. Kislak, J. W.: The susceptibility of *Bacteroides fragilis* to twenty-four antibiotics, J. Infect. Dis. **125:**295, 1972.
7. Leake, D. L.: Bacteroides osteomyelitis of the mandible, Oral Surg. **34:**585, 1972.
8. Nastrow, L. J., and Finegold, S. M.: Bactericidal activity of five antimicrobial agents against *Bacteroides fragilis,* J. Infect. Dis. **126:**104, 1972.
9. Shires, G. T., editor: Care of the trauma patient, New York, 1966, McGraw-Hill Book Co.
10. Sparling, P. F.: Diagnosis and treatment of syphilis, N. Engl. J. Med. **284:**642, 1971.
11. Sutherland, V. C.: A synopsis of pharmacology, Philadelphia, 1970, W. B. Saunders Co.
12. Syphilis: A synopsis, Public Health Service Pub. no. 1660, Washington, D.C., 1968, U. S. Government Printing Office.
13. Tracy, O., Gordon, A. M., Moran, F., Love, W. C., and McKenzie, P.: Lincomycins in the treatment of bacteroides infections, Br. Med. J. **1:**280, 1972.

CHAPTER 11

Acute infections of the oral cavity

Sanford M. Moose
Keith J. Marshall

The subject of acute infections of the oral cavity could in itself occupy a sizeable volume if descriptions of the diagnosis and treatment of all acute infections found in the oral cavity were included.

Many of the acute inflammatory processes manifest in the oral cavity provide evidence of acute infection by microorganisms. However, inflammatory conditions of the oral mucosa are also among the cardinal symptoms of dermatologic disease and other systemic disorders that are beyond the scope of a discussion of acute infections of the oral cavity. It is important therefore to realize that the oral and other mucous membrane surfaces of the body may provide early visible signs of disease other than primary infections of oral tissues. Many exanthematous diseases of childhood have primary lesions in the oral cavity that may become acutely inflamed as well as secondarily infected as a result of disruption of the integrity of the defense mechanisms provided by an intact mucous membrane.

Any primary systemic condition capable of adversely affecting the oral mucous membrane may play an important part in the etiology of oral infection as well as present a symptom complex manifested in inflammatory changes of oral mucosal surfaces.

Lesions of immunopathological origin are seen often in oral mucous membranes.[1,17] As the frequency and complexity of drug administration in the treatment of disease states have increased, so the variety and incidence of mucosal lesions caused by untoward reactions to these agents have increased. Food allergy has been identified as important in the genesis of oral lesions. Autoimmune disease mechanisms affecting oral tissues have been implicated in the production of alterations of mucosal surfaces. It has been recognized for a long time that nutritional deficiency diseases may give rise to ulceration and other changes of oral mucosa, either affecting surface epithelium or underlying connective tissue.

The Occupational Safety and Health Administration of the United States Department of Labor and the United States Department of Agriculture are important sources of information on nutrition and also for information regarding chemical poisons that may cause oral lesions.

Diseases that alter the body's defense mechanisms frequently result in secondary oral infections. Suppression of the immune system, either by diseases that affect the hemopoietic tissues or by steroids and other immunosuppressive agents administered in the treatment of disease states, may be responsible ultimately for the development of oral infections and other alterations of oral mucosa. Malignant diseases themselves or the iatrogenic diseases generated in their treatment always are important considerations in the evaluation of oral lesions.

Local diseases may play an important role in the production of acute infections of the oral and maxillofacial apparatus. Odontogenic tumors and cysts may escape detection until an acute inflammatory lesion becomes superimposed. Acute infection may be the ultimate lesion of the maxilla or mandible, but invasion of adjacent soft tissues of the cheek, lips, tongue, and soft palate is not infrequent. Less common, but certainly significant, are more distant extensions of infection by metastasis, which may result in mortality or permanent injury.

When considering the panorama of etiologic factors contributing to the production of acute infections of the oral cavity, the practitioner must be alert to suspect obscure causes rather than to jump to obvious but possibly incorrect conclusions on the basis of superficial appearances and insufficient investigation. While visual inspection is indispensable in the evaluation of oral lesions, a carefully elicited history often reveals the information required for an accurate diagnosis, and unfortunately this is one of the elements most apt to be neglected.

ACUTE INFECTIONS OF THE JAWS
Periapical abscess

The periapical abscess, commonly called an acute alveolar abscess, usually begins in the periapical region and is caused by a necrotic pulp. It may occur almost immediately after injury to the pulpal tissues, or, after a long latent period, it may suddenly flare into an acute infection with the symptoms of inflammation, swelling, and fever.

Factors that cause some periapical lesions to suddenly become acute are not understood, although many theories have been advanced regarding this transition. The fact simply remains that a nonsymptomatic tooth today may cause extreme distress requiring definitive treatment at any time in the future.

Although the symptoms producing distress are often confined to the immediate region of the tooth, occasions arise when toxins released by interaction of the infective agent and host defense mechanisms produce a systemic reaction sufficient to render a patient generally ill. Periapical abscesses may confine themselves to the osseous structures and during the early period of abscess formation may cause excruciating pain without any observable swelling. However, even though many cases may start initially in this manner, the abscess may burrow through the cancellous and cortical bone until it reaches the surface and invades the soft tissues in the form of either a subperiosteal or supraperiosteal abscess.

Prior to actual abscess formation, however, the infection is capable of producing a cellulitis in the soft tissues of the region involved (Fig. 11-1). The palpable soft tissues

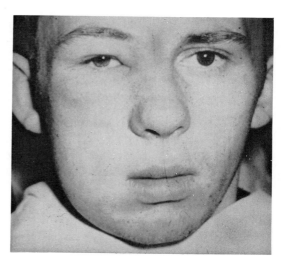

Fig. 11-1. Infraorbital cellulitis from infected tooth. (Walter Reed Army Hospital.)

of the oral and maxillofacial area appear hard and dense. This brawny condition is known as induration. Until the infectious process becomes well circumscribed in the form of an abscess, the patient is usually in extreme discomfort.

Treatment should be directed toward localizing the infection during the period of induration, confining the infection to the region of onset, and eliminating the etiology of the infection. Early employment of appropriate antibiotic therapy in adequate dosage may be extremely important in a severe and life-threatening infection. Localization of the infection may be aided by using warm compresses and warm mouth rinses at frequent intervals. It is only when localization takes place that an abscess should be surgically incised and drained. Physiologically, it is at this time that nature has constructed a barrier around the abscess, walling it off from the circulation and making it possible to palpate the presence of fluid purulent material within the abscess cavity. The deeper the abscess forms within tissue, the more difficult it is to palpate.

An early decision should be made on the most desirable disposition of a tooth or teeth involved in the development of an acute infection. After such teeth have been carefully evaluated, if their retention is indicated, the necrotic pulp canals should be opened in an effort to relieve the pressure generated within a closed chamber. If this fails to achieve the desired relief, the offending tooth should be extracted. The sooner this is accomplished the more rapidly may the symptoms be expected to subside.

The philosophy of never extracting a tooth in the presence of an acute infection has long been abandoned. It should be realized that frequently the best route through which the abscess can be drained is through the alveolus from which the tooth is extracted. The alveolar bone in such cases is so dense and resistant to further penetration of the abscess that the infectious process is confined, increasing the symptoms until ex-

traction is the only recourse. Under such circumstances, pus is usually observed flowing from the alveolus immediately after the extraction. If the extraction is delayed, a possibility exists that the infection will diffuse into tissues remotely located from the original site, and that septicemia or osteomyelitis or both will develop.[5]

When definitive action is indicated in the presence of acute infection, the patient should be protected by the administration of adequate doses of an antibiotic to ensure a rapid and sustained blood level. Selection of the appropriate antibiotic should be made, whenever possible, on the basis of identification of the microorganism and its sensitivity to available antibiotics. When time does not permit complete culture and sensitivity determination, the clinical and gram-staining characteristics of the organisms, if any specimen can be obtained, provide a better basis for antibiotic selection than purely empirical selection. Multiple extractions or extensive surgery should be postponed until the remission of acute symptoms.

When an abscess has formed or is induced to localize and the infectious process invades the extra-alveolar tissues, it should be incised simultaneously with the extraction of the tooth. If the tooth is to be retained, the palpable abscess should be incised and drained simultaneously with the opening of the pulpal chamber. If a fluctuant localized abscess is palpable intraorally and is in the region of the maxillary or mandibular buccal vestibule, then the choice of drainage incision should be at a point below the most fluctuant portion of the abscess. On the other hand, if the abscess should localize or point subperiosteally or supraperiosteally on the palate or on the lingual surface of the mandible, then the site of incision should be chosen in deference to the neurovascular structures found on these surfaces.

When the presence of important anatomical structures becomes a hazard, then the incision should be made with a sharp scalpel through only the superficial tissues, followed by blunt dissection with a hemostat into the abscess cavity and down to the bony surface. With the hemostat closed, the point is forced through the incised surface into the abscess cavity and then opened, and the aperture is dilated to permit the installation of adequate-sized drainage material. Small openings for the purpose of draining abscesses are entirely unsatisfactory and do not permit adequate drainage. A large opening for the drainage of most abscesses should permit the end of the gloved index finger to be admitted to the bony surface from which the abscess has emerged.

Pericoronal infections

Although pericoronal infection may occur at any time throughout life, pericoronal infections occur commonly during infancy, childhood, and young adulthood. Pericoronal infection in infancy is associated with tooth eruption, when the supradental tissue involving the superior portion of the follicle and overlying mucoperiosteum may become inflamed and ultimately develop into a fluctuant abscess. Occasionally these abscesses may develop into a cellulitis, causing not only local but systemic reactions associated with fever. When fluctuance can be visibly and digitally ascertained, incision and drainage followed by warm saline mouth rinses held over the area at frequent intervals usually give prompt relief so that no further treatment is necessary. Similar conditions may occur at any time during the eruption period of permanent teeth and should be managed in the same manner.

The type of pericoronal infection less frequently encountered occurs in late adult life in an edentulous ridge. For some reason a tooth has failed to erupt, and a denture has been constructed for the patient, either because the existence of the unerupted tooth was not known or in the belief that the tooth could remain asymptomatic in the edentulous jaw.

It is generally believed that the cause of

the acute infection associated with such teeth is the result of pressure from the denture over a period of years. At the onset of a patient's denture wearing, such embedded teeth are in all probability a sufficient distance from the surface to be unaffected by the pressure reaction from the denture. However, as time goes on, with the resultant resorption of the ridge, the bone and soft tissue between the denture and the embedded tooth is ultimately subjected to the inflammatory influences of denture pressure and motion.

When an acute infection occurs under these circumstances, a different course of treatment is indicated. If a fluctuant abscess occurs, overlying the crown of this embedded tooth, it should be incised and drained and a sufficient time allowed for the acute condition to become subacute. At this later time, surgical removal of the unerupted tooth is indicated.

The most common type of pericoronal infection is the one found around the mandibular third molar (Fig. 11-2). This occurs most frequently in adolescents and young adults. Symptoms accompanying this type of pericoronal infection are variable, and it is not unusual for patients to experience their only symptoms in the peritonsillar region. For this reason they seek the ser-

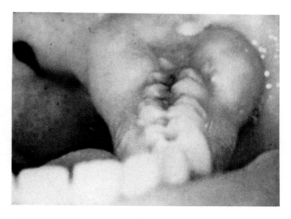

Fig. 11-2. Pericoronal abscess around third molar. (Walter Reed Army Hospital.)

vices of a physician, believing they have a sore throat or tonsillitis. The interesting aspect of this type of pericoronal infection is that it actually does have peritonsillar symptoms marked enough that visual symptoms lead to the diagnosis of peritonsillar abscess or streptococcal sore throat, for which the patient is not infrequently hospitalized and treated accordingly. Repetition of these symptoms may occur for several years before an unerupted third molar is finally diagnosed as the offender.

The most typical symptoms of pericoronal infection of the third molar are submandibular lymphadenopathy, trismus, pain in the region of the third molar, and a general condition of malaise not infrequently attended with a moderate elevation of temperature. These symptoms vary in degree from mild to extreme to a point at which the patient may suffer extreme pain and may develop a cellulitis capable of producing difficulty in swallowing, extreme tenderness to palpation extraorally and intraorally, and edema visible both in the submandibular and pharyngeal regions. When symptoms of this type occur, the tooth or a surface of the unerupted tooth is usually close to the surface. A visible portion of the tooth may be exposed to the oral cavity. The communication to the oral cavity may be so obscured by edema and the general inflammatory process that this communication may be ascertained only by the use of a probe.

More frequently than not, this communication permits the probe to be advanced along the buccal aspect of the unerupted tooth. Careful palpation with the probe permits entry into an expanded follicular space. After dilation of the aperture of entrance, the evacuation of pus and other septic material is made possible. If the aperture can be dilated sufficiently to permit drainage, the insertion of a 6-mm wide drain made from rubber dam material or Penrose drain or a 6-mm strip of iodoform gauze moistened with eugenol or guaiacol and olive oil should permit continuous drainage and provide adequate analgesia. The patient should be instructed to use warm saline mouthwashes for 5 minutes at half-hour intervals until retiring. If adequate localization of the infection has not occurred, antibiotic therapy is indicated immediately in a dosage and by a route of administration sufficient to assure a rapid, adequate blood level. This should provide prompt relief from the acute symptoms, and as soon as a subacute condition exists, definitive treatment may be instituted.

Definitive treatment, of course, will depend on the judgment concerning the final disposition of the unerupted tooth. If the third molar is impacted, surgical removal should be performed as soon as symptoms become subacute. If the tooth is not impacted but has been recurrently troublesome without eruption and it is ascertained that insufficient room exists for adequate eruption space in the patient's mouth, then extraction is also indicated.

If, however, the first molar is missing or has a poor prognosis and the second molar similarly may not be a suitable abutment tooth for prosthetic replacement of missing teeth anterior to the second molar, then the third molar assumes a more important potential role. If marginally adequate space for eruption exists, such a third molar may be permitted to erupt while under other circumstances extraction would be the treatment of choice. Consideration should be given to the persistent or recurrent nature of inflammatory episodes as well as their severity and to possible serious hazards to a patient's oral and general health prior to elective retention. If retention is elected, it may be necessary to excise inflamed or fibrotic tissues overlying and surrounding the occlusal portion of the tooth.

If excision of the overlying tissues is decided on, it should be done adequately. All overlying tissues should be thoroughly excised, and the occlusal portion of the unerupted tooth should be completely exposed. After excision has been completed the wound should be packed with a surgical dressing. This should be allowed to remain approximately 7 days.

The time for the employment of a definitive surgical procedure has been a controversial subject for a number of years, but since the advent of the chemotherapeutic and antibiotic era, patients can be protected from violent postoperative systemic reactions, acute cellulitis, and osteomyelitis by the use of antimicrobial agents. Delay of surgery is believed to play a significant role in permitting an osteomyelitic infection to become established. Consequently, discretion should be employed in the selection of a suitable time for surgical action. In the presence of acute, fulminating infection, antibiotic therapy and early incision and drainage is the method of choice, followed by definitive surgical treatment of the condition as soon as it becomes subacute.

The maxillary third molar can be a contributing factor to pericoronal infections of an unerupted mandibular third molar. In the examination of a patient with a pericoronal infection associated with a mandibular third molar, it is imperative that the region of the maxillary third molar be examined to see whether it has erupted, whether it is in malalignment, or whether it has supererupted as a result of the delayed eruption of the mandibular third molar. It must be determined whether room is present in the mandibular retromolar area of the patient's jaw for the eruption of the mandibular third molar and if the presence of the maxillary third molar is a continuous source of trauma to the soft tissue in the mandibular retromolar area during the eruption period of the mandibular third molar.

On occasion it is found desirable to retain the mandibular third molar even when recurrent infectious episodes persist from the traumatic influence of the erupted maxillary third molar. In such cases it is desirable to remove the maxillary third molar if its presence is a continual source of trauma. Pericoronal infections occur less frequently around an erupted or unerupted maxillary third molar, but when they do, the same procedure should be employed as the one described for the management of the mandibular third molar.

Dissecting subperiosteal abscess
(Fig. 11-3, *A*)

A certain type of subperiosteal infection may occur several weeks after an apparently uneventful healing of a mandibular third molar wound. This may present itself primarily as an indurated swelling in the mucoperiosteal tissue as far forward as the first molar or second bicuspid. It may become progressively edematous and indurated and finally develop into a fluctuant, palpable, and visible subperiosteal abscess

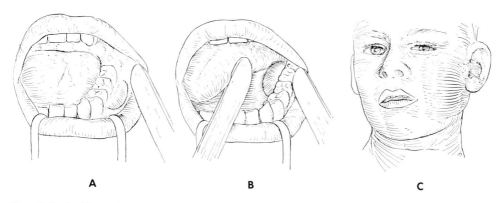

A   **B**   **C**

Fig. 11-3. A, Dissecting subperiosteal abscess. **B,** Medial mandibular angle postoperative abscess. **C,** Acute infected emphysema.

that has migrated from the original third molar wound beneath the periosteum to the point of fluctuance. When the diagnosis is made, antibiotic therapy should be initiated, and as soon as the fluctuance is palpable, the abscess should be incised and drained. This condition may be externally visible and palpable as a swelling of the cheek in this region.

The drainage incision should start from the point of origin, which is the third molar region deep in the buccal vestibule, and extend anteriorly to the point of fluctuance. The incision should be made through the mucoperiosteum down to the bone. Tissues on either side of the incision should then be expanded with a hemostat, and the wound, along the length of its entire course, should be packed open with iodoform gauze impregnated with a suitable analgesic, antiseptic, lubricating agent (equal parts balsam of Peru and castor oil) or other suitable agents having similar properties. This type of packing material should not be changed daily but should be allowed to remain, thereby keeping the wound expanded and permitting the purulent material to drain out around it. It should be observed at 48-hour intervals, and the dressing should be allowed to remain in place for approximately 7 days. If the dressing is expelled from the wound during this period by action of the muscles of mastication, it should be replaced so that the wound remains saucerized and therefore will heal by granulating from the depth of the wound.

Killey and co-workers[11] have published a comprehensive in-depth study on various types of subperiosteal infectious invasions and their treatments and end results.

Medial mandibular angle postoperative abscess (Fig. 11-3, B)

A medial mandibular angle postsurgical abscess may occur several days after the surgical removal of a mandibular third molar. It is accompanied by extreme discomfort, trismus, and difficulty in swallowing. The symptoms become progressively worse until it is with great difficulty that the patient is able to open his mouth for adequate examination. Whenever symptoms of this type are present and no symptoms are visible on the facial or occlusal surface of the wound, one may suspect this lingual type of abscess. It therefore becomes necessary either by persuasion under adequate sedation or by application of force to open the mouth sufficiently to permit digital examination of the medial surface of the angle of the jaw.

Inspection will reveal an extremely tender swelling of the tissues. The pain is severe. When fluctuance is determined, a small, curved, closed hemostat should be forced down through the wound of the third molar. It is introduced between the periosteum and the lingual surface of the bone, and, by sliding along the bone, the hemostat is advanced inferiorly and posteriorly until an abscess cavity is encountered. At this point the hemostat should be opened widely to dilate the tract through which the infection has descended into this region. If surgical intervention is correctly timed, pus will immediately be seen emerging from the cavity after withdrawal of the hemostat. A small, round-tipped brain-type aspirator may now be inserted into the cavity to aspirate additional amounts of pus that may be present. A gentle compression of the soft tissue under the angle of the jaw may also expel pus through the intraoral aperture.

After this, a small piece of Penrose drain or rubber dam material may be inserted deep into the region of the abscess with the end protruding slightly into the third molar wound, where it may be sutured without occluding the aperture. Whenever possible, a foreign material that may become dislodged should be secured to prevent aspiration and possible serious respiratory sequela, including death through respiratory obstruction or respiratory infection. Antibiotic therapy initiated as early as possible may be an important adjunct to the surgical incision and drainage, but it is no substitute for indicated surgical intervention.

Acute infected emphysema (Fig. 11-3, *C*)

Acute infected emphysema is usually caused by the indiscreet use of air-pressure syringes or atomizing spray bottles activated by compressed air. In drying out a root canal with a compressed air syringe, septic material may be forced through the apical foramen into the cancellous portion of the alveolar process and ultimately out through the nutrient foramina into adjacent soft tissues, resulting in formation of a septic cellulitis and emphysema.

A similar condition can be induced by the use of a compressed-air spray bottle for irrigation of wounds, particularly in the retromolar region. If enough pressure is applied, it is possible to force air and septic materials through the fascial planes into the surgical spaces, which, after being forced open, remain in communication with this septic region. It is safer to use a hand-activated syringe when irrigating wounds or drying root canals since it is unlikely that an emphysema would be produced under these circumstances. Similarly it is important to avoid the use of any air-driven dental handpiece that exhausts compressed air within the oral cavity if a soft tissue wound is present. Conventional air-driven contraangle handpieces with air or air-water spray devices are totally unsatisfactory as surgical handpieces and may be very dangerous.

Periodontal abscess

Acute periodontal abscesses (Fig. 11-4) are usually the culmination of a long period of chronic periodontitis. This type of infection usually starts in the gingival crevice at the surface and extends down one or more surfaces of the roots, frequently as far as the apical region. Acute episodes usually have a sudden onset with extreme pain, and they are associated with swelling of the soft tissues overlying the surface of the involved root. For some

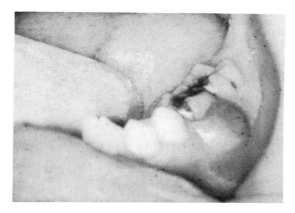

Fig. 11-4. Periodontal abscess.

unknown reason the tissues apparently seal themselves off at the gingival surface, impeding the drainage of the abscess and causing the distention and discomfort that is usually the patient's first indication of this condition.

A periodontal abscess may or may not be associated with nonvital teeth or traumatic injury, either external or occlusal. It may, however, be induced by the traumatic influence of a partial denture. The primary treatment for relief of acute symptoms is incision of the fluctuant abscess from the depth of the abscess cavity to the gingiva. The incision should extend through the soft tissues to the root surface, which has been previously denuded by the presence of the infectious process. If one or more surfaces of the root of such a tooth have been denuded to a point beyond the apical third of the tooth, extraction is indicated. If a third or more of the investing bone appears normal, then an evaluation of the potential usefulness of such a tooth should be made by considering all factors involved, including the general condition of the patient's health and his regenerative and resistance capacity.

Definitive treatment by debridement of root surface and removal of granulation tissue and treatment for new attachment and tissue regeneration should be deferred until the acute phase of the infection has subsided.

A lateral periodontal abscess can produce an infection capable of diffusing from the original offending tooth through the alveolar bone to involve several teeth on either side of the offender, rendering them extremely mobile and tender. Frequently this can baffle the most astute diagnostician and make identification of the primary offending tooth difficult. Radiographs are, of course, a primary aid to diagnosis. Frequently, however, the lateral surface of the root involved is so obscured by the tooth structure that a radiograph contributes little toward the ultimate diagnosis.

ACUTE CELLULITIS

When infection invades tissues, it may remain localized if the host resistance factors in the region are capable of walling off the infection and preventing it from spreading. In such cases, a physiological barrier is formed around the nidus of infection and it is either resolved and drained off in the lymphatic circulation or suppuration occurs, at which time surgical drainage is indicated.

Occasionally the bacterial infection is overwhelming, or the bacteria are either extremely virulent or resistant to antibiotic therapy. The resistance of the host tissues may be minimal, and bacterial invasion under these circumstances is unimpeded as it progresses through surrounding tissues to areas remote from the original site of infection. When physiological response fails to control the invasion of infection and therapeutic agents prove futile, then death ensues.

An acute cellulitis of dental origin usually is confined to the general area of the jaws. Tissues become grossly edematous and often hard to palpation. At this period the infection has not localized, and, during this stage, suppuration has not occurred.

The patient may show a severe systemic reaction to the infection. The temperature is usually elevated, the white cell count is increased, and the differential count may be altered. The erythrocyte sedimentation rate is usually increased, and the pulse rate is accelerated. The electrolyte balance is changed, and the patient frequently experiences malaise.

When the invasive process is overwhelmed by the physiological defense, resolution is achieved. Frequently, a specific antibiotic can complete resolution of the process, and either no pus is formed or the small amount present can be removed by the lymphatic circulation. Usually, however, a massive cellulitis will ultimately suppurate, particularly if the bacteria are staphylococci or other pus-producing organisms rather than streptococci. Since pus indicates localization of the infection, early literature referred to it as "laudable pus."

Purulent material may burrow its way toward the surface, where it may evacuate spontaneously or be intercepted by surgical intervention (incision and drainage). Depending on its location and the proximity of anatomical structures that guide its progress, pus may evacuate into the nose, maxillary sinus, oral vestibule, floor of the mouth, face, or the infratemporal fossa (Fig. 12-2). It can burrow into the cranial vault by bony resorption, or it can go through the numerous foramina into the base of the skull.* Haymaker[6] reported cases in which death occurred after extension of infection into the cranium, usually by means of a bacteremia. Progress in this direction is difficult to diagnose, and neurological signs form the basis for such diagnosis. Every deep infection of long standing must be observed closely for such signs.

TREATMENT

Surgical evacuation of pus will reduce the absorption of toxic products, thereby allowing the patient to recover. It will pre-

---

*See references 8, 13, 18, and 23.

vent further burrowing of the purulent mass in an attempt toward spontaneous evacuation. Antibiotics may control further infection, but they will not evacuate pus.

The optimum time for incision and drainage may be difficult to determine. No difficulty in timing is encountered when a large cellulitis develops a superficial erythematous spot, which is pathognomonic of pus near the surface. Bimanual palpation will reveal a body of fluid material. One finger pressing down on one side of the mass will convey a fluid movement to a finger placed on the other side of the mass. This mass should be incised immediately and a drain inserted. When no superficial red spot is present, fluctuance is more difficult to determine, particularly if deep pus is suspected, and the palpation must be accomplished through superficial indurated tissues. Incision into an unlocalized cellulitis in an erroneous search for pus can disrupt the physiological barriers and cause diffusion and extension of the infection.

It is often difficult to determine by manual palpation the presence or localization of fluid. Under such indefinite circumstances, aspiration may prove to be a valuable diagnostic aid. Needle aspiration may be used as a diagnostic aid or to evacuate deep fluctuant areas. A large 13- to 16-gauge needle is used to penetrate the area after the superficial skin or mucosa is properly prepared. Pus is aspirated into a syringe and transferred into suitable transport containers for delivery to the microbiology laboratory. Special containers are available for both aerobic and anaerobic laboratory identification procedures. Anaerobic infections, which in prior years escaped diagnosis, may now be more easily detected because of improved technology in the microbiology laboratories, but it is essential that the techniques of specimen collection and transport be given careful attention. A negative report from the laboratory may only be a result of failure of organisms to survive the transfer of the specimen from patient to laboratory, and it will be of little value in arriving at an accurate diagnosis. Aspiration is by far the most suitable method of collecting a specimen when anaerobic organisms are involved. Such infections are becoming more frequently reported in the literature.[14,16,20]

Surgical incision and drainage is performed when the presence of pus is diagnosed (Fig. 11-5). Surgical drainage of deep fascial spaces is usually done in the hospital with the patient under general anesthesia. However, large fluctuant masses can be incised for an ambulatory clinic or office patient under either general or local anesthesia. The skin is prepared in an aseptic manner, and the prepared area is draped with sterile towels. If a local anesthetic is used, a ring block of peripheral skin wheals is made for skin anesthesia. No attempt is made to make a deep injection. The knife is introduced into the most inferior portion of the fluctuant area. A small hemostat is introduced into the wound in closed position and then opened in several directions when introduced into the abscess cavity. A rubber drain is placed in the deepest portion of the wound so that 1 cm remains above the skin surface. It is then sutured in place, and a large dressing is applied.

In areas involving considerably more infection, a through-and-through Penrose drain is introduced. A skin incision is made near the anterior extension of the mass. A large Kelly clamp is used to traverse the fluctuant area to its posterior border. Another skin incision is made over the emerging point of the clamp. The rubber drain is placed in the jaws of the clamp, which is withdrawn to the primary incision, leaving the drain in the tissue tunnel. Two centimeters of drain is left on each end outside of the tissue. A sterile safety pin is placed on each end of the drain so that it cannot be lost, and a heavy dressing is applied.

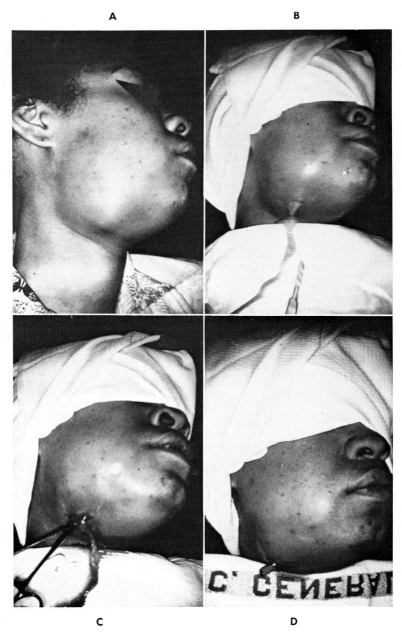

Fig. 11-5. A, Fluctuant cellulitis. Note shiny area (which is red), indicating that the abscess is ready for incision. **B,** Incision. **C,** Hemostat opened in abscess cavity. **D,** Rubber tube affixed in wound by skin suture to maintain drainage. (Courtesy Dr. Arthur Merril.)

Fascial planes

In addition to timing, another problem of surgical evacuation of pus is to determine its exact location and extent. The region of the jaws and mouth is well compartmented by fascial layers. Shapiro[19] states that "The fascial spaces are potential areas between

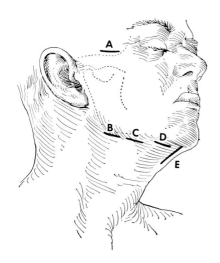

Fig. 11-6. Incisions for drainage of various fascial spaces: *A,* Temporal pouches; *B,* masticator space; *C,* submandibular space; *D,* sublingual space; *E,* submental space.

layers of fascia. These areas are normally filled with loose connective tissue, which readily breaks down when invaded by infection."

Infection started in any area is automatically limited by tough fascial layers, although it may extend by lymphatic or blood vessel routes. The infection fills the immediate fascial space and is contained therein unless physiological factors cannot limit its activity. If the infection becomes massive, it breaks through a nearby fascial barrier into the next fascial space. The infection can be contained here, or it can erode through into contiguous spaces until it reaches the carotid space or the mediastinum, which is infrequent.

To treat acute invasive infections it is necessary to have a thorough practical understanding of these anatomical routes.[22] A systematic survey of the various potential spaces will determine the extent of the infection, and from this knowledge and a knowledge of the optimum place of incision for the evacuation of each fascial space, the location of the incision is determined (Fig. 11-6).

An excellent discussion of the fascial compartments of the head and neck in

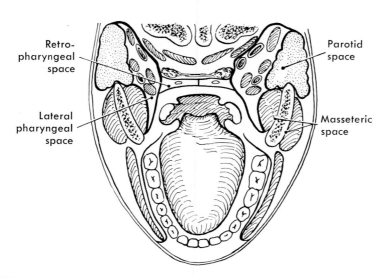

Fig. 11-7. Fascial spaces situated near the jaws. (Courtesy Dr. O. Solnitzky.)

relation to dental infections, taken from an article by Solnitzky,[21] follows:

The most common dental sources of infection are infections of the lower molar teeth. Such infections tend to spread particularly to one of the following compartments: the masticator space, the submandibular space, the sublingual space and temporal pouches [Fig. 11-7]. Infections of the maxillary teeth are less frequent and tend to spread to the pterygopalatine and infratemporal fossae. In either case the spreading suppurative process may involve secondarily the parotid space and the lateral pharyngeal space. In fulminating cases the infection may spread through the visceral space into the mediastinum.

THE DEEP CERVICAL FASCIA

The deep cervical fascia consists of the following parts: (1) a superficial or investing layer; (2) the carotid sheath; (3) the pretracheal layer; and (4) the prevertebral layer.

The superficial or investing layer surrounds the whole neck. It is attached above to the mandible, zygomatic arch, mastoid process, and the superior nuchal line of the occipital bone. Inferiorly it is attached to the spine of the scapula, the acromion, the clavicle, and the sternum. Anteriorly it blends with the same layer of the opposite side and is attached both to the symphysis menti and the hyoid bone. Posteriorly it is attached to the ligamentum nuchae and the spine of the seventh cervical vertebra. This layer splits to enclose two muscles; the sternocleidomastoid and trapezius; and two glands, the submandibular and parotid. It also splits above the manubrium sterni to form the suprasternal space. The investing layer is associated with three fascial compartments important in the spread of dental infections: the submandibular, the submental, and the parotid spaces.

The carotid sheath is a tubular sheath surrounding the common and internal carotid arteries, the internal jugular vein, and the vagus nerve. It blends with the investing layer where the latter splits to enclose the sternocleidomastoid. Near the base of the skull the carotid sheath is especially dense and is here also attached to the sheath of the styloid process.

The pretracheal layer extends across the neck from the carotid sheath of one side to that of the opposite side. It forms an investment for the thyroid gland. It is attached above to the thyroid and cricoid cartilages of the larynx. Inferiorly it continues into the thorax, where it becomes continuous with the fibrous pericardium.

The prevertebral layer lies in front of the vertebral column and the prevertebral muscles. Laterally it blends with the carotid sheath and also forms the fascial floor of the posterior triangle of the neck lying between the trapezius and the sternocleidomastoid muscles. Inferiorly it sends a tubular prolongation about the axillary vessels and the brachial plexus into the axilla.

Between the pretracheal and prevertebral layers is a large space, the visceral space, which is directly continuous with the mediastinum of the thorax. In the upper part of this space are the pharynx and the larynx; in the lower part are the esophagus and trachea, which of course are continued downward into the mediastium. This space can be reached by dental infections, with a resulting mediastinitis.

THE MASTICATOR SPACE

Anatomy. The masticator space includes the subperiosteal region of the mandible and a fascial sling containing the ramus of the mandible and the muscles of mastication. This space is actually formed by the splitting of the investing layer of the deep cervical fascia, the splitting occurring as the fascia becomes attached to the lower border of the mandible. The outer sheath of the fascia covers the external surface of the mandible, the masseter and temporal muscles, while the inner sheath covers the internal surface of the mandible and the medial and lateral pterygoid muscles. The fascial sling is not only attached to, but also reinforces, the periosteum of the mandible along its inferior border. Anterior to the masticator space the deep cervical fascia also helps to form the space for the body of the mandible. Hence the space of the body of the mandible and the masticator space are continuous with each other subperiosteally. Due to the fact that the mandibular periosteum is firmly attached inferiorly, infection follows the line of least resistance, which is posteriorly from the molar region into the masticator space. The firm periosteal attachment also prevents extension of infection inferiorly into the neck.

Posteriorly the masticator space is bounded by the parotid space laterally and the lateral pharyngeal space medially. Superiorly it is continuous with the superficial and deep temporal pouches.

Infections. Infections of the masticator space are practically always of dental origin, particularly the lower molar region. It is the masticator space that is involved in the well-known phlegmonous swelling of the lower jaw following dental extraction, which subsides within a few days without suppuration, the swelling resulting from an inflammatory reaction of the contents of the masticator space [Fig. 11-8].

It is important to remember, both from the standpoint of diagnosis and treatment as well as prognosis, that abscesses of the masticator space often simulate infection of the lateral pharyngeal space. As a matter of fact, abscess of the masticator space is not infrequently mistaken for abscess of the lateral pharyngeal space. It is very important to differentiate these two conditions since both the prognosis and treatment are different.

Infections of the masticator space have a great tendency toward localization. Unless properly drained such infections may spread to the superficial and deep temporal pouches, the parotid space, and even to the lateral pharyngeal space.

Masticator space infections usually result from one of the following:

(1) Infections of the last two lower molars, especially the third molar
(2) Nonaseptic technique in local anesthesia of the inferior alveolar nerve
(3) Trauma to the mandible: external, or fracture into the socket of diseased third molar

Pathologically, infection of the masticator space is characterized by mandibular subperiosteal abscess and cellulitis of the mandible. The masseter and medial pterygoid may also be involved. If the abscess lies more anteriorly, it may involve also the body of the mandible. In some cases osteomyelitis of the ramus of the mandible may set in, particularly if proper drainage of the abscess is not instituted in time.

Clinically the picture of masticator space infection is dominated by trismus, pain, and swelling occurring within a few hours following a molar extraction or trauma to the mandible. The clinical signs increase rapidly to reach a peak in 3 to 7 days. The trismus is likely to be particularly severe because of irritation of both the masseter and medial pterygoid. It may be so intense that the incisors can be opened only to the extent of about half a centimeter. The pain may be excruciating and radiate to the ear. While some rise in temperature is present, chills do not occur as a rule. Dysphagia may be present.

The swelling associated with masticator space infections may be internal, external, or both. As

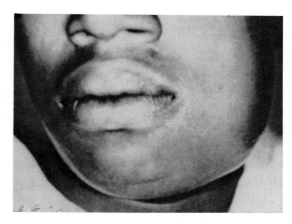

Fig. 11-8. Masticator space infection. (Walter Reed Army Hospital.)

a rule the swelling is both external and internal. The external swelling consists of a brawny induration over the ramus and angle of the mandible. The swelling may extend below the mandible and cross the midline to the opposite side. The subangular space is usually at least partially obliterated to palpation. At the same time constant tenderness occurs along the ramus of the mandible and in the subangular space. In the case of external swelling the mandibular subperiosteal abscess has reached the masseter along the lateral border of the mandible. Internal swelling may predominate in some cases. Such swelling involves the sublingual region and the pharyngeal wall. The pharyngeal swelling pushes the palatine tonsil toward the midline. However, the lateral pharyngeal wall behind the palatine tonsil is not swollen. This feature is important in differentiating a masticator space infection from an infection of the lateral pharyngeal space. In the latter the lateral pharyngeal wall is swollen also behind the palatine tonsil. The pharyngeal swelling in masticator space infection is somewhat lower and more anterior than in lateral pharyngeal or peritonsillar infections. The sublingual region adjacent to the involved portion of the mandible is also swollen and prevents satisfactory depression of the posterior portion of the tongue. The sublingual swelling may give the impression that the condition is a beginning Ludwig's angina.

Since masticator space infections tend to become localized, it is wisest to treat the condition conservatively for several days. If spontaneous drainage has not occurred, surgical drainage

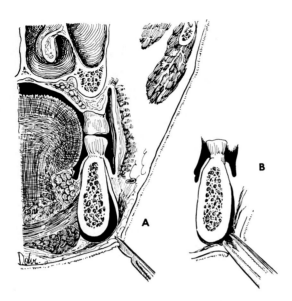

Fig. 11-9. A, External incision for drainage of pus in masticator space. **B,** After incision through skin and superficial fascia. A blunt dissection with a hemostat is the safest method of avoiding important structures while advancing until bone is contacted for drainage of a subperiosteal abscess.

should be employed. Spontaneous drainage is apt to occur if the swelling is exclusively or predominantly internal and if dysphagia is a prominent symptom. Spontaneous intraoral drainage when it occurs usually takes place between the fourth and eighth day. The point of spontaneous drainage is consistently from the lingual border of the mandible near the base of the tongue. Chemotherapy alone is of no avail in the presence of a suppurative process.

The surgical approaches to the masticator space are both internal and external. The internal approach is not satisfactory except in cases where the swelling is exclusively internal.

The internal approach consists of an incision in the mucobuccal fold opposite the third molar, which is extended posteriorly to the ascending ramus of the mandible. The incision is made down to bone. A curved hemostat is then introduced into the incision and directed medial to the ramus into the masticator space behind the angle of the mandible.

The external surgical approach to the masticator space is essential if the swelling is external or both external and internal. The incision for drainage should be made just below and parallel to the angle of the mandible [Fig. 11-9]. As a result of brawny induration it may be difficult to determine the exact line for incision. Because of the swelling, the distance between the angle of

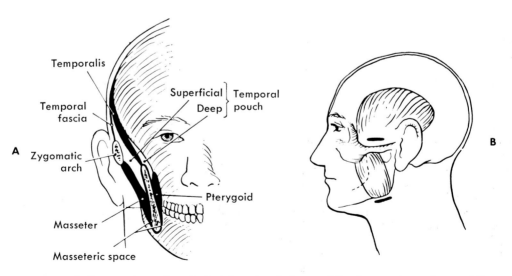

Fig. 11-10. A, Temporal pouches. **B,** Incisions for drainage of the temporal pouches and the masticator space. (Courtesy Dr. O. Solnitzky.)

the mandible and the skin may be greatly increased above normal. In any case the incision must be carried deeply until the bone is actually reached. Since the pus lies subperiosteally, it is imperative that the incision be carried through the periosteum to the bone. Through the external incision at the mandibular angle both the lateral as well as the medial aspects of the ramus of the mandible can be explored for pus.

If surgical drainage is postponed, osteomyelitis of the mandible is apt to occur. At the same time the danger is present of extension of the infection from the masticator space to the temporal pouches, parotid and lateral pharyngeal spaces. Osteomyelitis of the mandible may occur following curettage of the tooth sockets. In the presence of osteomyelitis, drainage may continue for months. It must also be remembered that osteomyelitis of the mandible may set in before the invasion of the masticator space becomes evident.

THE TEMPORAL POUCHES

Anatomy. The temporal pouches are fascial spaces in relation to the temporalis muscle. They are two in number: the superficial and deep [Fig. 11-10].

The superficial temporal pouch lies between the temporal fascia and the temporalis muscle. The temporal fasica consists of a very strong aponeurotic layer, which is attached above to the superior temporal line. Below, it splits into two layers, which are attached to the lateral and medial margins of the superior border of the zygomatic arch. The temporalis muscle arises from the whole of the temporal fossa. Its fibers pass downward, deep to the zygomatic arch, through the gap between the zygoma and the side of the skull, and insert into the coronoid process and ramus of the mandible. The deep temporal pouch lies deep to the temporalis muscle, between the latter and the skull. Below the level of the zygomatic arch the superficial and deep temporal pouches communicate directly with the infratemporal and pterygopalatine fossae.

Infections. Infections of the temporal pouches are usually secondary to primary involvement of the masticator, pterygopalatine, and infratemporal spaces.

Clinically, pain and trismus are present. Externally, swelling over the temporal region may or may not be apparent.

Surgical drainage of the temporal pouches is effected through an incision above the zygomatic

arch, carried through skin, superficial fascia, and the temporal fascia. This incision reaches the superficial temporal pouch. To reach the deep temporal pouch the incision is then carried through the temporalis muscle.

THE SUBMANDIBULAR AND SUBLINGUAL SPACES

The term submandibular space includes the submandibular and submental spaces. Since these spaces communicate with each other, they will be described together.

Anatomy. The submental space lies in the midline between the symphysis menti and the hyoid

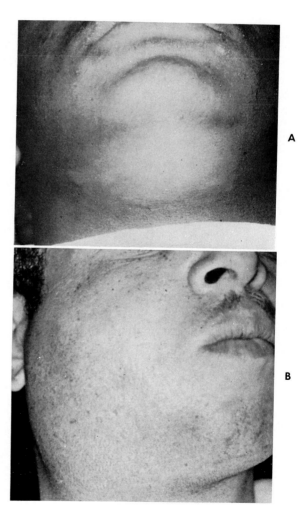

Fig. 11-11. A, Submental abscess. (Walter Reed Army Hospital.) **B,** Parotid space abscess. (Courtesy Dr. George Morin.)

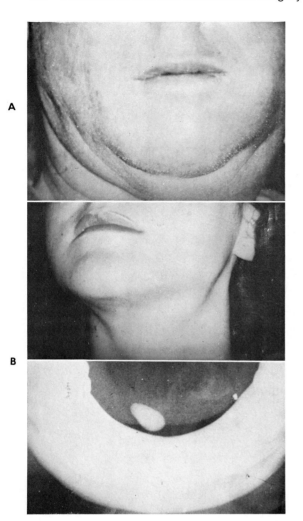

A

B

Fig. 11-12. A, Submandibular space abscess. **B,** Swelling of the submandibular salivary gland secondary to calculus in the duct. Salivary gland involvement must be differentiated from fascial space involvement. (Walter Reed Army Hospital.)

bounded posteroinferiorly by the stylohyoid muscle and the posterior belly of the digastricus, anteroinferiorly by the anterior belly of the digastricus, and above by the lower border of the mandible. Its floor is formed by the mylohyoid and the hyoglossus muscles. This space is enclosed by the investing layer of the deep cervical fascia, the superficial layer being attached to the inferior border of the mandible and the deep layer to the mylohyoid line. Elsewhere the two layers fuse around the periphery of the submandibular gland and become continuous with the fascia covering the mylohyoid and the anterior belly of the digastricus. The submandibular space contains as its major structure the superficial part of the submandibular gland, the deep portion of the gland continuing around the posterior border of the mylohyoid into the sublingual space. Deep to the gland is the facial artery, the nerve to the mylohyoid and the mylohyoid vessels. The facial artery gives off the following branches in this space: the ascending palatine, the tonsillar, the glandular, and the submental. Superficial to the gland is the facial vein. This space also contains the submandibular lymph nodes.

The sublingual space lies above the mylohyoid. Its roof is formed by the mucous membrane of the floor of the mouth. Laterally it is bounded by the inner surface of the body of the mandible above the mylohyoid line. Medially it is limited by the geniohyoid and the genioglossus muscles. The floor is formed by the mylohyoid muscle. It contains the sublingual gland, the submandibular duct, the deep portion of the submandibular gland, the lingual and hypoglossal nerves, and the terminal branches of the lingual artery.

Infections. The most serious infection involving the sublingual, submandibular, and submental spaces is Ludwig's angina. . . .

THE LATERAL PHARYNGEAL SPACE

Anatomy. The lateral pharyngeal space is also known as the parapharyngeal space. . . . It is a deeply situated fascial space lying lateral to the pharynx and medial to the masticator, submandibular, and parotid spaces. It extends from the base of the skull to the level of the hyoid bone. It is bounded medially by the superior constrictor muscle of the pharynx, laterally by the mandible, medial pterygoid muscle, and retromandibular portion of the parotid gland, anteriorly by the pterygomandibular raphe, posteriorly by

bone [Fig. 11-11]. It is bounded laterally by the anterior belly of the digastricus. Its floor is formed by the mylohyoid muscle, while its roof is formed by the suprahyoid portion of the investing layer of the deep cervical fascia. In this space the anterior jugular veins originate. It also contains the submental lymph nodes that drain the median parts of the lower lip, tip of the tongue, and floor of the mouth.

The submandibular or digastric space lies lateral to the submental space [Fig. 11-12]. It is the apposition of the prevertebral and visceral layers of the deep cervical fascia, superiorly by the petrous portion of the temporal bone with the foramen lacerum and jugular foramen, and inferiorly by the attachment of the capsule of the submandibular gland to the sheaths of the stylohyoid muscle and posterior belly of the digastricus.

This space is subdivided into two compartments by the styloid process: an anterior and a posterior compartment. These two compartments are not completely separated from each other. However, infections can and do involve each compartment singly. Often the two compartments are involved simultaneously. The anterior compartment contains lymph nodes (part of the deep cervical group), the ascending pharyngeal and facial arteries, and loose areolar connective tissue. The posterior compartment contains the carotid sheath with the internal carotid artery, internal jugular vein, and vagus nerve as well as glossopharyngeal, accessory, and hypoglossal nerves and the cervical sympathetic trunk. No lymph nodes are found in the posterior compartment.

Infections. Infections of the lateral pharyngeal space are very serious and often are a direct threat to life. While this space is most often involved by infections of the palatine tonsil, mastoid air cells, parotid gland, the retropharyngeal space, and deep cervical lymph nodes, it may also be involved directly or indirectly by infections of dental origin. . . .

This space is most often involved in dental cases by the spread of infection from the masticator space.

Pathologically, most often infections of the lateral pharyngeal space are represented by abscesses. However, sometimes the infection is a rapidly spreading cellulitis similar to that of Ludwig's angina. Fortunately this latter pathological picture is not frequently seen.

The clinical picture is marked by a rapid onset following infections of the upper third molar, accompanied by a rapid rise in temperature. Chills occur if septicemia exists. Marked trismus is present from irritation of the medial pterygoid muscle as well as severe pain resulting from the great tension produced by the accumulation of pus between the medial pterygoid and the superior constrictor muscle of the pharynx. Dysphagia may be marked. Dyspnea, while not so prominent a feature as in Ludwig's angina, may be present.

If the infection is confined to the anterior compartment, external swelling occurs anterior to the sternocleidomastoid muscle. This swelling is first seen at the angle of the mandible and in the submandibular region. It may obliterate the angle of the mandible. The external swelling also extends upward over the parotid region. Internally the anterior part of the lateral pharyngeal wall is swollen and pushes the palatine tonsil together with the soft palate toward the midline. The trismus and pain are particularly severe in infections of the anterior compartments. On the other hand, usually no evidence of septicemia is present.

With infections of the posterior compartment the clinical picture is apt to be dominated by septicemia. Usually little or no trismus and little pain are present. External swelling is apt to be less extensive than with involvement of the anterior compartment. The internal swelling involves the lateral wall of the pharynx behind the palatopharyngeal arch.

As previously mentioned, the lateral pharyngeal space may be the site of a rapidly spreading cellulitis. The clinical picture is grave, being marked by evidence of septicemia and respiratory embarassment due to edema of the larynx. Externally there is a brawny induration of the face above the angle of the mandible. This induration may extend downward to the submandibular region as well as upward to the parotid region and the ipsilateral eye.

The complications of lateral pharyngeal space infections are particularly serious, especially if the infection involves the posterior compartment. These complications include:

(1) Respiratory paralysis resulting from acute edema of larynx
(2) Thrombosis of the internal jugular vein
(3) Erosion of the internal carotid artery

Of these complications perhaps the most dramatic is erosion of the internal carotid artery. Occasionally the erosion may involve the ascending pharyngeal or facial arteries. Such hemorrhages may prove rapidly fatal unless heroic measures are promptly taken.

Since most infections of the lateral pharyngeal space, secondary to dental conditions, have a tendency to localization with abscess formation, it is wisest to wait for such localization before instituting surgical treatment. Prompt surgery is always indicated in the presence of septicemia or hemorrhage.

The surgical incision for drainage may be external or internal.

The external incision is to be preferred for easy access to the carotid arteries in case of hemorrhage. The incision is made along the anterior border of the sternocleidomastoid muscle, extending from below the angle of the mandible to the middle third of the submandibular gland. The fascia behind the submandibular gland is incised, and a curved hemostat is then introduced and carefully directed medially behind the mandible as well as superiorly and slightly posteriorly until the pus cavity is reached. A drain is then inserted.

The internal surgical approach is to be avoided as much as possible since in the presence of erosion of the internal carotid artery the resulting hemorrhage may be massive and uncontrollable. However, if no evidence of such a contingency is found, the internal approach consists of passing a curved hemostat through the pterygomandibular raphe along the surface of the mandible, medial to the medial pterygoid and just lateral to the superior constrictor of the pharynx. The instrument is then directed posteriorly into the pus pocket. . . .

Edema of the larynx is a complication that may arise with great suddenness with lateral pharyngeal space infections. Unless treated promptly by tracheostomy, the issue may be fatal. Hence preparations for immediate tracheostomy should always be made in the presence of such an infection.

THE PAROTID SPACE

Anatomy. The parotid space is a compartment formed by the splitting of the investing layer of the deep cervical fascia. It contains the parotid gland as well as extraglandular and intraglandular parotid lymph nodes. The fascia covering the external surface of the gland is very thick and sends septa into the interior of the gland, subdividing it into lobules. The internal layer of the fibrous capsule is thin and often incomplete superiorly where it may communicate with the lateral pharyngeal space. Posteriorly the parotid space is also in close relation with the middle and external ear. Inferiorly the fascia is reinforced, presenting a strong band called the stylomandibular ligament, which very effectively separates the parotid from the submandibular space.

Infections. While this space is not usually involved by infections of dental origin, sometimes dental infections may extend up the ramus of the mandible and invade it. This may occur particularly in improperly treated masticator space infections.

In the presence of infection in this space a hard, smooth swelling occurs over the parotid region in front of and below the external ear. The swelling gradually becomes more intense. This may be accompanied by fever and chills. The swelling may extend over the entire side of the face with edema and closure of the eye on the affected side.

The surgical approach to the parotid space is made by an incision in front of the external ear, extending from the level of the zygoma to the angle of the mandible. The skin and subcutaneous fascia are reflected over the external surface of the gland. Since the parotid fascia is firmly attached to the skin, this reflection must be done carefully. After exposure of the gland transverse incisions are made into the gland superficially. The gland and abscess should then be opened by blunt dissection in a direction parallel to the branches of the facial nerve. However, since the branches of the facial nerve lie deep to the superficial part of the parotid gland, they are not very likely to be injured by this procedure. Drains are then inserted.

THE PTERYGOPALATINE AND INFRATEMPORAL FOSSAE

These two spaces are usually involved by infections of the upper molar teeth.

Anatomy. The pterygopalatine fossa lies behind the maxillary sinus, below the apex of the orbit, lateral to the muscular plate of the pterygoid process of the sphenoid bone and deep to the temporomandibular joint. The pterygopalatine fossa communicates with the infratemporal fossa through the pterygomaxillary fissure. At its upper end the pterygomaxillary fissure is continuous with the inferior orbital fissure, which leads from the pterygopalatine fossa into the orbit. The inferior orbital fissure contains the infraorbital nerve, the continuation of the maxillary nerve. The infraorbital nerve gives off the anterior and middle superior alveolar nerves, which pass through canals in the bony wall of the maxillary sinus to be distributed to the upper incisor, canine, and premolar teeth, and the mucous membrane of the upper gums. The pterygopalatine fossa also communicates with the pterygoid canal, which transmits the nerve of the pterygoid canal (Vidian). The Vidian nerve is made up of the great petrosal nerve from the facial, transmitting preganglionic parasympathetic fibers to the pterygopalatine ganglion, and the deep petrosal nerve conveying postganglionic sympathetic fibers from the superior cervical sympathetic ganglion by way of the internal carotid artery. The pterygopalatine fossa contains part of the maxillary nerve, the pterygopalatine ganglion, and the terminal part of the maxillary artery. Superiorly the pterygopalatine fossa is closely related to the abducens nerve and the optic nerve. Both of these nerves may become involved in infections of the pterygopalatine fossa.

The infratemporal fossa lies behind the ramus of the mandible below the level of the zygomatic arch. It is bounded medially by the lateral plate of the pterygoid process and the lateral wall of the pharynx, represented here by the upper part of the superior constrictor, and the auditory tube covered by the tensor veli palatini muscle. Posteriorly the fossa is limited by the parotid gland, which overlaps here into it. Anteriorly the infratemporal fossa is limited by the maxilla, superficial to which the fossa extends forward into the cheek superficial to the buccinator muscle. The buccal pad of fat plugs this space and extends for some distance between the buccinator and the ramus of the mandible. Superiorly the roof of the infratemporal fossa is formed, as far as the infratemporal crest, by the infratemporal surface of the greater wing of the sphenoid, perforated by the foramen ovale, which transmits the mandibular nerve, and the foramen spinosum, which transmits the middle meningeal artery. Lateral to the infratemporal crest the infratemporal fossa is continuous with the temporal pouches. Inferiorly the infratemporal fossa is continuous with the region deep to the body of the mandible that above the mylohyoid line forms part of the wall of the mouth and below the mylohyoid line constitutes part of the submandibular region.

Infections. Infections of the pterygopalatine and infratemporal fossae are comparatively rare.

Primary infections of these fossae usually result from:

(1) Infections of the molar teeth of the maxilla, especially the third molar

(2) Local infiltration of the maxillary nerve

Clinically, marked trismus and pain occur. Externally, swelling is evident in front of the exter-

nal ear over the temporomandibular joint and the zygomatic arch. The swelling soon extends to the cheek. In severe and untreated cases the swelling involves the whole side of the face. The eye is closed and proptosed. Abducens paralysis may be present. The swelling may also extend into the neck. In such severe cases optic neuritis may also develop.

At the same time osteomyelitis of the maxilla may set in. The osteomyelitis is usually confined to the alveolar process. The osteomyelitis of the maxilla may lead to secondary involvement of the maxillary air sinus.

The pterygopalatine and infratemporal fossae may also become involved secondarily from infections of the masticator, parotid, and lateral pharyngeal spaces.

Infections of the pterygopalatine and infratemporal fossae have a great tendency to later abscess formation.

These spaces may be reached surgically by two approaches. The external approach consists of an incision made just above the zygomatic arch. The underlying fibers of the temporalis muscle are then spread and a curved hemostat is introduced and directed downward and medialward beneath the zygomatic arch into the abscess cavity. The internal approach consists of an incision made in the buccolabial fold lateral to the upper third molar. The incision is made down to, but not including, the periosteum of the maxilla. A curved hemostat is then introduced carefully behind the tuberosity of the maxilla and then directed medially and superiorly into the abscess cavity. A drain is then inserted.

Surgical drainage should not be delayed if sepsis is present.*

Ludwig's angina

Ludwig's angina[2,4,12] may be described as an overwhelming, generalized septic cellulitis of the submandibular region (Fig. 11-13). Although not seen often, Ludwig's angina, when it does occur, usually is an extension of infection from the mandibular molar teeth into the floor of the mouth, since their roots lie below the attachment of

---

*Reprinted with minor changes (approved by author) from Solnitzky, O.: Bull. Georgetown Univ. Med. Center **7:**86, 1954.

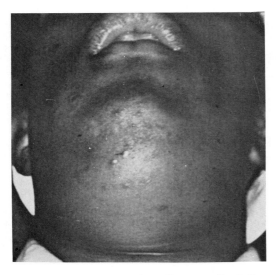

Fig. 11-13. Ludwig's angina. (Courtesy Dr. Arthur Merril.)

the mylohyoid muscle. It is usually observed after extraction.

This infection differs from other types of postextraction cellulitis in several ways. First, it is characterized by a brawny induration. The tissues are boardlike and do not pit on pressure. No fluctuance is present. The tissues may become gangrenous, and when cut, they have a peculiar lifeless appearance. A sharp limitation is apparent between the involved tissues and the surrounding normal tissues.

Second, three fascial spaces are involved bilaterally: submandibular, submental, and sublingual spaces. If the involvement is not bilateral, the infection is not considered a Ludwig's angina.

Third, the patient has a typical open-mouthed appearance. The floor of the mouth is elevated, and the tongue is protruded, making respiration difficult. Two large potential fascial spaces are at the base of the tongue, and either or both are involved. The deep space is located between the genioglossus and geniohyoid muscles; the superficial space is located between the geniohyoid and mylohyoid muscles. Each space is divided by a median septum. If the

tongue is not elevated, the infection is not considered a true Ludwig's angina.

The infection is often caused by a hemolytic streptococcus, although the infection may be a mixture of aerobic and anaerobic organisms, which may account for the presence of gas in the tissues. Chills, fever, increased salivation, stiffness in tongue movements, and an inability to open the mouth herald the infection. Thickness is found in the floor of the mouth, and the tongue is elevated. Tissues of the neck become boardlike. The patient develops a toxic condition, and respiration becomes difficult. The larynx is edematous.

Treatment consists of massive antibiotic and other supportive therapy. In the acute stage tracheostomy must be considered, and if the respiration becomes embarrassed, this procedure should be done to maintain an airway. If there is no change for the better in a matter of hours, surgical intervention is necessary for two reasons: the release of tissue tensions and the provision for drainage. Although in the classic case little pus is present, in other cases a large amount is found, even though fluctuance cannot be palpated through the induration. The small pocket of pus is usually found not in the midline but near the medial aspect of the mandible on the side where the infection originated.

The radical surgical approach in acute cases takes the form of an incision made under local anesthesia parallel and medial to the lower border of the mandible, which may be difficult to find. The incision is extended upward to the base of the tongue in the submandibular area. In the submental area the incision extends through the mylohyoid muscle to the mucous membranes of the mouth. The tissues are probed for a pus pocket. To obtain maximum release of tissue tension the surgeon makes no attempt to suture.

Cavernous sinus thrombosis

Infections of the face can cause a septic thrombosis of the cavernous sinus. This

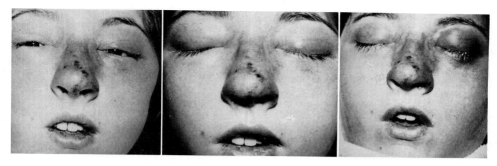

Fig. 11-14. Cavernous sinus thrombosis with fatal termination in spite of massive antibiotic therapy. (Courtesy Dr. I. D. Fagin.)

was almost always fatal before the advent of antibiotics. Furunculosis and infected hair follicles in the nose are frequent causes. Extractions of maxillary anterior teeth in the presence of acute infection and especially curettage of the sockets under such circumstances can cause this condition. The infection is usually staphylococcal. The antibiotic to which the organism is most susceptible is given in large doses. Occasionally the antibiotics will not adequately resolve the septic thrombus, and death ensues (Fig. 11-14).

The infected thrombus ascends in the veins against the usual venous flow. This is possible because of the absence of valves in the angular, facial, and ophthalmic veins.

The diagnosis of cavernous sinus thrombosis is made in the presence of the following six features, according to Eagleton[3]: (1) a known site of infection, (2) evidence of bloodstream infection, (3) early signs of venous obstruction in the retina, conjunctiva, or eyelid, (4) paresis of the third, fourth, and sixth cranial nerves resulting from inflammatory edema, (5) abscess formation in the neighboring soft tissues, and (6) evidence of meningeal irritation.

Clinically one eye experiences early involvement. Later the other eye may be involved. Empirical antibiotic therapy followed by specific antibiotic therapy based on blood or pus culture is the treatment.

Surgical access through eye enucleation has been suggested.

GENERAL MANAGEMENT OF PATIENT WITH ACUTE INFECTION

The care of the patient with an acute infection is directed toward two ends—to destroy or inhibit the bacterial growth and to encourage the physiological defense mechanisms by means of active attention to the patient's physiological needs.

Immediate empirical use of an indicated antibiotic in adequate doses is the preferred treatment for bacterial infections unless contraindicated by a history of allergy.

In severe or fulminating infections, blood should be drawn for a blood culture for later laboratory analysis, and immediate empirical antibiotic therapy should be initiated after the blood is drawn. In general, antibiotics used empirically should be selected based on the belief that penicillinase-producing organisms may be involved. Therefore, and antibiotic that is effective against both penicillinase-producing and nonpenicillinase-producing organisms is desirable. Gram-negative organisms, although less likely, may be responsible, and therapy directed at these organisms should be employed whenever they are strongly suspected. Maximal doses of the selected antibiotics should be employed. As well as providing maximum therapeutic effect, this approach makes diagnosis less confusing if favorable results are not obtained. Time is not wasted by resorting to trial of higher levels of the same antibiotic if, in fact, that antibiotic is not effective against the infecting organisms. Unless extremely rapid deterioration of the patient's condition occurs, another antibiotic regimen based on laboratory identification and antibiotic sensitivity may be instituted within a short time. If such time is not available then a change of antibiotics may be necessary.

For hospitalized patients, intravenous therapy may be used to produce high therapeutic levels of antibiotic drugs rapidly and to maintain them effectively during the acute phase.

Patient care is important. Dehydration alone can account for an increase in temperature of a degree or two. Fluid in several forms should be continually urged on the patient. In severe cases an input-output record is kept. Hospitalized patients benefit from intravenous fluid therapy and other aids to help them achieve an adequate fluid balance. Adequate nourishment is essential, in liquid or soft form if necessary. A laxative can be suggested if needed. Complete rest is necessary. Analgesics and sedatives will relieve pain and anxiety.

The use of heat and cold applications has been predicated on tradition. In general, moderate heat has been found to supply an analgesic effect and to be beneficial in localizing infection.[15] Ice compresses applied intermittently for short intervals in an early postoperative period may inhibit the edema occurring after traumatic operative procedures, but they have no other therapeutic value. Excessive or prolonged use of ice compresses may impede healing by inhibition of normal defense processes, which function best at normal body temperature. When heat is used for therapy, it should be in the form of moist dressings. A washcloth placed under tap water as warm as the wrist can stand, wrung out, and folded in fourths is applied to the face, which has been protected from dehydration with cold cream. The face, with washcloth in place, is covered with a dry Turkish towel and a hot-water bag placed over this. The compress is maintained for 30 minutes, removed for 30 minutes, and then reapplied. Flaxseed poultices hold the heat better but are not in common use.

OSTEOMYELITIS

Acute osteomyelitis occurs more frequently in the mandible than in the maxilla. It starts with an infection of the cancellous or medullary portion of the bone, which usually enters by way of a wound or an opening through the cortical plate of bone (for example, the alveolar socket), admitting an infection into the central structure. This infection may enter as a result of a periapical or pericoronal infection prior to any surgical intervention, or it may be introduced through a needle puncture, particularly if pressure methods have been employed or interosseous anesthesia has been a method employed.

The infection may be localized, or it may diffuse through the entire medullary structure of the mandible or maxilla, and it may be preceded by an acute infection. It can be preceded by septic cellulitis, or it can follow what was apparently a simple extraction of an infected tooth.

The onset of an osteomyelitis is evidently associated with the lack of resistance of an individual patient to the particular organisms that invade the osseous structure.[10] Prior to the advent of chemotherapeutic and antibiotic agents, osteomyelitic infection was not uncommon. It most frequently followed an invasion through a third molar wound. Since the employment of antibiotic therapy at the first sign of septic postoperative sequelae, osteomyelitis is rarely seen. On infrequent occasions, however, this disease still occurs,[9] and the use of antibiotics has but little impeding effect on its progress.

Symptoms include a deep persisting pain, occasionally accompanied by intermittent paresthesia of the lip. An edema of the overlying soft tissues and an accompanying periostitis is usually present. The patient may ultimately experience malaise and an elevation in temperature. The condition may persist to a state at which the infection breaks through the cortical bone and invades the soft tissues, and induration followed by abscess formation becomes evident (Fig. 11-15).

Since wide variations in radiographic evidence or clinical symptoms occur, early diagnosis sometimes is difficult. The osteomyelitic process originates within the cancellous structure of the bone, and destruction of the cancellous structure occurs with much less resistance than that of the cortical bone. The cortical bone is dense, and the destructive process may progress before it can be revealed in the the radiograph because of the superimposition of the denser cortical bone. In the more aggressive or rampant types, destruction may occur rapidly and the cortical bone may be invaded so that radiographic evidence becomes visible at an early date. This destructive process has no definite pattern. A radiolucent area seen in the radiograph is often described as having a wormy appearance.

In the invasive or rampant nonlocalized type, all teeth in the section of the mandible or maxilla may become mobile or tender, and pus may be observed around the necks of the teeth and interproximal spaces. Multiple perforating sinuses may be draining pus into the oral vestibule or burrowing into the overlying musculature and forming abscesses, which, if not incised and drained, will spontaneously rupture to the surface. If this latter condition is permitted, an ugly, indented scar results.

Treatment. The earlier a diagnosis can be made and definitive treatment started, the greater is the opportunity of impeding the progress of the infection. Even before purulent material can be obtained for culture, it is advisable to begin administering an antibiotic in high doses. Of course this may make it difficult to obtain a culture when suppuration begins, but time is the important factor, and the earlier antibiotic therapy can be started, the better is the chance of therapeutic control. As soon as it is possible to obtain a culture, the antibiotic that the laboratory finds to be most efficacious may be given.

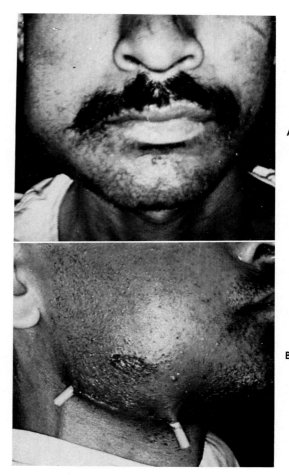

Fig. 11-15. **A,** Acute osteomyelitis. **B,** Drainage tube in position. The portion of the tube lying in the tissues is perforated by a series of holes for irrigation and drainage. (Courtesy Dr. Arthur Merril.)

Edema and induration should be observed closely for the first indication of fluctuance so that at the earliest possible moment a liberal incision can be made down to the bony surface for the early evacuation of pus, thereby preventing the pus from elevating the periosteum. If induration extends beyond the limit of the incision after the primary drainage, then the incision should immediately be extended.

The destructiveness of osteomyelitis is caused by the pressure and lysis of suppurative material in a confined space. A staphlococcus is usually the cause. If the bacteria are killed or their growth is stopped by the antibiotic, resolution of the infection occurs without the need for surgery beyond the extraction of the offending tooth (if the infection is odontogenic in origin). If the bacteria are resistant to antibiotics (for example, a "hospital staphyloccus") or if a massive collection of pus has formed before effective antibiotic therapy can be instituted, then portions of the bone become devitalized because their blood supply has been cut off by thrombosis of the vessels. The island of dead bone thus formed becomes a convenient place for precipitation of the ionized calcium that has been mobilized by the surrounding osteolytic process, and therefore this sequestrum appears as a radiopaque shadow on the radiograph (Fig. 11-16). Nature tends to expel the sequestrum, although occasionally a small sequestrum is lysed during long, effective antibiotic therapy.

The pattern for treatment, then, is (1) effective antibiotic therapy, (2) drainage of purulent material if and when pus forms in spite of antibiotic therapy, (3) a period of supportive therapy during which the drainage area is kept open by dressings and the antibiotic therapy is continued, and (4) sequestrectomy.

The sequestrum should not be removed too early. It should be clearly outlined on the radiograph. If the infection has been controlled, the sequestrum is lifted gently out of its soft tissue bed, or involucrum. This bed is not curetted. Occasionally the overhanging margins of cortical bone are ronguered back to cortical bone that rests on intact medullary bone. This is called saucerization.

The treatment pattern can be interrupted at any of the four stages if normal healing occurs. The antibiotic should be continued for a minimum of 4 to 6 weeks after drainage has ceased.

If clinical and radiographic evidence of rampant invasion of the medullary structure of the bone is found and the cortical plate has not been perforated by the infectious process, holes may be drilled through the inferior border of the mandible to permit drainage of the cancellous structure. This latter procedure is controversial and depends on the judgment and discretion of the

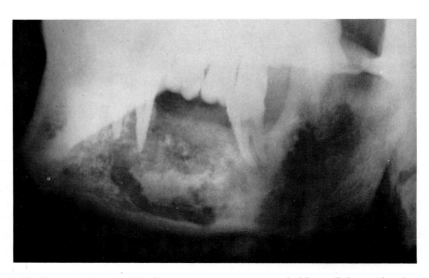

Fig. 11-16. Chronic osteomyelitis. Note sequestrum surrounded by radiolucent involucrum.

surgeon, who will have to evaluate the case according to its behavior pattern.

Decortication has been employed with satisfactory results. Intraoral decortication with immediate soft tissue closure followed by pressure bandages places vascular tissue in contact with the decorticated medullary bone that has been deprived of its physiological blood supply. In reestablishing an available blood supply, antibiotic therapy may be expected to be of greater value. Hjorting-Hansen[7] has described in detail decortication of the mandible in the treatment of osteomyelitis.

The decision whether or not to extract excessively mobile teeth in the segment of the jaw where suppuration is visible around the gingiva is another point of controversy and one that requires the keenest discretion and judgment. Some of the most spectacular suppurative and rampant cases can apparently reach a crisis, at which point symptoms will subside and regeneration begin without the extraction of mobile teeth. The offending tooth, of course, is usually extracted.

Drainage incisions for osteomyelitis have a tendency to proliferate large amounts of granulation tissue, which will expel artificial drains from the wounds. Unless retained with mattress sutures over the dressings, drainage gauze that is packed into the wound may become extruded. Suturing of the drainage material may be necessary to maintain its position so that the wound remains saucerized. This procedure pertains to both intraoral and extraoral wound dressings. The retention of dressings that maintain saucerization of the wound for intervals of 5 to 7 days without replacement is recommended unless clinical symptoms indicate intervention.

REFERENCES

1. Bickley, H. C.: A concept of allergy with reference to oral disease, J. Periodontol. **41:**302-312, 1970.
2. Crystal, D. K., and others: Emergency treatment in Ludwig's angina, Surg. Gynecol. Obstet. **129:** 755-757, 1969.
3. Eagleton, W. P.: Cavernous sinus thrombophlebitis and allied septic and traumatic lesions of the basal venous sinuses. A clinical study of blood stream infection, New York, 1926, The Macmillan Co.
4. Fein, S., and Mohnac, A. M.: Ludwig's angina infection: report of case and associated systemic complications, J. Oral Surg. **31:**785-787, 1973.
5. Gold, R. S., and Sager, E.: Pansinusitis, orbital cellulitis, and blindness as sequella of delayed treatment of dental abscess, J. Oral Surg. **32:**40-43, 1974.
6. Haymaker, W.: Fatal infections of the central nervous system and meninges after tooth extraction, Am. J. Orthodont. Oral Surg. (Oral Surg. Sect.) **31:**117, 1945.
7. Hjorting-Hansen, E.: Decortication in treatment of osteomyelitis of the mandible, Oral Surg. **29:** 641, 1970.
8. Hollin, S. A., Hayashi, H., and Gross, S. W.: Intracranial abscesses of odontogenic origin, Oral Surg. **23:**277, 1967.
9. Khosla, V. M.: Current concepts in the treatment of acute and chronic osteomyelitis: review and report of four cases, J. Oral Surg. **28:**209-214, 1970.
10. Killey, H. C., and Kay, L. W.: Acute osteomyelitis of the mandible, J. Int. Coll. Surg. **43:**647, 1965.
11. Killey, H. C., Kay, L. W., and Wright, H. C.: Subperiosteal osteomyelitis of the mandible, Oral Surg. **29:**576, 1970.
12. Marks, R. B., and others: Ludwig's angina: report of case, J. Oral Surg. **32:**462-464, 1974.
13. Marlette. R. H., Gerhard, R. C., and Conley, J.: Brain abscess of dental origin: report of case, J. Oral Surg. **28:**134-137, 1970.
14. Monaldo, L. J., and others: Bacteroides infection of the mandible with secondary spread to the neck, J. Oral Surg. **32:**370-372, 1974.
15. Moose, S. M.: The rational therapeutic use of thermal agents with special reference to heat and cold, J. Am. Dent. Assoc. **24:**185, 1937.
16. Quayle, A. A.: Bacteroides infections in oral surgery, J. Oral Surg. **32:**91-99, 1974.
17. Rickles, N.: Allergy in surface lesions of the oral mucosa, Oral Surg. **33:**744-754, 1972.
18. Rockoff, P. R., and others: Meningitis as a result of a postextraction infection: report of case, J. Oral Surg. **30:**687-689, 1972.
19. Shapiro, H. H.: Applied anatomy of the head and neck, Philadelphia, 1947, J. B. Lippincott Co.
20. Sharp, P. M., Meador, R. C., and Martin, R. R.: A case of mixed anaerobic infection of the jaw, J. Oral Surg. **32:**457-459, 1974.
21. Solnitzky, O.: The fascial compartments of the head and neck in relation to dental infections, Bull. Georgetown Univ. Med. Center **7:**86, 1954.
22. Spilka, C. J.: Pathways of dental infections, J. Oral Surg. **24:**111, 1966.
23. Tatoian, J. A., and others: Meningitis and temporal lobe abscess of dental origin, J. Oral Surg. **30:**423-426, 1972.

CHAPTER 12

Chronic periapical infections

James A. O'Brien

When trauma or caries causes a tooth to die, the pulp cavity and canals become repositories for necrotic pulp tissue. This degenerating tissue (with or without bacteria) produces periapical irritation through the apical foramina. The body attempts to combat this irritation by an inflammatory response. If a virile organism is responsible for the infection, the process is likely to be acute. On the other hand, if the organism is not virile or if the irritation is produced by toxins of the necrotic pulp, the process is likely to be chronic (Fig. 12-1).

TYPES OF CHRONIC PERIAPICAL INFECTION
Chronic alveolar abscess

An abscess, by definition, is a localized collection of pus in a cavity formed by the disintegration of tissues. The chronic alveolar abscess may be the aftermath of an acute periapical infection, or it may be produced by a chronic periapical infection. In either case periapical bone is destroyed by a localized osteomyelitis, and the resultant cavity is filled with pus. The inflammatory process walls off the area. If the chronic irritation continues, the abscess will expand until it drains itself by perforating the gingiva (''gumboil'') or the skin (Fig. 12-2).

If the source of the irritant is removed,

either by extraction of the tooth or by means of a root canal filling, the abscess cavity will drain itself and be replaced by granulation tissue, which then will form new bone.

Granuloma

A granuloma is, literally, a tumor made up of granulation tissue. However, the term dental granuloma is used to designate the situation in the periapical region in which an abscess or a localized area of osteolysis is replaced by granulation tissue.

The chronic irritation from the dental pulp results in destruction of periapical bone. The body's attempt to repair the defect consists of an ingrowth of capillaries and immature connective tissue that, were it not for the continued irritation from the dental pulp, would rebuild the bone tissue. However, the continued irritation causes a mixture of this reparative tissue with the inflammatory exudate, and this makes up the dental granuloma.

Microscopically, the granuloma is made up of organizing connective tissue with numerous capillaries, with a fibrous capsule that has collagenous fibers running parallel to the periphery, and with evident inflammatory exudate (principally lymphocytes and plasma cells). The radiograph usually

208

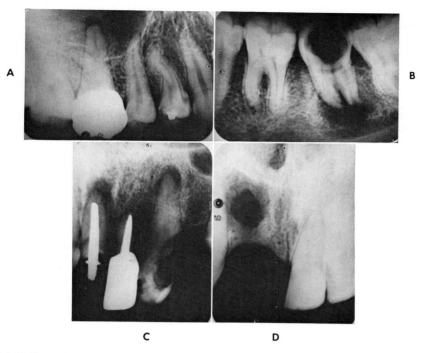

Fig. 12-1. A, Break in lamina dura at apex of palatal root, first molar. This disturbance can lead to an acute infection or grow slowly into a chronic lesion without an acute phase. **B,** Chronic alveolar abscess. The margins of the lesion are indistinct, the roots show slight resorption, and a condensing osteitis is demonstrated. **C,** Granuloma. The lesion on the cuspid, in particular, is rounded. Frequently the granuloma stays attached to the extracted tooth. **D,** Residual defect of bone after loss of both palatal and labial plates of bone through surgery or disease. In the absence of clinical symptoms this defect should not be reopened.

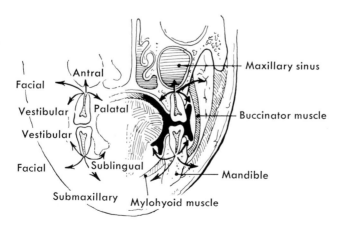

Fig. 12-2. Possible pathways for spontaneous eruption of pus from dental infections. Note that the buccinator and mylohyoid muscle attachments determine whether the pus will erupt intra-orally or through the skin.

demonstrates a discrete, rounded lesion, which is difficult, if not impossible, to differentiate from a cyst.

A granuloma may contain epithelial cell rests of Malassez. These cell rests have the potential to form a cyst if the granuloma remains in the bone, even if the tooth is removed.

Periapical cyst

A cyst is defined as a sac that contains a liquid or semisolid. The periapical cyst is an epithelium-lined sac containing liquid or semisolid inflammatory exudate and necrotic products. The periapical cyst is considered to originate from the dental granuloma. The epithelial cell rests of Malassez entrapped in the granuloma are stimulated to proliferate. A central area of breakdown forms, and the proliferating epithelium becomes an encapsulating membrane. Cellular disintegration within the cyst causes diffusion of additional fluid into the cystic cavity and resultant pressure. This increased pressure causes the peripheral bone to resorb and the cyst to enlarge. An inconstant radiographic finding is a radiopaque line around the cyst cavity (Fig. 12-3). The mechanism of cyst growth or the reason one cyst becomes larger than another is still not clearly understood. As a rule, the periapical cysts, which are always considered to be infected, do not grow as large as the follicular cysts, which are not infected unless contamination occurs.

A periapical lesion may be large without showing radiographic evidence of bone destruction. This is because osteolytic lesions in cancellous bone cannot be detected radiographically; it is only when a portion of cortical bone is destroyed that the radiograph demonstrates it.[1,10,11]

TREATMENT

Chronic periapical pathological conditions, such as chronic alveolar abscess, granuloma, or periapical cyst, may undergo acute exacerbations. Treatment of the acute phase, particularly when severe, is described in Chapter 11. However, treatment of localized exacerbation requires the following additional considerations.

1. If the tooth is a useless one, removing it is the simplest and best treatment, subject to other factors considered in Chapter 11.

2. If the tooth is a useful one, conservation should be the prime goal. Therefore the treatment should consist of opening the pulp chamber and removing a major part of the contents of the canals to obtain drain-

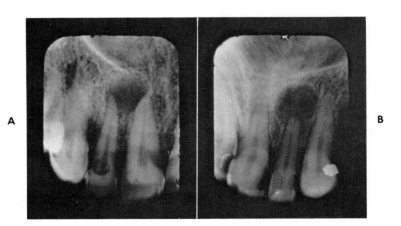

Fig. 12-3. A, Periapical cyst. No white line encircles it; therefore it cannot be differentiated radiographically from a granuloma. **B,** Periapical cyst, well defined. (From Stafne, E. C.: Oral roentgenographic diagnosis, Philadelphia, 1958, W. B. Saunders Co.)

age. If drainage by this route is inadequate, an incision for drainage may be necessary. Antibiotic therapy is discussed in Chapter 9.

When the exacerbation has subsided, root canal treatment should be carried out. Most endodontists report a success rate of 90% or better without recourse to surgery. Investigators have demonstrated that approximately 43% of periapical lesions are cysts.[3,5] It seems evident then that most small cysts will heal without surgical enucleation if the root canal filling is adequate. However, surgical intervention in the periapical area is a relatively simple procedure, and there are several indications for it:

1. In a case that cannot be followed postoperatively for whatever reason. Surgical curettement of the periapical area assures a result that is no longer endangered by debris from the endodontic procedure or by epithelial elements.

2. In a case in which there is a suspicion of an unfilled accessory canal orifice or a severely curved root end. Apicoectomy will remove the unfilled portion of the canal.

3. In procedural accidents, removal of broken root canal instruments or filling material may require periapical surgery.

4. Necessity for retrograde filling of a canal. Extremely large ("blunderbuss") canals cannot be filled adequately by insertion of points or pastes or both; they must be obliterated by amalgam at the apex. Retrograde fillings are also useful to close a canal in a tooth that cannot be treated in the usual manner because of a porcelain jacket or some other obstacle (for example, limitation of mandibular movement, preventing access through the crown of the tooth).

5. Persistent postoperative discomfort after root canal filling. Periapical curettage and apicoectomy will frequently eliminate the symptoms.

Technique of apicoectomy

1. Make a radiograph after the root canal filling has been completed to determine the level at which the root should be amputated. This level should be such as to remove any unfilled portion of root canal, and it should also facilitate access to the periapical cyst or granuloma to ensure its complete removal.

2. Design the mucoperiosteal flap with three considerations in mind (Fig. 12-4): (a) Be sure blood supply and tissue mass are adequate to avoid necrosis and poor healing. Incisions sharply made perpendicular to bone are important. (b) Make the flap

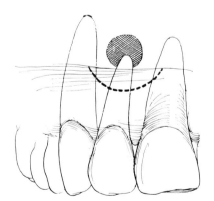
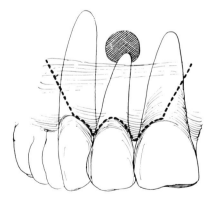

Fig. 12-4. Two types of incision for apicoectomy.

large enough to provide good access. (c) Make the flap extend well beyond the bony defect so that the soft tissue will be supported by bone when it is replaced.

3. After the mucoperiosteal flap has been raised, make an opening into the periapical bony defect using a surgical bur or chisel if the granuloma or cyst has not already perforated the labial plate of bone. Extend the opening in the labial plate with bur, chisel, or rongeurs to obtain good access to the limits of the defect.

Then, with a fissured cylindrical bur, amputate the root at the level determined with the aid of the radiograph. The cyst or granuloma should be enucleated, preferably in toto, by means of small curets.

4. Control hemorrhage within the defect by crushing bleeding points in bone, by pressure, or by cotton pledgets dipped in epinephrine (Adrenalin).

5. Suture the mucoperiosteal flap with a small cutting needle and No. 4-0 silk or catgut.

6. After closing, maintain firm pressure over the area for 10 minutes to avoid formation of a hematoma.

7. Obtain an immediate postoperative radiograph to check the level of root amputation and for future comparison.

Retrograde filling

Retrofilling is sometimes a very useful procedure when complete filling of a canal is impossible by coronal approach or when symptoms persist following filling of the canal. Several points are important to success:

1. Bevel the root surface in the apicoectomy so you have very good visualization of the apical foramina.

2. In the "cavity preparation" for the retrograde filling, undercut only toward the lingual side of the canal. On that side you will have enough dentine apical to the undercut; on the labial side, attempting to undercut just chips out the wall (because of the bevel of the apicoectomy).[4]

3. A small suction tip is essential. Of great help has been the use of a 16-gauge needle that fits on the end of a standard suction tip. With several of these needles at hand, your assistant can use the regular tip to pick up larger debris (including amalgam fragments) and quickly place or remove the needle tip as needed.[4]

4. Zinc-free amalgam is the most commonly used retrofilling material. Gutta percha also has been used with success.

Other aspects of periapical radiolucencies

In this discussion the term, cyst, will be used to include granulomas as well.

It is a cardinal point that a periapical cyst is not the cause of radiolucency if the tooth is vital. If the tooth is vital, the periapical radiolucency has some other basis, and the fact that the root of the tooth lies within the apparent cyst is no indication for extracting it or for root canal therapy. Also, lack of vital response, without symptoms and without radiographic changes, is not an indication for extraction or root canal therapy.[3]

If the tooth is extracted, the small periapical cyst usually can be enucleated through the socket. A small curet is inserted with the sharp edge against bone and the convex surface against cyst membrane (Fig. 12-5). By careful dissection the cyst can be separated from the bone and lifted out in toto. If it fails to come out intact, the wall of the defect must be curetted carefully to remove all remnants of the cyst.

For larger cysts the technique consists of raising a mucoperiosteal flap similar to the apicoectomy flap, removing the overlying bone by means of bur, chisels, or ronguers, and enucleating the cyst by means of currets. Again, "shelling-out" a cyst is best accomplished by using the back side of the curet. That is, the concave side of the curet is toward bone and the convex side is against the cyst. In this way, the cyst is removed without tearing the cyst wall, and therefore the chance of leaving epithelial cells that might reproduce the cyst is lessened. After the cyst has been removed, the

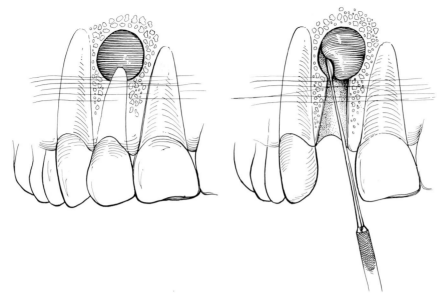

Fig. 12-5. The back of the curet is employed to remove a small periapical cyst through the socket.

mucoperiosteal flap is replaced and sutured and pressure is maintained on the area for 10 minutes.

If a large periapical cyst is accessible and does not involve vital teeth or the maxillary sinus, it is usually best treated by enucleation. Primary closure of a large defect, however, can result in the accumulation of a pocket of necrotic material if the large, unsupported blood clot breaks down. Therefore if the defect is more than 15 mm in diameter, it is good practice to pack the void with petrolatum gauze (¼ or ½ inch) or Adaptic strip, bringing the end out through the line of closure. This packing prevents the accumulation of a pool of blood in the defect. The packing is removed after approximately 5 days.

When a large periapical cyst involves the roots of adjacent vital teeth or approximates the antral wall, treatment consists of exteriorizing the cyst, thus removing the central pressure that causes the expansion of the cyst. With this central pressure removed, the periphery will slowly fill in, gradually decreasing the size of the defect.

This process can be allowed to continue until the defect is obliterated, but this may take many months. The period of treatment can be shortened by enucleating the cyst after it has been reduced to a size that does not threaten the adjacent teeth and the antrum.

Two basic methods of exteriorizing a cyst are available:

1. The entire cyst can be unroofed. The epithelized cystic membrane lining the cavity is then sutured to the mucosa immediately adjacent to it around the periphery. In effect the cyst wall is made a part of the oral mucosa. This is the Partsch procedure of marsupialization.

2. The other method of exteriorizing is based on the same principle but differs in practice. Instead of removing the entire roof of the cystic cavity, a window is cut into the cavity. The fluid contents of the cyst are removed by aspiration. No attempt is made to remove the cyst wall. The cavity is then packed with iodoform gauze. The end of the gauze is brought out through the window in the mucoperiosteum. The iodo-

form gauze is removed after 5 days. Then an obturator is constructed to fit the window (Fig. 12-6). The patient is instructed to remove the obturator daily and to irrigate the defect. Frequently, the obturator can be constructed so that irrigation can be carried out with it in place. As the defect fills in, it is necessary to reduce the size of the obturator periodically. A piece of rubber or plastic catheter or tubing makes a useful obturator; the external end is simply ligated to an adjacent tooth with wire.

Treatment of chronic periodontal infection

Chronic periodontal infection, or chronic periodontitis, can be a debilitating condition. In the past it was common to simply extract the teeth in such cases. But in modern practice, treatment of the disease is directed toward salvaging the teeth in most cases. Since this is not a textbook of periodontics, suffice it to say that care of the periodontium by dentist, hygienist, and patient can often restore a severely diseased mouth to health.

When a tooth is to be removed from an area of periodontal infection, however, it is wise to take certain precautions. A small curet should be passed firmly down the root surfaces of the involved tooth before extraction to detach the tooth; the adjacent gingiva can be torn severely if the tooth is not separated from it. Be careful to avoid leaving crushed calculus in the wound. The surrounding alveolar bone is conserved as much as possible so that an alveolar ridge can be formed by the healing process. Isolated bony projections can be removed to form an even ridge, but conservatism should be paramount. If a question of judgment arises regarding alveoloplasty, the area can be allowed to heal without further surgery for 3 weeks. Then the need for alveoloplasty, if present, will become more apparent, and it can be done at that time. A localized periodontal lesion may have formed secondarily to a periapical lesion. If the cause of the periapical lesion is corrected by root canal therapy, the secondary periodontal lesion should clear.

Removal of broken needles

In spite of all precautions a needle may break and disappear in the oral tissues. The removal of a broken needle may be a difficult procedure and should not be attempted unless the operator is thoroughly familiar with the technique and anatomy involved.

Location of the needle by means of radiographs made from several different angles is an important aid, particularly after insertion of another needle, which can be detached from the syringe and left in the tissues for purposes of orientation. The technique in locating the needle varies with the anatomical site, but the following principle holds true for all techniques: do not

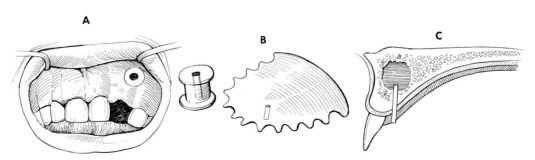

Fig. 12-6. Obturators used for exteriorizing a cyst. **A,** Acrylic button placed through labial wall. **B** and **C,** Plastic tube attached to acrylic partial denture, acting as obturator as well as prosthesis. See Fig. 14-20, p. 266.

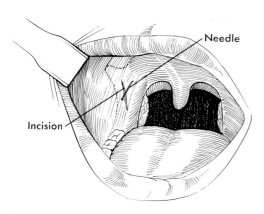

Fig. 12-7. Incision for removal of broken needle.

search in the direction that the needle was inserted but, rather, in a direction perpendicular to the direction of insertion. For example, if the needle was broken while blocking the mandibular nerve through an insertion near the pterygomandibular raphe, the incision for searching is not made at the site of insertion of the needle, but a vertical incision is made just medial to the anterior border of the ramus, and then the dissection is carried medially and posteriorly; that is, the needle is approached from a direction perpendicular to it (Fig. 12-7). If the anesthesia technique consisted of insertion immediately adjacent to the ramus rather than at the pterygomandibular raphe, the incision for searching should be made near the raphe and the dissection then

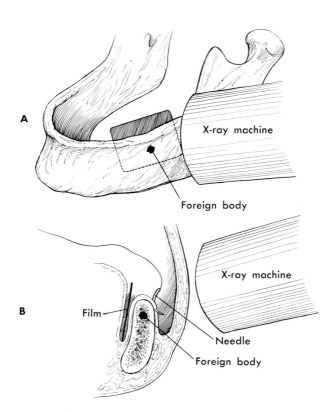

Fig. 12-8. Localization of a foreign body.

carried laterally. When the blade of the scalpel or blunt dissector comes in contact with the needle, it can be readily felt. The tissues are retracted to this depth, and when the needle comes into view, it can be grasped with a hemostat and removed. It is important in this procedure that good assistance be available so that it is unnecessary for the operator to look away from the operative site (for example, to pick up an instrument) once dissection has started.

The removal of a broken needle is not an acute surgical emergency. However, it is advisable to remove it as soon as possible to relieve the patient's anxiety. Actually, broken needles have been left in place permanently without complication, so that failure to retrieve one is not a catastrophe.

The removal of other foreign bodies from oral tissues presents problems in localization. If teeth are present in the area, localization is simply a matter of obtaining radiographs on which one can measure the distance from tooth to foreign body. In addition to the panograph and the ordinary lateral radiograph, a vertically directed view, such as an occlusal film, is often helpful.

Where no other landmarks are available for reference, a threaded suture needle can be placed through the mucosa in the approximate area (Fig. 12-8). After the radiographs have been taken, the needle is pulled on through the tissues and the suture loosely tied to show the former position of the needle.

Once the foreign body has been localized on radiographs, its removal is performed exactly the same as removal of a root tip.

A question of whether foreign bodies should be removed sometimes arises. If the patient is completely asymptomatic and no radiographic evidence of tissue reaction is found in the area, small fragments of amalgam and other metallic foreign bodies may be ignored. However, if pain or any other symptom appears that might be produced by the foreign body, removal is advised. In general, it is also good practice to remove any foreign body if a denture is to be placed over the area.

REFERENCES

1. Bender, I. B., and Seltzer, B.: Roentgenographic and direct observation of experimental lesions in bone, J. Am. Dent. Assoc. **62**:26, 1961.
2. Bhaskar, S. N.: Periapical lesions—types, incidence and clinical features, Oral Surg. **21**:657, 1966.
3. Bhaskar, S. N., and Rappapport, H. M.: Dental vitality tests and pulp status, J. Am. Dental Assoc. **86**:409, 1973.
4. Harris, M. H.: Personal communication, 1977.
5. Healey, H. J.: Endodontics, St. Louis, 1960, The C. V. Mosby Co.
6. Ingle, J. I.: Endodontics, Philadelphia, 1965, Lea & Febiger.
7. Lalonde, E. R.: A new rationale for the management of periapical granulomas and cysts: an evaluation of histopathological and radiographic findings, J. Am. Dent. Assoc. **80**:1056, 1970.
8. Lalonde, E. R., and Luebke, R. G.: The frequency and distribution of periapical cysts and granulomas, Oral Surg. **25**:861, 1968.
9. Patterson, S. S., Shafer, W. G., and Healey, H. J.: Periapical lesions associated with endodontically treated teeth, J. Am. Dent. Assoc. **68**:191, 1964.
10. Priebe, W. A., Lazansky, J. P., and Wuehrmann, A. H.: The value of the roentgenographic film in the differential diagnosis of periapical lesions, Oral Surg. **7**:979, 1954.
11. Wuehrmann, A. H., and Manson-Hing, L. R.: Dental radiology, St. Louis, 1965, The C. V. Mosby Co., p. 264.

See also references of Chapter 14.

CHAPTER 13

Hemorrhage and shock

Charles C. Alling III

The ancient Greek words for "blood" and "to burst forth" are the derivations of the modern English word "hemorrhage" and serve as a graphic definition of the subject of this chapter. Included will be the various types of hemorrhage from that expected during surgery, through an annoying oozing during the postoperative phases, to exsanguination. This chapter will discuss the appropriate classifications, etiologies, prevention, and direct treatment of hemorrhages associated with the oral cavity.

BLEEDING AND CLOTTING PHENOMENON

Hemostasis is the spontaneous or the induced cessation of the flow of blood from

Sincere appreciation is extended to Dr. Victor J. Matukas, Associate Dean and Professor of Dentistry, University of Alabama School of Dentistry, Birmingham, Alabama, for the continuing unselfish sharing of his knowledge by contribution of the section on shock. Other major contributions to this chapter were illustrations prepared by the Medical Media Production Service, Veterans Administration Hospital, Birmingham, Alabama and the exemplary support of the manuscript preparation by Mrs. Linda Widener. My gratitude is extended to all of these friends of oral surgery. A very special pleasure was found in sharing with Dr. Jeri Vitek, Diagnostic Radiology Service, University of Alabama Hospital, his enthusiasm and research for head and neck anatomy as seen through radiography; special thanks are extended to Dr. Mary Lynne Hartselle for her thorough analysis of the arteriograms that came from Dr. Vitek's research.

ruptures in the integrity of the vascular system. Spontaneous or controlled cessation involves overlapping considerations of intravascular factors, which include the blood platelets, calcium, and coagulation protein; extravascular factors, which include the general metabolism, organ systems, connective tissues, and mucosal and cutaneous tissues; and the vascular factors, which include the general metabolism and the type, size, and location of the blood vessels.

Intravascular factors

Platelets, with their functions of adhesion and aggregation, form a hemostatic plug in small vessels. In large vessels another function of platelets, clot retraction, plays a necessary role in closing an opening or a break in blood vessels (Fig. 13-1). The intravascular clot of platelets does not endlessly propagate itself, and thereby produce serious consequences, because of the conversion of soluble fibrinogen to insoluble fibrin, which absorbs the thrombin produced from prothrombin during blood coagulation. Once hemostasis is established and wound repair begun, the ubiquitous platelets have still another function, the lysis and removal of fibrin.[12]

Blood coagulation.[17] There is an international classification of 13 blood moieties (12 protein and one ionic calcium) that partic-

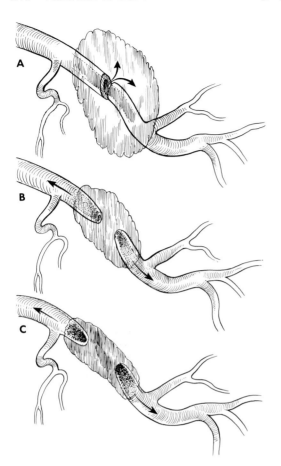

Fig. 13-1. Bleeding time from, **A,** the time of severing a blood vessel, to, **B,** the time hemorrhage stops as a result of retraction, contraction, and, **C,** platelet-fibrin plugging of the vessel.

Table 13-1. Coagulation factors

Factor	Descriptive terms and synonyms
I	Fibrinogen
II	Prothrombin
III	Thromboplastin
IV	Calcium
V	Proaccelerin, accelerator, globulin, labile factor, thromboplastin cofactor, Owen's factor
VI	No longer used
VII	Proconvertin, serum prothrombin conversion accelerator (SPCA), stable factor, prothrombin accelerator
VIII	Antihemophilic factor (AHF), antihemophilic globulin, thromboplastinogen
IX	Plasma thromboplastin component (PTC), Christmas factor
X	Stuart-Prower factor
XI	Plasma thromboplastin antecedent (PTA)
XII	Hageman factor, contact factor
XIII	Fibrin-stabilizing factor (FSF), Laki-Lorland factor

ipate in the coagulation of blood (Table 13-1). These coagulation factors are designated by Roman numerals I through XIII, representing the order in which they were identified, not the order in which each plays a role in blood coagulation.

The objective of the first stage of coagulation is concerned with the activation of thromboplastin by the rapid extrinsic tissue system and by the slower-acting intrinsic or extravascular system, which both contribute to a common pathway to produce activated thromboplastin. With regard to the extrinsic system, essentially all tissues contain a complex of materials known as thromboplastin (Factor III) that is activated by the enzymatic reaction of the B-globulin, preconvertin (Factor VII), and free calcium (Factor IV). Production of Factor VII by the liver is dependent on vitamin K.

The intrinsic system is initiated by the activation of the Hageman factor (Factor XII) by contacting roughened intima or collagen. (Contact with a glass slide likewise will initiate the blood coagulation and permit in vitro studies.) Following the activation of Factor XII, there is a sequential series of activations in which each step initiates the next. Factor XII activates plasma thromboplastin antecedent (PTA) (Factor XI); Factor XI activates plasma thromboplastin component (PTC) (Factor IX); Factor IX activates the antihemophilic factor (AHF) (Factor VIII). The activation of Factors IX and VIII requires the presence of ionic calcium ions (Factor IV).

After both the extrinsic and intrinsic systems have begun the activation of thromboplastin, a final pathway common to both systems is activated. Stuart-Prower factor (Factor X), proacceleren or Owen's factor (Factor V), a platelet factor, and the

Table 13-2. Screening tests for deficiencies in coagulation factors

Defect	Clotting time	Prothrombin time	Partial thrombo-plastin time	Thromboplastin generation time
I	N/P*	N/P	P	N
II	N/P	P	P	N
V	N/P	P	P	P (plasma only)
VII	N	P	N	N
VIII	P	N	P	P (plasma only)
IX	N/P	N	P	P (serum only)
X	N/P	P	P	P (serum only)
XI	N/P	N	P	P (serum and plasma)
XII	P	N	P	P (serum and plasma)
XIII	N	N	N	N
PF3†	N	N	N	P (substitution of platelets)

*N is normal; P is prolonged.
†Platelet factor 3.

ionic calcium factor (Factor IV) contribute, in the order given, to the final activation of thromboplastin.

The objective of the second stage is to convert the inactive enzyme prothrombin (Factor II) to thrombin by means of the thromboplastin generated in stage one in the presence of calcium ion. Adequate amounts of Factors V, VII, and X are necessary for this conversion to take place; therefore, a deficiency of any of these factors will result in a prolonged prothombin time.

The objective of the third stage of the coagulation system is to convert soluble fibrinogen (Factor I) to insoluble fibrin. Fibrinogen, by action of thrombin, is converted to a fibrin monomer that aggregates to form fibrin polymers. Small amounts of the fibrin-stabilizing factor (Factor XIII), which is activated by thrombin and the ever-present calcium ion, produce cross-linking of the fibrin polymers, producing the fibrin clot.

The degree of hypocalcemia that would prolong blood coagulation, less that 2.5 mg per 100 ml, is not compatible with life, therefore lack of calcium is not a cause of aberrant coagulation time.

Extravascular factors

The extravascular factors involved in hemostasis depend on the state of health, the tonicity, and the tautness of mucosa,

submucosa and cutaneous, subcutaneous, muscular, and other tissues that surround and support the blood vessels. Disorders that lead to atrophy of subcutaneous tissues (purpura senilis), fragility of skin (Cushing's syndrome), or degeneration of elastic tissues (pseudoxanthoma elasticum) may produce benign purpura and may not be as severe as disorders produced by defective intravascular factors.

Vascular factors

Disorders of the vessels themselves, from capillaries to arteries and veins, may produce a group of vascular purpuras. The etiologies vary from scurvy, caused by a deficit of vitamin C that causes a defect in the intercellular cement of small vessels, to purpuras resulting from infection, chronic renal diseases, and allergies. As a rule, the mechanisms of these purpuras are not well understood.

LABORATORY TESTS AND ANALYSIS OF HEMORRHAGIC DISORDERS[17]

The studies of the greatest clinical value in analyzing the coagulation factors are prothrombin time, partial thromboplastin time, thromboplastin generation time (Table 13-2), and platelet count and clot retraction. To provide an estimate of the integrity of the extravascular and vascular factors, the bleeding time and the tourniquet tests are used.

Prothrombin time (PT) test

In the PT test, plasma that has been rendered incoagulable by an anticoagulant is added to a mixture of equal amounts of active tissue thromboplastin and calcium ion. Thromboplastin activates the prothombin to form thrombin, which converts fibrinogen (Factor I) into insoluble fibrin. Since fibrin is the end point of prothombin time, adequate amounts of Factor I must be present to produce a normal finding of 11 to 12.5 seconds with this test. The PT measures only certain factors in stages 2 and 3 of coagulation; stage 1 is bypassed. Deficiencies of Factors I, II, V, VII, and X will result in prolonged PT. Normal PT may be obtained when deficiencies exist in Factors VIII, IX, XI, XII, and XIII and in the phospholipid of platelet factor 3.

Partial thromboplastin time (PTT) test

The PTT test is a measure of the integrity and activation of the intrinsic system and common pathways of thromboplastin generation by the addition of a lipid form of thromboplastin. The integrity of stage 2 of coagulation and the adequacy of Factor I (fibrinogen) in stage 3 are measured. Deficiencies of Factors VII and VIII and the phospholipid of platelet factor 3 are not detected. There are different ranges of normal for PTT depending on the specific type of PTT test being performed in a given medical laboratory.

Thromboplastin generation time (TGT) test

The TGT test is based on the development of potent thromboplastin activity during the incubation of absorbed normal

Table 13-3. Normal values of coagulation test results

Test	Normal value	Measures
Clotting time	5 to 15 min	Stage I and Stage III (abnormal in heparin therapy)
Prothrombin time (PT)	70% to 100% of normal, 11 to 12.5 sec	Prothrombin Factors V, VII, and X (abnormal in liver disease, vitamin K deficiency, and warfarin [Coumadin] therapy)
Partial thromboplastin time (PTT) (activated)	30 to 45 sec	All factors except platelets and Factor VII (abnormal in hemophilia)
Thromboplastin generation time	8 to 12 sec	
Platelet count	150,000 to 300,000/cu mm	
Clot retraction	Clot from normal individual will decrease to one-half original mass within 1 hour after clotting and is completely contracted by 24 hours	Platelet function
Bleeding time	2.5 to 9.5 min	Vascular platelet function
Tourniquet test	Up to five petechiae in 3.25 cm circle after 5 min of pressure midway between systolic and diastolic pressures	Vascular platelet function
Fibrinogen	170 to 410 mg/100 ml	Low concentration in disseminated intravascular coagulopathy and primary fibrinolysins
Dilute whole blood clot lysis	No lysis within 2 hours	Circulating fibrinolysins
Euglobulin lysis test	No lysis within 2 hours	Circulating fibrinolysins

plasma, normal serum, and normal plasma in the presence of ionic calcium. Rates of development of thromboplastin activity are measured and compared to rates obtained when the patient's plasma, serum, or platelets are substituted for their normal counterparts in additional mixtures. Thus differentiations as to factor deficiencies may be interpreted because normal serum contains Factors VII, IX, X, and XII and lacks Factors I, II, V, VII, and XIII; absorbed plasma includes Factors I, V, VIII, XI, XII, and XIII and platelet factor 3; absorbed normal plasma lacks Factors II, VII, IX, and X. Based on these facts, the practical applications may be seen in Table 13-3.

Platelet count

Platelet count gives a quantitative result not the qualitative aspect of platelet functions in the coagulation mechanisms. Since multiplication factors are used, a difference of only 10 in the counting could result in a difference of 10,000 to 50,000 platelets on the report. Of great value is the description of the platelets and the morphological examination of the blood smear.

Clot retraction

Clot retraction depends on the quantity and quality of platelets necessary to influence the completeness of retraction of the coagulum produced by nonanticoagulated whole blood in a test tube rinsed in normal saline. Multiple variables that do not help to pinpoint the etiology (for example, poor clot retraction as seen in thrombocytopenia, multiple myeloma resulting from viscosity of plasma, and polycythemia caused by an over abundance of erythrocytes) may affect this test.

Bleeding time

The bleeding time test measures the vascular response to hemostasis or the ability of small vessels to contract and retract and achieve a fibrin plug following injury. The test measures the time from injury to ces-

sation of hemorrhage caused by a puncture wound. The test is performed either by an earlobe puncture or by three uniform punctures in the ventral surface of the forearm, respectively, the Duke and the Ivy methods; the time is measured from puncture to cessation of hemorrhage and, in the Duke method, ranges from 1½ to 4½ minutes. The test is influenced by the general state of extravascular factors of age and nutrition and by the microphysical factors of the skin and subcutaneous tissues. Prolonged times will be seen in thrombocytopenic states and pseudohemophilia, that is, von Willebrand's disease, in which there is a deficiency to some degree of Factor VIII plus prolonged bleeding time.

Tourniquet test

The tourniquet test, also termed the Rumpel-Leede test or the capillary fragility test, measures the response of the arteriole-venule junction to internal stresses. Providing the systolic pressure is above 100 mm of mercury, a constant 100 mm of recovery is maintained for 5 minutes. The appearance of multiple petechiae distal to the blood pressure cuff denotes a positive result and may indicate scurvy, thrombocytopenia, and certain purpuras.

Microhematocrit test

The microhematocrit test is a standard procedure in many offices wherein general anesthesia or deep sedation is used with ambulatory outpatients. Obviously, the reason for the test is to obtain an estimate of the quantity of erythrocytes available for transporting oxygen. As Westwood, Tilson, and Margeno-Rowe[28] pointed out, microhematocrit examination is not a substitute for the coagulopathy tests mentioned previously, but it may be indicative of conditions that predispose the patient to hemorrhage. For example, resting on top of the packed erythrocytes following centrifuging is the buffy coat layer that is composed mostly of leukocytes. A large buffy coat may suggest the presence of an infection or a blood dyscrasia such as a leukemia. The plasma layer is above the buffy coat, and a yellow color may indicate various normal metabolic as well as diseased states: a high vegetable diet, liver disease, or diabetes. The preceding are observations and indications that may or may not be present in any given patient, but observation of the hematocrit is part of the total ongoing inspection of the patient that is made by dedicated doctors.

CLINICAL ABNORMALITIES OF BLOOD COAGULATION*

The clinical manifestations of abnormalities of blood coagulation may be categorized and summarized according to the following outline:

A. Acquired
  1. Impaired synthesis
    a. Liver disease
    b. Renal insufficiency
  2. Development of circulating anticoagulants
    a. Disseminated intravascular coagulopathy (DIC)
    b. Fibrinolysis
  3. Pharmacotherapeutic agents
    a. Administration of warfarin (Coumadin). Note: Surgery is contraindicated if PT activity is greater than two times the control. The PT test should be performed on the day of surgery.
    b. Heparinized patients
    c. Quinine
    d. Acetylsalicylic acid
    e. Oral contraceptives
    f. Citrate salt agents, as in blood preservatives in blood transfusions
B. Genetically inherited
  1. First stage of coagulation deficiencies
    a. Factor VIII deficiency (classical hemophilia)
      (1) Sex-linked recessive disorder
      (2) Female is carrier with no clinical signs or symptoms.

---

*From Frommeyer, W. B., Jr.: Blood coagulation. In Menaker, L., editor: Biologic basis for wound healing, New York, 1975, Harper & Row, Publishers, pp. 19-41.

(3) No sons of hemophiliac would have disorders; half of daughters would be carriers.
(4) Unusual bleeding at an early age as a result of trivial trauma
(5) Bleeding into joints is frequent, also skin and gastrointestinal (GI) and genitourinary (GU) tracts.
(6) Treatment
  (a) To control hemorrhage, either fresh blood or fresh plasma or cryoprecipitated and glycine-precipitated concentrate is administered.
  (b) Preoperatively, a minimum level of 35% of normal concentration of Factor VIII should be maintained by infusions of human Factor VIII concentrates.
(7) Majority of hemophiliacs have had hepatitis; thus precautionary measures should include autoclave sterilizing of instruments.[15]
b. Factor IX deficiency (Christmas disease or hemophilia B)
  (1) Sex-linked recessive transmission as with Factor VIII deficiency. The recessive gene may express itself to the degree that symptoms may appear in female heterozygotes.
  (2) Hemorrhage may first appear at birth from the umbilical cord or following circumcision.
  (3) In later life, bleeding into GI and GU tracts, bone and joint, and skin but less than with Factor VIII deficiency; however, hemorrhage following exodontics and other surgery may be as excessive and persistent as with Factor VIII deficiencies.
  (4) Treatment
    (a) A concentrate may be used that contains Factors II, VII, IX, and X.
    (b) Usually plasma or whole blood is administered and should be used if doubt exists as to the specific deficiency.
c. Factor XI deficiency
  (1) Transmitted as an autosomal dominant trait, not sex linked.

Therefore, either male or female has a 50% chance of passing the disorder to offspring.

(2) Bleeding is not as frequent nor as severe as with Factor VIII and IX deficiencies.

(3) Rarely, in comparison with Factor VIII deficiencies, is there GI and GU tract, bone and joint, and skin hemorrhage.

(4) Following minor surgery such as exodontics, hemorrhage is usually as severe as with Factor VIII and IX deficiencies.

(5) Treatment

  (a) Preoperatively, 50% level of Factor XI should be maintained using infusions of Factor XI concentrate. Usually, 4.5 ml frozen plasma per kg of body weight will raise level 10%.

  (b) Level should be replenished every 2 or 3 days postoperatively even though half-life of Factor XI in blood is 60 hours.

d. Factor XII deficiency

  (1) No clinical symptoms of hemorrhagic diathesis; therefore, patients will withstand surgery in a normal manner.

  (2) Disorder usually is found by accident when preoperative studies reveal normal PT but extremely prolonged clotting time.

2. *Either* first or second stage disorders

a. Factor II deficiency

  (1) Genetic disorder—very rare autosomal trait with mild manifestations

  (2) Acquired form

    (a) Liver disease

    (b) Iatrogenic disturbance of vitamin K metabolism, sterilizing drugs in GI tract, and coumarin class of antiprothrombin drugs

    (c) Manifestations are hemorrhage from gingival tissues, nasal passages, GU and GI tracts, and skin—rarely hemarthrosis.

(3) Treatment

  (a) Plasma infusions

  (b) Concentrate of Factors II, VII, IX, and X plus vitamin K, usually intramuscularly 25 to 50 mg at a rate of less than 5 mg per minute.

b. Factor VII deficiency

  (1) Inherited codominantly, and onset of hemorrhage in infancy may be from umbilical cord. GI tract hemorrhages, epistaxis, and bruising are common.

  (2) Acquired form is seen with liver disease and administration of coumarin drugs.

  (3) Treatment is with concentrates of Factors II, VII, IX, and X, and a level of Factor VII at 15% to 20% will control spontaneous hemorrhage as well as hemorrhage resulting from surgery. If deficiency is induced by coumarin drugs, treatment is administration of natural vitamin K.

EXTRAVASCULAR HEMORRHAGE

Extravascular hemorrhage may be classified according to the type of vessels involved and the time of the hemorrhage.[20]

Type of vessels

The character of hemorrhage will depend on the type of vessels severed—arteries, veins, or capillaries. *Arterial hemorrhage* will be distinguished by its pulsating character, vigor of the flow, and bright red coloration of the blood. *Venous hemorrhage* may not have a pulsating quality, the flow will be slightly less rapid, and there will be a darker red coloration. In the head, neck, and maxillofacial tissues, the lack of valves in the veins and the short connections between the jugular system and the terminal branches often will permit awesome surges of venous blood when a major vein is severed. *Capillary bleeding* will be oozing, nonpulsating in character, and an intermediate red, a color between the bright red of arterial blood and the darker red of venous blood.

Capillary bleeding may be quite aggressive in the oral and maxillofacial region as a result of the strong arterial pulse on one side of the capillaries and the open, direct, nonvalved access to the jugular system on the venous side. Classifiable as capillary hemorrhage is the vigorous bleeding encountered during procedures in the vascular shunt area posterior to the mandibular condyle.[22]

Time of hemorrhage

Primary hemorrhage occurs as a normal part of surgery as well as from lacerations incurred in trauma. In most intraoral operations, for example, exodontics and alveoloplasty surgery, the normal bleeding time will provide reasonable hemorrhage control (Fig. 13-1). The application of pressure dressings in the form of gauze packs, immediate dentures, or splints will control the primary hemorrhage; also, the vasoconstrictors in local anesthetic solutions will help to control primary hemorrhage. In some cases in intraoral surgery, clamping and tying or electrocoagulation may be necessary to control bleeding; the latter modalities are, of course, routinely used in extraoral surgical approaches.

Secondary hemorrhage occurs during the postoperative phase. Some doctors use the phrases "intermediate hemorrhage" to describe the unexpected hemorrhage that occurs in the first 24 hours postoperatively and "secondary hemorrhage" for the hemorrhage that occurs after the first 24 hours. Regardless of the time phases, secondary hemorrhage following intraoral surgery is most often associated with the presence of foreign bodies in an alveolus. This may be a splinter of bone, a fleck of enamel, or a piece of dental restorative material that causes repeated, delayed organization of a blood coagulum. The result may range from an aggressive oozing hemorrhage of blood that continually fills the oral cavity, to a liver clot, to mere blood-tinged saliva that causes alarm to the uninformed patient (Fig. 13-2).

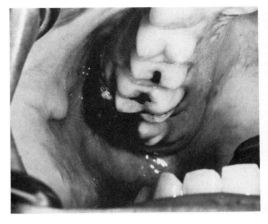

Fig. 13-2. Mass of clotted blood, a so-called liver clot, produced by repeated or continuous hemorrhages.

If the secondary hemorrhage is from a metabolic or blood intravascular coagulopathy, definitive care must include managing the general systemic problem.

Prevention of extravascular hemorrhage from dentoalveolar areas

Following surgery, from simple exodontics to extensive alveoloplasties, the surgical sites are irrigated with normal saline and cleansed with suctioning. It is reasonable for the doctor to take the suctioning device and inspect all aspects of the surgical site while the oral surgical nurse irrigates with normal saline.

The postoperative pack is a 10 by 10 cm gauze that is dampened with saline and molded over the surgical site. The saline decreases the tendency of the clot to become embedded in the gauze mesh. The molding of gauze is designed so that the tongue is presented only with smooth folded margins, the free edges being toward the cheek. The gauze is tailored so that none of it protrudes from the oral cavity when the lips are closed; for anterior extraction sites it may be necessary to use 5 by 5 cm or 7.5 by 7.5 cm gauzes to ensure that the material will not protrude from the lips and produce unsightly extraoral excretions.

The postoperative instructions are given by the doctor to either the patient or a responsible adult. The instructions are delivered in a deliberate, concerned manner and include impressing on the patient that the gauze must stay in place and that talking, eating, and expectorating should not be done for 2 or 3 hours. An allegory is made to the patient that pressure bandages are frequently taped or wrapped over the site following surgery elsewhere on the body; however, the only way a pressure bandage may be placed in the patient's mouth is by the cooperation of the patient in closing firmly on the gauze for 2 or 3 hours. The time the gauze may be removed is *written* on the instruction sheet.

Each patient is telephoned in the evening to reinforce, among other things, that blood-tinged saliva is normal and should not be confused with hemorrhage.

This regimen, each step of which is critically important, has been highly successful in controlling postoperative problems produced by secondary hemorrhage. Incidentally, when elective surgical procedures are performed only in patients in whom there are no oral and *pharyngeal* infections, there has been a significant reduction in postoperative localized osteitis and other infections. It is logical that deft, delicate surgery performed in an area free of infections and well protected by a vitalized blood coagulum would decrease untoward sequelae.

Extravascular hemorrhage control

Coagulation may be delayed by deficiencies of factors described previously, and this was termed intravascular hemorrhage. However, given a normal coagulation system, the control of extravascular hemorrhage is primarily dependent on a normal vessel contraction, retraction, and fibrin plug. During a surgical procedure, positive control of hemorrhaging vessels is possible with various procedures and agents. It is a sound and a fundamental surgical principle that one leaves a dry field,

that is, an area with no macroscopic hemorrhage, at the conclusion of an operation. This prevents hematoma formation that may dissect to involve other areas, such as the airway, or may serve as a bed in which microorganisms can flourish. Extravascular hemorrhage control must be effective, also, to stem aggressive and sometimes life-threatening effusions.

Assuming the patient has a normal coagulation time, the agents and methods for control of extravascular hemorrhage are pressure, direct occlusion with hemostats, coagulation of the hemorrhaging point by the precipitation of proteins, occlusive dressings, production of an artificial clot, provision of an artificial fibrin network, hastening of the coagulation mechanism to produce vasoconstriction, production of an adherent, protective bonding between the coagulum and the surrounding tissues, and administration of general systemic agents that are calculated to decrease hemorrhage.[11]

Pressure will control most hemorrhages. This may be direct occluding of a pressure point of a major vessel leading to the hemorrhaging site. Pressure points are located between the mandibular gonial angle and the sternocleidomastoid muscle to control the external carotid artery, over the mandibular notch (premasseteric incisure) to control the facial artery, and between the tragus of the ear and the zygomatic process of the temporal bone to control the temporal artery. Pressure may be exerted by pooling of escaped blood that tamponades the ruptured vessels. In a negative sense, the lack of pressure manifested in shock may decrease hemorrhage. Obviously, the best method of control would be directly at the hemorrhage site, and according to surgical circumstances, this may be pressure with intraoral gauzes or splints and extraoral bandages.

Direct occlusion of bleeding vessels is obtainable by the application of mosquito hemostats, so named because of their delicate, fine points. The hemostats may be curved or straight; the curved ones are more versatile and more readily lend themselves to the application of ties.

The ties may be nonabsorbable black silk, 3-0 or 4-0, usually placed on named vessels, that is, vessels large enough to be noted by an anatomical name. Smaller vessels are tied with 3-0 or 4-0 plain gut or polyglycolic acid sutures. These absorbable sutures will persist for varying lengths of time. Plain gut will persist the shortest time (measured in weeks), the polyglycolic acid the longest (measured in months). The usual technique involves placing two hemostats on a vessel, points curved to the area to be divided; the vessel is cut, and with the points directed upwards, the ties are placed. Stick ties are those in which sutures are placed in the soft tissues lateral to the free end of the vessel that has been clamped; the knot is drawn tight to occlude the vessel by compression from the surrounding tissues when the hemostat is removed (Fig. 13-3).

Coagulation of the hemorrhaging point may be produced by a variety of modalities

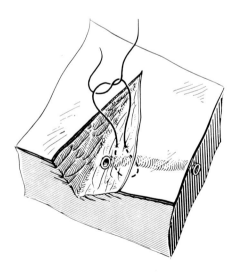

Fig. 13-3. Use of the "stick-tie" method of ligating a vessel that lies within a deep recess and cannot be clamped. The vessel and surrounding tissue are ligated.

that precipitate proteins. Electrocoagulation and cryotherapy are controlled, destructive techniques that produce occlusion of vessels. Styptic and astringent agents have been employed for hundreds of years; among the most popular have been ferric subsulfate, in the form of Monsel's solution, and tannic acid, a home remedy in the form of tea bags. In general, the chemical agents have been replaced by the use of thrombin and absorbable gelatin sponge for the control of intraoral secondary hemorrhages.

Bone wax (beeswax and salicylic acid) may be used in small amounts to occlude bony canals that bear hemorrhaging vessels. These vary from walls of dental alveoli to foramina through which the neurovascular bundles have been avulsed.

An artificial clot may be produced by oxidized cellulose (Novacell, Oxycel) and regenerated oxidized cellulose (Surgicel). Oxidized cellulose attracts erythrocytes and thus produces an artificial clot. The material should be used dry, and, in the absence of infection and in areas where bone repair is not necessary, it provides rapid control of capillary and venous oozing hemorrhages. The material may be placed over, not in, an alveolus and maintained with a pressure gauze to help control primary hemorrhaging. Remnants of the gauze may be removed by flushing with normal saline or an alkaline solution.

An artificial fibrin network that will disrupt platelets is created by application of an absorbable gelatin sponge (Gelfoam). The combined action of the platelets and the gelatin will control capillary hemorrhage and may be enhanced by the addition of thrombin.

Thrombin, used as a *topical agent,* directly clots fibrinogen to produce rapid hemostasis. Gelatin sponges moistened with thrombin provide very effective coagulation of hemorrhages from small veins and capillaries. In dental alveoli, particularly in mandibular posterior regions, gelatin sponges may absorb oral microorganisms and cause alveolar osteitis, a painful condition that will delay repair.

The vasoconstriction of bleeding beds may be produced by the use of epinephrine, either topically or in combination with local anesthetic solutions. The topical solution, 1:1,000, may produce blood pressure responses nearly equal to those resulting from an intramuscular injection. Minimal concentration should be used to avoid untoward reactions. In most instances, another modality, such as thrombin or regenerated oxidized cellulose, should be used in oral surgery to control capillary and venule hemorrhages. In some cases, the injection of 1.8 ml of local anesthetic solution containing 1:100,000 epinephrine will suffice to control annoying primary hemorrhages.

Cyanoacrylate adhesive monomers are under animal laboratory investigation for use as hemostatic agents following surgery in the oral cavity* and these agents have had some controlled clinical applications.[4,14] Polymerization of the monomer occurs extremely rapidly in the oral environment and bonds to oral tissues as well as to the coagulum (Fig. 13-4). This produces a protective, hemostatic dressing for surgical sites. Controlled clinical investigations will probably produce approval and

---

*See references 7, 8, 16, and 25.

acceptance of this modality of hemostasis in oral surgery.

Agents given systemically are reported from time to time for use in otherwise normal individuals to control postoperative hemorrhage. Aside from the fact that these agents have effectiveness that ranges from none to varying, the manipulation of an entire biological system does not seem warranted to control the normal physiologic response of bleeding and coagulation.

ORAL AND MAXILLOFACIAL ARTERIES

The external carotid arteries are the major arterial supply to the oral and maxillofacial tissues. Pressure on these arteries should stem the flow from hemorrhaging peripheral arteries. Anastomosing arterial networks from the opposite side (Fig. 13-5) as well as the rich venous bed may make pressure to the external carotid arteries only partially effective in controlling hemorrhage. Following consultations and transfers, if appropriate, the external carotid artery is controlled as follows.[18,26] The patient is placed in a supine position with the head rotated and the neck slightly extended towards the contralateral side. An incision is made through the skin and superficial fascia overlying the anterior slope of the sternocleidomastoid muscle and is centered over the hyoid bone. Variations in the direction of the incision through the skin are

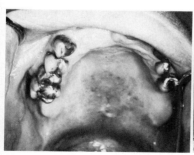 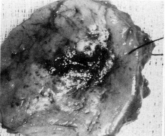 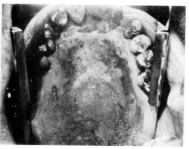

| A | B | C |

Fig. 13-4. Hyperkeratotic lesion, produced by prolonged use of tobaccos. **A,** Preoperative view; **B,** specimens; **C,** surgical area sprayed with a cyanoacrylate, producing instant hemostasis.

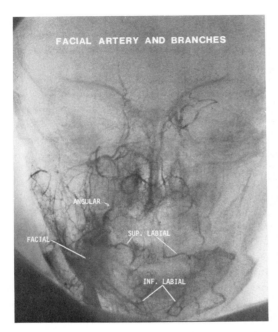

FACIAL ARTERY AND BRANCHES

ANGULAR

FACIAL

SUP. LABIAL

INF. LABIAL

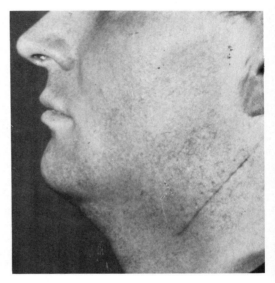

Fig. 13-5. Arteriogram illustrating anastomosing and filling of vessels on the contralateral side of the face following injection of the facial artery.

Fig. 13-6. Incision line from a surgical approach to the external carotid artery to control a severe hemorrhage of the inferior alveolar artery. (Courtesy Dr. D. B. Osbon.)

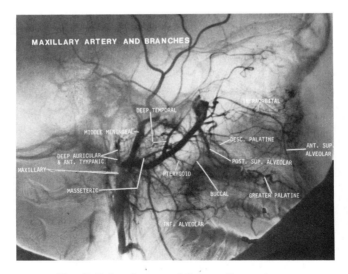

MAXILLARY ARTERY AND BRANCHES

DEEP TEMPORAL

INFRAORBITAL

MIDDLE MENINGEAL

DESC. PALATINE

ANT. SUP. ALVEOLAR

DEEP AURICULAR & ANT. TYMPANIC

MAXILLARY

PTERYGOID

POST. SUP. ALVEOLAR

MASSETERIC

BUCCAL

GREATER PALATINE

INF. ALVEOLAR

Fig. 13-7. Arteriogram of the maxillary artery.

seen; however, the hyoid bone landmark is about the level of the common carotid artery bifurcation and allows access to its branches. Blunt dissection will expose the carotid triangle and its contents, the blue jugular vein, yellow vagus nerve, and the red common carotid and external and internal carotid arteries. An umbilical tape is secured around the external carotid artery to assess the effect of occluding the artery. If indicated, permanent ties are placed and the artery is sectioned (Fig. 13-6).

Temporal arterial hemorrhage is readily accessible to identification of bleeding points, hemostatic control, and ties. A pressure point exists over the root of the

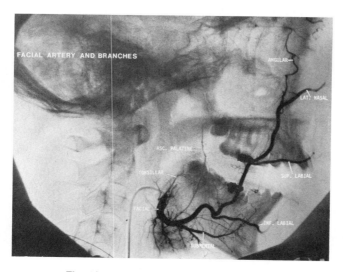

Fig. 13-8. Arteriogram of the facial artery.

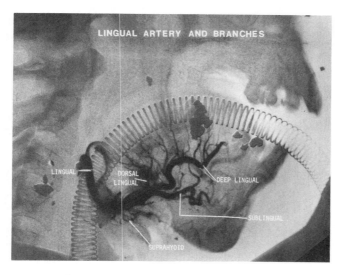

Fig. 13-9. Arteriogram of the lingual artery.

zygomatic process of the temporal bone that will give hemostatic control to temporal arterial hemorrhages.

In the event of a scalping injury of the cranium, the freely anastomosing subcutaneous arteries may produce a profound, aggressive hemorrhage. Treatment should include direct ligation or electrosurgical coagulation and pressure bandages.

The maxillary artery is a direct continuation of the external carotid artery (Fig. 13-7). Injuries to this artery result in massive and, possibly, life-threatening hemorrhages. Control may be difficult if the injury to the artery is in a fairly deep wound, such as on the medial side of the condylar neck when approached by a preauricular incision. Tight packing of the wound and pressure and ties of the external carotid artery are indicated. In hemorrhages from the maxillary artery, blood replacement and prevention of shock become of paramount importance.

The masseteric artery, traversing the sigmoid notch from the maxillary artery to the masseteric muscle, will produce a copious hemorrhage if torn by either retraction or by cutting during procedures performed on either the medial side of the mandible, such as a midsagittal split of the ramus, or on the lateral side of the ramus, such as oblique osteotomies when approached either intraorally or extraorally. Because of the depths of and limited access to the surgical sites, pressure from gauzes soaked in hot saline maintained for 10-minute increments has been effective.

The facial artery (Fig. 13-8) has a pressure point at the premasseteric incisure, the mandibular notch, or the antigonial notch as it is variously termed. Digital pressure should stem distal hemorrhage flows. However, other arteries that contribute to the nourishment of the facial tissues—infraorbital, mental, transverse facial, and buccal—and anastomosing flows from the opposite side may make the application of pressure futile. In any case the accessibility of the facial tissues to inspection and identification of hemorrhaging points makes the usual treatment of choice the application of hemostats and subsequent ties and coagulation methods. Though dramatic, facial lacerations and hemorrhages are not in themselves usually life threatening. Blood from a through-and-through buccal laceration may pool in the airway and produce a truly emergent condition of airway embarrassment.

In the event of lingual hemorrhage (Fig. 13-9) that cannot be directly controlled, one may need to resort to approaching the carotid triangle to ligate either the external carotid or the lingual artery. The lingual artery is approachable, according to textbooks, through Lesser's triangle. Many oral surgeons, head and neck general surgeons, and emergency room general surgeons queried stated that none had ever exposed the lingual artery by way of this triangle. However, the approach is described as a curvilinear incision from the gonial angle to the mental region of the mandible, extending inferolaterally to overlay the hyoid bone.[18] Exposure of the anterior and posterior bellies of the diagastric muscle and the hypoglossal nerve completes the triangle. Within the triangle the vertical fibers of the hypoglossus muscle are separated, revealing, at least in cadaver dissections, the lingual artery, which may then be clamped.

Fig. 13-10. A, The course of the, *A,* maxillary division of the trigeminal nerve as it enters the foramen rotundum, *B,* pterygopalatine fossa, *C,* posterior superior alveolar nerve, and, *D,* anterior superior nerve. The radiograph shows, *C,* the anterior alveolar nerve canal and, *D,* the bony depression of the posterior superior alveolar nerve. (**B,** From Dolan, K. D., and Hayden, J.: Maxillary "pseudofracture" lines, Radiology **107:**321, 1973.)

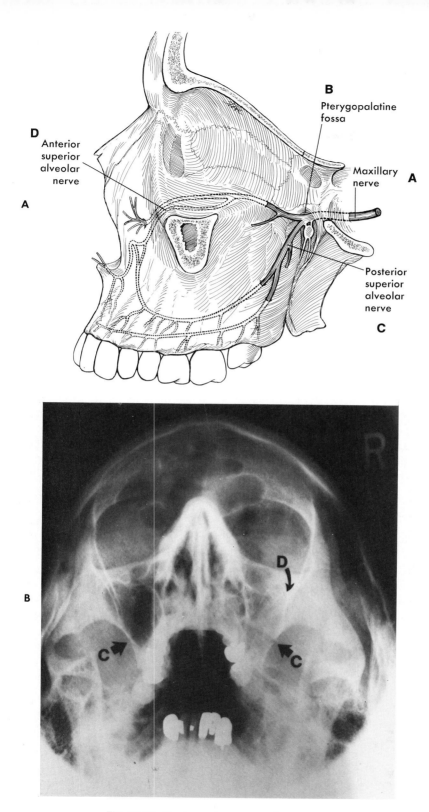

Fig. 13-10. For legend see opposite page.

To repeat, positive control of the lingual artery may be achieved at its origin from the carotid artery. The exposure of the external carotid is as described above; the lingual artery is the second anterior branch above the bifurcation of the external and internal carotid arteries. Even though clamped, the peripheral hemorrhage may go on unabated as a result of the rich venous blood supply and the anastomosing arteries from the opposite side. The best control of lingual hemorrhage, though difficult, is directly at the injured site, with due regard, of course, for the challenges to the airway of accumulated blood and from expanding hematomas.

The posterior superior alveolar artery may be bound by periosteum to the posterolateral wall of the maxillary tuberosity, and occasionally it may produce an osseous depression* (Fig. 13-10). In these instances, the artery cannot move away from a local anesthesia injection needle and, if lacerated, will produce a rapidly expanding hematoma. Treatment consists of ice bag pressure packs and reassurances to the patient. As a general rule, the planned surgical or other intraoral procedure should be deferred.

ORAL AND MAXILLOFACIAL VEINS

The abundant veins of the head and neck, devoid of valves, provide a generous vascular bed for movement of the massive quantities of blood required by the brain and the oral and maxillofacial tissues. Although the arteries are often implicated in the untoward sequelae in facial and related hemorrhages, it is the veins that often are the more dangerous structures in terms of risk and more difficult in terms of control. Whereas one may ligate the external carotid artery to help control an arterial hemorrhage, a laceration of, say, the retromandibular vein may not be approachable for ligation *above* the injured site. In a like manner, massive basilar skull fractures may open venous sinuses and channels of hem-

*See references 1, 3, 13, and 27.

orrhage that will rapidly lead to hypovolemic shock. Furthermore, the lack of valves may help provide direct communication for the passage of infections in a retrograde direction to the cavernous sinuses or other intracranial areas.

The pterygoid plexus of veins, with its rather far-reaching extensions, envelops the origins and the spaces between the medial pterygoid muscle and the anterior heads of the lateral pterygoid muscle. Local anesthetic injections to the inferior alveolar foramen may pass through and lacerate the delicate venule channels and permit a pooling of blood in the inverted pyramidal-shaped pterygomandibular space at the site of the foramen. Aspiration will pick up this pooled blood and give the impression of an intravascular placement of the needle tip.[2,3]

Local anesthetic injections for the posterior superior alveolar nerve are frequently accompanied by a rapidly developing hematoma. As mentioned previously, this hematoma is probably associated with laceration of the posterior superior alveolar artery and not, as sometimes described, the pterygoid plexus of veins. Pressure gradients within the veins, especially the small veins, probably are not sufficient to produce an expending hematoma in the plexus area.

The sublingual, or the ranine, vein may be a direct contributor to the jugular vein or it may contribute first to the lingual vein. In either case, opening of this vein provides a direct, explosive outlet for the jugular veins. Suctioning, clamping, and pressure dressings may control this effusion that could follow frenoplasty for ankyloglossia or a laceration. A lingual artery hemorrhage possibly may be controlled with ligation of the external carotid artery, but one is not able to approach in a reasonable manner the jugular vein superior to the injured site.

The sizeable posterior facial vein, the retromandibular vein, is especially vulnerable to closed and semiclosed operations that pass cutting and stripping instruments posterior to the ramus of the mandible (Fig.

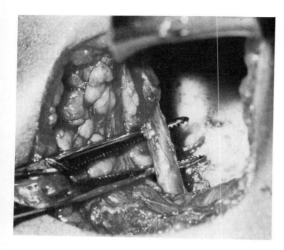

Fig. 13-11. Posterior facial vein noted during an angle of the mandible surgical approach to the ramus of the mandible.

13-11). Also, it is conceivable that hemorrhages following a midsagittal split of the ramus may be produced by sharp bony margins that could lacerate this vein. The first treatment would be directed toward packing the area with gauze dampened with hot saline and applying pressure.

OTHER MAXILLOFACIAL VESSELS

The inferior alveolar neurovascular bundle contains the named vessels most likely to be damaged by oral surgical procedures. The inferior alveolar canal is an actual bony canal with perforations, in dentate individuals, for the passage of dental neurovascular structures. When a tooth is removed, these structures are severed and the bony canal, in time, closes over the perforations. Thus in an edentulous individual the canal becomes a smooth bony tube that traverses the mandible from the inferior alveolar foramen to the mental foramen. In some cases, the bony canal is not distinct in either the edentulous or dentulous individual. In these instances the clinical impression that one gains when performing body of the mandible ostectomy procedures is that there are multiple filaments and strands of neurovascular bundles passing through the body of the mandible.

The mandibular third molar area is where the inferior alveolar vessels are most likely to be damaged during surgery. The location of the inferior alveolar canal may be ascertained by shifting intraoral radiographs; in this case the shifts should be vertical rather than horizontal, which is usual. In general the neurovascular bundle will be located buccal to the apical area of the third molars. Obviously, if the inferior alveolar canal is in juxtaposition to the area of proposed surgery, the patient should be informed and consent obtained because of this special surgical hazard.

If encountered during surgery, the hemorrhage from the inferior alveolar vessels may be quite brisk. Though dismaying to the doctor and the team, this hemorrhage will not be life threatening if adequately treated. Direct treatment includes controlling the hemorrhage by clearing the excess blood by aspirating and then packing the site with oxidized cellulose and injecting the area and reinjecting the inferior alveolar foramen area with vasoconstrictors in local anesthetic solutions.

Following these procedures, a saline-dampened sponge should be placed over the area and held in place for at least 10 minutes. If on reinspection the hemorrhage should recur, one may repeat the entire procedure. Then, if on reinspection the hemorrhage should again recur, one may wish to pack a gelatin sponge containing thrombin over the oxidized cellulose, suture the overlying mucoperiosteum, place a 3-hour intraoral pack, and either give the patient another appointment for continuation of the surgical procedure in 7 days or refer the patient to an oral surgeon. If on a subsequent appointment the hemorrhage should again be present or if there have been intermittent recurring bouts of hemorrhage, then one may be faced with a scalped vessel, a vessel that has been partially severed, and the remaining attachments of the vessel prevent its retraction and contraction. In this case, the area should be cut with a curet to ensure severance of the vessel and then treated as a new surgical site.

The buccal vessels may be encountered in reflection of flaps from the area of the mandibular second molars to the retromolar trigone. Although the sudden velocity of blood is somewhat surprising, the problem is quickly remedied by hemostats followed by ties, electrocautery, cryotherapy, or injection of vasoconstrictors in local anesthetic solutions.

The mental vessels emerging from the mental foramen are predictably located 10 to 12 mm above the base of the mandible.[10] Thus in individuals with either normal or elongated alveolar processes, there is only a slight possibility of encountering these vessels during usual intraoral surgery. In the event that the neurovascular bundle is likely to be encountered, great care should be taken to prevent its severance because of the possibility of a paresthesia or anesthesia in the inferior lip. The hemorrhage problem is managed handily by pressure dressings to avoid clamping filaments of sensory nerves to the lips, by hemostat controls, or, if the vessel has been severed at the foramen, by packing gelatin sponges or oxidized cellulose into the foramen.

Hemorrhage may occur from the mylohyoid vessels in the mandibular first molar area back to the third molar area. The bleeding may follow flap elevation or fracture of the medial alveolar bone, especially in the second and third molar regions. Control by pressure or by hemostats is usually effective and must be maintained for at least 10 minutes. Since the vessels are bound to the bony canal, ties are nearly impossible to place, and electrosurgical cauterization may be necessary. If a destructive modality such as electrosurgery or cryotherapy is employed, it should be precise to avoid damage to the lingual nerve, which is located just medial to this area. Secondary hemorrhage of the mylohyoid vessels could produce a dissecting hematoma in the sublingual and submandibular spaces. Poste-

rior extensions of hemorrhage in the lateral pharyngeal space may lead to a series of worsening problems. Therefore, accurate treatment of the primary hemorrhage is of fundamental importance.

The palatine vessels, occupying the canal made by opposing grooves in the maxillary and palatine bones, may produce troublesome hemorrhage during orthognathic surgery wherein osteotomies are performed to move the middle facial skeletal segments (Fig. 13-7). Attention given to using sharp chisels, placing lines of cleavage, and being prepared with adequate light, suctioning, and clamping instruments will make hemorrhage from the descending pallatine arteries and veins an insignificant incident in the course of an orthognathic surgical procedure.

Hemorrhage may be encountered from the anterior or the greater palatine artery during the elevation of palatal mucoperiosteal flaps, and control may be difficult to obtain because of poor visibility. When compared to the visibility available with buccal and labial flaps, the lines of sight into the palatal vault, either direct or indirect through a mirror, are more difficult for the operating team, especially if uncontrolled blood is flooding the region, the rotated tissue is thick and dense, and the flap is rotated toward the doctor, not away as in the case with flaps lateral to the dentoalveolar processes. Control of the anterior or greater palatine artery hemorrhage may be directed toward clamping, followed by either tying or coagulation by electrical techniques. For the clamping and subsequent procedures to be accomplished, the flap may need to be further elevated anteriorly and toward the midline to clearly uncover the offending vessels. If a definite bleeder cannot be isolated, then the doctor may resort to the use of pressure and deep sutures or stick ties.

The nasal palatine vessels seldom contribute to troublesome hemorrhage. The passage of arterial blood may be from either the palatal towards the nasal or vice versa or both. The low pressure gradients in these vessels, which are near the end of the maxillary artery, minimize complicating hemorrhage. If these vessels are severed in the raising of a palatal flap, a piece of gelatin sponge may be placed in the canal to minimize postoperative hematoma formation.

HEMORRHAGIC LESIONS

There are two entities that constitute absolute contraindications to exodontics: arterovenous or sinusoidal aneurysms and central hemangiomas. Removal of teeth in situations in which the root structures are involved with one of these lesions may produce death by one of several modalities. The patient may exsanguinate, develop shock, or aspirate the high velocity and volume of blood.

Identification of these lesions may be fairly simple. There may be a history of hemorrhage from the gingival cuffs around the teeth, loosening of teeth accompanied by hemorrhage, mobility of teeth, a palpable thrill over the lesion, or a bruit noted by stethoscopic auscultation, or endless blood, sometimes under pressure, may be aspirated from the area. Roots of teeth may be eroded, as noted on radiological examination, overlying tissues may have color and contour changes, and pain or paresthesia may be present. On the other hand, any or all of these findings may be absent.

Radiological interpretation is not reliable. There appear to be no consistent findings of radiodensities, margins, locations, trabeculations, or presence of calcific bodies. Obviously, if there are otherwise clinically healthy teeth in an area of radiolucency, then further investigation is indicated to diagnose the radiolucent lesion. Nonrestorable, diseased teeth may be situated adjacent to an area that is a potentially devastating central hemangioma or aneurysm. Therefore, one should consider aspirating central radiolucent lesions prior to performing invasive surgical procedures including simple exodontics.

In the event a tooth is removed and an otherwise undiagnosed central vascular lesion is exposed, the tooth may be replaced immediately in the alveolus as a stopper. The patient should be transferred to an inpatient facility without delay for evaluation and definitive care. When performing a biopsy of a central lesion of the mandible, one should consider aspiration before opening widely into an unknown area. If the bone is too thick to permit passage of a needle for aspiration, it may be thinned with a round bur and thus permit perforation with the aspirating needles.

Management of central aneurysms and hemangiomas includes surgical excision (Fig. 13-12),[23] irradiation,[21] curettage,[6] and embolization.[19] If resection is performed,

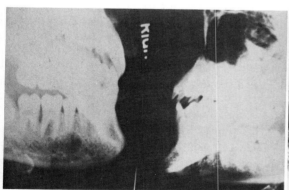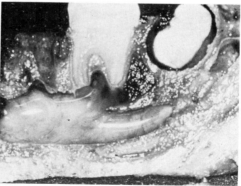

B

Fig. 13-12. Arteriovenous aneurysms seen by radiograph and surgical excision (pathological specimen). (From Moose, S. M.: Sinusoidal aneurysm of the mandible, J. Oral Surg. **15:**246, 1957.)

Moose pointed out that the section removed may be replaced as an autogenous bone graft.[24] Angiographic techniques have led to embolization capabilities that may precisely occlude the major feeding vessels to a hemorrhagic lesion.

Occasionally lakes of blood with large feeders are encountered in central areas in the maxillofacial skeleton. These may be managed by occlusive packing of a strip of 1-cm–wide gauze, perhaps following moistening with thrombin. These packs may be left in place for a week; on removal there usually is a bed of granulation tissue without the vascular challenge.

Hemorrhages from soft tissue hemangiomas may be anticipated in most instances (Fig. 13-13). Hemangiomas have camouflaged themselves as ranulas and mucoceles, and therefore, bluish- and reddish-colored soft tissue lesions should be aspirated, as with the central lesions. However, palpation, resultant blanching, and then rapid refilling often constitute differential physical examination points for diagnosing isolated peripheral hemangiomas.

Treatment of soft tissue hemangiomas and aneurysms consists of cryotherapy, introduction of fibrosing solutions such as sodium morrhuate, and resection or combinations of these modalities. Multiple treatments with cryotherapy or by fibrosing with sodium morrhuate are usually necessary before the lesion is reduced enough in size to permit its excision.

Operations on bone underlying soft tissue hemangiomas may not pose a problem, although, obviously, precautions should be considered to include typing and crossmatching the patient's blood and having several units on standby.

Lymphangiomas usually do not constitute a hemorrhagic threat. These compressible, asymptomatic (except for their presence) lesions may be reduced in size or excised by surgical resection or by cryotherapy.

CLINICAL MANAGEMENT OF TYPICAL SECONDARY HEMORRHAGE

The treatment in a clinic of an extravascular secondary hemorrhage originating from an intraoral source would begin by separating the patient from the usual retinue of relatives and friends and calming the patient. The oral cavity is cleansed with suctioning and mouth rinses, the hemorrhaging source identified, regional anesthesia obtained, and treatment performed according to the etiological and anatomical factors.

Preoperative considerations in management of dentoalveolar secondary hemorrhage include patient cooperation and an adequate light. Patient cooperation may be enhanced with the use of a sedative or a minor tranquilizer. A headlight or fiberoptic-illuminated instruments should be considered. The area is cleansed by suctioning with a large tonsillar suction tip. The standard preanesthetic injection preparation of drying and painting with an antiseptic solution is followed by injection of regional anesthesia solution without vasoconstrictors, for example, 3% mepivacaine. While the local anesthetic is taking effect, a 10 by 10 cm gauze is placed in the oral cavity over the hemorrhaging site, and the patient is asked to close firmly on the gauze without talking or expectorating. Following the onset of local anesthesia, a radiograph is made of the area. Assuming the area is free

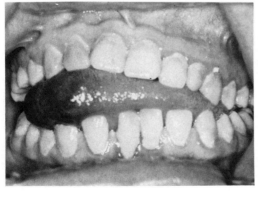

Fig. 13-13. Fibrohemangioma of the tongue causing distortion of the alveolar process.

of foreign bodies based on clinical and radiographic examinations, the mouth is irrigated with normal saline and the hemorrhaging site cleared and cleansed with a small tip suction device. Inspection and palpation are used to determine if the alveolar bony walls are intact, including bone in the bifurcation and trifurcation areas. In the event there is a fracture of the dentoalveolar process, the bone should be removed, even if a soft tissue flap needs to be raised, and the site treated as though it were a new surgical site.

Although the hemorrhage may be diminished by the local anesthetic that does not contain a vasoconstrictor and by the pressure gauze, one may usually detect where the primary bleeding site was, either local mucoperiosteal gingival tissues, alveolar bony wall, or apical vessels.

Gingival and mucoperiosteal hemorrhaging sites may be treated by local anesthetic injections with vasoconstrictors, for example, lidocaine with 1:100,000 epinephrine and the placement of sutures under tension to provide long-term pressure over the bleeding site. In some instances, mosquito hemostats will be necessary to control the hemorrhage. The hemostat can serve its usual role in tying bleeders, it may be used to conduct an electrocoagulating current, or it may be left in place for an extended period of time, for example, 30 minutes, and then removed to ascertain if the crushing of the offending vessel by the hemostat was effective in occluding the vessel.

Alveolar bone surrounding the tooth socket has passages to accommodate the vessels that bring nutrients to the periodontal ligament as well as an opening in the apex for the passage of the dentoalveolar neurovascular bundle. The vessels in these osseous canals may or may not have sufficient lateral hydrodynamic pressures, as do vessels in soft tissues, to ensure their contractible state, and recurrent hemorrhages may occur as the vessels relax. Nutrient canals are in all areas of the alveolar process and may contain vessels that have the capability of producing troublesome primary or secondary hemorrhages in the same manner as the vessels that pass through lamina dura to the alveoli. Burnishing the bleeding bone or crushing the areas with hemostats are time-tested methods of controlling alveolar process hemorrhages. Bone wax may be pressed into the osseous bleeding sites; in situations in which the hemorrhage from the alveolar process bony areas is unusually aggressive, the socket may be packed with gelatin sponge that was moistened with thrombin. In every case, the patient will be required to hold a 10×10 cm gauze in the mouth for 2 hours postoperatively.

To summarize the management of the usual secondary hemorrhage from a dentoalveolar surgical site, the following steps should be considered:

1. Instruct the patient to place a large gauze sponge, linen cloth, or handkerchief (never absorbent cotton) over the hemorrhaging site, close firmly, and then come to the responsible doctor's clinic for evaluation and indicated treatment.

2. With only the doctor and nursing assistant in attendance, prepare and drape the patient as for oral surgery.

3. Cleanse the area with a tonsillar suction device and 10×10 cm gauzes.

4. Obtain an effective light; consider a head light or fiberoptic-illuminated retractors.

5. Prepare the oral cavity and administer a local anesthetic without a vasoconstrictor.

6. Obtain a radiograph of the area.

7. If indicated, administer a simple sedative (50 mg secobarbital [Seconal], intravenously) or a minor tranquilizer (10 mg diazepam, [Valium] intravenously). (If the doctor has had training, experience, and current competence in general anesthesia or deep sedation modalities, additional intravenous or inhalation agents could be administered as indicated.)

8. If the general physical status indicates dehydration and a fasting state, begin an

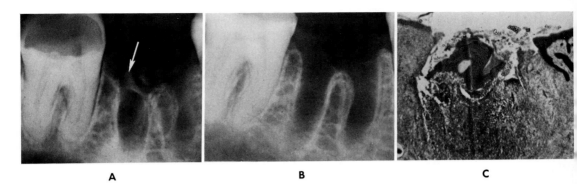

Fig. 13-14. A, Preoperative and, **B,** postoperative radiographs of a bony spicule (arrow) that produced a secondary hemorrhage from a dental extraction site. **C,** The photomicrograph shows inflammation and increased cellularity and vascularity produced by a bony fragment.

intravenous infusion of 5% dextrose in water.

9. Ascertain the source of the hemorrhage.

    a. If present, the foreign body or fractured bone should be removed (Fig. 13-14).

    b. If from soft tissue, local anesthesia with vasoconstrictor injection, clamping, clamping and tying, electrocoagulation, or cryotherapy may be used; sutures under tension may be placed over the offending tissues.

    c. If in bone, crushing of bone and small amounts of bone wax may be indicated.

    d. If generalized from the alveolus, packing the socket with gelatin sponge gauze moistened with thrombin may be indicated.

10. Suture the mucoperiosteum, and then place a pressure gauze in the mouth with instructions to close on it for 2 hours.

SHOCK*

In the past, shock was defined and identified almost solely with hypotension. While a decrease in arterial blood pressure usually accompanies the shocklike state, current thinking defines shock at the cellular level.

*By Victor J. Matukas, D.D.S., Ph.D., M.D.

A suitable definition would then be "inadequate blood flow to vital organs or failure of the cells of vital organs to utilize oxygen." Thus, strictly speaking, one can produce shock with normal or increased blood pressure but with poor compensation with decreased flow to vital organs or with a generalized metabolic state whereby cell damage occurs and oxygen cannot be appropriately utilized.

Traditionally shock has been classified as hypovolemic, cardiogenic, septic, and neurogenic. Decreased volume and pump failure are still valid causes of shock but the latter two classifications can perhaps be better defined as peripheral pooling with decreased venous return and decreased cellular uptake resulting from such states as sepsis. Regardless of its pathogenesis, shock produces a cycle of events that, if not interrupted, will ultimately lead to uncompensated declining homeostasis and death (Fig. 13-15).

Thus in this context the common denominator is either poor oxygen delivery or poor oxygen utilization at the cellular level. The net result is a shift from aerobic to anaerobic metabolism by the cells with the resultant production of lactic acid from pyruvate. This assumes significant clinical importance as studies have shown that there is a direct relationship between mor-

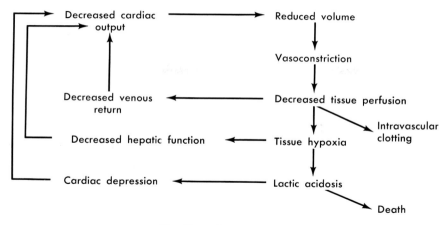

Fig. 13-15. Shock cycle.

tality as a result of irreversible shock and serum lactate levels. The accumulation of the latter will be reflected in altered blood gases, usually indicating a pattern of primary metabolic acidosis with a compensatory respiratory alkalosis.

The above cycle of events not only leads to increased serum lactate levels but to a wide variety of cellular events that, if not treated early, lead to irreversible cellular changes. Poor energy utilization with attending membrane instability is the best known phenomenon. Electrolyte balance is dependent on cellular work and active transport. In shock, passive equilibration tends to occur with ensuing passing of sodium and water into cells and potassium into the serum. The attending electrolyte and water shifts further aggravate any preexisting volume losses. Thus if vascular volume is depleted by blood loss or dehydration, fluid from the extracellular space shifts to the vascular compartment to compensate for this reduced volume; the actual depletion of the extracellular space is greater than the volume loss because of coincident passive movement of water intracellularly produced by the previously mentioned cellular shifts.

The shifts of fluid previously mentioned are the rationale for the use of crystaloid solutions in the primary therapy of shock,

prior to blood replacement. Often a proportionately larger amount of fluid must be used to restore homeostasis than the amount lost. This is partially caused by intracellular shifts of fluid and partially caused by the fact that vascular volume must be replaced to maintain cardiac output but crystaloids rapidly equilibrate between the vascular and interstitial space. Since the vascular space is about 5% and the total extracellular space about 20% of the body weight, a fourfold increase over blood loss is often necessary to restore vascular volume if crystaloid is used. It is obvious that this is a temporizing measure, and lost blood should be replaced with whole blood or component blood therapy. This measure does assume great importance, however, when the volume deficit is caused by dehydration or loss of body fluid other than blood. Dextrose and water alone has no place in the treatment of shock since this fluid will equilibrate with the intracellular space and little will remain in the vascular space to maintain cardiac output.

Assessment

The recognition of shock and assessment of its severity depend largely on awareness of the compensatory mechanisms that act to maintain homeostasis. These can be noted as clinical signs and symptoms. Uncompensated shocklike states lead to death. The compensatory mechanisms with different types of shock are similar, but the oral surgeon will most often have to deal with hypovolemic shock. The following events occur in compensation for shock and are usually easily recognized:

1. Decreased cardiac output—A decrease in cardiac output is based first on decreased venous return in hypovolemic shock. If the condition persists, decreased cardiac nutrition occurs and primary pump failure may result.

2. Cool clammy extremities—Vasoconstriction to skin and other nonvital organs occurs with resultant shunting of blood to brain, heart, and kidneys. There is a preferential shifting of fluids from the skin first, the gastrointestinal system next, and the renal, brain, and heart systems last. Thus cool clammy skin and adequate urine flow indicate early compensated shock.

3. Tachycardia and tachypnea—Both represent a compensatory increase in oxygen delivery to combat hypoxia. Both are early symptoms of shock. Tachypnea may be aggravated by the metabolic acidosis with a compensatory excretion of carbon dioxide. However, these symptoms may also be present with anxiety.

4. Arterial blood pressure—Blood pressure may be maintained in the supine position in early shock, but decompensation occurs on standing. Postural hypotension is often the most sensitive sign of early hypovolemic shock and should be a routine portion of the early examination.

5. Central venous pressure—In hypovolemic shock the central venous pressure will be decreased because of poor venous return and a depleted vascular volume. If shock progresses to pump failure, the central venous pressure will rise. Thus an isolated reading is of less value than serial determinations to assess the status of the patient. A clinical estimate may be made of central venous pressure on the basis of evaluation of neck veins in the supine and sitting state.

6. Arterial blood gases—Modern therapy of shock dictates the use of arterial blood gas determinations. Serial gas studies may be necessary to monitor the effects of treatment. Basically the degree of hypoxia and the acid-base status of the patient are important. The oxygen partial pressure (pO_2) should not be allowed to drop beyond 60 if possible. Fair reserve exists with pO_2 levels of 60 to 90, but as a result of the shape of the hemoglobin dissociation curve, small changes in pO_2 after 60 lead to large changes in oxygen saturation and decompensation may occur with minor changes in clinical conditions. In addition, because of lactic acidosis, the pH may be low and the bicarbonate radical (HCO_3) and carbon dioxide partial pressure (pCO_2) decreased, representing compensated metabolic acidosis.

7. Renal function—In early shock, renal blood flow is maintained at the expense of skin and the gastrointestinal system. As further shock occurs renal blood flow decreases with a concomitant fall in glomerular filtration rate and urine output. Thus decreased urinary output (less than 20 ml per hour) indicates fairly advanced shock. In addition, if decreased renal perfusion is allowed to continue over a long enough period of time, ischemia and tubular necrosis may ensue. Therefore, at this stage, therapy should be prompt and vigorous.

8. Hematocrit—Changes in hematocrit will vary according to the cause of shock and the stage. In early blood loss no change occurs and a drop in hematocrit does not become manifest until transcapillary refill occurs from the interstitial space. This may go on for 12 to 24 hours after blood loss. On the other hand, if volume depletion is associated with dehydration, then the hematocrit will be proportionally high because there has been no loss of red cell mass. Serial hematocrit determinations are most useful in assessing the progress of shock and monitoring for continuing blood loss.

Principles of treatment

1. Assure oxygen exchange—Good oxygen exchange is mandatory, and ways to assure it may range from relief of obstruc-

tion to oxygen therapy to assisted ventilation by way of an endotracheal tube. A tracheotomy under emergency conditions is rarely indicated and, if necessary, should almost always be done under controlled conditions after endotracheal intubation.

2. Ensure homeostasis—Any ongoing bleeding should be controlled until definitive therapy can be rendered. This may be accomplished by pressure, tourniquets, or direct ligation of severed vessels.

3. Maintain homeostasis—One and sometimes two large indwelling catheters should be placed, one preferably central. Initial therapy should be directed toward replenishing the vascular volume and the depleted extracellular space. One to two liters of Ringer's lactate or equivalent solution may be helpful after the patient is typed and crossmatched for blood therapy. If the cause of shock is blood loss, further therapy should be either fresh whole blood or component blood therapy. The latter is preferable if five or more units are needed since citrate intoxication, clotting factor depletion, and platelet depletion are minimized. There are numerous regimens, but an accepted one is packed red cells and plasmanate supplemented by three units of fresh frozen plasma with every ten units and six platelet packs with every 20 units. The above regimen minimizes bleeding, transfusion reactions, and electrolyte imbalance. Volume should be restored on a one-to-one

basis with appropriate attention paid to monitoring all systems. As mentioned previously there is no place for glucose and water and little indication for artificial plasma expanders such as dextran in modern hospital practice.

4. Position—The preferred patient position is with the legs elevated and the body supine. With the head down or body tilted, impingement of the abdomen contents on the diaphragm may occur and cause poor respiratory function (Fig. 13-16). In addition, the patient should be kept warm and dry, but the use of excess cover should be discouraged.

5. Relief of symptoms—Early wound care and relief of pain and anxiety is important. Wounds should be dressed and sutured and fractures set as soon as possible. Assurance and appropriate use of pain medication is also desirable to prevent neurogenic shock. Only enough medication should be used to control pain without depressing respiration. It is probably wiser to use small doses of intravenous narcotic (morphine) than unpredictable larger doses of intramuscular medication.

6. Monitor—Several parameters should be noted at appropriate intervals to assess the state of the patient.

 a. Vital signs—Blood pressure should remain stable and orthostatic changes disappear during treatment. Both tachypnea and tachycardia should di-

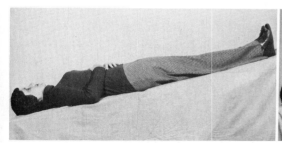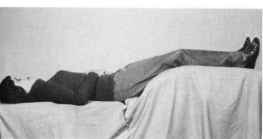

Fig. 13-16. A, Head down position permits abdominal contents to impinge on the diaphragm and interfere with respiration; also circulation within the head and neck may be compromised by a pooling effect. **B,** With the head, heart, and trunk horizontal, there will be more effective circulation in the head and neck and respiration will be improved.

minish as well. Worsening of these conditions indicate ongoing or inadequately treated shock.

   b. Renal flow—Urine flow should be greater than 20 ml per hour and preferably greater than 30 ml per hour. If renal flow is adequate and the urinary specific gravity greater than 1.020, then the patient is in early shock and still has some reserve available. Decreasing urinary output may mean either inadequate volume replacement or early renal failure. This distinction is important and must be made on the basis of such parameters as urine sodium and specific gravity and other clinical and historical clues.

   c. Arterial blood gases—The goal is maintenance of sufficient pO_2 (greater than 60) and normal or reasonable acid-base balance. Fluid replacement usually corrects the metabolic acidosis and rarely is bicarbonate therapy necessary.

   d. Central venous pressure—A low central venous pressure may indicate decreased venous return and vascular depletion while elevated central venous pressure may indicate fluid overload or cardiac failure. Thus the response to therapy shown by serial measurements is of more value than an isolated value.

   e. Hematocrit—As mentioned previously, in case of blood loss, changes in hematocrit are delayed until transcapillary refill occurs. Thus early hematocrit readings may be normal and not reflect volume depletion. Serial hematocrit measurements are valuable in estimating total original blood loss or monitoring ongoing loss. It is not necessary to restore the hematocrit to normal levels, but values should be kept above 30 to assure adequate oxygen exchange at the tissue level.

7. Drugs—The use of drugs in shock resulting from hypovolemia has a very limited role. Pain should be relieved by appropriate medication, antibiotics prescribed for contaminated wounds, and tetanus prophylaxis given. If signs of cardiogenic shock are present, the use of digitalis may be considered.

Controversy still exists regarding the role of steroids and vasopressors. While not conclusive, current thinking regarding steroids is that they have limited value in the absence of adrenal insufficiency or septic shock. If the former is present, prompt response to relatively small doses of intravenous steroids usually occurs. With the latter, massive doses are indicated and are considered adjunctive. Vasopressors are also of limited value in early compensated shock, since usually the body is already in maximum sympathetic tone. They may be useful if volume is restored and decompensation of peripheral vasculature or cardiac output occurs.

It is thus clear that the successful management of shock lies in recognizing and treating the state during the compensatory stage and prior to irreversible cellular dysfunction. This requires meticulous attention to detail in diagnosis and assessment and intelligent therapeutic intervention.

CONCLUSION

In medicine, gathering and organization of information is possible by taking the history and performing a physical examination. If the history is taken and physical examination performed, nearly every one of the conditions described in this chapter, many of which are awesome in their manifestations and consequences, will be prevented. The history and the physical examination, augmented by selected radiographic and laboratory studies, are basic.

REFERENCES

1. Allen, W. E., III, Kier, E. L., and Rothman, S. L. G.: The maxillary artery: normal arteriographic anatomy, Am. J. Radiol. **118:**517, 1973.
2. Alling, C. C.: Local anesthesia. In Clark, J. W., editor: Clinical dentistry, vol. 1, New York, 1976, Harper & Row, Publishers, chapter 24, pp. 1-10.
3. Alling, C. C., and Christopher, A.: Status report

on dental anesthetic needles and syringes, J. Am. Dent. Assoc. **89:**1171, 1974.

4. Alling, C. C., and Davis, B. P., Jr.: Compound, comminuted complex maxillofacial fractures, J. Oral Surg. **32:**415, 1974.

5. American College of Surgeons: Manual of preoperative and postoperative care, Philadelphia, 1971, W. B. Saunders Co.

6. Battersby, T. G.: Cavernous hemangioma of the mandible, Br. Dent. J. **103:**347, 1957.

7. Berkman, M. D., and others: Pulpal response to cyanoacrylate in human teeth, J. Am. Dent. Assoc. **83:**140, 1971.

8. Bhaskar, S. N., and Frisch, J.: Use of cyanoacrylate adhesives in dentistry, J. Am. Dent. Assoc. **77:**831, 1968.

9. Condon, R. E., and Nyhus, L. M., editors: Manual of surgical therapeutics, Departments of Surgery, The Medical College of Wisconsin and University of Illinois, Boston, 1975, Little, Brown and Co.

10. Cook, W. A.: The mandibular field and its control with local anesthetics, Mod. Dent. **22:**11, 1955.

11. Council on Dental Therapeutics: Hemostatics, styptics, and astringents. In Accepted dental therapeutics, ed. 34, Chicago, 1971, American Dental Association, pp. 194-201.

12. Dempsey, H.: Hemostasis. In Menaker, L., editor: Biologic basis for wound healing, New York, 1975, Harper & Row, Publishers, pp. 1-5.

13. Dolan, K. D., and Hayden, J.: Maxillary "pseudofracture" lines, Radiology **107:**321, 1973.

14. Eklund, M. K., and Kent, J. M.: The use of isobutyl 2-cyanoacrylate as a postextraction dressing in humans, J. Oral Surg. **32:**264, 1974.

15. Evans, B. E., editor: Dental care in hemophilia, New York, 1977, The National Hemophilia Foundation, p. 3.

16. Ewen, S. J.: Periodontal uses of a tissue adhesive, J. Periodontol. **38:**138, 1967.

17. Frommeyer, W. B., Jr.: Blood coagulation. In Menaker, L., editor: Biologic basis for wound healing, New York, 1975, Harper & Row, Publishers, pp. 19-41.

18. Hollinshead, W. H.: Anatomy for surgeons. vol. 1. The head and neck, ed. 2, New York, 1968, Harper & Row, Publishers, pp. 520-522.

19. LaDow, C. S., and Tatoian, J. A., Jr.: Treatment of central hemangioma of the maxilla by embolization, J. Oral Surg. **34:**622, 1976.

20. Lapeyrolerie, F.: Management of dentoalveolar hemorrhage. In Alling, C. C., editor: Symposium on dental emergencies, Dent. Clin. North Am. **17:**523-532, 1973.

21. Macansh, J. D., and Owen, M. D.: Central hemangioma of the mandible, J. Oral Surg. **30:**293, 1972.

22. Mahan, P. E., and Kreutziker, K. L.: Diagnosis and management of temporomandibular joint pain, Oral Surg. **40:**165, 297, 1975.

23. Moose, S. M.: Sinusoidal aneurysm of the mandible, J. Oral Surg. **15:**245, 1957.

24. Moose, S. M.: Personal communication, 1977.

25. Ochstein, A. J., Hansen, N. M., and Swenson, H. M.: A comparative study of cyanoacrylate and other periodontal dressings on gingival surgical wound healing, J. Periodontol. **40:**515, 1969.

26. Osbon, D. B.: Management of surgical complications. In Clark, J. W., editor: Clinical dentistry, vol. 3, New York, 1976, Harper & Row, Publishers, chapter 39, pp. 8-9.

27. Watson, J. E.: Some anatomic aspects of the Gow-Gates technique for mandibular anesthesia, Oral Surg. **36:**328, 1973.

28. Westwood, R. M., Tilson, H. B., and Margeno-Rowe, A. J.: The diagnostic significance of the microhematocrit as an office screening test, J. Oral Surg. **33:**698, 1975.

CHAPTER 14

Cysts of bone and soft tissues of the oral cavity and contiguous structures

Leroy W. Peterson

A cyst is a cavity occurring in either hard or soft tissue with a liquid, semiliquid, or air content. It is surrounded by a definite connective tissue wall or capsule and usually has an epithelial lining. The contained substance is a predominant feature in proportion to the size of the entire mass of tissue.

CLASSIFICATION

Congenital, developmental, and retention types of cysts occur within the oral cavity and about the face and neck. Cysts of dental origin are by far the most common. In the combined grouping of these cystic lesions, the following classification, modified from that given by Robinson and Thoma and others,[1] is offered for discussion.

A. Congenital cysts
   1. Thyroglossal
   2. Branchiogenic
   3. Dermoid
B. Developmental cysts
   1. Nondental origin
     a. Fissural types
       (1) Nasoalveolar
       (2) Median
       (3) Incisive canal (nasopalatine)
       (4) Globulomaxillary
     b. Retention types
       (1) Mucocele
       (2) Ranula
   2. Dental origin
     a. Periodontal
       (1) Periapical
       (2) Lateral
       (3) Residual
     b. Primordial (follicular)
     c. Dentigerous
     d. Keratocysts

Killey and Kay[9] include the solitary bone cyst, idiopathic bone cavity cyst, and aneurysmal bone cyst in their classification of cysts of the jaws. These lesions are well described in their text, and their review of other classifications is comprehensive.

Neoplasms that may appear to be cystic are not included in the previous classification. These tumors are discussed elsewhere, but the most common ones encountered are the ameloblastoma and the mixed salivary gland tumor. The ameloblastoma, a true dental neoplasm, may have no clinical characteristics other than appearing to be a cystic lesion. This neoplasm involves bone primarily, with displacement of the adjacent soft tissue by erosion and expansion.

Other than the parotid area, the mixed cell, salivary neoplasms appear more often on the hard and soft palates than in any part of the oral cavity except perhaps the cheek. They occur rarely in the lips, where they form a palpable swelling and appear similar to a mucocele.

Various benign tumors of the soft tissues of the oral cavity that may have the clinical appearance of a cyst include the fibroma, lipoma, myoma, hemangioma, lymphangioma, and papilloma.

Additional neoplasms and dysplastic conditions of bone may appear roentgenographically as cystic lesions. These neoplasms include the giant cell tumor, fibrous dysplasia, ossifying fibroma, metastatic and invasive carcinoma, osteolytic sarcoma, other rare primary bone tumors, and multiple myeloma.

Metabolic or systemic dysfunctions that may give rise to lesions having the radiographic appearance of a cyst are osteitis fibrosa cystica (hyperparathyroidism) and the diseases of the reticuloendothelial system (histiocytosis X).

Hemorrhagic or traumatic bone cavities (Fig. 14-14, *A*) as well as the idiopathic bone cavities (Fig. 14-14, *B*) described by

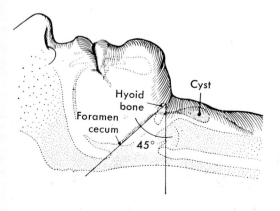

Fig. 14-1. Thyroglossal cyst. (From Copeland, M. M., and Geschickter, C. F.: Am. Surg. **24:**321, 1958.)

Stafne[19] and others may also enter into the differential diagnosis of true cysts of the jaws.

Congenital cysts

Thyroglossal duct cysts. Thyroglossal cysts (Fig. 14-1) may arise from any portion of the thyroglossal duct. They are therefore in a midline position and are usually of dark color. They may be so vascular as to resemble hemangiomas. One frequent important symptom is hemorrhage into the mouth, resulting from the rupture of the overlying veins.

The thyroglossal duct lies in the line between the thyroid gland and the foramen cecum on the tongue. A cyst or sinus tract derived from this structure is located in the midline at any point between the thyroid isthmus and the base of the tongue. The tract is usually attached to or in close relationship with the hyoid bone. The cyst may be asymptomatic or may cause symptoms as a result of pressure on other structures. Swallowing will cause the mass to move upward.

Because of the thyroglossal duct the cyst may become infected. If so, the lesion may drain spontaneously but also may be incised. Ideally, it should be removed before infection occurs or after acute symptoms have subsided. Complete excision of the tract to the base of the tongue, frequently including a portion of the hyoid bone, is necessary for a cure.

Branchiogenic cysts. Several theories have been advanced concerning the origin of branchiogenic cysts (Fig. 14-2), but most of the evidence supports the belief that they arise from persistencies of the second branchial cleft. They are characteristically located along the anterior border of the sternocleidomastoid muscle at any level in the neck. A fistulous tract may extend up to the digastric muscle and terminate in the tonsillar fossa. These cysts or tracts are lined with ciliated and stratified squamous epithelium and contain a milky or mucoid fluid. An external fistula may be present.

Treatment consists of complete surgical excision.

Dermoid cysts. Dermoid cysts (Fig. 14-3) are relatively uncommon in the oral cavity. The dermoid cyst consists of a fibrous wall lined with stratified squamous epithelium. The cyst frequently contains hair, sebaceous and sweat glands, as well as tooth structures. They may occur on the hard and soft palates, on the dorsum of the tongue, or more commonly in the floor of the mouth. They cause swelling in the same location as the sublingual retention cysts and must be differentiated from them. They do not give the vesicular appearance of the ranula. The dermoid cyst (Fig. 14-3, *B*) may be located either above or below the geniohyoid muscle. Dermoids usually occur in the midline but may be displaced laterally during development and, as such, must be differentiated from cysts of branchial origin.

Dermoid cysts are not easily discovered unless they cause swelling beneath the chin or up into the floor of the mouth. On palpation, these cysts have a rubberlike sensation. They generally contain a yellow cheesy material. This yellow color aids sometimes in differentiation of the dermoid cyst from the ranula, which has a bluish hue. X-ray examination may be helpful in distinguishing a dermoid cyst from other lesions of similar nature because of their contents, which frequently include radiopaque objects.

Treatment is the surgical removal of the entire tumor.

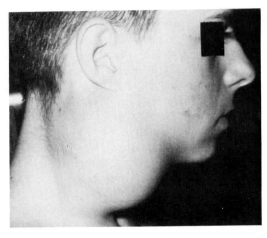

Fig. 14-2. Branchiogenic cleft cyst. (Courtesy Washington University School of Medicine, Division of Plastic Surgery, St. Louis, Mo.)

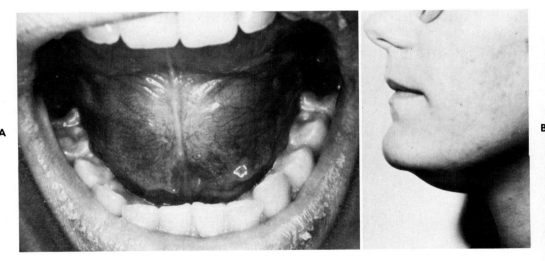

A   B

Fig. 14-3. A, Dermoid cyst occurring above floor of mouth. **B,** Dermoid cyst occurring below floor of mouth. (Courtesy Dr. John Delfino, Washington University School of Dental Medicine, St. Louis, Mo.)

Developmental cysts
Nondental origin

Nasoalveolar cysts. A nasoalveolar cyst (Fig. 14-4) forms at the junction of the globular, lateral nasal, and maxillary processes. It produces a swelling at the attachment of the ala of the nose, and as it expands it encroaches on the nasal cavity. Since these cysts are not central bony lesions, x-ray findings are negative. The cysts are usually lined with nasaltype epithelium but may also contain some stratified squamous cells. On clinical observation they may be mistaken for cysts of dental

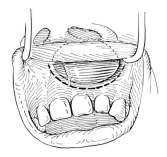

Fig. 14-4. Nasoalveolar cyst. This cyst presents no radiographic change. It usually bulges into the floor of the nose. It is removed intraorally.

origin or dental alveolar abscesses on the maxillary anterior teeth.

Treatment consists of complete surgical excision. The nasoalveolar cyst is usually removed intraorally by carefully incising the overlying mucous membrane and enucleating the cyst.

Median cysts. The median cyst (Fig. 14-5) is a bone cyst that forms in a median fissure of the palate from embryonic remnants. Median alveolar cysts have also been described. Robinson[1] maintains that these are not true median cysts since the bones uniting in these areas have their origin deep within mesenchymal tissue with no chance for inclusion of epithelial rests. Robinson presumes that they are primordial cysts of supernumerary tooth buds. Median cysts of the mandible have been described; they are extremely uncommon.

Median cysts are differentiated from incisive canal cysts primarily by their location, since they usually occur more posteriorly in the palate. X-ray findings are often misleading because of the overlapping shadows of the paranasal sinuses. Injection of a radiopaque material will definitely outline this cyst (Fig. 14-14, *D*).

Surgical excision of these cysts is the preferred treatment, although the Partsch

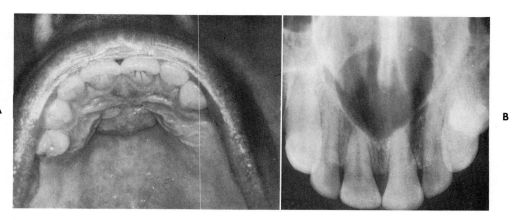

A   B

Fig. 14-5. Median cyst of palate. **A,** Clinical view showing expansion through palatal bone. **B,** Radiographic view.

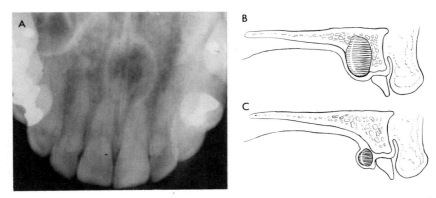

Fig. 14-6. A, Incisive canal cyst. In the edentulous maxilla the cyst may appear to be at the crest of the alveolar ridge. **B,** Diagram of cross section of incisive canal cyst. **C,** Diagram of cross section of cyst of the palatine papilla. Although a similar amount of clinical enlargement of the palatine area may be present, this cyst does not involve bone. This cyst is rare.

method may be used. Frequently, these cysts have to be approached by reflecting a mucoperiosteal flap from the labial aspect of the maxilla as well as from the palate. These cysts are in close proximity to the floor of the nose and bulge into the nasal cavity. The median cyst has a connective tissue sac lined by squamous epithelium. Like other cysts, cholesterol crystal spaces may be surrounded in some instances by foreign body cells.

Incisive canal cysts (nasopalatine cysts). Cysts located in the center of the bone are named incisive canal cysts (Fig. 14-6). Occasionally a soft tissue cyst forms in the palatine papilla. These cysts do not expand inside the bone, nor do they alter significantly the overlying mucosa. They are called cysts of the papilla palatini and are differentiated from a bone cyst by x-ray and surgical examination.

The radiograph is of great value in diagnosis of incisive canal cysts. However, the size of the incisive canal is by no means constant, and many a large canal and foramen may give the appearance of a cyst. In edentulous jaws, because of resorption, the cyst may appear closer to the surface. Differential diagnosis from radicular cysts is necessary to prevent devitalization or extractions of these teeth.

These cysts usually give no clinical symptoms unless they become secondarily infected. A persistent discharge, or pus escaping under pressure, may be noted. Probing or puncturing the area will usually allow the accumulation of fluid to escape, but swelling will recur unless the cyst is removed surgically. For the surgical approach to these cysts, a palatal flap is usually retracted after incising along the lingual gingival margins. By careful elevation of the flap, the continuity of the nerves and vessels, which lie in the foramen and emerge at the papilla, can be preserved. Frequently, the nerves and vessels must be interrupted for better access to the cystic tissue. This does not cause any undesirable sequelae. Usually the cyst can then be teased away gently from the soft tissue or the bony bed, as the case may be. Nasopalatine cysts usually contain a thick membrane of connective tissue. The lining of the lumen varies in type from squamous to transitional to ciliated columnar epithelium. In many cases marked inflammatory infiltration takes place as a result of secondary infection from the oral cavity.

Globulomaxillary cysts. Globulomaxillary cysts (Fig. 14-7) are epithelial-lined sacs formed at the junction of the globular and maxillary processes between the lateral in-

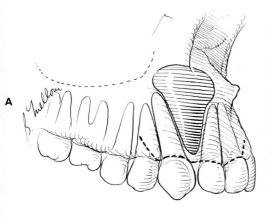

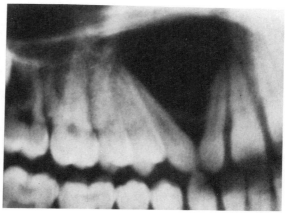

Fig. 14-7. **A,** Globulomaxillary cyst. Typical pear-shaped appearance on the radiograph. The adjacent lateral incisor and canine teeth, which have been pushed aside by the cyst, are vital. The wound is closed with drainage if it is secondarily infected. **B,** Radiographic appearance. (Courtesy Dr. Peter Pollon, Washington University School of Dental Medicine, St. Louis, Mo.)

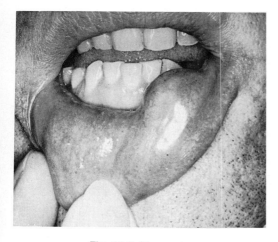

Fig. 14-8. Mucocele.

cisor and canine teeth. They usually cause a divergence of the roots of these teeth and appear as pear-shaped radiolucencies on x-ray film. As is true with other cysts of the oral cavity, they become secondarily infected and undergo acute inflammatory changes.

Diagnosis of the globulomaxillary cyst depends almost entirely on its location between the lateral incisor and canine plus a clinical evaluation of the adjacent teeth to differentiate it from one of dental origin. These teeth usually respond favorably to vitality tests. The cyst consists of a connective tissue membrane lined with stratified squamous epithelium. Treatment is surgical and consists of careful excision, although the Partsch method (p. 266) may be used. Generally the adjacent teeth need not be disturbed if the operation is planned and carried out properly. A mucoperiosteal flap must be reflected from the labial bone so that adequate access to the pathology may be obtained and the cyst carefully enucleated. The majority of these incisions heal by first intention, and primary closure can be obtained without the use of dressings or other substances to obliterate the cavity.

Mucoceles. Mucocysts or mucoceles (Fig. 14-8) result from the obstruction of a glandular duct and are commonly located in the lip, cheek, and floor of the mouth. They may also be found on the anterior portion of the tongue, where glands are located at the inferior surface. These are small, round or oval, translucent swellings, sometimes having a bluish color, and may be mistaken for a hemangioma. The mucocele is freely movable and usually found right underneath the mucosa. Occasionally it may be punc-

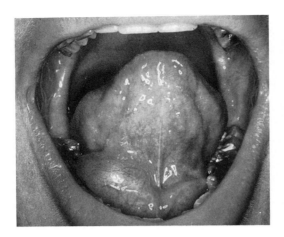

Fig. 14-9. Ranula.

tured accidentally or will rupture spontaneously, only to recur. The preferred treatment is complete excision. If the mucocele is incompletely removed, it has a marked tendency to recur, but the lesion is not known to become malignant.

Ranulas. A ranula (Fig. 14-9) is a cyst forming in the floor of the mouth, generally from a sublingual gland. The ranula forms in a manner similar to the mucocele but develops to a much larger size.

When it attains a large size, the mucosa is thinned out, and the cyst assumes a bluish color. It is a nonpainful lesion, but the tongue may be raised and its motion hindered, thus impairing mastication and speech. The ranula is subject to rupture when injured, with escape of a mucoid fluid that reaccumulates as the area heals.

The size of the ranula cannot be determined from the appearance within the mouth. It is tense and fluctuant but does not pit on pressure. The ranula seldom causes any external swelling and rarely becomes infected. It is painless and contains a stringy, mucoid fluid. A ranula is much more firm than the angioma occasionally found in the floor of the mouth. Dermoid cysts have a doughy feeling on pressure and occur more often in the median line. Lipomas are more firm. Cysts of the submandibular duct usually cause swelling in the

gland. They develop more rapidly than the true ranula and are associated with pain and other symptoms of inflammation. The best treatment for a ranula is surgery in the form of marsupialization.

Dental origin (odontogenic cysts)

Harris and Toler[8] recognize three major types of odontogenic cysts and state that they have distinct developmental identities. Periodontal or inflammatory cysts appear to be a lymphoepithelial barrier to the spread of periapical infection and may possibly regress with the removal of the causative agent. Disturbances in the eruptive process, including formation of clefts in the enamel epithelium and reduction of this tissue before tooth eruption, may give rise to follicular and dentigerous cysts. Keratocysts appear to arise from submucosal cells that have the features of dental lamina rests. These rests could have a role in normal tooth formation and eruption.

According to the classification being discussed in this chapter, the following types of cysts are important.

Periodontal cysts. A periodontal cyst (Fig. 14-10) is formed from epithelial rests or remnants in the periodontal membrane. These cysts are all of inflammatory origin. The usual location is at the apex of the tooth, where they are termed radicular cysts, but they also may be formed along the lateral surface and are then termed lateral cysts. Cysts of inflammatory nature in edentulous areas are termed residual. These result from incomplete surgical removal of pathological tissue at the time an infected tooth is extracted.

Inflammatory cysts are a result of dental infection, with necrosis of pulpal tissue and resultant degeneration into granulomas or cysts. All epithelial granulomas do not develop into cysts. The formation of a cyst depends, first, on the dissolution of the central part of the granuloma and, second, on transudation of fluid through the epithelium-lined connective tissue sac into the lumen. These cysts are commonly lined by strati-

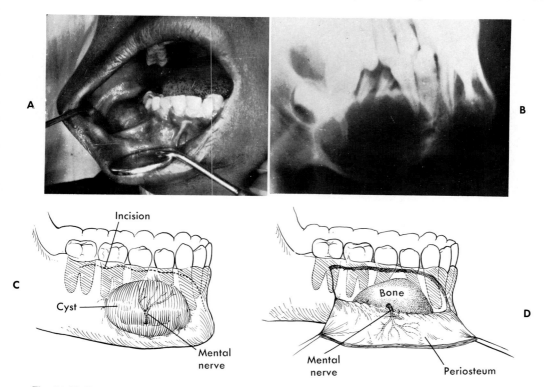

Fig. 14-10. Periodontal cysts. **A,** *Periapical (radicular) cyst.* Clinical appearance. **B,** Radiographic appearance. **C,** Incision for reflecting mucoperiosteal flap. The buccal cortical plate is thin because of the expansion of the cyst. **D,** The continuity of the mental nerve is preserved within the flap during the surgical dissection.

Continued.

fied squamous epithelium. Round cell infiltration and other signs of chronic inflammation are usually found. The periodontal cyst, being primarily inflammatory in nature, will not show any progression toward neoplastic formation of the epithelial cells lining the cyst wall.

The small periodontal cyst can often be enucleated through the alveolar socket after removal of the involved tooth. However, it is frequently much better to elevate a surgical flap and remove the cyst by the labial or buccal approach. This ensures better visibility of the pathological region and allows for more definite removal of all the cyst tissue.

Large periodontal cysts usually appear to involve several teeth, and it is extremely important that vital teeth not be removed

unnecessarily. This overlapping as visualized on the x-ray film may extend buccally, labially, or palatally to the apparently involved teeth, and, as such, access to and removal of the cyst can be gained by sacrificing sound dental structures. In these large cystic areas the Partsch method of treatment is preferred if adjacent teeth are in danger of damage.

Many of these inflammatory cysts become chronically infected and form fistulas through the alveolar bone to the overlying mucoperiosteum. In some instances, expansion of the cyst is great enough that all overlying bone has disappeared, and the cyst wall is adherent to the mucoperiosteum. In these instances the dissection involved in reflecting a mucoperiosteal flap becomes somewhat tedious, and care must

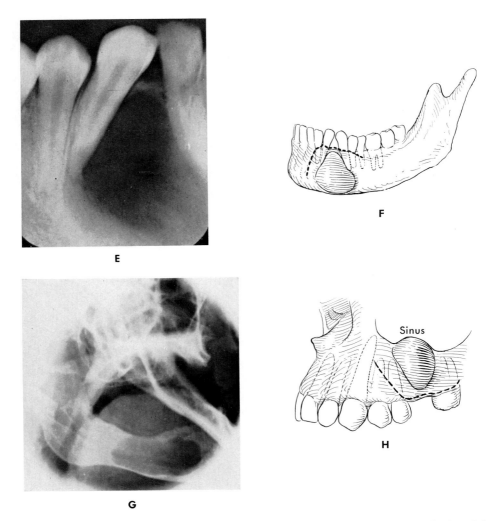

Fig. 14-10, cont'd. E, *Lateral cyst.* In this particular case the adjacent teeth are displaced. **F,** Incision for removal of lateral cyst. **G,** *Residual cyst.* The cyst may be treated by enucleation or the Partsch method. The continuity of the mental foramen structures can be preserved either way. **H,** Residual cyst from previously extracted first molar tooth. Radiopaque material could be injected to confirm the fact that the maxillary sinus is not involved if differential diagnosis is doubtful. The cyst should be enucleated carefully.

be taken to strip the cystic lining cleanly from the soft tissue covering the bone.

Tooth roots that protrude into a bone cavity after enucleation of a cyst should be amputated after proper root canal therapy has been instituted, or the teeth should be extracted. Complete removal of cystic tissue in inaccessible areas is difficult, since often the involved region cannot be too clearly visualized or approached surgically, because of tooth root interference.

Residual periodontal cysts cannot be diagnosed from x-ray findings alone and are often verified only on microscopic examination. Treatment in all cases, however, is either by enucleation or marsupialization.

Primordial cysts (follicular). Primordial cysts (Fig. 14-11) differ from periodontal

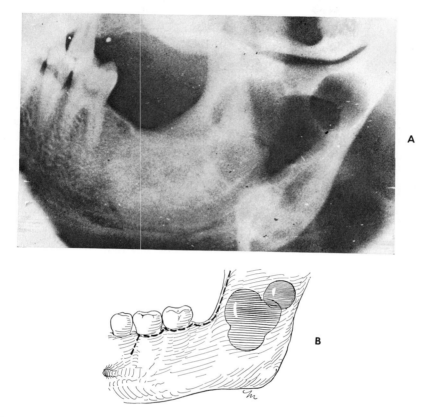

Fig. 14-11. A, Multilocular primordial cyst forming from tooth bud of third molar that never developed. **B,** Incision for intraoral removal of cyst.

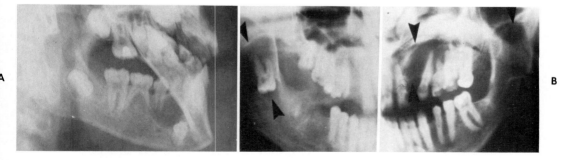

Fig. 14-12. A, The dentigerous cyst was removed and the unerupted tooth retained in this case. The tooth should continue to erupt. The Partsch method of treatment may be used because sometimes it is difficult to dissect the cyst free without displacing the unerupted tooth. **B,** Multiple dentigerous and follicular cysts in basal cell nevus syndrome.

and dentigerous cysts in that they contain no calcified structures. The term follicular has often been applied to this type of lesion and can be used synonymously with it. In primordial cysts the retrogression of the stellate reticulum in the enamel organ takes place before any calcified tooth structure is formed. The word primordial means most simple and most undeveloped in character. These cysts are lined by stratified squamous epithelium and may be either locular, multilocular, or multiple. Odontogenic cysts, such as primordial and dentigerous cysts, are formed from primitive oral epithelium and are therefore closely related to each other and to the ameloblastoma, a true dental neoplasm. In these cysts, epithelial cells have a definite potential of developing into a neoplasm.

Except for the absence of dental structures resulting from the period in development when cystic changes took place, these primordial and dentigerous cysts are basically identical in all respects so far as surgical treatment is concerned, and their differential diagnosis, to a large degree, is purely academic.

Dentigerous cysts. A dentigerous cyst (Fig. 14-12) contains a crown of an unerupted tooth or dental anomaly such as an odontoma. These cysts develop after deposition of enamel and are probably a result of degenerative changes in the reduced enamel-forming epithelium. The fact that the epithelium of a dentigerous cyst is attached to the neck of the tooth is fairly strong evidence that in most cases the cyst is formed by the enamel organ and not independently of it.

If cysts form when a tooth is erupting, they are called eruption cysts (Fig. 14-13). These cysts interfere with normal eruption of the teeth. Eruption cysts are more commonly found in the child and young adult and may be associated with any tooth. If treatment is indicated, simple incision or "deroofing" is all that is needed.

Enlarged dentigerous cysts can cause a marked displacement of teeth. Pressure of accumulated fluid usually displaces the tooth in an apical direction, and, frequently, the root formation becomes stunted. Dentigerous cysts may be found anywhere in the mandible or the maxilla but are more frequently located at the angle of the jaw, the cuspid regions, maxillary third molar areas, the antral cavity, and also in the floor of the orbit.

Cysts may be produced by several tooth germs acting together in their formation, giving a multiple follicular-type appearance. The tooth bud given off from the dental lamina or outer epithelial layer of the enamel organ of the tooth may branch and form a number of follicles. Each follicle may form a cyst, causing a formation of

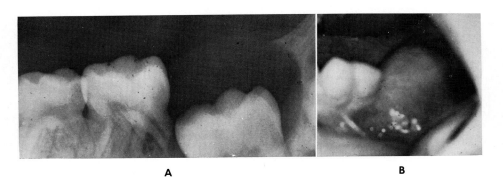

A   B

Fig. 14-13. A, Eruption cyst associated with a permanent first molar tooth. **B,** Intraoral swelling associated with eruption cyst.

so-called daughter cysts, which necessitate careful exploration at the time of surgery. It should be remembered that the primordial or dentigerous cyst is a potential ameloblastoma. The formation of buds at the basal layer of the epithelium and papillary outgrowth into the lumen may be the beginning of this dental tumor.

Keratocysts. Many follicular and dentigerous cysts contain keratinizing material and are known as keratocysts.[17] Keratocysts differ from other odontogenic cysts in their microscopic appearance and clinical behavior. They may resemble periodontal, primordial, or follicular cysts. Usually they cannot be distinguished radiographically. The term odontogenic keratocyst was first used by Phillipsen in 1956. Pindborg and Hansen in 1963 described the essential features of this cyst. Stoelinga and Peters[20] report a histological study of six keratocysts. Their findings strengthen the idea that oral mucosa plays an important role in the origin of keratocysts. As a result of this study it is advocated that wide excision of overlying mucosa in the area where the cyst wall is adhered to mucosa is a treatment of choice. Nonkeratinized cysts increase in size primarily because of degenerative characteristics of the lining. Keratocysts increase in size principally by a process of epithelial cell multiplication and have a greater tendency toward recurrence.

Basal cell nevus syndrome.

Multiple cysts are a common finding in basal cell nevus syndrome (Fig. 14-12, *B*). The cyst may be follicular, primordial, or periodontal in nature, with all types of histological variations in the epithelial linings. There is a preponderance of the keratocyst type.

The basal cell nevus syndrome[24] is a hereditary complex embracing various manifestations of cutaneous and skeletal abnormalities. Congenital cysts generally develop earlier than the skin lesions. Therefore, the dentist may be the first to encounter and identify this syndrome when he or she discovers multiple cystlike radiolucencies in the jaws. Multiple conventional jaw cysts occur more frequently than do those of basal cell nevus syndrome. In these cases of multiple cystic lesions one must be aware, however, that the other associated skeletal and cutaneous lesions may develop later to tie in with the syndrome.

• • •

Developmental cysts have a marked tendency to recur. Frequently, cysts with thickly epitheliated linings are more likely to recur than cysts with a thin layer of epithelium, especially if they are multiple.

Complete enucleation of the cyst sac is indicated in developmental dental cysts. A partial excision is dangerous, and any small part left behind may contain the potential of developing into a true dental tumor. When, because of anatomical considerations, combined Partsch and enucleation techniques are used, multiple biopsies should be taken from the area and the postoperative course thoroughly followed with x-ray examination every 6 months. Any pathological tissue that is removed should not be discarded. It should be placed in a bottle of 10% formalin and prepared for complete microscopic examination. Carcinomas have been reported as developing in the epithelial cells of this type cystic lesion.[15]

Many of these cysts give no clinical symptoms until noticeable asymmetry of the face develops. These cysts can reach rather large proportions to involve the entire body or ramus of the mandible as well as a large portion of the maxilla, displacing the orbital and paranasal sinus cavities rather than invading them. Many times, radiographs will show marked expansion of bone so that the overlying cortical plate is paper thin.

Treatment of choice, even in the extremely large cystic lesions, is careful enucleation. If one cortical plate of bone is entirely destroyed by expansive pressure, the periosteal tissue is left intact, which serves as an excellent aid for regeneration of bone. When marked expansion and asymmetry have occurred, in the repair process, nature will reestablish normal jaw contour and complete regeneration of bone if the surgery is adequate and no recurrence of the cystic lesion takes place.

Each case presents its own individual problems in diagnosis and treatment, but if both are adequate, the prognosis should be excellent and complications kept to a minimum. The patient must be given every consideration, and he should have as good an understanding of the surgeon's problems as the surgeon has of the patient's concern for a satisfactory prognosis.

GENERAL CONSIDERATION OF CYSTIC LESIONS

This discussion will include problems in differential diagnosis, x-ray examination, surgical technique, postoperative treatment, and complications of surgery.

Diagnosis

Diagnosis in each individual case should rest on a combination of physical findings, history, x-ray evaluation, and tissue biopsy. Histological examination is desirable and often essential to establish a correct diagnosis, but other clinical laboratory studies are often necessary. A patient should not be subjected to biopsy immediately to eliminate other studies; biopsy should be deferred until indications for it are clear. Clinical symptoms are generally absent unless the cyst reaches large proportions and causes a facial deformity. Pain may be caused by the pressure of a cyst on a nerve, and, likewise, paresthesia or numbness may be a clinical complaint. Cysts may be multiple, each from a separate anlage, but, conversely, multiple cysts may be indicative of systemic disease.

Because cysts of soft tissues in the neck are often tense, the differentiation between cystic and solid tumors may be difficult. The presence of inflammation and tenderness on pressure is a better sign of a cyst than of a tumor because cysts become secondarily infected more frequently. However, the tenderness of a cyst and mobility of the neck structures frequently make fluctuation of fluid an unreliable sign. Location, mobility, fixation, consistency, regional changes, and associated diseases are the most important factors in diagnosis.

In large, cystic, bony defects that produce facial asymmetry, expansion takes place usually along the line of least resistance in bone and generally in one direction. A true neoplasm will usually grow and expand in and through bone in any and all directions. Structures such as nerves, blood vessels, and paranasal sinuses are usually displaced by the pressure exerted by the fluid contents of the cyst; a neoplasm invades and surrounds these tissues.

X-ray findings

The x-ray examination gives information about the location and extent of a bone cyst and involvement of other teeth. Overlying shadows may be misleading when many teeth appear involved in a cystic area, and a thorough clinical examination, including vitality tests, should be made. Pressure of the cystic fluid within the cavity may cause the formation of a compact layer of bone in which the cyst sac is contained. This dense lamina is seen on the x-ray film as a thin white line outlining the area containing the radiolucent cyst. A diagnosis can never be made positively from the x-ray findings, since many neoplastic and metabolic diseases appear radiographically cystic. The jaws have been frequently referred to as an area of surgical romance because of the complexity of disease entities they contain, all of which present a problem in differential diagnosis. (See Fig. 14-14, *A* and *B*.) Cysts usually have a smooth, rounded, lobular outline and may be multilocular in appearance (Fig. 14-14, *C*). However, if secondary infection exists, the margins can be irregular.

Cysts occurring in the maxilla are often difficult to visualize because of the overlapping shadows cast by the paranasal

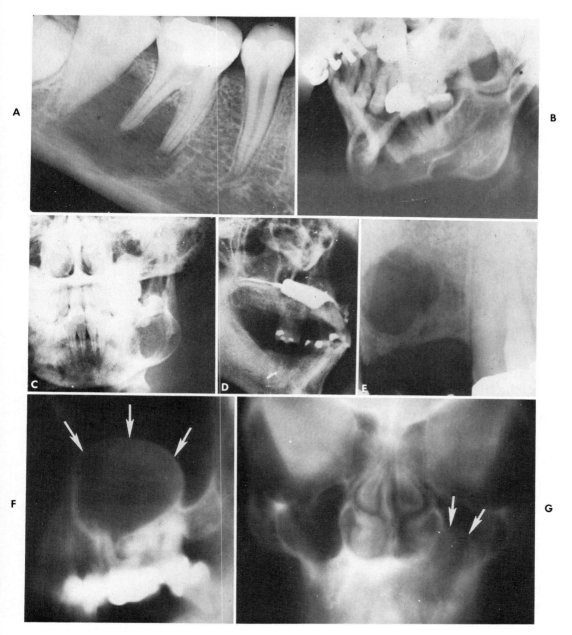

Fig. 14-14. A, Hemorrhagic or traumatic bone cavity. The presence of an intact lamina dura and a positive vitality test indicate that the lesion is not of odontogenic origin. **B,** Lateral jaw radiograph showing latent bone cavity near inferior border of mandible. **C,** A characteristic cystic lesion showing expansion and thinning of the cortical bone. **D,** Maxillary cyst outlined by the injection of a radiopaque material. **E,** Radiographic appearance of a healed postoperative defect in which both labial bone and palatal cortical bone were lost in the removal of the original cystic lesion. **F,** Lateral laminagram showing cystic lesion of dental origin involving but not invading sinus (arrows). **G,** Anterior-posterior laminagram outlining the cystic lesion (arrows). **(F** and **G** Courtesy Mallinckrodt Institute of Radiology, Washington University School of Medicine, St. Louis, Mo.)

sinuses on x-ray examination. A radiopaque substance such as iodized oil (Lipiodol) may be injected into the cystic cavity (Fig. 14-14, *D*) after aspiration of the cystic contents. A large 19- or 20-gauge needle is used on a 3 or 5 ml Luer syringe. After the fluid is aspirated from the cyst, the syringe is removed from the needle, which is left in place, and another Luer syringe containing iodized oil attached to it. The opening made for entry into the cavity must be immediately stopped with a hemostat or sponge and the x-ray film taken as soon as possible to avoid escape of the fluid. This technique can also be used to visualize soft tissue cysts and sinus tracts that otherwise would not be outlined on the x-ray film. Dermoid cysts may contain radiopaque objects.

Newer x-ray machines and technology have made possible the taking of laminagrams of the head and neck area. This is a series of exposures by a machine that has the ability to focus in on a small area and clearly delineate the location of the pathological lesion (Fig. 14-14, *F* and *G*). By review of the series of films and comparison of associated anatomical landmarks, the nature and extent of the lesion can be determined readily. This is helpful in planning a surgical procedure and frequently predetermines the need of a nasal antrostomy when the cyst occurs in the maxillary sinus area.

Occasionally a radiolucent, irregularly outlined, small, punched-out type of area seen radiographically is mistaken for a recurrence of a cystic lesion. This radiographic appearance results when both cortical plates of bone are involved in the cystic defect or else removed during surgical excision of the lesion (Fig. 14-14, *G*). Complete regeneration of these cortical plates rarely occurs, and the defect will always be seen on the x-ray film. Here a history of previous surgery or treatment is important. It is wise to inform a patient of this finding so that it can be explained if he is examined by another dentist, thereby avoiding further and needless operations on these areas.

Surgical technique

Regardless of the etiology, nature, or location of the cyst, two methods of treatment are generally accepted:

1. Enucleation of the cystic sac in its entirety
2. The Partsch operation or marsupialization, by which the cyst is uncovered or "deroofed" and the cystic lining made continuous with the oral cavity or surrounding structures

In either case the surgical procedure must be based on sound fundamental principles —preservation of the blood supply to the area, avoidance of undue trauma to nerve filaments and nerve trunks in the region, control of hemorrhage, aseptic technique, atraumatic handling of the soft tissues, planning of a surgical flap so that adequate relaxation may be obtained to allow good access to a cystic area, avoidance of important anatomical structures such as muscle attachments and large blood vessels, and proper suturing and readaptation of the soft tissues. A sharp, clean incision planned so that the soft tissues are readapted over a firm bony bed will always heal better with less postoperative discomfort than when tissue is torn, lacerated, or sutured directly over a bone defect.

All excised lesions should be examined microscopically. When a neoplasm is noted on pathological examination, more aggressive surgery may be necessary.

The discussion on surgical technique will include the treatment of both soft tissue and bone cysts.

Soft tissue cysts

Soft tissue cysts include those of congenital origin, which occur primarily in the neck, and the retention-type cysts, mucoceles and ranulas, which occur primarily in the oral cavity. The surgical techniques described for the treatment of congenital cysts are presented primarily to indicate correct procedure rather than to describe the detailed dissection frequently necessary in the structures of the neck.

Congenital cysts. Congenital cysts occur usually in the neck and submandibular and submental regions. They are benign entities, but thorough dissection and excision are necessary for a cure.

THYROGLOSSAL CYSTS. Thyroglossal duct abnormalities should be treated by surgical excision. Repeated lancing of the cyst, except to alleviate an acute inflammatory condition, is ineffective. The use of sclerosing agents and irradiation is also contraindicated.

Surgical excision is accomplished through a transverse incision over the cyst (Fig. 14-1). Overlying tissues are carefully separated and the fibrous tract identified and followed by further dissection. Injection of a dye to more definitely outline the sinus tract has one disadvantage—the dye frequently spills over and stains other tissues, obscuring the operative field. Usually the fibrous tract can be followed without this additional aid. To facilitate exposure the hyoid bone is separated to aid in dissecting above this point and allow excision of the foramen cecum, which is the terminating point of the thyroglossal duct.

In closing the wound the musculature of the tongue is brought together with interrupted silk or chromic sutures, the severed edges of the hyoid bone are approximated with sutures through periosteum or adjacent fascia, and a small rubber tube drain is placed deep in the muscles of the tongue and through the skin incision.

BRANCHIOGENIC CYSTS AND FISTULAS. In excising branchiogenic fistulas, a radiopaque substance such as iodized oil (Lipiodol) or iophendylate (Pantopaque) is used to identify the extent and location of the fistula and sinus tract. A probe may also be passed in the tract to aid in identification as the dissection proceeds. A stepladder technique, as developed by Bailey, aids in following the sinus tract to its termination in the pharyngeal wall. This two-step procedure minimizes resultant scar formation.

The tract is ligated with fine silk or catgut at its entrance into the pharynx, and the wounds are closed in the usual manner with dependent drainage. The drain is usually removed in 2 or 3 days.

The best approach to a branchiogenic cyst is through an incision centered over the most prominent part of the cyst and parallel to the anterior border of the sternomastoid muscle (Fig. 14-2). The cyst may have attachments to important nerve trunks and vessels, and it is therefore necessary to have adequate exposure in visualizing the

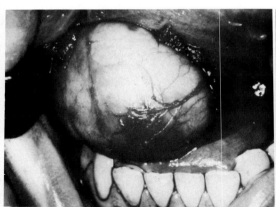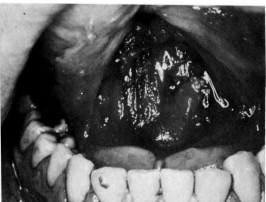

B

Fig. 14-15. **A,** Dermoid cyst avulsing after midline incision in floor of mouth. **B,** Resultant surgical "bed" after dermoid cyst is enucleated. (Courtesy Dr. John Delfino, Washington University School of Dental Medicine, St. Louis, Mo.)

cyst. Care must be taken to prevent rupture of the cyst during the dissection. Any epithelium left behind will give rise to a recurrence. The wound is closed in layers and skin sutured in such a manner as to give the best cosmetic result. A small drain is left in the wound for 1 or 2 days.

DERMOID CYSTS. Dermoid cysts (Fig. 14-3) are as a rule more superficial to the brachiogenic cleft cysts and are not attached to the lateral pharyngeal wall. They can occur either above or below the mylohyoid muscle. Surgical removal is the treatment of choice in either case. The sublingual dermoid cysts (Fig. 14-15) are usually excised intraorally. Those occurring below the floor of the mouth are usually excised extraorally.

Retention cysts. Retention cysts are generally located in the oral cavity and are treated by simple excision or marsupialization, depending on their size and location.

MUCOCELES. The preferred treatment is complete surgical excision (Fig. 14-16). An incision must be carefully made through the thin, overlying epithelium, which is usually stretched tight over the underlying mucous cyst. An alternate incision (Fig. 14-16, C) preserving the overlying mucous membrane, to aid in grasping tissue during enucleation of the mucocele, sometimes facilitates dissection. Usually the mucous cyst will tend to pop out of its soft tissue bed and can be carefully teased free, using blunt dissection with a small curved hemostat, curet, or periosteal elevator. Care must be taken not to rupture the sac, since then the dissection becomes more difficult and one cannot be positive that the cyst has been removed in its entirety. Recurrences of

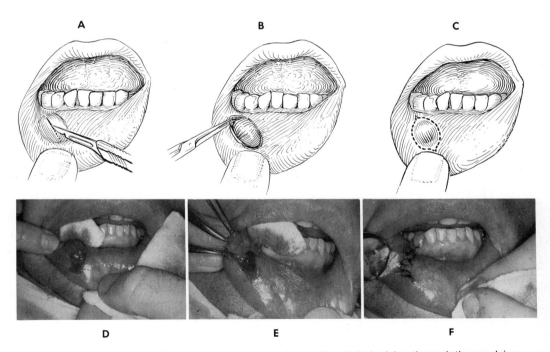

Fig. 14-16. A, Removal of mucocele, showing scalpel making light incision through the overlying mucous membrane. **B,** Fine scissors to free cyst wall from surrounding tissues. **C,** Alternate method: an eliptical incision leaving the mucous membrane intact over the cyst membrane may aid in dissecting the mucocele. **D,** Mucocele "popping out." **E,** Cyst grasped with tissue forceps and dissected free. **F,** Bleeding controlled and incision sutured.

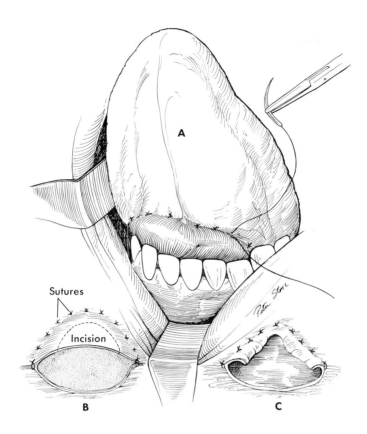

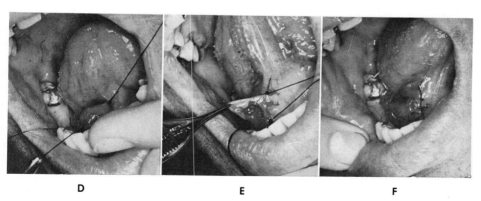

Fig. 14-17. A, Marsupialization of a ranula, showing sutures being placed through mucous membrane and underlying cyst wall. **B,** Cross section. **C,** Window cut and contents of cyst aspirated. The floor of the cyst becomes part of the floor of the mouth. **D,** Clinical view of first stage, showing placing of sutures. **E,** Mucous membrane overlying cyst, and superior wall of cyst grasped with tissue forceps and cut free with scissors inside of sutures. **F,** Additional sutures placed. The floor of the cyst, which is now a portion of the floor of the mouth, can be seen.

these lesions is common. Shira[18] has described a technique in which he aspirates the contents of the mucocele and injects a thin mix of alginate or rubber-base impression material. This hardens and clearly outlines the entire extent of the lesion and aids in the dissection.

RANULAS. Simple incision and drainage of the ranula always results in its recurrence. Enucleation of a ranula without rupturing the thin cystic wall is practically impossible and fraught with considerable complications. Once a cyst ruptures, it is difficult to pick up the continuity of a lining, and if all is not thoroughly removed, the ranula is likely to recur. A seton in the form of a wire loop may be used to attempt to reestablish an epithelial-lined duct opening, but this frequently fails. The use of radium for

treatment of ranulas is known to be effective.

The Partsch operation or marsupialization of a ranula is generally agreed on as the best surgical procedure. This consists of excising the superior wall of the ranula and suturing the cystic lining to the mucous membrane of the floor of the mouth to make it continuous with the oral cavity.

The following technique is used (Fig. 14-17). A series of sutures is placed around the peripheral margins of the cyst. The sutures go through the normal mucosa of the floor of the mouth and the cyst lining. When the cyst outline is well marked with sutures, the superior wall is excised just inside the sutures. The bottom of the cyst then elevates into a normal position, with escape of the fluid contents, and becomes continuous

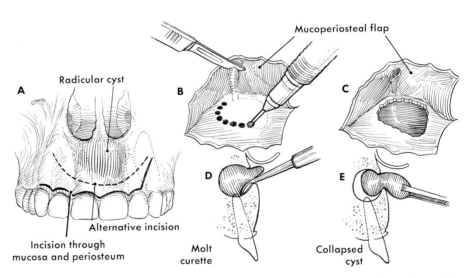

Fig. 14-18. Cyst enucleation. **A,** Incision is made either at the gingival margins or in semilunar form above the margins, and a large mucoperiosteal flap is raised. The central incisors are nonvital in this case. **B,** Note the fibrous attachment of the cyst wall to the mucoperiosteum because of chronic fistula. The attachment must be dissected free. Perforations may be made carefully with a bone bur through the cortical plate to outline the cystic cavity. The bone chisel can be used equally well, or a rongeur will suffice if the bony perforation is large enough for initial entrance. **C,** The overlying bone has been removed. The anterior portion of the cyst wall is seen. **D,** The back of a curet is used to lift the cyst wall from the sides of the bony cavity. **E,** Gentle traction on the cyst wall with tissue forceps and concomitant release of the deeper portion of the cyst wall from the bone with the curet will deliver the cyst. The devitalized teeth must have root canal therapy with apicoectomy or else be extracted. A gauze dressing is placed in the defect and brought out through the alveolar socket or through a stab incision in the flap if the teeth are retained. The wound is sutured.

with the floor of the mouth. The cystic membrane undergoes transformation and assumes the characteristics of the adjoining structures.

Some operators like to remove a small portion of the superior wall, aspirate the contents of the cyst, and outline the defect by filling it with sterile, selvage-edged gauze. The dissection of the superior cyst wall is then completed, and peripheral sutures are placed. This procedure is best done using a local anesthetic with lingual nerve block. Supplemental local infiltration is generally unnecessary. If the swelling occurs across the midline, bilateral block is necessary.

Catone and co-workers[6] recognized that some ranulas are deeper in origin than others and that often it is necessary to remove the associated sublingual gland. They emphasized that logical surgical care is based on pathogenesis and pathological anatomy of the lesion and that a dogmatic approach to the treatment of cystic lesions of the floor of the mouth is not justified.

Bone cysts

Access to a bone cyst must be gained by incising and reflecting the mucoperiosteum. The nature of the surgical approach is governed by the location and extent of the cyst. Whether a bone cyst is completely enucleated or treated by the Partsch method or its modifications depends more

on its size and location than on the actual diagnosis of the cyst.

When enucleation is the method of choice, overlying bone must be removed with chisels, rongeur forceps, or bone bur. Many times the bone is of tissue paper thickness and can be removed readily with a hemostat. Frequently, the bone is entirely eroded through, and the cystic membrane becomes attached to the periosteum or soft tissue covering and has to be cleanly dissected from it. This is further complicated by secondary infection on occasions, with the formation of a fistulous tract and considerable scar tissue. The cystic sac must be well exposed so that it can be carefully teased from its bony bed (Fig. 14-18).

Moose[13] has advocated the use of an osteoperiosteal flap in operating on large tumors and cysts of the jaw that exhibit thin cortices (Fig. 14-19). This technique consists essentially of incising through the mucoperiosteum and the thin cortical plate of bone at the same time. This may be done with a knife if the bone is thin or by placing a sharp chisel on the flap outline and carefully tapping it so that the chisel penetrates the bone. The bone is then reflected, adherent to the mucoperiosteum, to expose the cystic area. This procedure is best carried out on the labial and buccal sides of the maxilla and mandible. After removal of the lesion the flap is returned to its original position and sutured. The preservation of this

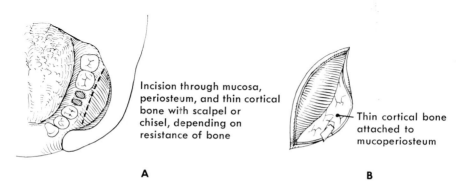

Incision through mucosa, periosteum, and thin cortical bone with scalpel or chisel, depending on resistance of bone

Thin cortical bone attached to mucoperiosteum

A   **B**

Fig. 14-19. Osteoperiosteal flap. **A,** Line of incision. **B,** Flap retracted. The underlying cyst wall can be seen.

bone attached to the periosteum increases the osteogenic surface of tissues surrounding the blood clot filling the cystic cavity. This enhances the possibility of primary healing and also forms a better nucleus for regeneration of bone. Fractures occurring in this thin bone as the flap is reflected are not important as long as the pieces do not become entirely detached from the periosteum. If they do become detached, they are removed and discarded.

A thin-blade curet is a suitable instrument for removing a cystic lining from bone. The largest curet that can easily be placed in the defect should be used. The concave side of the curet is usually placed against the bone as the thin blade is teased in between the cyst wall and the bone cavity (Fig. 14-18, D). Care must be utilized to avoid tearing the cystic sac and allowing escape of the fluid contents if possible. Good lighting and direct vision are essential so that it can be determined that the entire cystic sac is removed from bone. Frequently, in large cysts a suction tip can be used in dissecting the cyst free from its bony bed. In large defects, nerves and vessels are usually found pushed to one side, and they should not be traumatized unduly. The bony edges of the defect should then be saucerized and smoothed before the soft tissues are reapproximated with sutures and the wound is closed. This may be done with a rongeur, antrum bur, or bone file. Local antibiotic therapy in the form of dusting the walls lightly with topical drugs may aid in wound healing. Systemic antibiotic medication is favored in the presence of inflammation or infection. Any local use of an antibiotic drug should be augmented by systemic therapy.

The size and location of the cyst usually governs whether primary closure is attempted or the resultant cavity is packed with gauze, Gelfoam, bone chips, or other substitutes to obliterate the defect. There is a marked trend toward primary closure, with bank bone being the material of choice for placing in the defect. Dressings of any kind tend to control bleeding, prevent hematoma formation, control septic drainage, and at the same time promote healing.

Van Doorn[22] discusses results and problems encountered in primary closure of large bone cysts. The smaller cyst up to 15 to 20 mm in size usually heals by primary intention with no complications. An organized blood clot forms in the cavity, which leads to proliferation of young connective tissue and ultimate new-bone formation. In the larger cavity the wound heals by secondary intention, with gradual apposition of tissue obliterating the defect. If primary closure is the method of choice, hemorrhage and oozing must be well controlled, and the wound must be free from infection. Bone edges must be well saucerized to allow mucoperiosteal flaps to collapse into the cavity. The use of a closed system continuous suction is helpful in controlling hematoma formation. Either the Hemovac or Jackson Pratt system may be used.

Generally, in large cysts a substitute dressing in the form of gauze, resorbable cellulose products such as Gelfoam and Surgicel, bone chips, plaster of paris, and other anorganic substitutes have been utilized.

When a gauze dressing is used, 12- to 24-mm selvage iodoform or plain gauze with a medication such as balsam of Peru incorporated in it is satisfactory. This gauze is well placed in the cavity to exert pressure against any points that may show some tendency toward bleeding and is usually removed, either entirely or partially, on the fifth to seventh postoperative day. If considerable bleeding is encountered at the time of surgery, it is usually best to loosen the dressing gradually and remove it in sections over a period of 10 to 12 days. The defect can be carefully irrigated when the dressing is removed, and these areas are usually redressed twice a week until healing takes place over the bony walls where the cyst has been removed. This time interval usually involves 15 to 20 days.

The large cystic area may also be packed with bone chips obtained from the bone bank. Freeze-dried bone in small fragments suitably prepared from cancellous or cortical bone can be packed into the bony crypt.[4] Cancellous bone is preferred. Antibiotics or sulfa drugs may be incorporated into the mass before replacing the soft tissue flap and carefully suturing the wound closed. Occasionally some of the small chips may act as foreign bodies and be exfoliated. However, the great majority of the chips will remain to serve as a supporting structure for the blood clot. Also some stimulation of the young connective tissue seems to occur, increasing fibroblastic and osteoblastic activity and further enhancing the rate of healing.

The Oral Surgery Service at Mount Sinai Hospital in Detroit[16] had been utilizing cancellous bank bone from the head of the femur as a scaffolding on which the repair process could carry out remodeling of the defect. The marrow was curetted and rongeured from the femur and placed in a solution containing 5 million units of penicillin and about 30 ml of saline solution. The wound was irrigated thoroughly with penicillin solution prior to packing the defect with as much bank bone as possible. An attempt was made to obtain watertight closure of the mucosa, utilizing a continuous, horizontal mattress suture and an overlying and running baseball stitch.

Various bone substitutes have been used to obliterate cystic cavities after removal of the pathological tissue. None of these has proved as satisfactory as freeze-dried or preserved bank bone. For example, heterogenous processed bone has been given extensive trial.[11] Plaster of paris has been used to obliterate bone cavities.[5] Bahn[3] has published a review of the literature and reported many clinical cases in which results have been favorable.

The search continues for a suitable bone substitute that can be used to fill large cystic cavities in bone so that the overlying tissues can be sutured tightly without the need for packing and removing gauze strips. The substitute ideally should be made from lower species' tissue to be commercially available. It should be treated in such manner that the immune reaction will not cause graft rejection, and still it should be capable of stimulating host osteoclastic and osteoblastic activity.

The marsupialization technique as previously described for surgical treatment of ranula is also applicable to bone cysts. This cyst is "deroofed" and the surrounding mucoperiosteum sutured to the margins of the cyst wall or held in place with dressings. This, in effect, makes the cyst wall continuous with the oral cavity (see Fig. 14-21).

After reflecting the oral mucoperiosteal flap, the bone overlying the cyst is carefully removed, taking care not to penetrate the cyst. When the periphery of the cavity is reached, a sharp pair of scissors can be used to cut out the exposed membranous wall. This tissue is sent to the laboratory for histological examination. After the contents of the cyst are evacuated, the mucoperiosteum is allowed to fold into the defect and is sutured to the lining of the cyst. Apposition is maintained by pressure, using gauze dressings.

If gauze dressings are used, they may be removed in about 7 to 10 days, although it may be necessary to change the dressings in the interim. If a large opening has been made in the marsupialization of the cyst, usually nothing more is necessary as healing progresses. If only a small window is made to gain access to the cystic cavity, it sometimes becomes necessary to construct an acrylic plug that can be drilled and made hollow to maintain drainage in the area and also keep the opening patent as healing progresses (Fig. 14-20). The wound can be kept irrigated and clean through this opening.

With the release of fluid pressure in bone, regeneration occurs beneath the defect, and the cystic epithelial lining is transformed into normal mucous membrane by evagination from adjacent areas. The tube drainage technique of treating large cysts, as advo-

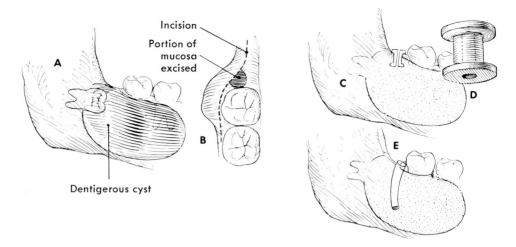

Fig. 14-20. Modified marsupialization technique. **A,** Dentigerous cyst around unerupted third molar. **B,** A window is cut in the mucosa to receive the obturator. The third molar is removed, and a portion of the cyst wall is removed for microscopic study. Developmental cysts that have the potential of histological cell change must be carefully observed postoperatively. **C** to **E,** An acrylic button or a plastic or metal tube is used to keep the wound open, maintain drainage, and provide access for irrigating the cystic defect to keep the wound clean. These devices are removed when radiographic examinaton shows that new bone has formed up to them.

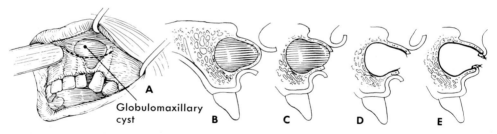

Fig. 14-21. Marsupialization technique. **A,** Enucleation of the globulomaxillary cyst in this case might endanger the adjacent teeth. **B,** Incision made through mucoperiosteum. The central portion of the flap is removed. **C,** The bone overlying the cyst is removed generously to correspond with the outline of the underlying cavity. **D,** The exposed portion of the cyst wall is excised and submitted for microscopic examination. **E,** The mucosa is sutured to the cyst wall, with the mucoperiosteal flap folded in. The cavity is packed with selvaged gauze for 5 days. The gauze may be changed once or twice before removing it entirely.

cated by Thomas,[21] is also a modification of the Partsch method (Figs. 14-20 to 14-22). A small opening is made into the defect, and a soft metal or polyethylene tube is inserted and held in place by ligation to adjacent teeth to maintain drainage. Either tube is easily adapted to the cyst opening. This relieves pressure from inside the cyst, and gradual obliteration of the cavity occurs by apposition of soft and bony tissue to close the defect. Periodic irrigation of the cavity is accomplished through the tube. The tube may be shortened as healing progresses.

Indications for marsupialization of a cyst include those conditions in which adjacent vital structures such as teeth may be in-

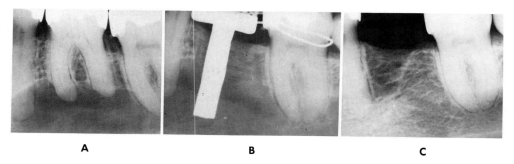

Fig. 14-22. A, Inflammatory cyst arising from nonvital molar and extending to adjacent teeth. **B,** Extraction of involved molar and tube drainage established. **C,** Cystic lesion healed with normal bone regeneration and good support of adjacent teeth for a dental prosthesis.

volved if the cystic contents are completely enucleated, or danger exists of entering adjacent paranasal sinuses, or a marked bone defect is to be avoided. The possible occurrence of paresthesia from surgical trauma or severance of a nerve is also eliminated.

This technique is applicable to a large number of cysts occurring in the oral cavity. However, it must be used with some reservation in those cystic lesions that have potential to develop into tumor. In these instances adequate exposure should be made so that the cyst lining can be thoroughly examined clinically, and in many cases biopsy should be taken from any suspicious section. This type of lesion should be followed closely postoperatively with clinical and x-ray examination.

Archer[2] has long been an advocate of the marsupialization technique for treating large cysts of the jaws to prevent the loss of involved teeth and other complications that result in the so-called dental cripple. He offers statistics to support his contention that few benign or malignant tumors occur in retained cystic membranes.

Olson and co-workers[14] have reported the successful treatment of a large odontogenic keratocyst by the Partsch operation and delayed enucleation. In 4 years of observation there was no evidence of recurrence.

Some operators will remove the cystic or epithelized lining in a second operation when enough bone apposition has occurred after relief of pressure from the cystic lesion. This eliminates the danger sometimes encountered in primary enucleation but submits the patient to a second surgical procedure and does not materially affect the final outcome of treatment.

In the Partsch operation the actual filling in of a bone defect may take a longer period of time. However, in most instances no contraindication exists for not going ahead with whatever prosthetic restoration might be necessary. Maintenance of good oral hygiene and care in keeping the area clean should be all that is necessary after normal epithelization of the defect has occurred.

Postoperative complications

Complications that may result after enucleation or marsupialization of congenital and developmental cysts include swelling, infection, hematoma formation, sensory and motor nerve injury, primary or secondary hemorrhage, oral fistula, fracture of bone, and obstruction of the airway. Motor nerve injury and airway obstruction occur primarily in removal of lesions involving dissections in the neck and submandibular areas.

The best way to avoid complications is to prevent them by thorough diagnostic study, good surgical judgment, and proper surgical technique. However, complications will occur, and it is well to know how to treat them when they develop.

Postoperative edema is normal and physiological after most surgical procedures on the jaws. Most of this surgery is of a traumatic nature, and prolonged retraction of tissues adds to the interference of normal lymphatic drainage of the area. This, coupled with inflammatory reaction, is bound to produce edema and swelling. The patient should be advised of this beforehand. The height of the swelling should be reached about the second postoperative day, with gradual subsidence if no secondary infection or hematoma formation develops. The immediate application of cold is of doubtful benefit but may be used for the first 8 to 10 hours postoperatively. Antiinflammatory agents such as corticosteroid drugs and animal and plant enzymes may be helpful in certain instances in controlling postoperative edema. These agents must be administered with a complete knowledge of possible side effects and contraindications.

The possibility of infection can be minimized by antibiotic therapy, good surgical technique, and strict adherence to rules of asepsis. Any acute infection occurring in these lesions should be well controlled before surgical intervention is done. Antibiotics must be carefully chosen and administered in therapeutic dosage, either empirically or by organism sensitivity tests.

Hematoma formation can be prevented by controlling the bleeding initially and by the additional use of dressings and applied pressure. Large blood vessels should be tied off, but most of the bleeding that might be encountered comes from areas inaccessible for ligation, and pressure is utilized for its control. Soft tissue flaps should be well sutured and adequate external pressure placed on the operative area for the first few postoperative hours.

A persistent hematoma that is readily accessible should be aspirated and drained. Otherwise a breakdown of the blood clot will occur, with septic drainage. The use of enzyme therapy, such as hyaluronidase, might be of some value in early hematoma formation but should be avoided if any question of secondary infection is present. This substance, injected into the tissues, opens up the interstitial spaces and promotes a more rapid absorption and diffusion of fluids from an involved area.

Sensory nerve trunks are usually displaced by cystic lesions, and many times the cyst linings are stripped free of this nerve by careful dissection. When a sensory nerve trunk is exposed in a cavity, a paresthesia usually results. This may be of unknown duration, since the rate of recovery to nerve injury varies considerably. However, large nerve trunks are usually not severed in careful surgical procedures, and return of sensation almost universally occurs. Small nerves that are sacrificed in these surgical areas usually have some cross innervation so that the immediate effect is not noticed by the patient. The patient should be thoroughly forewarned of this complication; he then is able to accept the resultant numbness much more graciously. One should carefully explain that possible fifth nerve injury involves sensation only and not any motor function, so that no outward changes to the appearance of the face will occur. However, in soft tissue dissection the anatomy of the facial nerve must be thoroughly understood. Injury to this motor nerve will result in muscle paralysis.

Primary hemorrhage must be controlled at the time of surgery. Secondary hemorrhage usually occurs in those cases in which injury to a large vessel has occurred at the time of surgery. It can also occur by inadvertent trauma of newly proliferated blood vessels during removal of surgical dressings. This complication is usually again controlled by pressure. Care should be taken to remove large blood clots and determine the site of bleeding before applying pressure in the correct manner. Occasionally a blood vessel can be identified and tied off with a ligature.

Oronasal or oroantral fistulas sometimes result from injudicious choice of surgical procedure or human error in surgical technique. They can also result from a normal anatomical relation of pathology to existing structures. This complication can often be avoided by careful dissection, and often cystic linings can be carefully peeled from other membranous linings without penetration into nasal or antral cavities. Use of the Partsch method of treatment, if applicable, may be helpful. If small openings occur, proper healing can usually be attained by careful attention to wound closure and detailed instructions to the patient. Postoperative care is of paramount importance in many instances in preventing permanent fistula formation, which necessitates secondary closure. Secondary infection should also be prevented. The patient should be cautioned about excessive sneezing and coughing and instructed to keep his mouth open, should these episodes occur, to equalize the pressure in the paranasal sinuses and prevent undue force on the area where the wound communicates with the oral cavity.

Bone is weakened by the presence of a cyst, with the exact amount of weakening dependent on the size and extent of the pathology. Usually the possibility of fracture occurring during surgery is remote unless undue trauma is exerted on the jaw or both cortical plates are excessively thin. Trauma in the form of a twisting movement producing torque is much more likely to fracture bone than is direct pressure. Because of the nature of a cyst, which expands primarily in a single direction, one cortical plate of bone is likely to be intact. This preserves the continuity of the jaw. Prevention again is the best form of treatment, and careful surgical technique must be used, particularly in those cysts in which unerupted teeth are present and difficult to remove. Should a fracture occur, proceed with the enucleation of the cyst, and then pack the defect well with suitable gauze dressings or bone chips to maintain the position of the fragments and prevent un-

necessary displacement. The jaw should also be immobilized. A patient with a large cystic involvement of the jaws should be cautioned to avoid any undue trauma, both preoperatively and postoperatively, since a blow is more likely to cause fracture in a weakened jaw than in a normal one.

Postoperative airway obstruction may follow surgical procedures involving the jaws, tongue, and tissues of the neck. Massive edema, hematoma formation, and infection are contributing factors. Should signs of labored breathing and inadequate respiratory exchange be evident, tracheostomy must be done. This should, so far as possible, be an elective procedure rather than an emergency one.

Proper postoperative care is just as important a part of the patient's overall problem as the diagnosis and surgical treatment.

REFERENCES

1. Archer, W.: Oral surgery, ed. 4, Philadelphia, 1966, W. B. Saunders Co.
2. Archer, W. H.: Transactions of the Second Congress International Association, Conference on Oral Surgery, Copenhagen, 1967, Munksgaard-Copenhagen, p. 152.
3. Bahn, S. L.: Plaster, a bone substitute, Oral Surg. **21:**682, 1966.
4. Boyne, P. J.: Clinical use of freeze dried homogenous bone, J. Oral Surg. **15:**236, 1956.
5. Calhoun, N. R., Neiders, M. E., and Greene, G. W., Jr.: Effects of plaster of paris implants in surgical defects of mandibular alveolar processes of dogs, J. Oral Surg. **25:**122, 1967.
6. Catone, G. A., Morrill, R. G., and Henny, F. A.: Sublingual gland mucus-escape phenomenon—treatment by excision of sublingual gland, J. Oral Surg. **27:**774, 1969.
7. Gorlin, R. J., and Goldman, H. M.: Thoma's oral pathology, St. Louis, 1970, The C. V. Mosby Co.
8. Harris, M., and Toller, P.: The pathogenesis of dental cysts, Br. Med. Bull. **31:**159, 1975.
9. Killey, H. C., and Kay, L. W.: Benign cystic lesions of the jaws, Baltimore, 1966, The Williams & Wilkins Co.
10. Kreuz, F. P., and others: Preservation and clinical use of freeze dried bone, J. Bone Joint Surg. **33A:**803, 1951.
11. Lyon, H. W., and Boyne, P. J.: Host response to chemically treated heterogenous bone implants, J. Dent. Res. I.A.D.R. Abstracts **42:**83, 1963.
12. Martin, H.: Surgery of head and neck tumors, New York, 1957, Hoeber-Harper.

13. Moose, S. M.: Osteoperiosteal flap for operation of large tumors and cysts of jaws, J. Oral Surg. **10:**229, 1952.

14. Olson, R. E., Thomsen, S., and Li-Min, L.: Odontogenic and keratocysts treated by the Partsch operation and delayed enucleation: report of a case, J. Am. Dent. Assoc. **94:**321-325, 1977.

15. Pindborg, J. J., and James, P.: Variations in odontogenic cyst epithelium, Transactions of the Second Congress International Association, Conference on Oral Surgery, Copenhagen, 1967, Munksgaard-Copenhagen, pp. 121, 127, 135-140.

16. Rotskoff, K.: Personal communication, Department of Oral and Maxillofacial Surgery, Sinai Hospital of Detroit, 1972.

17. Shafer, W. G., Hine, M. K., and Levy, B. M.: Textbook of oral pathology, ed. 3, Philadelphia, 1974, W. B. Saunders Co., pp. 247-251.

18. Shira, R. B.: Simplified technic for the management of mucoceles and ranulas, J. Oral Surg. **20:**374, 1962.

19. Stafne, E. C.: Developmental defects of the mandible. In Stafne, E. C., and Gibilisco, J. A.: Oral roentgenographic diagnosis, ed. 3, Philadelphia, 1969, W. B. Saunders Co.

20. Stoelinga, P. J. W., and Peters, J. H.: A note on the origin of keratocysts of the jaws, Int. J. Oral Surg. **2:**37-44, 1973.

21. Thomas, E.: Saving involved vital teeth by tube drainage, J. Oral Surg. **5:**1, 1947.

22. Van Doorn, M. E.: Enucleation and primary closure of jaw cysts, Int. J. Oral Surg. **1:**17, 1972.

23. Ward, G. E., and Hendrick, J. W.: Diagnosis and treatment of tumors of the head and neck, Baltimore, 1950, The Williams & Wilkins Co.

24. Wood, N. K., and Goaz, P. W.: Differential diagnosis of oral lesions, St. Louis, 1975, The C. V. Mosby Co., pp. 404-407.

CHAPTER 15

Diseases of the maxillary sinus of dental origin

Phillip Earle Williams

DESCRIPTION

The maxillary sinus is generally larger than any of the other sinuses and lies chiefly in the body of the maxilla. It is also called the antrum of Highmore because this antrum, meaning a cavity or hollow space especially found in bone, was first described by Nathaniel Highmore, an English anatomist of the seventeenth century. It is actually present as a small cavity at birth, starting its development during the third fetal month and usually reaching its maximum development in early adult life about the eighteenth year. The capacity of the average adult antrum is from 10 to 15 ml, and its complete absence is rare. Often subcompartments, recesses and crypts, are present, being formed by osseous and membranous septa. Fig. 15-1 shows x-ray films that reveal this condition.

The maxillary sinus is pyramidal in shape with its base at the nasoantral wall and its apex in the root of the zygoma. The upper wall or roof in the adult is thin; it is situated under the orbit and is the orbital plate of the maxilla. This plate usually possesses a bony canal for the infraorbital nerve and vessels. The floor of the sinus is the alveolar

process of the maxilla. In front the antero-lateral or canine fossa wall is the facial part of the maxilla. The posterior or spheno-maxillary wall, which is of lesser importance, consists of a thin plate of bone separating the cavity from the infratemporal fossa. The nasal wall separates the sinus from the nasal cavity medially. The nasal cavity contains the outlet from the sinus, the ostium maxillae, which lies just beneath the roof of the antrum. The location of this opening precludes the possibility of good drainage when the individual is in a vertical position.

The sinus is lined with a thin mucosa, which is attached to the periosteum. The ciliated epithelium aids in the removal of excretions and secretions that form in the sinus cavity. The cilia hold foreign material at their tips much as twigs or leaves are held on the surface of many blades of grass. Waves of ciliary action carry the material from one ciliated region to another toward the ostium. These waves could be compared to gusts of wind indenting a wheat field from one side to the other. Only a pathological membrane that has deficient ciliary action or is devoid of cilia in whole

271

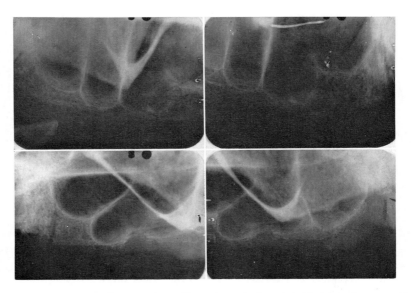

Fig. 15-1. Osseous septa in normal maxillary sinus. Left and right sides of same patient.

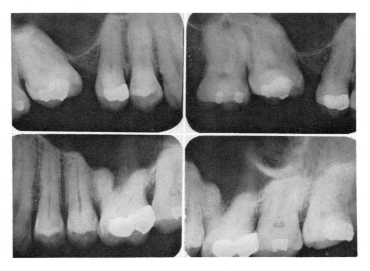

Fig. 15-2. Large sinus (left and right) with thin bony wall separating the floor from the apices of the teeth.

or in part will allow foreign materials to rest on its surface.

The thickness of the sinus walls is not constant, especially the roof and floor. The walls may vary in thickness from 2 to 5 mm in the roof and from 2 to 3 mm in the floor. Edentulous areas in the alveolar ridge vary

from 5 to 10 mm. In the event that the posterior wall is penetrated, causing entrance into the infratemporal fossa, care must be exercised in any operative procedure because of the presence of large vessels such as the maxillary artery and vein. Infraorbital and superior alveolar vessels are frequently ruptured in midfacial fractures, giving rise to the formation of hematomas in the antrum.

Below the floor are found the deciduous and permanent teeth, and often the roots of the permanent molar or premolar teeth may extend into the sinus itself. In children and infants the floor of the sinus is always higher than the floor of the nose so that better drainage is readily obtainable from window operations, which will be described later. In adults the reverse is true; the floor of the sinus is lower than the nasal floor.

The nerve supply is from the maxillary branch of the fifth cranial nerve, the posterosuperior alveolar branch of this nerve supplying the lining of the mucous membrane. Its blood supply is derived from the infraorbital artery, a branch of the maxillary artery. Some collateral supply is derived from the anterosuperior alveolar artery, a branch of the same vessel. The lymphatic supply is abundant and terminates into the submandibular nodes.

The functions or purposes of the paranasal sinuses are as follows: (1) to give resonance to the voice (note the change in the sounds of words of persons with colds), (2) to act as reserve chambers to warm the respired air, and (3) to reduce the weight of the skull. During inspiration the suction through the nasal cavity draws some warmed air from the sinuses. The sinuses are connected with the nasal cavities by openings or channels so that the mucous membrane of the sinuses is continuous with that of the nose. Because of this, ventilation and drainage of the sinuses are made possible.

Frequently, radiographs reveal unusually large sinuses, with the root ends residing directly in the floor (Fig. 15-2). This may be confusing, resulting in an erroneous suspicion of a pathological condition. Intraoral views are obtained of the opposite side, and comparison is made; if the bony architecture is the same, then a diagnosis of no apparent pathological abnormality is readily made. The taking of skull films is to be encouraged because a study of them is most revealing, and comparison of all the anatomical structures may be made readily. Of all the diagnostic aids used in the study of the maxillary sinus, the radiograph is the most dependable. Fig. 15-3 shows a skull film of normal, healthy sinuses.

In this connection, any time that the usual intraoral radiographs reveal the absence of a tooth in the arch and no history of previous extraction of that tooth is found, then extraoral views should be made. Many times the absent tooth will be shown to be aberrant and residing high in the superior part of the maxillary sinus. Figs. 15-4 and 15-5 show preoperative and postoperative views of this condition. Often these teeth will be the cause of headaches or neuralgias, and on the removal of the displaced tooth and associated pathological abnormalities, these unpleasant conditions will disappear.

Toothache is frequently a symptom of maxillary sinus infection. The superior alveolar nerves run for a considerable distance in the walls of the antrum. They are contained with small blood and lymph vessels in narrow, sometimes anastomosing canals. Progressive expansion of the sinus in older persons invariably causes resorption of the inner walls of one or more of these canals, and thus the connective tissue covering the structures in the canals is brought into direct contact with the connective tissue of the mucoperiosteum of the sinus. This will cause involvement of dental nerves if sinus inflammation occurs. The quality of the pain sometimes resembles that of pulpitis. Examination of the teeth by cold stimulation will reveal, however, that not one but an entire group of teeth, sometimes all of the teeth in one maxilla, are hypersensitive.

DISEASES

Maxillary sinusitis occurs in acute, subacute, and chronic forms. A careful diagnosis is important, since the cure of the disease depends on the removal of the

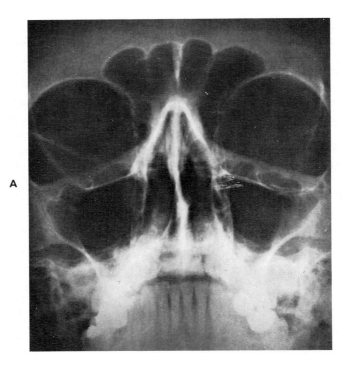

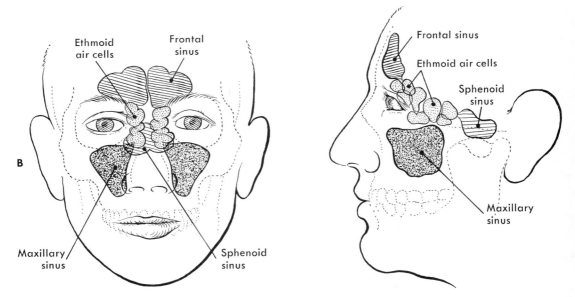

Fig. 15-3. A, Radiograph of normal healthy sinuses. **B,** Diagram of frontal view of paranasal sinuses. **C,** Diagram of lateral view.

cause. It is important to determine whether any other nasal sinuses are involved. In many instances the maxillary sinus remains infected from the ethmoids or from the nose itself.

The symptoms of *acute* maxillary sinus-

itis depend on the activity or virulence of the infecting organism and the presence of an occluded ostium. The main symptom is severe pain, which is constant and localized. It may seem to affect the eyeball, cheek, and frontal region. The teeth in that

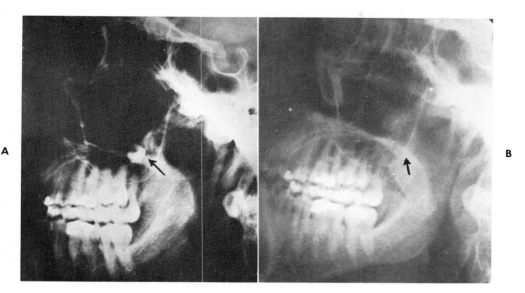

Fig. 15-4. A, Unerupted third molar residing half in and half out of the sinus. No apparent pathology of the antrum. **B,** Postoperative view. Removal of tooth was accomplished by exposure made through tuberosity approach so that the sinus was not involved.

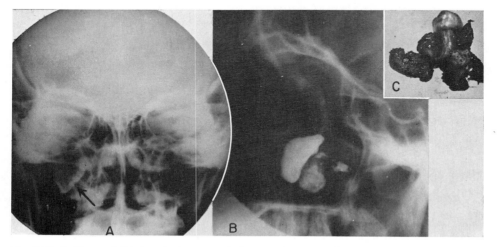

Fig. 15-5. A, Aberrant third molar located within maxillary sinus. **B,** Lipiodol in sinus disclosing presence of cyst. **C,** Surgical specimen showing tooth with cyst attached. The tooth and cyst were removed by means of a Caldwell-Luc approach.

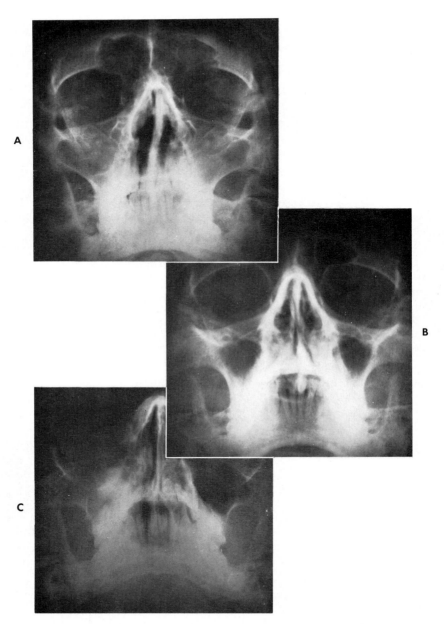

Fig. 15-6. A, Marked clouding of each maxillary sinus. **B,** Thickening of the mucosal lining associated with chronic maxillary sinusitis. **C,** Clouded right antrum produced by trauma that caused fracture of the right infraorbital rim.

area may become extremely sore and painful. Any unusual motion or jarring may accentuate the suffering. The nasal discharge may at first be thin and watery and serous in character, but soon it becomes mucopurulent in form, dripping into the nasopharynx and causing a constant irritation. This produces spitting, swallowing, and a constant clearing of the throat. In the type of sinusitis that develops from infected teeth the secretion has a very foul odor. General toxemia develops with the disease, producing chills, sweats, elevation of temperature, dizziness, and nausea. Difficult breathing is common.

Subacute sinusitis is devoid of the symptoms associated with acute congestion such as pain and generalized toxemia. Discharge is persistent and is associated with nasal voice and stuffiness. Throat soreness is common. The patient feels run down, tires easily, and often cannot sleep well because of an irritating cough that keeps him awake. The diagnosis is based on the symptoms, rhinoscopy, transillumination, x-ray examination, sinus lavage, and a history of a persistent head cold or sinus attack of a few weeks' or months' duration.

Subacute sinusitis may be the interim stage between acute and chronic sinusitis, and many cases continue on to a stage of chronic suppuration. Proper medical and surgical treatment is important to prevent the acute case from ultimately becoming a chronic one. The relief may come on slowly or suddenly, but it usually takes place soon after improvement of drainage from the sinus reaches the point that secretions are able to leave the cavity as rapidly as they form.

Chronic maxillary sinusitis is produced by the following factors: (1) repeated attacks of acute antritis or a single attack that has persisted to a chronic state, (2) neglected or overlooked dental focus, (3) chronic infection in the frontal or ethmoid sinuses, (4) altered metabolism, (5) fatigue, (6) overindulgences, worries, dietary deficiencies, and lack of sleep, (7) allergies, and (8) endocrine imbalances and debilitating diseases of all kinds.

The fundamental pathological change in chronic sinusitis is that of cellular proliferation. The lining is thick and irregular. Fig. 15-6 shows the characteristic appearance of chronic antritis radiographically. In some cases the lumen of the cavity may be almost occluded by the thickened membranes. This edematous process involves the ostium, causing a complete blockage so that drainage ceases. Medical treatment is of little value in chronic sinus disease. Roentgen-ray therapy and shortwave diathermy are advocated but are of questionable value without the establishment of proper sinus drainage. This can best be done by performing an intranasal antrostomy or creating an antral window. Conditions conducive to early repair are supplied by the establishment of adequate drainage. The success obtained by this procedure along with other conservative measures properly carried out has practically eliminated the need of radical procedures on the maxillary sinus.

PATHOLOGY

It is generally estimated that from 10% to 15% of the pathological conditions involving the maxillary sinus is of dental origin or relationship. This includes accidental openings in the floor of the antrum during the extraction of teeth, the displacement of roots and even entire teeth into the antrum during the attempted removal of teeth, and infections introduced through the antral floor from abscessed teeth, either of the apical or the parietal variety. Usually infections are most likely to occur in those cases in which the roots of the teeth are separated from the floor of the antrum by a thin lamella of bone, but many cases are reported in which this bone is thick and heavy.

Empyema of the sinus may occur as a result of too active curettage of root sockets after extractions. This procedure, of course, is frowned on, and only light and gentle curettement, if any, should ever be employed. The blind and indiscriminate use of the curet is to be condemned, since it is the means of spreading infection into bone and soft tissues in any part of the mouth. However, it is possible at times for the infection to involve the sinus for no apparent reason.

Dentigerous cysts are often found in the sinus. Other pathological entities include cysts of the mucosa of the sinus, benign and malignant neoplasms, osteomyelitis, antral rhinoliths, and polyps. Angiomas, myomas, fibromas, and central giant cell tumors seldom invade the sinus. Cystic odontomas may encroach on the sinus. They are usually incapsulated and can be shelled out readily without involving the antrum. The osteoma, a benign tumor, is often treated radically when it invades this area. If it obliterates the sinus, it often causes mechanical constriction to vital structures so that a hemimaxillectomy is necessary.

Ameloblastoma invading the sinus causes marked expansion of both facial and nasal walls. X-ray studies usually disclose the character of the lesion. Mixed tumors undergo malignant changes and result in rapid growth and invasion of this area. Connective tissue lesions such as fibrogenic and osteogenic sarcomas seldom involve the sinus. If they do occur, it is usually in childhood, and they offer a poor prognosis. Unfortunately, characteristic symptoms of malignant tumors develop in this region when the disease has reached an inoperable stage.

Epidermoid carcinoma of the antrum is more common than sarcoma. These conditions may be present for some time without producing clinical evidence. The teeth may become loose, and pain develops. If extraction of the teeth is done, the sockets fail to heal. Metastases to vital organs may cause death before local extension occurs. Often swelling of the face is the chief reason for seeking medical advice. In the interest of early diagnosis, close attention should be given to persistent or recurrent pain in the teeth or face without clear-cut dental cause. Early diagnosis is pertinent whether the dentist assumes the responsibility of the treatment of the disease or not.

Trauma such as fractures of the maxilla with associated crushing of the sinus region sometimes occurs. Occasionally, after traumatic zygoma impactions, the zygoma is forced into the sinus. An acute sinus infection may follow because of the retention of an accumulation of blood in the sinus.

TREATMENT
Accidental openings

If information is obtained from the preoperative radiographs that root ends of the teeth to be extracted penetrate the floor of the sinus and if this condition is suspected after exodontics is completed, the patient is instructed to compress the nares with the fingers and blow the nose gently. If an opening has occurred through the membrane lining the sinus, the blood that is present in the tooth socket will bubble.

If this opening is small and great care is exercised, such as the avoidance of the use of irrigations, vigorous mouth washing, and frequent and lusty blowing of the nose, then in the majority of cases a good clot will form and organize and normal healing will occur. At no time should these sockets be packed with gauze, cotton, or other materials because in most instances these procedures will perpetuate the opening rather than serve as a means of causing it to close. Probing of the sockets with instruments must be avoided as much as possible so that infection will not be introduced into uncontaminated areas.

If the floor of the antrum is completely disrupted and portions of the bone remain on roots of the teeth after their removal and inspection reveals a large patent opening, then immediate closure should be done. Primary closure reduces the possibility of contamination of the sinus by oral infections and diseases. Such immediate closure circumvents pathological changes of the sinus, which may persist for some time and require considerably more effort to manage and cure. It often prevents the formation of an oroantral fistula, which would require subsequent surgery of a more difficult and extensive nature.

A simple procedure that yields good results for the closure of large, accidental sinus openings is described as follows: The mucoperiosteum is raised both buccally and lingually, and the height of the alveolar ridge is reduced at the site of the opening substantially. Edges of the soft tissue that is to be approximated are freshened so that raw surfaces will be in contact with each other. Relaxing incisions are made as illustrated in Fig. 15-7. Suturing may then be done without tension. The edges are drawn together with mattress sutures and reinforced with multiple, interrupted black silk sutures, No. 3-0 (Fig. 15-8). This type of material is preferred to the absorbable type (for example, catgut) because it obviates the possibility of the sutures coming out too soon, which could possibly limit the success of the closure. The sutures are left in place from 5 to 7 days. Nose drops are prescribed

to shrink the nasal mucosa and promote drainage.

The anatomical proximity of the roots of the molar and bicuspid teeth to the floor of the sinus leads to potential infection of the sinus, either by direct extension of an apical abscess or through the accidental perforation of the sinus floor during exodontics. A fractured root apex that is separated from the floor of the sinus by a paper-thin lamina of bone can easily be pushed into the sinus and inoculate it with virulent bacteria. Unless the operator is skillful in the removal of such an accidentally displaced root tip, manipulation and trauma will usually be followed by an acute infection. If a short, precise primary endeavor to remove the root tip is unsuccessful, it should be abandoned and the wound encouraged to heal. If the wound is large, the buccal and palatal mucoperiosteum should be approximated.

The patient should be informed of the existence of the displaced root fragment. The surgical approach for removal of a root in the maxillary sinus should not be made through the alveolus after the primary at-

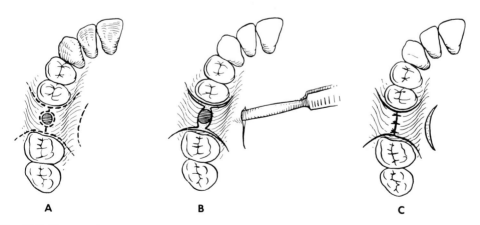

Fig. 15-7. Closure of large accidental sinus opening in the dentulous arch. **A,** Incisions are made around teeth and across opening. A relaxing incision is made on the palate, avoiding the palatine artery. The buccal and lingual alveolar walls are reduced with a rongeur. **B,** Mucosal edges on the ridge are freshened, and flaps are raised. A periosteal elevator raises the palatal mucoperiosteum so that approximation of mucosal edges is made possible. **C,** Flaps are sutured. Healing should take place by primary intention. The palatal wound is left open.

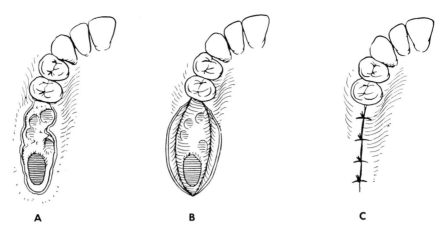

A   B   C

Fig. 15-8. Closure of large accidental sinus opening in edentulous areas (loss of maxillary tuberosity). **A,** Sinus opening immediately after extraction. **B,** Reduction of buccal and lingual walls to allow coaptation of buccal and lingual soft tissue flaps. The soft tissue flaps are trimmed conservatively to form a somewhat even line. **C,** Flaps sutured.

tempt to recover the root has been done. It should be made through a Caldwell-Luc incision, which will permit adequate visualization of the entire sinus.

Occasionally during the procedure for removal of an impacted upper third molar tooth, it will suddenly disappear. The tooth could have been residing in the floor or in the distal portion of the maxillary sinus, or it could have formed a part of the wall. It may have been dislodged from its crypt in the maxillary bone to slide into the infratemporal fossa.

No effort at recovery should be instituted until the exact location of the tooth is determined by careful clinical and radiographic examination. It is traumatic to the patient, if under local anesthesia, and to the operator to suddenly find that he or she is working in the wrong area.

The employment of stereoscopic and panographic radiographs will definitely assist in the location of the aberrant tooth. If, on probing the area where the tooth had previously resided, the instrument goes directly into the antral cavity, and if a nosebleed occurs immediately after tooth loss (produced by blood escaping from the sinus through the natural ostium into the nose), then the tooth is certainly in the maxillary sinus. The approach for its removal is the Caldwell-Luc procedure.

In the event that the tooth is not in the sinus cavity and definitely in the soft tissues, then a practical and careful approach is most important. The cause of loss may have been inadequate exposure by not having a proper flap reflected. For example, when pressure was applied by means of an elevator to remove the tooth from its socket, the tightness and elasticity of the mucoperiosteal flap propelled the tooth out of sight into the soft tissues. At this time the flap should be more liberally extended and raised so that the tissue may be explored for the lost tooth. Often the buccal fat pad will be exposed and opened, and this further conceals the tooth. Do not persist in exploring and probing after a few minutes of careful effort.

The patient should be informed of the problem and the search should be abandoned for a period of 5 or 6 weeks. Most patients will react favorably to a complete and proper explanation of the situation.

The law of gravity is a law that cannot be

broken. There will be some movement toward a dependent position, and after awhile the tooth will become fibrosed and will not move around when removal is attempted. Incision is made directly to the tooth, and it can be recovered with minimal effort.

Preoperative considerations

Anesthesia for operation on the maxillary sinus may be either local or general, depending on the operator's choice and the type especially indicated for the case concerned. If general anesthesia is to be employed in the hospital, then, of course, that becomes the responsibility of the anesthesiologist.

In the event that local anesthesia is to be employed, this may be obtained satisfactorily in the following manner: The patient is premedicated with 100 mg of pentobarbital sodium and 0.4 mg of atropine about 30 minutes prior to operation. Then a pledget of cotton saturated with cocaine (5% to 10% solution) or tetracaine (Pontocaine), 2% in ephedrine, is carefully applied just above and below the inferior turbinate. This is left in place 10 to 15 minutes. An anterior infraorbital nerve block or a second division block then is administered, using any local anesthetic agent of choice.

It should be stressed strongly that any patient who receives the application of cocaine to the oral or nasal mucosa should not be left alone but should be constantly observed by someone trained to recognize the symptoms of sensitivity and shock that may occur in those individuals who are sensitive to the drug. When an idiosyncrasy is present, positive and immediate steps must be instituted, including the intravenous injection of agents such as thiopental sodium (Pentothal) and the employment of oxygen therapy. This may be lifesaving, and delay or failure to recognize symptoms may precipitate a crisis that may lead to a fatality. These conditions are rare, and, if they are suspected, tests for sensitivity may be made. The ophthalmic test is easy to do and consists of dropping some of the substance

that is to be used into one of the patient's eyes. This will produce a conjunctivitis within 5 minutes if the patient is sensitive to the drug; no harm will occur to the eye otherwise.

The skin test may be used in the patient suspected of an idiosyncrasy. It is done by making a wheal or bleb with the drug between the dermis and epidermis; if a marked erythema develops within 5 minutes, that particular drug should not be used. These tests require only the expenditure of a few minutes of time but may be the means of saving hours of worry and confusion or even the individual's life. Definitive tests are made by an allergist.

Closure of the oroantral fistula

Closure of the oroantral fistula, especially in the case of a large opening, may be accomplished well by employing the palatal flap method (Fig. 15-9). A pedicle flap raised from the palate is thick and has good blood supply, so that the chances of success are definitely enhanced. The design of the flap can be determined by a trial or practice procedure prior to surgery. A cast of the maxilla showing the defect or opening is made, and a soft acrylic palate is formed on this cast. The flap is outlined on the acrylic, the incision made, and the flap turned, covering the defect. This provides a preview of results that should be obtained. The material may be sterilized and placed in the mouth for use at the time that the incisions are made through the mucoperiosteum of the palate. This procedure will show that the flap to be raised will be adequate to cover the opening.

With a No. 15 blade, the tissue is incised and the flap is raised. A V-shaped section of the tissue may be excised at the region of greatest bend to prevent folding and wrinkling. The pedicle is raised with the periosteum and of course should contain a branch of the palatal artery. The margins of the fistular defect are freshened and the edges undermined. The flap is then tucked under the undermined edge of the buccal

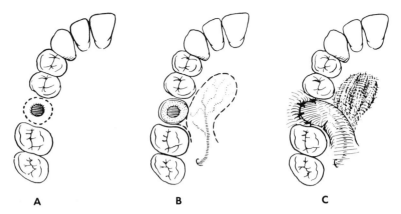

Fig. 15-9. Palatal flap to close chronic oroantral fistula. **A,** The hard and soft tissues surrounding the fistula are freshened. The buccal tissue is undermined. **B,** A mucoperiosteal flap is designed and raised. It must contain the artery. **C,** The flap is swung over the defect, tucked under the buccal flap, and sutured to place. Note V of tissue removed on lesser curvature to minimize folding. The donor area is packed with gauze or surgical cement.

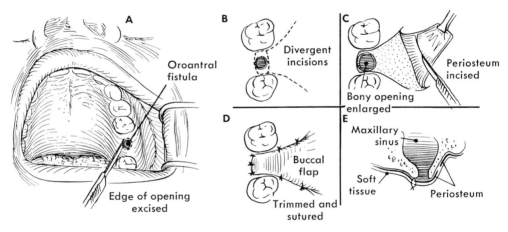

Fig. 15-10. Berger's sliding flap technique for oroantral closure. **A,** Edge of opening excised. **B,** Two divergent incisions carried from the opening into the mucobuccal fold. **C,** Flap elevated and bony opening made large enough for inspection and cleansing of sinus. Several horizontal incisions are made through the periosteum on the underside of the flap, which allows the flap to be extended. **D,** Flap trimmed to meet palatal tissue and closed with mattress sutures followed by interrupted sutures. **E,** Cross-sectional view of closure, showing stretching of flap allowed by incised periosteum.

flap. This procedure permits two raw or fresh bleeding surfaces to be in contact. With mattress sutures the tissues are drawn in good contact, and the margins are sutured with multiple interrupted sutures. Catgut is not used because it may not hold for a sufficient length of time for healing to occur. The silk or Dermalon sutures should be left in position for 5 to 7 days. The exposed bone at the donor site on the palate may be covered with surgical cement or a gauze strip saturated with compound tincture of benzoin.

Berger, a dentist, described in 1939 a satisfactory method of closing oroantral openings by obtaining tissue from the buccal or cheek area (Fig. 15-10). The tissues that form the rim of the fistula are incised. From the extreme edges, diagonal incisions are made through the mucoperiosteum to the bone. The incisions are carried upward into the mucobuccal fold. The flap is elevated, exposing the bone defect. In the undersurface of the flap the periosteum is incised horizontally at different points, care being taken to incise the periosteum only so that there will be no interference with the blood supply. The incision in the periosteum lengthens the flap so that it may slide down over the opening. Mattress sutures are then introduced over the area, and definite coaptation is secured. The edges are sutured with multiple black silk sutures, which are allowed to remain in place for 5 to 7 days.

The Berger technique can be combined with the Caldwell-Luc operation. Chronic antral infection, so often present in the patient with a persistent fistula, must be eradicated and antral polyps removed before healing can occur. To obtain good access to the antrum in the combined technique, the anterior limb of the flap used in the Berger technique is extended forward in the sulcus from its upper end, making a separate Caldwell-Luc incision unnecessary.

Another method of closure that is simple and has been successful was described by Proctor. He places a cone-shaped piece of preserved cartilage into the defect. The tooth socket is prepared by curettement, and the cartilage is wedged into place. It is important to have the cartilage of sufficient size so that it can be definitely wedged into place. If loose fitting, it may become dislodged and drop out before the membrane grows over it or it may pass upward into the sinus and become a foreign body.

Gold disks, or 24-karat, 36-gauge gold plate, have been used most successfully by many oral surgeons over the country.[2] The procedure is practical, effective, and uncomplicated. The involved sinus is thoroughly cleaned and adequately exposed. It is imperative that the sinus be as free from infection as possible. The bone is prepared for the reception of the metal, and then the metal is placed over the opening and maintained there by suturing the soft tissue flaps over it. The patient is placed on an antibiotic to reduce the possibility of an antral or soft tissue infection. A nasal spray is advised to maintain good nasoantral drainage and avoid stasis over the gold implant.

Autogenous bone disks have been advocated for closure of the oroantral fistula combined with a Caldwell-Luc procedure and nasal antrostomy.[1]

The possible closure of oroantral fistulas by means of free, full-thickness transplants obtained from the opposite side of the palate or from the mucobuccal fold is an approach that should not be overlooked. It is feasible and uses tissue that is not foreign to the mouth, since it is a transfer of tissue from one part of the mouth to another. The donor site heals readily, being protected initially by the application of compound tincture of benzoin or sedative dressings.

Causes of failure in the closing of an oroantral fistula may be listed as follows:

1. Complete elimination of all infection within the antral cavity prior to closure not accomplished. This may be done by lavage or antibiotics that have been proved effective against the bacteria present or both.

2. The patient's general physical condition not adequately explored and treated. Such diseases as diabetes, syphilis, and tuberculosis can influence adversely the normal healing of wounds.

3. Flaps placed over the opening with too much tension, and failure to provide a fresh or raw surface at the recipient site of the flap

The best insurance for a successful closure is the obtaining of good drainage from the sinus to the nose by the establishment of an intranasal antrostomy prior to making any attempt to close the chronic fistula. This may be performed in the following manner: A cotton pledget with 2% tetracaine (Pontocaine) in ephedrine 1% solution, is applied to the inferior meatal wall and the inferior turbinate. After anesthesia is established, the wall is penetrated with a punch or trocar, which will make a sufficiently large opening to admit cutting forceps. The window is enlarged in all directions until a diameter of at least 2 cm is obtained at its narrowest point. It is important to lower the nasoantral ridge to the floor of the nasal cavity. If any of the ridge is left standing, it might defeat the entire purpose of the new opening, which is to permit a free flow of secretions from the sinus into the nose.

Caldwell-Luc operation

Indications for the Caldwell-Luc radical sinus operation are many, including the following:

1. Removal of teeth and root fragments in the sinus. The Caldwell-Luc operation eliminates blind procedures and facilitates the recovery of the foreign body.

2. Trauma of the maxilla when the walls of the maxillary sinus are crushed or when the floor of the orbit has dropped. This type of injury is best corrected by the approach furnished by this operation.

3. Management of hematomas of the antrum with active bleeding through the nose. The blood may be evacuated and the bleeders located. Hemorrhage is arrested with epinephrine packs or hemostatic packs.

4. Chronic maxillary sinusitis with polypoid degeneration of the mucosa

5. Cysts in the maxillary sinus

6. Neoplasms of the maxillary sinus, which are best removed by this technique

The surgical procedure employed is described as follows: With the use of the anesthetic best suited for the patient, the mouth and face are prepared in the usual manner. If the patient is asleep, he will be intubated and the throat packed along the anterior border of the soft palate and tonsillar pillars. The upper lip is elevated with retractors. A U-shaped incision is made through the mucoperiosteum to the bone. Vertical incisions are made in the cuspid and second molar areas from points just above the gingival attachment up to and above the mucobuccal fold. A horizontal line connecting the two vertical incisions is made in the alveolar mucosa several millimeters above the gingival attachments of the teeth. The tissue is elevated from the bone with periosteal elevators, going superiorly as high as the infraorbital canal. Care is exercised here to prevent injury to the nerve. An opening is made into the facial wall of the antrum above the bicuspid roots by means of chisels, gouges, or dental drills, and this is enlarged by means of bone-cutting forceps to a size that permits inspection of the cavity. The size ultimately obtained is about the size of the end of an average index finger.

The opening should be made high enough to avoid the roots of the teeth in that area. The purpose of the operation (for example, the removal of root ends or foreign bodies) is readily accomplished. Seldom is the radical removal of the entire sinus mucosa required, but if it is deemed advisable, this is readily done by means of periosteal elevators and curets. The cavity is cleansed, and the soft tissue flap is replaced and sutured over the bone with multiple, interrupted black silk sutures. These are allowed to remain for a period of 5 to 7 days. Fig. 15-11 illustrates the approach in the Caldwell-Luc operation.

Anesthesia of the cheek and teeth may follow injury to the infraorbital nerve or nerves of the teeth during chiseling of the bony wall. Swelling of the cheek is common but usually disappears in a few days. The prognosis is good, and the development of severe conditions is rare.

Modern techniques of orthognathic surgery, performed so frequently today, often violate the integrity of the maxillary sinus. Complete control or eradication of latent or incipient infection is important. The most effective antibiotic may be determined preoperatively by bacterial sensitivity tests on material obtained from the antrum. This precaution will reduce or avoid potential complications. Nasal decongestants are

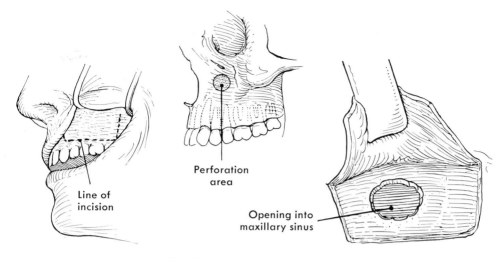

Fig. 15-11. Caldwell-Luc operation.

recommended preoperatively and post-operatively to shrink the mucous membrane, thereby preventing the development of gross edema.

SUMMARY

Intimate juxtaposition of the antrum and roots of the teeth with their surrounding alveolar bone is complicated by occasional maxillary sinusitis of dental origin. Teeth and roots that are to be removed from the alveolus sometimes slip above the thin bony plate separating the alveolus from the sinus. Sometimes they lodge between the bone and the antrum membrane. Frequently, they enter the antrum, in which case the problem of the opening in the antrum cavity is complicated by an opening into the mouth as well as residual dental infection in the alveolus. The operator is then faced with the problem of deciding how far to probe through the alveolus for a lost root or tooth, whether the buccal plate of the alveolus should be opened at that site, or whether a Caldwell-Luc operation is indicated.

The oroantral fistula is a problem that requires detailed attention to the management of a flap in the mouth. However, in all these conditions the problem of antral infection is potential or real. For the sake of obtaining the best results and to give the patient the benefit of mutual or specialized knowledge, a close liaison between the otolaryngologist and the oral surgeon and the unhesitating call for consultation, if needed and available, are certainly to be encouraged.

REFERENCES

1. Anderson, M. F.: Surgical closure of oroantral fistula: report of a series, J. Oral Surg. **27**:862, 1969.
2. Fredrics, H. S., Scopp, I. W., Gerstman, E., and Morgan, F. H.: Closure of oroantral fistula with gold plate: report of case, J. Oral Surg. **23**:650, 1965.

CHAPTER 16

Tissue transplantation

Philip J. Boyne

Research achievements in immunology and related disciplines combined with sophisticated improvements in surgical techniques have made possible innovative organ and tissue transplantation procedures in many different surgical specialties. These scientific advancements have produced the successful application of improved techniques of bone, tooth, and skin grafting to oral and maxillofacial surgical practice. Many oral surgeons have adapted these new grafting principles in the development of more efficient procedures in preprosthetic surgery, in the treatment of congenital defects and orthognathic deformities, and in the reconstruction of jaws after oncological surgery. These developments have made possible a health care service that gives every indication of increasing in significance in the future.

Of the various types of transplantable tissues available, *bone* is the most commonly utilized in oral surgical procedures, although skin grafting is becoming increasingly popular in some areas of preprosthetic surgery and in postoncological restorative procedures. Cartilage, fascia, and dura mater are more rarely used as tissues grafts in oral surgical procedures.

In the grafting of intact *organ systems,* oral surgeons have adapted immunological research to the transplantation of viable teeth with incompletely formed roots. (The grafting of endodontically treated nonviable teeth constitutes a *tissue* rather than an organ transplant inasmuch as such teeth do not function as viable organs after surgical transplantation.) Although the viable tooth bud graft constitutes the principal organ transplant system with which oral surgeons are concerned, it should be remembered that the grafting of fresh autogenous marrow within a cancellous bone graft constitutes an intact organ system, with the marrow organ being involved in the process of hemopoiesis as well as osteogenesis.

In an organ- or tissue-grafting procedure, the transplanted substances are classified according to their immunologic origins:

1. Autogenous grafts composed of tissues taken from the same individual
2. Allogeneic grafts (allografts) or implants composed of tissues taken from an individual of the same species who *is not* genetically related to the recipient
3. Isogeneic grafts or implants (isografts or syngenesioplastic grafts) composed of tissues taken from an individual of the same species who *is* genetically related to the recipient
4. Xenogeneic implants (xenografts that

are composed of tissues taken from a donor of another species, for example, animal bone grafted to man)

Generally, the term "implant" applies to the tranplantation of nonviable tissues. The term "graft" is usually reserved for a true transplantation of living tissue with the success of the grafting procedure depending on the survival of the transplanted cells.

IMMUNOLOGICAL CONCEPTS APPLIED TO ORAL SURGICAL TRANSPLANTATION PROCEDURES

The various methods of transplanting living *autogenous* tissues, although frequently presenting surgical and technical problems, do not as a rule involve immunological complications. However, graft rejection phenomena must be given serious consideration when allografts or xenografts of bone and cartilage are used in oral surgery. The basis for these rejection phenomena is reviewed in the following discussion to more fully identify the clinical response to various graft materials.

The immune response

The process by which the host rejects foreign graft material is a manifestation of an immunologically specific tissue reaction called the *immune response*. In the past it has been customary to explain the immune process within the context of disease susceptibility. The human body does not possess a natural immunity to many types of invading organisms. The immune process is initiated by exposure of the human host to invading bacteria, viruses, or parasites. The initial invasion of the host by these agents results in the production of specific substances in the tissues and body fluids that are capable of reacting with and destroying the invading agents.[27] The invading agent causing the initiation of the immune response is called an *antigen*. The specific protein developed in the body in response to the antigen is called an *antibody*, or an *immune body*. This specific protein antibody is available to combine with the ini-

tiating antigen should it again invade the host organism. This reaction between the antigen and the antibody, which occurs on subsequent exposure or invasion by the antigenic substance, is called the *immune response*.

Tissue immunity and humoral immunity

Two types of immunity are described in relationship to the mechanism of antibody release in the host. The cell most often implicated in antibody production is the plasma cell. Large lymphocytes and reticulum cells are also known to produce moderate amounts of antibody. These cells are capable of releasing their formed antibody into the circulatory body fluids; hence the name *humoral immunity*.

Other cells of the invaded host may also respond to foreign antigens. These cells, however, do not release antibody into the intercellular fluids of the host but do react, often violently, with foreign material containing the antigens, giving rise to the so-called *tissue immunity,* which as the name implies operates at the cellular level.[27,44] Humoral immunity lasts only as long as the specific antibody persists in the body fluids. Tissue immunity may last indefinitely.

Immune response applied to tissue transplantation

Because there is a tendency to think of the immune response in terms of infectious disease processes, it is not always appreciated that organic material taken from one person as part of a tissue graft may be foreign to another individual. The rejection of tissue grafts made between unrelated members of the same species is called an *allograft response*. This rejection of a living homogenous or allogeneic graft is the result of the cellular reaction of the host to the transplanted antigens. Such rejection is not immediate, however, and an allogeneic homograft transplanted into a normal animal enjoys an immunological latent period during which its healing is indistinguishable from that of an autograft.[27,44]

The length of this latent period depends on the disparity between donor and host, that is, the genetic relationship of the two. Genetic similarity between the donor and recipient of a transplanted tissue appears to be the major factor responsible for the success of the graft.[2] For example, skin allografts transplanted between closely related mice (isografts in inbred strains) may remain in place for over a month; skin allografts between different lines of mice may, on the other hand, be destroyed in an acute inflammatory reaction within a few days.

The second set response

The destruction of a tissue allograft leaves the recipient host in a specifically immune state, which is a condition of heightened resistance that may last for months. A second allograft from the same donor transplanted within this period is destroyed much more rapidly than its predecessor; indeed, these second transplants (the so-called white grafts) are even rejected with little or no evidence of beginning revascularization. This is called a *second set* reaction and has been demonstrated in most tissue transplants, including bone and teeth.[44]

All available evidence at present indicates that humoral or circulating antibodies do not play a significant part in solid tissue homograft rejection.[53]

Methods used to attenuate the immune response in grafting

In attempting to solve problems of incompatibility in grafting from one individual to another, three approaches have been used.[4,27] One approach attempts to modify the host's immune mechanisms to block the rejection of the graft. Various methods have been used to effect this modification in experimental animals, including thymectomy, the use of high and low dosages of antigen, the use of irradiation, and the employment of immunosuppressive drugs. A second approach attempts to alter the inherent graft antigenic properties so that normal immune defenses of the host will not be stimulated.[4] (For example, irradiation, freezing, and freeze-drying tend to diminish graft antigenicity of bone.[4,22,29]) A third method of attenuating or altering the antigenic properties of a graft by storage of the transplant organ in an intermediary host has been used experimentally. (Kidneys, for example, have been stored in intermediary host animals that have been given immunosuppressive drugs for the storage time period. The organ is then retrieved and transplanted into a third animal recipient.)

The first of the approaches just listed has been used largely in the form of immunosuppressive drugs in major organ transplants (for example, kidney and heart). This type of treatment has not been used clinically in oral surgical transplantation procedures. The second method of pretreating the graft material to alter its antigenicity has, however, been used successfully in the storage and preservation of allogeneic bone and cartilage[4] for use in oral surgery. The third method remains highly experimental.

Tissue typing procedures by which individual donors may be identified as having tissues histocompatible with a given recipient have produced marked advancement in certain organ transplant surgery such as kidney transplantation. Characterization of HL-A locus in genetic distribution and the matching of this genetic material, particularly in lymphocyte cytotoxicity testing, and other serological techniques have produced effective laboratory procedures for histocompatibility evaluation.[32,55,56]

BONE GRAFTING

Historically attempts have been made for centuries to employ bone graft materials in surgical procedures. In 1668 Van Meekren is recorded as having successfully transplanted heterogenous bone from a dog to man in restoring a cranial defect.[21] Hunter conducted experiments in the eighteenth century on the host response to bone grafts, noting the phenomena of resorption and remodeling of the graft matrix. The first successful autogenous bone graft was reported by Merrem in 1809.[44] Macewen reportedly transplanted allogeneic bone successfully in clinic patients in 1878.[21,39]

Various forms of devitalized bone from an animal source (xenografts) have been used clinically during the past half century. Orell[42] in 1938 produced a graft material from bovine bone by the use of strong alkalies. Boiling and defatting procedures have been employed in the treatment of animal bone prior to its use in xenogeneic grafting.[5,42] Bovine osseous tissue grafts treated with chemicals such as ethylenediamine,[36] hydrogen peroxide,[38] and strong detergents[3] have also been used clinically.

Attempts have been made to preserve allogeneic bone by the use of chemical agents. Thimerosal (Merthiolate) coagulation was employed for some time as a method of storing bone taken at autopsy.[48] The drastic treatment of human (allogeneic) bone by physical or chemical agents, however, is now generally thought to be an inferior method of preservation in comparison to cryogenic methods of tissue preservation. Cryobiological methods of storage were first employed by Inclan,[31] who is credited with developing the first modern bone bank in 1942. Following the use of refrigeration (above-freezing temperatures) for the preservation of bone, Wilson[59] developed a bone bank using freezing techniques.

Criteria used in bone graft evaluation

In evaluating the clinical and histological effectiveness of various bone graft materials, the following criteria are usually employed:

1. The graft must be biologically acceptable to the host (that is, it must not elicit an adverse immunological response).

2. The graft must *actively* or *passively* assist osteogenic processes of the host.

3. The graft material or its accompanying metallic or nonosseous supporting implant should withstand mechanical forces operating at the surgical site and contribute to internal support of the area.

4. Ideally the graft ultimately should become completely resorbed and replaced by host bone.

Allogeneic bone
Storage and preservation of allogeneic bone for grafting

The most successful tissue storage methods used in the banking of allogeneic bone have been cryobiological in nature, that is, by use of cooling, freezing, or freeze-drying environments.[4,22,29] Bone grafts preserved by cryogenic methods are more rapidly and completely revascularized, resorbed, and remodeled than are allografts that have been deproteinized, boiled, or otherwise drastically treated.

The application of cryobiological techniques to bone preservation is predicated on the unique histological nature of osseous tissue. Unlike many soft tissue and organ systems having large cell populations, bone and cartilage are composed of relatively small numbers of living cells with large amounts of calcified and noncalcified intercellular matrix, which is considered to be nonviable. Since the survival of the cells of an allogeneic bone graft is not necessary or even desirable because of the previously discussed immunological factors, a method of storage that will bring about this cellular death without deleteriously altering the remaining osseous structure of the graft material is considered to be essential for the development of an effective graft substance. This is accomplished by freeze-drying[29] and by most controlled methods of freezing to low temperatures. Since cells of a cryobiologically preserved bone graft do not survive, the assistance on the part of the graft to osteogenic processes of the host is purely *passive*. No active osteogenic stimulation is expected of these grafts. Such grafts offer their extracellular matrix as a system of absorbable surfaces over which new bone of the host may grow to reconstruct the grafted defect.

Although clinical evaluation of freeze-dried allogeneic bone has indicated that implants preserved in this manner are highly acceptable allografts, disadvantages associated with freeze-drying techniques have interfered with a more generalized use of this osseous material. These disadvantages relate to equipment costs and to the relatively large personnel requirements necessary for the performance of aseptic autopsies and for the processing and storing of the bone product. Efforts to minimize these disadvantages have been directed toward eliminating the need for aseptic autopsies by sterilization of the bone after its procurement by less time-consuming, nonsterile procedures. Sterilization methods employed have been in the form of irradiation from cathode and cobalt sources and chemical sterilization with such agents as ethylene oxide and betapropiolactone.[8]

Clinical use of allogeneic banked bone

Freeze-dried and frozen allogeneic bone can be produced in various anatomical forms to conform to the needs of different oral surgical procedures.

Cancellous iliac crest bone can be ground into particles having a diameter of approximately 2 to 10 mm for use in confined intrabony defects after cyst enucleation (Fig. 16-1). Smaller cancellous particles may be

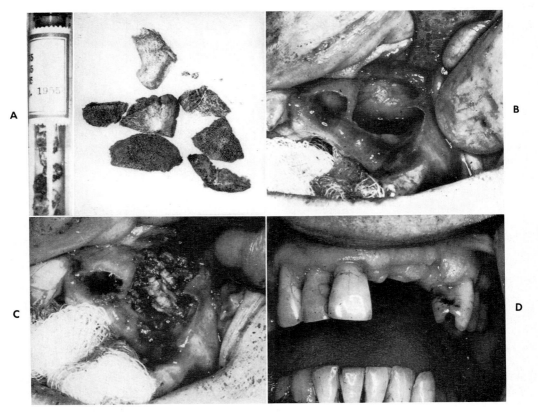

Fig. 16-1. A, Freeze-dried allogeneic cancellous bone prior to implantation in an intrabony cystic defect. **B,** Osseous defect after enucleation of a radicular cyst involving maxillary anterior teeth. **C,** Intrabony defect is filled with freeze-dried allogeneic bone particles. **D,** Three weeks postoperatively the alveolar ridge is well healed with acceptable width and contour restored.

used in periapical areas after curettage, and larger cancellous chips may be used in recontouring procedures of the alveolar ridge. Some surgeons[49] have also utilized cancellous allogeneic freeze-dried chips in the treatment of nonunion of fractures of the mandible.

Frozen or freeze-dried, split-rib grafts may be used as onlays to improve *width* and *contour* of deficient edentulous ridges[12] (Fig. 16-2) and to cosmetically restore other facial bone deficiencies (Fig. 16-3). Although freeze-dried allogeneic allografts of bone may be used in recontouring procedures to improve the width of deficient edentulous alveolar ridges, autogenous iliac crest bone is recommended for rebuilding the *height* of deficient ridges. (See section on autogenous bone grafts.)

It may appear paradoxical that banked allogeneic bone will at times produce a better recontouring onlay implant for rebuilding deficient mentum areas than will an autogenous graft. The slow remodeling rate of the allogeneic bone in comparison to the fresh cancellous autograft permits the onlay graft to maintain the desired contour for longer periods of time postoperatively. Fresh autogenous bone grafts placed in this

area are not infrequently resorbed rapidly with no accompanying replacement of the graft by host osseous tissue to maintain the correct contour. The disadvantage of using banked allografts in the mentum area, of course, relates to the slow acceptance and slow bonding to the host bone, thus prolonging the postoperative period when slight trauma could completely dislodge the graft from the host bone, leading to failure of the procedure.

Although considered to be second-rate graft materials, cryobiologically preserved bone allografts are used in the surgical treatment of the indicated minor defects and can be used in selected cases as substitutes for larger autogenous bone transplants in patients for whom the operation necessary to obtain an autogenous graft is contraindicated.

A recent application of banked cryologically preserved allogeneic bone has been in certain orthognathic surgical sites following osteotomy procedures. If the surrounding musculature is conducive to good revascularization of the host bone and the graft recipient site, a banked bone implant will accomplish the desired surgical result as readily as an autogenous fresh graft. Such

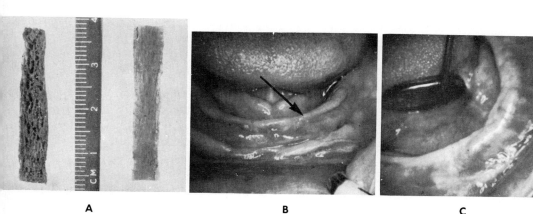

A   B   C

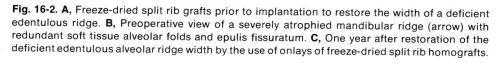

Fig. 16-2. A, Freeze-dried split rib grafts prior to implantation to restore the width of a deficient edentulous ridge. **B,** Preoperative view of a severely atrophied mandibular ridge (arrow) with redundant soft tissue alveolar folds and epulis fissuratum. **C,** One year after restoration of the deficient edentulous alveolar ridge width by the use of onlays of freeze-dried split rib homografts.

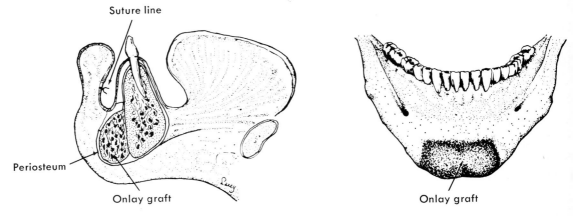

Fig. 16-3. Restoration of deficient mentum with an onlay of freeze-dried allografts of split rib.

favorable orthognathic surgical sites primarily are in the ramus where the pterygomasseteric sling affords good vascularity to both the medial and the lateral aspects of the ramus and to any graft placed in this area. Additionally, allogeneic bone has been placed in Le Forte I osteotomy sites along the lateral aspect of the horizontal osteotomy and in the maxillary tuberosity–pterygoid space. It appears clinically that such banked implants do as well as fresh autogenous bone, and the application in the future for this type of implant-grafting procedure appears to be most promising.[34]

Experimentally, allogeneic bone has been used in the attempted reconstruction of edentulous ridges; however, at this time the long-term effect of prosthetic function over such osseous restorations has not substantiated the ability of such grafts to withstand resorptive forces.

Another experimental way in which allogeneic banked bone has been used is as an interpositional graft after splitting the body of the mandible and raising the superior portion of the alveolar ridge, interposing the allogeneic graft between the raised superior portion of the ridge and the base of the mandibular bone.[54] Again, the long-term response of such implant-grafts after the clinical application of prosthetic forces has not been determined. These types of procedures indicate the interest of surgeons in finding new applications and more effective procedures for bone grafts and implants in orthognathic surgery and in maxillofacial reconstruction.

Banked allogeneic bone may be subjected to various surface decalcification procedures as well as enzymatic treatment in order to render the surface of the graft more amenable to remodeling and eventual replacement with new host bone. The use of surface decalcified allogeneic bone appears to have application at the clinical level. The effect of such surface treatment generally is to enhance the graft's acceptance through increasing the chance of resorption and remodeling of the surface-altered matrix of the osseous implant.[43,45,46]

Clinical use of allogeneic banked cartilage

Cryobiologically preserved allogeneic cartilage has been utilized in restoring contour defects of facial bones. If the cartilage allograft is placed supraperiosteally within a soft tissue pocket (as in the mentum area), fibrous encapsulation and a prolonged resorption of the implant occur. This host reaction in certain soft tissue implant areas restoring facial defects is considered to be advantageous, since the cartilage graft will remain in place for longer periods of time, maintaining the desired postsurgical contour.

Cartilage placed subperiosteally that is well immobilized will unite with the underlying bone by the formation of reactive osseous tissue.[12] Such grafts are so slowly revascularized, however, that they are subject to complete rejection and loss if only a slight dehiscence of the overlying soft tissue occurs postoperatively. Normally, the cartilage implant in such a recipient site will gradually be replaced with host bone.[12] The bone replacement rate as well as the revascularization of cartilage onlays placed subperiosteally on edentulous alveolar ridges is generally slower than that of similarly implanted bone grafts. Thus in the selection of the graft material to be used in these areas, the disadvantage of the slow remodeling and replacement of subperiosteally placed implants of allogeneic cartilage must be weighed against the advantage of ease of manipulation of the cartilaginous tissue as opposed to the more rigid allogeneic bone graft material.

Xenogeneic bone
Attempted preparation of xenogeneic bone for grafting

Although properly preserved hard tissue allografts have a place in oral surgical procedures, the expense of preparing allogeneic bone in an acceptable manner has not been conducive to the widespread establishment of tissue banks in hospital centers. For this reason a continuing effort has been made through the years to develop an acceptable xenogeneic bone graft material.

As one would expect, cross-species bone and cartilage transplants stimulate an immune response on the part of the host. Studies have shown that in the case of bone allografts the main antigens are associated with nucleated marrow and bone cells contained in the transplant, whereas in the case of xenografts the osseous matrix and the serum proteins are also potentially highly antigenic.[4] As a result the problem of rendering animal bone acceptable to the

human host becomes increasingly difficult. Since the major antigenic component of animal bone is contained within the organic fraction of the tissue, this portion of the bone must either be altered or removed to render the product acceptable to the human host.

The problem of cross-species antigenicity in bone xenografting procedures has been approached for the most part by treating animal bone material with vigorous chemical measures to remove, alter, or destroy the organic portion of the osseous tissue. Consequently, although many chemical techniques have been described in the literature for processing of xenografts, relatively few reports have appeared describing the use of freezing and freeze-drying in xenogeneic bone preservation and storage.[26]

As previously mentioned, the treatment of bovine bone by boiling in water,[5] boiling in alkalies (such as potassium hydroxide),[42] macerating in hydrogen peroxide,[38] and extracting with ethylenediamine[36] has been used in the past to render potentially antigenic xenografts acceptable to the host (Fig. 16-4). The preservation of beef bone by storage in alcohol and in ether also has been described. However, extensive clinical and histological evaluations of most of these methods have indicated serious disadvantages that preclude the clinical use of these materials.

Attempts to produce an acceptable xenograft from calf bone, using a process that included treatment with chemical detergents and freeze-drying, resulted in a product that, although acceptable as a space-occupying implant in certain minor osseous defects, did not develop into an effective substitute for autogenous or even preserved allogeneic bone.[14]

Animal cartilaginous tissue treated by various means has also been investigated as a xenogeneic implant material. Such materials have not enjoyed significant clinical acceptance.

Various organic extracts of animal bone

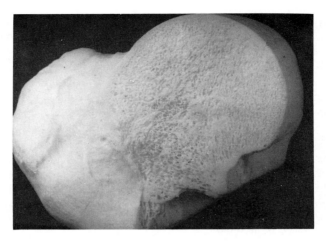

Fig. 16-4. View of a specimen of ethylenediamine-treated bovine bone demonstrating the effect of removal of all organic material from osseous tissue. The cancellous spaces are exposed and cleared of all organic material.

have been used in the past in an effort to produce an inductor substance that would stimulate bone formation. Such studies have involved evaluation of the properties of the mucopolysaccharide fraction of bone and effects of chondroitin sulfates on bone repair.[40] Results of these studies have been at best equivocal, and, to date, no clinical application is apparent.

Thus research efforts have not at the present time produced a clinically acceptable xenogeneic bone graft material.

Autogenous grafts

It is obvious that the most optimal type of bone graft material should be autogenous in origin. While there is general agreement among surgeons that autogenous bone is a superior graft material, there has been considerable disagreement as to the optimal anatomical form that this type of graft should take. Autogenous grafts are usually employed to restore large areas of lost mandibular bone following surgery or trauma. Restoration of the traumatically avulsed or the surgically resected mandible has been of paramount clinical concern for many years. Of all the facial bones resected in oncological surgery, the mandible is the most frequently removed. It is paradoxical

that the most frequently resected facial bone is also the most difficult to reconstruct surgically. The constant movement of the mandible in swallowing and in speech and the unprotected contours of the mandible in the facial skeleton coupled with the relative paucity of blood supply to the area and the minimal amount of muscular tissue surrounding the structure make the mandibular bone one of the most difficult to esthetically and functionally reconstruct through osseous grafting. Reconstruction procedures are not only technically difficult but their prognosis is most uncertain. Since the degree of surgical difficulty attending the restoration of a resected or lost mandible is great, it is appropriate that the determination of maximum effectiveness of any graft material in maxillofacial surgery should be based on its ability to reconstruct this particular facial bone.

Some surgeons have preferred to use rib grafts for spanning such large defects, fabricating the transplant to the desired shape by notching and cutting the rib in order to bend the graft to the appropriate contour of the maxillofacial defect. Rib grafts also may be placed in an onlay position overlaying the host bone, either on a decorticated or nondecorticated recipient site. For production of angle grafts to replace a disarticulated mandible, a costochrondral rib graft may be employed with the cartilaginous portion simulating the temporomandibular joint and condyle. The overall postoperative results of the use of rib grafts in large discontinuity defects of the mandible in general have not been consistently rewarding. Autogenous ribs, however, may be used to reconstruct smaller missing segments of the mandible with a fair degree of success.

Other surgeons have preferred to take solid, one-piece grafts from the iliac crest, cutting these to desired form and shape. Many types of mortising "carpentry" are performed to make the graft interface with the host bone in an onlay, inlay, or combination of forms of attachment with the remaining host bone fragments. The iliac crest graft also can be cut to simulate the angle of the mandible.

Additionally, a cut from the inner table of the iliac crest may give a curvature that, to a limited extent, simulates that of a mandibular hemisection. Such grafts, however, during the first 3 postoperative months tend to resorb at the interface between the grafts and the host bone. Such resorption leads to immobilization problems. Grafts utilized in this manner have a tendency to become mobile, displaced from their anatomical sites, and to undergo extensive resorption. In the use of solid one-piece grafts, care must be taken by the surgeon to effect maximal intermaxillary immobilization to avoid failure caused by the phenomenon of interface resorption.

Particulate autogenous marrow-cancellous bone grafting

Recently, experimental studies have demonstrated the marked osteogenic potential of hemopoietic marrow. Marrow taken from the iliac crest can be transplanted autogenously to effect new bone formation in various types of osseous defects. Autogenous hemopoietic marrow and autogenous cancellous bone containing marrow

appear to be the only types of bone graft material that are capable of actively inducing osteogenesis. (As mentioned previously, properly preserved allogeneic bone in certain graft sites can passively assist the osteogenic process of the host, but this type of graft material is not actively osteogenic.)

The clinical exploitation of the marked osteogenic potential of hemopoietic marrow and cancellous bone has been impeded in the past by the lack of development of a satisfactory method of containing the graft within the surgical site and of preventing the ingrowth of fibrous tissue, which has a tendency to insinuate between the individual particles of the graft material, producing a fibrous union. Recent studies, however, have developed a technique whereby these particulate marrow grafts may be applied to many areas of oral surgical treatment. The technique that has been developed is one in which autogenous bone and marrow taken from the iliac crest is placed in a metallic chrome-cobalt or titanium mesh implant (Fig. 16-5, A and B). The metallic mesh serves to span the discontinuity defect of the mandible or maxilla, contain the graft material, and immobilize the host bone fragments.

The use of autogenous rib grafts (Fig. 16-6) in restoring similar large areas of lost mandibular bone has not been particularly successful. Massive resorption of the rib grafts frequently results. In cases in which the surgeon can be confident of having a complete intraoral closure of healthy mucosa a cellulose acetate filter may be placed within the troughlike metal implant. The filter serves to further contain the graft and to prevent ingression of fibrous tissue into the graft area (Fig. 16-5, C).[10] The use of this type of autogenous graft material in the surgical system described was found to have several advantages over the solid one-piece autograft in the regeneration of large discontinuity defects of the mandible.

This technique has been used successfully in restoring large areas of the mandible, including the entire body of the man-

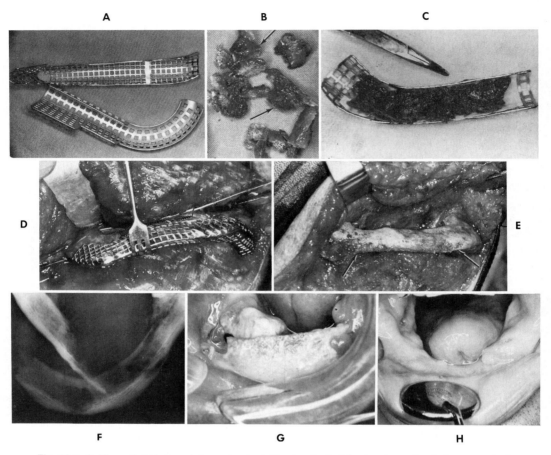

Fig. 16-5. A, View of metal mesh bone implant. The implant at the top is made of chrome-cobalt. The lower implant is composed of pure titanium. The metal implant in each case is used to contain the marrow bone graft. **B,** View of the autogenous graft material used in this system, that is, marrow and cancellous bone taken from the iliac crest. The bone particles contain a high percentage of marrow (arrows). This type of particulate graft material offers maximum osteogenic efficiency. **C,** A cellular acetate porous filter may be used to line the metal mesh implant. Such a filter serves to further retain the graft material within the surgical site and to prevent ingression of fibrous connective tissue into the grafted area. The filter is not used, however, in cases presenting with intraoral communication or areas in which intraoral dehiscence is probable. **D,** Use of the metal implant marrow bone graft system in restoring a hemisectioned mandible is demonstrated here. The metal implant extends from the midramus to the opposite parasymphysis. The implant will be filled with the particulate marrow bone graft. **E,** Eight months after grafting, the metallic mesh has just been removed, revealing the completely restored mandible from angle to symphysis. The mandible has not only regenerated but has also remodeled to form a thick outer cortex of lamellated bone (arrows). **F,** One of the advantages of the use of particulate marrow and cancellous bone in restoration of the lost mandibular bone is that the graft material may be utilized in areas involved by postirradiation osteomyelitis. The radiograph depicts osteoradionecrosis 2 years following irradiation for a carcinoma of the floor of the mouth. The mandible is necrotic and fractured with loss of considerable osseous structure. **G,** Intraoral view shows the exposed necrotic bone and the fractured mandible overriding to the right side. **H,** After proper debridement and sequestrectomy, the patient had a graft using particulate marrow and cancellous bone that resulted in complete restoration of continuity of the mandible and the alveolar ridge.

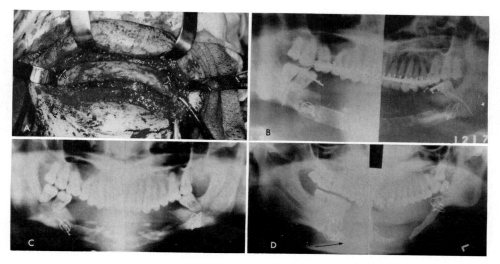

Fig. 16-6. A, An autogenous rib graft has been inserted to restore an avulsed body of the mandible. The rib is fixed to the host fragments with stainless steel wire. **B,** Radiograph of the rib transplant shown in **A** taken immediately after surgery. **C,** Radiograph of the same case 10 months after grafting. Massive resorption has occurred, and movement at the host-graft interface is clinically detectable. **D,** A case similar to that shown in **C.** The patient in this case had undergone a resection of the mandible for an ameloblastoma and had an autogenous rib bone graft placed. Two years after surgery the radiograph shown here reveals almost complete resorption of the rib graft (arrow) and a complete lack of bony continuity.

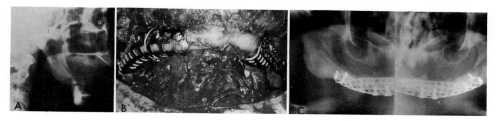

Fig. 16-7. A, Radiograph of a bilateral nonunion of 10 years' duration of an atrophic edentulous mandible in a 48-year-old woman. Note the inferior displacement of the anterior mandibular fragment. **B,** The bilateral nonunion is treated with a marrow cancellous bone graft and bilateral titanium mesh bone implant. **C,** View of a similar case of bilateral fracture nonunion treated with a marrow cancellous bone graft and a single titanium mesh implant.

dible in cases of traumatic loss after gunshot wounds and other types of injuries.[9] More recently the technique has been applied to the reconstruction of resected mandibles after oncological surgery (Fig. 16-5, *D* to *H*).[19,41,47] The procedure is also used for the treatment of nonunion of the body of the mandible, particularly in cases of old nonunion or malunion of *atrophic* edentulous mandibles (Fig. 16-7). The procedure may additionally be used for smaller traumatic or surgical defects (Fig. 16-8).

The procedure of using autogenous particulate marrow in this system has the following advantages:

1. The particulate graft of marrow and cancellous bone is easily obtained by making only a small opening along the lateral

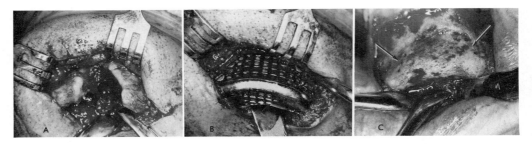

Fig. 16-8. A, View of a moderately large osseous defect of the mentum and inferior border of the mandible resulting from a gunshot wound. **B,** View of the defect being grafted with a cast chrome-cobalt implant made to conform to the curvature of the mentum. The mesh implant has been lined with the filter membrane and has been filled with an autogenous marrow bone graft. **C,** Six months after grafting the metallic mesh is removed transorally, demonstrating the regenerated symphysis with a completely remodeled and reformed outer bone cortex (arrows).

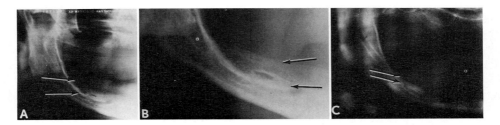

Fig. 16-9. A, Radiograph of a deficient edentulous alveolar ridge 2½ years after grafting with a particulate graft of marrow and cancellous bone. The restored area is seen between arrows. Approximately 30% of the original graft has resorbed. **B,** A close-up view of the regenerated alveolar ridge of the mandible in **A.** The restored area is indicated by arrows. **C,** Radiographs of a rib graft placed to restore a deficient edentulous alveolar ridge. Approximately 50% of the graft has resorbed 3 years after surgery.

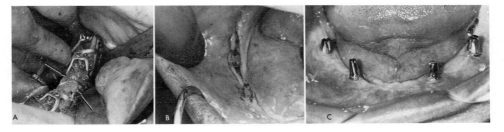

Fig. 16-10. A, View of the surgical site of an atrophic mandible after placing the specially constructed subperiosteal implant over a graft of marrow cancellous bone. The mucoperiosteum will now be closed over the implant and graft. Screws have been placed in the area of the implant normally containing posts. These screws will be removed 5 weeks postoperatively, and the semiburied posts will be inserted. **B,** Five weeks after surgery single incisions are made in the mucosa overlying the screws in the buried implant. The screws are removed, and posts are then inserted into the implant to receive the newly constructed denture. **C,** The posts have been inserted, and the patient is ready for the construction of an implant denture superstructure.

surface of the iliac crest rather than taking a large portion of the ilium or a rib to effect the desired surgical result.

2. Complete healing of the grafted defects with viable bone is more rapid than when the solid one-piece autograft is used.

3. The need for intermaxillary fixation can be greatly reduced because of the rapid spanning and osseous regeneration of the defect by new bone and because immobilizing support of the host bone fragments is provided by the metal implant itself.

Treatment of the edentulous atrophic alveolar ridge. The use of surgical procedures to correct atrophied, deficient, alveolar ridges has included both soft tissue, ridge-extension–type surgery and the use of bone graft material to increase the osseous alveolar base. A technique employing the marrow-cancellous bone graft system has been utilized to extend the height of atrophic deficient alveolar ridges.[11] It was found in a long-term, follow-up study of these types of grafts in clinical human patients that approximately 35% of the alveolar height restored at surgery was resorbed at the end of a 3-year period. It is believed that this technique compares favorably with the use of rib grafts to restore the edentulous alveolar ridge, in which, based on my experience and the observations of others, approximately 50% of the graft is lost during this same 3-year period.[33] Neither of these two types of autografting procedures would appear to be completely feasible for the long-range treatment of the deficient edentulous alveolar ridge (Fig. 16-9).

A more recent application of the marrow grafting principle to the treatment of deficient edentulous alveolar ridges has been the combination of marrow cancellous bone grafts with a subperiosteal metal implant used for the attachment of semiburied posts for implant denture construction.[35] This new technique has resulted in a clinical application that has been used initially with considerable success. The patients are being observed on a long-term basis to determine whether the usual stresses transmitted directly through the posts to bone by way of the subperiosteal metal implant will produce the same degree of resorption as the mucosally transmitted forces of the conventional denture (Fig. 16-10).

Treatment of maxillary clefts. Another application of the autogenous marrow and cancellous bone particulate graft has been in the secondary grafting of residual clefts of the alveolar ridge and the palate in congenital cleft palate cases.[17,18] It was found that in children between the ages of 8 and 12 with residual osseous clefts of the alveolar ridge and anterior palate, the autogenous cancellous bone graft may be used effectively. It was found that the permanent cuspid and lateral incisor teeth on either side of the previously existing cleft may be moved into the cleft area orthodontically within 2 or 3 months of the time of grafting (Fig. 16-11). Additionally, the maxillary arch may be expanded orthodontically to improve the occlusion after the bone grafting of the clefts. Thus the responsiveness of the viable marrow graft to changes in function is well demonstrated by this particular grafting technique. It has been shown in the past that rib grafts in the same types of residual clefts were not successful because teeth could *not* be moved into the grafted area postoperatively, and considerable constriction of the lateral expansile growth of the maxilla sometimes occurred.

It is clear that in areas of the oral cavity in which a viable graft is necessary to respond to the forces of function and orthodontic movement, the autogenous particulate marrow-cancellous bone graft is the transplant of choice.

More recently, autogenous marrow grafts have been used in periodontal therapy by the placement of grafts in intrabony pockets. The same type of graft material is used in these smaller defects, with the grafting material being taken by a trephine biopsy needle from the iliac crest while the patient is under local anesthesia. This technique of taking a small amount of the highly osteogenic graft material from the iliac crest

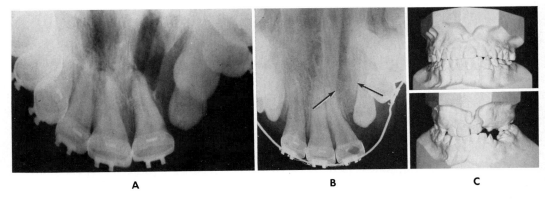

A **B** **C**

Fig. 16-11. A, Radiograph of a palatal and alveolar cleft in a 12-year-old patient demonstrating the extremely thin wall of bone along the distal aspect of the central incisor next to the cleft. The cuspid is erupting into the cleft and has no osseous tissue on its medial aspect. (The lateral incisor had previously erupted into the cleft and was lost.) **B,** Radiograph taken 3 months after grafting. The cuspid tooth is being actively moved into position in the arch through the viable graft area (arrows). A complete osseous and dental arch may be restored by this combination of surgical and orthodontic treatment. **C,** Pregrafting, postgrafting, and postorthodontic treatment casts demonstrate the effectiveness of the particulate marrow cancellous bone graft in restoring continuity to the osseous arch in order to establish the basis for definitive orthodontic therapy. The lower casts show the pregrafting arch with an open cleft into the nose, palatally displaced central incisor, and constricted maxillary arch. Following grafting of the cleft, closure of the oronasal opening, and return of a competent osseous arch, orthodontic therapy produced the results shown in the upper casts with a complete alignment of the teeth, expansion of the maxillary arch, and excellent occlusion. Approximately 25 of these cases have now been followed over 6 years, with the patients out of orthodontic retention and maintaining arch alignment and form without difficulty.

using local anesthesia offers a new opportunity for the oral surgeon to obtain a maximally osteogenic graft with a minimal amount of trauma and inconvenience to the donor.

The use of autogenous particulate marrow and cancellous bone grafts in areas adjacent to the roots of erupted teeth must be accompanied by the caveat that the highly cellular pluripotentiality of living marrow grafts may stimulate an adverse cellular response and result in a clinical failure even though the osseous defect itself may be regenerated. The cellular marrow graft has the capacity to form osteoclasts that have as their function the resorption of nonvital bone and hard tissue trabeculae. This resorptive process leads to remodeling and paves the way for viable osseous regeneration. Such osteoclasts, however, may also attack other hard tissue matrices such as the cemental surfaces of roots of adjacent teeth and cause massive root resorption leading to the exposure of the pulps and complete loss of the teeth. For this reason, in periodontal therapy, killed cell suspensions and nonvital allogeneic grafts that have been preserved by freezing usually are used instead of fresh marrow transplants.

The same precautions must be used in grafting in cystic areas next to the cervical portions of roots of adjacent teeth and in the use of marrow in palatal cleft grafting in adults. In cleft bone grafting, it does not appear that the placement of autogenous viable marrow against the roots of unerupted teeth in children leads to any resorptive process. In the adult patient, however, root resorption may occur in teeth located along the margins of the cleft after grafting.

Treatment of cystic bone cavities. Autogenous marrow and cancellous bone have

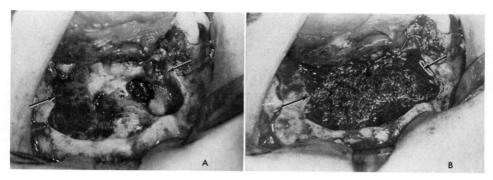

Fig. 16-12. A, View of the surgical site after removal of a large giant cell reparative granuloma in the mandibular symphysis of a 33-year-old woman. The restoration of the anterior aspect of the mentum area and the height of the alveolar ridge are of upmost importance in cases of this type. For this reason an autogenous graft of marrow and cancellous bone was used. **B,** Marrow and cancellous bone has been placed in the defect. The mucoperiosteum will now be closed. Complete restorations of the alveolar ridge can be effected in this manner.

also been utilized in large cystic cavities after the enucleation of keratinizing cysts or after removal of benign but locally aggressive tumors, such as ameloblastomas (Fig. 16-12). It is found that in large cystic areas, the autogenous graft produces a more rapid regeneration of the defect and a more acceptable postoperative result than the banked homograft. Banked, freeze-dried allografts, however, continue to remain an acceptable graft material in the treatment of moderately sized cystic bone defects.

Autogenous bone chips obtained at operation from the oral cavity are usually qualitatively and quantitatively poor. Little cancellous bone is present at the operative sites of common oral surgical procedures. Most osseous specimens obtained from alveolectomies, ostectomies, and osteotomies are composed of cortical or lamellated bone. Such cortical chips are of little osteogenic value. They may, however, be used as an acceptably banked allograft that would be employed to fill well-demarcated intrabony defects and to restore contour to deficient osseous areas.

Summary of graft evaluation

Based on both experimental laboratory procedures and clinical experience it is possible to offer an overall evaluation of the surgical use of most types of bone graft materials. The relative effectiveness of the most common types of graft materials is given in the following outline. This evaluation is based on repeated experiments with laboratory animals, using various test systems and extensive clinical observation.

First-rate grafts
1. Viable autogenous marrow
2. Viable autogenous cancellous bone
3. Viable autogenous osteoperiosteal grafts
4. One-piece, autogenous cortical-cancellous bone (iliac crest or rib)

Second-rate grafts
1. Autogenous cortical bone
2. Banked, allogeneic freeze-dried bone
3. Banked, allogeneic frozen bone

Third-rate grafts (unacceptable)
1. Detergent-treated, freeze-dried xenogeneic bone
2. Ethylenediamine-treated xenogeneic bone
3. Fat-extracted xenogeneic bone
4. Improperly preserved allogeneic bone

Composite allografts-autografts

Current research studies indicate that a promising graft material for intraoral and extraoral use may be some combination of an acceptably preserved allograft and autogeneous marrow. Marked osteogenic

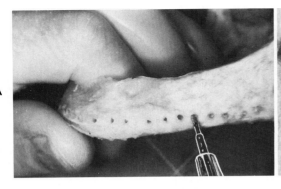
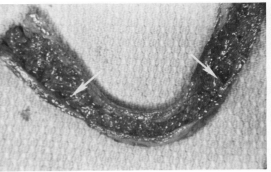

A

Fig. 16-13. A, View of a surface-decalcified, freeze-dried homogenous mandible being perforated with a bur after first removing the central portion of the graft. **B,** The central portion of the homograft shown in **A** has been filled with autogenous marrow and cancellous bone (arrows). The combined allograft-autograft will now be placed in the recipient patient to reconstruct the body of the mandible that had been previously resected for carcinoma.

properties have been observed with the use of this combination of tissues in experimental animals.[15,20]

The use of surface-decalcified allogeneic bone combined with autogenous hemopoietic marrow has produced an acceptable composite graft material.[43,45,46] The advantage of using such a composite allograft-autograft lies in the fact that the amount of autogenous graft tissue may be reduced to a minimum. With this combined graft, a much smaller extraction of marrow and cancellous bone from the iliac crest is necessary, with a lessening of postoperative complications. It was found that in the reconstruction of entire mandibles after oncological surgery for eradication of malignancies of the oral cavity, often an insufficient amount of hemopoietic marrow and cancellous bone could be obtained from one iliac crest. This necessitated the taking of autogenous marrow and cancellous bone from both ilia. In an effort to prevent the necessity of bilateral use of donor sites, a technique has been devised, utilizing a graft of allogeneic, surface-decalcified mandibular bone that has been "hollowed out" to enable the allograft to contain autogenous marrow within its troughlike structure (Fig. 16-13). Initial experimental work with this technique

has been most successful. It would appear to be an acceptable method of reducing the amount of autogenous graft material necessary to regenerate a given area of mandibular or maxillary bone.[16,45,46]

The combining of recently acquired knowledge about graft materials with results of present studies on osseous repair phenomena offers exciting areas for future surgical techniques.

Experimental studies related to bone graft procedures

Some promising bone grafting procedures in oral surgery have evolved from investigations of normal osseous healing mechanisms. By means of appropriate intravital labeling with tetracycline, it has been possible to delineate and predict areas of enhanced osteogenic activity after injury or surgical trauma to the facial bones.[7,13] These areas of osteogenic potential have been intensively investigated to determine the feasibility of utilizing these regions as sites for developing new oral surgical procedures and new bone-grafting techniques.

One area of enhanced osseous reparative response was found to occur along the lingual aspect of the mandible after removal of buccal or lateral osseous tissue in alveo-

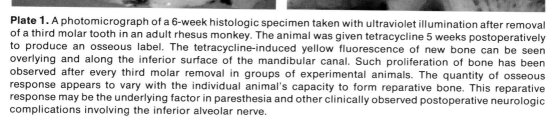

Plate 1. A photomicrograph of a 6-week histologic specimen taken with ultraviolet illumination after removal of a third molar tooth in an adult rhesus monkey. The animal was given tetracycline 5 weeks postoperatively to produce an osseous label. The tetracycline-induced yellow fluorescence of new bone can be seen overlying and along the inferior surface of the mandibular canal. Such proliferation of bone has been observed after every third molar removal in groups of experimental animals. The quantity of osseous response appears to vary with the individual animal's capacity to form reparative bone. This reparative response may be the underlying factor in paresthesia and other clinically observed postoperative neurologic complications involving the inferior alveolar nerve.

Plate 2. Photomicrograph taken with ultraviolet illumination after intravital labeling with tetracycline demonstrating homogenously transplanted incisor teeth in a dog. Yellow-fluorescing new bone formation can be seen entering the pulp chamber and replacing the normal pulpal tissue of the transplanted tooth bud on the left. The transplant on the right is not as yet exhibiting pulpal metaplasia.

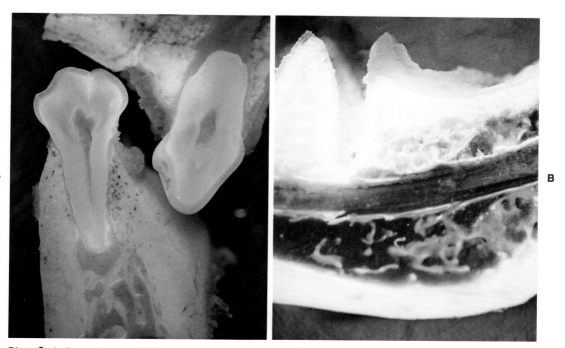

Plate 3. A, Transplanted, fully formed homogenous teeth in a dog after intravital labeling with tetracycline at 6 weeks postoperatively, demonstrating beginning resorption of the root of the transplant. Ultraviolet illumination reveals areas of tetracycline-induced yellow fluorescence indicating new bone formation surrounding the tooth. **B,** A photomicrograph taken with ultraviolet illumination demonstrating new bone formation that was labeled with tetracycline 27 weeks after extraction of the third molar. The second molar tooth was removed 1 week before the twenty-seventh–week (third molar socket) label. Therefore, fluorescence overlying the mandibular canal seen beneath the socket of the second molar represents new bone formation occurring 1 week after removal of that tooth. Such repair was also continuing beneath the third molar socket, the tooth of which had been extracted 27 weeks earlier, indicating that this type of bone repair can persist over a 4- to 5-month period.

lectomy procedures in dogs and monkeys. This subperiosteal lingual area has been found to be an excellent site for onlay implantation of grafts.

It has been found, however, that in experimental fractures of the body of the mandible in rhesus monkeys, callus formation in *endosteal* (marrow-vascular space) areas predominates over *subperiosteal* callus proliferation in effecting bony union. Experimental comparisons of gap-spanning grafts of the mandible placed in various positions in an effort to obtain the most optimal anatomical placement of grafts at surgery indicated that the best graft placement was in an onlay position adjacent to the marrow-vascular spaces of the host bone fragments and not in an overlapping onlay position.

Another aspect of the relationship of osseous repair to grafting procedures involves the optimal time for bone implantation. Important studies have been made of the histological effect of delayed grafting procedures in which bone implants were placed several days after an initial surgical trauma.[52]

An important peripheral application of the experimental studies of bone healing phenomena has been in understanding more fully the postsurgical osseous repair responses in the normal mandible and maxilla. Following surgical osteotomy of the alveolar crest or the removal of teeth or both, it was found that in addition to the proliferation of bone along the lingual subperiosteal aspect of the mandible, considerable bone formation occurred surrounding, and at the superior portion of, the underlying mandibular canal. Since this phenomenon was observed repeatedly in experimental animals, especially in fully adult rhesus monkeys, it is felt to be significant in explaining the occasional paresthesia that is observed following the removal of third molar teeth in clinical patients in whom no direct communication to the underlying mandibular canal was seen at the time of surgery. It is now believed that a normal healing response to the removal of third molar teeth is the formation of a certain amount of bone around the mandibular canal. In certain instances, representing possible individual variance, this formation of bone may be excessive. Such excessive bone formation may conceivably cause changes in the neurovascular bundle and result in paresthesia (Plates 1 and 3, *B*). Further work on these healing responses will undoubtedly elicit valuable information for the clinician in understanding and managing various postoperative complications.

Another important finding resulting from research of healing responses of the mandible has led to a more efficacious treatment of patients with osteoradionecrosis or postirradiation osteomyelitis requiring surgery and bone grafting procedures. It was found in experimental animals following irradiation and surgery, that of the two main areas of repair existing in the mandible, that is, the subperiosteal-lingual component of repair and the marrow-vascular repair component, the subperiosteal component of repair is the more severely damaged by the radiation process. With the passing of time after irradiation, the marrow-vascular component of repair returns partially with revascularization of the obtunded vasculature of the marrow-vascular spaces. However, the periosteum rarely regains its preirradiation capacity of osseous repair potential and does not form bone in response to a surgical procedure or assist in the acceptance of a bone graft. Therefore, the surgeon, in undertaking sequestrectomies, saucerization procedures, or bone grafting procedures in the postirradiated mandible, should develop surgical techniques that rely on the marrow-vascular component of the patient's remaining osseous structure to revascularize and to assist in the healing process. Procedures that rely on the subperiosteal component of repair, such as placing only one-piece onlay grafts along the lateral surface of an irradiated mandible, will result in failure because the patient's subperiosteal component of repair will not return following irradiation and, in the case of the onlay graft, no bonding of the graft to the host bed will occur. This is an extremely important point in undertaking osseous surgical operations or grafting procedures in the irradiated patient.

SKIN GRAFTS

Autogenous skin grafts have been used in oral surgery for some time. Recently, the use of split-thickness skin grafts in preprosthetic surgery has received additional emphasis with the development of more efficient surgical techniques. Skin grafts used in oral surgery may be of two types: full thickness and split thickness.

Full-thickness grafts are generally used in plastic surgical reconstruction of large facial defects and may be employed to line the oral or nasal cavities in such facial reconstruction procedures. However, for the most part, autogenous skin used in oral surgery is of the split-thickness type, ranging from 0.015 to 0.022 inch in thickness. When used in the oral cavity, such a graft survives and becomes an integral part of the mucosal surface. In addition to the use of such grafts in preprosthetic vestibuloplasty surgery (Fig. 16-14), split-thickness skin transplants may be used to cover a primary dressing over a stent after resection of various areas of the mandible or maxilla in eradication of tumors. The split-thickness skin graft is placed over a stent that is secured in place for approximately 7 to 10 days; at the end of this period, the obturator or stent is removed and the graft is trimmed. This graft material then serves as a soft tissue covering, supporting the surgical site. The split-thickness graft may later be reconstructed with a larger, thicker skin graft if necessary or with a composite bone and skin transplant procedure.

Allogeneic split-thickness skin obtained from the tissue bank and preserved by cryogenic means may be used as a *temporary* dressing for burns and skin abrasions. Oral surgeons have found this material an excellent dressing for facial abrasions contaminated with debris as a result of automobile accidents. After the debris-tattooed areas are vigorously scrubbed, the allogeneic skin is placed over the bleeding surface and kept in place for 7 to 10 days. Although these grafts later slough and are removed, they leave a clean, granulating surface, which is optimal for maximum epithelization.

TOOTH TRANSPLANTATION

During the past quarter of a century, research investigation of allogeneic tooth transplantation procedures has greatly in-

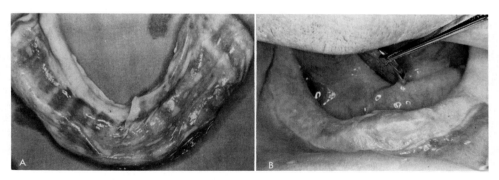

Fig. 16-14. A, An autogenous split-thickness skin graft has been taken from the thigh and placed over a compound lined splint. The skin graft will be carried to place over the surgically dissected mandibular surface and maintained in place for 7 to 10 days. **B,** Four weeks after grafting, the alveolar ridge is seen to have been extended by the combined procedure of vestibuloplasty and skin grafting. (The floor of the mouth has also been lowered in this case, giving additional room for the denture base.)

creased. This renewal of interest in the centuries-old surgical exercise of dental transplantation was occasioned by the advent of antibiotic therapy and the almost simultaneous development of tissue banking and histocompatibility testing procedures.[51,55,56]

Good evidence supports the view that teeth are capable of being antigenic.* The failure of tooth transplants to elicit overt immune responses may be the result of several factors. One interesting theory proposes to explain this lack of detectable immune response on the basis of the alveolus being a site of immunological privilege not subject to the usual laws of transplantation.[50] Further work has tended to disprove this reasoning, however.[23,24] The immune response phenomenon after tooth transplantation, although not of the same magnitude as that elicited by other types of tissues, may be evidenced by the following:

1. A chronic inflammatory infiltration of cells surrounding the transplant and infiltrating the pulpal tissue[23]
2. Failure of the pulp to function as a dentin-forming agent and failure to assist in the completion of the structure of the tooth root
3. Fibrous encapsulation and root resorption with replacement by osseous tissue[50]

It has been suggested that the following two phases are present in the immune response of the host to allogeneic homografts of teeth:

1. An early phase that is part of a reaction to the soft tissue portion of the transplant
2. A later, weaker phase in reaction to the less antigenic hard structure of the tooth[57]

Allogeneic tooth transplantation

Many attempts have been made to preserve tooth buds by refrigeration, by various freezing techniques, and by tissue culturing. In the final evaluation, these at-

*See references 23, 24, 31, 51, and 57.

tempts have generally been unsuccessful. Clinical acceptance without immediate rejection has been recorded after the transplantation of allogeneic teeth previously stored under these various conditions. However, no tissue culture or cryobiological method has been able to preserve the pulp so that it could assume a functional state subsequent to transplantation.[23] Necrosis of transplanted pulpal tissue invariably occurs after the storage of developing teeth by freezing and tissue culturing. Such necrosis results, of course, in a failure of further root development, and the pulp is gradually replaced by host fibrous and osseous tissue (Plate 2).

In the transplantation of pulpless, fully matured teeth from a homogenous allogeneic source, initial apparent acceptance has been obtained. However, ankylosis and progressive root resorption are the almost universal sequelae of such surgical procedures (Plate 3).

Although experimental work continues in evaluating the effects of histocompatibility testing of donor material,[51] the pretransplantation treatment of the root with fluoride and other agents,[51] and the cryobiological storage techniques of tooth banking, the present level of investigation does not support the extensive clinical use of homogenous allogeneic tooth transplantation.

Autogenous tooth transplantation

Although experimentation with tooth homografts has not been productive clinically, autogenous transplantation of teeth has during the past several years enjoyed a measure of success. A resurgence of clinical research in this area has occurred, with new surgical techniques developed in an effort to improve the transplantation success rate. A detailed surgical procedure has been described by Hale[28] and others[1,25] for the transplantation of developing third molars to the first molar position in the younger age groups. Proper patient selection is considered to be most important. Adequate mesiodistal width of the host implant site, absence of acute periapical or periodontal inflammatory states, and general oral health of the patient are emphasized.[28] The optimal root development of the tooth to be transplanted is approximately 3 to 5 mm of root growth apical to the crown.[28] The recipient site is prepared surgically by removing the interseptal bone with bur or rongeurs and by removing bone at the crest of the ridge to produce the proper size of alveolus to receive the transplant (Fig. 16-15, A). The transplant is removed from the donor site by elevator and forceps. In one technique the portion of the dental follicle surrounding the transplant may be re-

moved.[28] Damage to the soft tissue of the root sac, however, must be avoided (Fig. 16-15, B). The tooth is placed in the recipient site just below the level of occlusion and stabilized with stainless steel wire ligatures crossed over the occlusal surface of the transplanted crown (Fig. 16-16, A). Surgical cement is packed around the transplant and the crossed wire ligatures (Fig. 16-16, B). Some surgeons prefer to use an acrylic splint for stabilization. The surgical cement splint is usually allowed to remain in place for 14 days; acrylic splints may be employed for longer periods.

In another technique the developing third

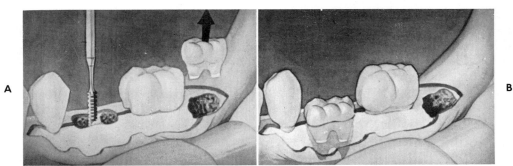

Fig. 16-15. A, The host site is prepared by removal of interseptal bone after the elevation of a mucoperiosteal flap from the retromolar to premolar area and after extraction of the first molar tooth. **B,** The third molar transplant is positioned below the level of occlusion in the recipient alveolus. (Courtesy Dr. Merle L. Hale.)

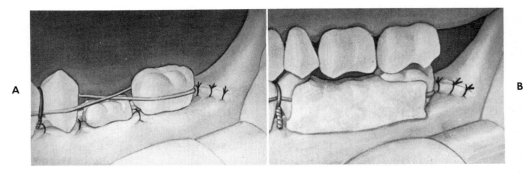

Fig. 16-16. A, A figure-of-eight stainless steel wire ligature is placed around the adjacent teeth to stabilize the transplant. **B,** A surgical cement pack is placed over the wire ligature and transplant. (Courtesy Dr. Merle L. Hale.)

molar tooth is removed with the operculum, gubernaculum, and follicle intact and transplanted to a first or second molar recipient site beneath a mucogingival flap.[1] An acrylic splint is also constructed in this procedure to maintain the intercoronal space and to prevent occlusal drift of the teeth mesial and distal to the transplant. As the transplant erupts into position, the splint is trimmed to permit proper tooth movement.

Various success rates using this procedure have been reported in the literature, with 5-year successes observed in 50% of cases.[1,28] Failure of complete root formation frequently occurs, and root resorption is not uncommon. The cause of such resorption has often been attributed empirically to damage to surrounding periodontal structures in the surgical transplantation procedure. Root resorption phenomena in autogenous tooth transplants have been studied by various techniques. Some investigators have found that the presence of periodontal ligament surrounding a transplanted tooth inhibits root resorption if a portion of the accompanying alveolar bone is implanted along with the grafted tooth.[58] Others have shown that the transplantation of teeth together with surrounding periodontal ligament and bone has resulted in an extensive root resorptive process.[37]

The autotransplantation of fully developed teeth has been attempted using various surgical techniques. The transplantation of fully matured, impacted maxillary cuspid teeth has been effected in a one-stage procedure. Initial attachment of the periodontal ligament after surgery can be demonstrated, and the transplanted tooth may be retained as a member of the dental arch for varying periods of time.[6,37] Root resorption eventually occurs, however, and rarely do these transplants remain in place for longer than 5 years postoperatively.

Reimplantation

Reimplantation refers to a dental procedure that is in reality a form of autogenous transplantation in which the avulsed or extracted tooth is returned to its original alveolus. Reimplantation of avulsed or partially avulsed teeth with incompletely formed roots and with or without a concomitant fracture of the surrounding alveolar bone may be undertaken in many cases. Proper splinting is essential in retaining the reimplanted tooth in the dental arch, although in some cases the reimplanted tooth can be digitally repositioned in such a manner as to make further mechanical splinting unnecessary. Root canal therapy may become necessary if revascularization of the pulpal tissue does not occur postoperatively.

Immediate endodontic therapy is necessary in reimplantation surgery involving completely avulsed teeth with fully formed roots and in all cases in which considerable time has elapsed between the accidental avulsion of the teeth and the institution of treatment.

Of the dental transplantation procedures used at the present time, the autogenous grafting of the developing third molar appears to be the most successful. Good evidence supports the autogenous transplantation of the third molar tooth as a practical procedure in well-selected cases.

SUMMARY

Current and projected investigations of bone and tooth transplantation are directed toward solving clinical oral surgical problems that are immunological, anatomical, and physiological in nature. Research in these problem areas must of necessity bring to bear the work of other disciplines in evolving new and effective clinical procedures. Root resorption after both homogenous and autogenous tooth transplantation, rejection of chemically treated osseous xenografts, the response of grafted areas to occlusal and prosthetic function, and the determination of the optimal time and anatomical location for grafting are all problems that must be solved to evolve more efficacious oral surgical transplantation procedures of the future.

REFERENCES

1. Apfel, H.: Autoplasty of enucleated prefunctional third molars, J. Oral Surg. **8:**289, 1950.
2. Bach, F., and Hirschhorn, K.: Lymphocyte interaction: a potential histocompatibility test in vitro, Science **143:**813, 1964.
3. Bassett, C. A. L., and Creighton, D. K.: A comparison of host response to cortical autografts and processed calf heterografts, J. Bone Joint Surg. **44-A:**842, 1962.
4. Bassett, C. A. L., and Rüedi-Lindecker, A.: Bibliography of bone transplantation, Addendum No. VI, Transplantation **2:**668, 1964.
5. Beube, F. E.: Periodontology, diagnosis and treatment, New York, 1953, The Macmillan Co., p. 571.
6. Boyne, P. J.: Tooth transplantation procedures utilizing bone graft materials, J. Oral Surg. **19:**47, 1961.
7. Boyne, P. J.: Osseous repair of the postextraction alveolus in man, Oral Surg. **21:**805, 1966.
8. Boyne, P. J.: Review of the literature on the cryopreservation of bone, Cryobiology **4:**341, 1968.
9. Boyne, P. J.: Restoration of osseous defects in maxillofacial casualties, J. Am. Dent. Assoc. **78:**767, 1969.
10. Boyne, P. J.: Autogenous cancellous bone and marrow transplants, Clin. Orthop. **73:**199, 1970.
11. Boyne, P. J.: Transplantation, implantation and grafts, Dent. Clin. North Am. **15:**433, April, 1971.
12. Boyne, P. J., and Cooksey, D. E.: The use of cartilage and bone implants in restoration of edentulous ridges, J. Am. Dent. Assoc. **71:**1426, 1965.
13. Boyne, P. J., and Kruger, G. O.: Fluorescence microscopy of alveolar bone repair, Oral Surg. **15:**265, 1962.
14. Boyne, P. J., and Luke, A. B.: Host response to repetitive grafting of alveolar ridges with processed freeze-dried heterogenous bone, International Association for Dental Research, Abstracts of the Forty-Fifth General Meeting, Abstract No. 51, March, 1967.
15. Boyne, P. J., and Newman, M. G.: The effect of calcified bone matrix on the osteogenic potential of hematopoietic marrow, Oral Surg. **32:**506, 1971.
16. Boyne, P. J., and Pike, R. L.: The use of surface decalcified allogeneic bone in full mandibular grafting, International Association for Dental Research, Abstracts of the Fiftieth General Meeting, Abstract No. 251, March, 1972.
17. Boyne, P. J., and Sands, N. R.: Secondary bone grafting of residual alveolar and palatal clefts, J. Oral Surg. **30:**87, 1972.
18. Boyne, P. J., and Sands, N. R.: Combined orthodontic surgical management of residual palatoalveolar cleft defects, Am. J. Orthod. **70:**20-37, July, 1976.
19. Boyne, P. J., and Zarem, H.: Mandibular reconstruction of the resected mandible, Am. J. Surg. **132:**49-54, July, 1976.
20. Burwell, R. G.: Studies in the transplantation of bone. VII. The fresh composite homograft-autograft of cancellous bone, J. Bone Joint Surg. **46-B:**110, 1964.
21. Carnesale, P. G.: The bone bank, Bull. Hosp. Spec. Surg. **5:**76, 1962.
22. Chalmers, J.: Transplantation immunity in bone homografting, J. Bone Joint Surg. **41-B:**160, 1959.
23. Coburn, R. J., and Henriques, B. L.: The development of an experimental tooth bank using deep freeze and tissue culture techniques, J. Oral Ther. **2:**445, 1966.
24. Coburn, R. J., and Henriques, B. L.: Studies on the antigenicity of experimental intraoral tooth grafts, International Association for Dental Research, Abstracts of the Forty-Fourth General Meeting, Abstract No. 103, March, 1966.
25. Fong, C. C.: Autologous and homologous tooth transplantation, Seminar of Dental Tissue Transplantation, School of Dentistry, San Francisco, November, 1965, University of California at San Francisco, pp. 2-8.
26. Guilleminet, M., Stagnara, P., and Perret, T. D.: Preparation and use of heterogenous bone grafts. J. Bone Joint Surg. **35-B:**561, 1953.
27. Guyton, A. C.: Textbook of medical physiology, Philadelphia, 1961, W. B. Saunders Co., p. 174.
28. Hale, M. L.: Autogenous transplants, Oral Surg. **9:**76, 1956.
29. Hyatt, G. W.: The bone homograft—experimental and clinical applications, Symposium on Bone Graft Surgery. In The American Academy of Orthopaedic Surgeons Instructional Course Lectures, vol. 17, St. Louis, 1960, The C. V. Mosby Co.
30. Inclan, A.: The use of preserved bone grafts in orthopaedic surgery, J. Bone Joint Surg. **24:**81, 1942.
31. Ivanyi, D.: Immunologic studies on tooth germ transplantation, Transplantation **3:**572, 1965.
32. Kissmeyer-Nielsen, F., and Thorsby, E.: Transplantation antigens (HL-A) and histocompatibility testing, Transplant. Rev. **4:**25, 1970.
33. Kline, S. N.: Personal communication, 1972.
34. Kline, S. N., and Boyne, P. J.: Personal communication, 1977.
35. Kratochvil, F. J., Boyne, P. J., and Bump, R. L.: rehabilitation of grossly deficient mandibles with combined subperiosteal implants and bone grafts, J. Prosthet. Dent. **35:**452-461, April, 1976.
36. Losee, F. L., and Hurley, L. A.: Successful cross-species grafting accomplished by removal of donor organix matrix, NM004006.09.01, Report, Naval Med. Res. Inst. **14:**911, 1956.
37. Luke, A. B., and Boyne, P. J.: Histologic responses following autogenous osseous-dental transplantation, Oral Surg. **26:**861, 1968.

38. Maatz, R.: Clinical tests with protein-free heterogenous bone chips, Bull. Soc. Int. Chir. **19**:607, 1960.

39. Merrem: Adnimadversiones quaedam chirurgicae experimentes in animalibus factur illustratae, Giessae, 1810. Cited by Peer, L. A.: Transplantation of tissues, Baltimore, 1955, The Williams & Wilkins Co., p. 152.

40. Moss, M., Kruger, G. O., and Reynolds, D. C.: The effect of chondroitin sulfate in bone healing, Oral Surg. **20**:795, 1965.

41. Nahum, A. M., and Boyne, P. J.: Restoration of the mandible following partial resection, Trans. Am. Acad. Ophthalmol. Otolaryngol. **76**:957, 1972.

42. Orell, S.: Surgical bone grafting with "os purum," "os novum" and "boiled bone," J. Bone Joint Surg. **19**:873, 1937.

43. Osbon, D. B., Gilly, G. E., Thompson, C. W., and Jost, T.: Bone grafts with surface decalcified allogeneic and particulate autogenous bone, J. Oral Surg. **35**:276-284, April, 1977.

44. Peer, L. A.: Transplantation of tissue, Baltimore, 1959, The Williams & Wilkins Co., vol. 2, p. 41.

45. Pike, R. L., and Boyne, P. J.: The use of composite autogenous marrow and surface decalcified allogeneic bone (SDAB) grafts in mandibular defects, J. Oral Surg. **31**:905-912, December, 1973.

46. Pike, R. L., and Boyne, P. J.: The use of surface-decalcified allogenic bone and autogenous marrow in extensive mandibular defects, J. Oral Surg. **32**:177-182, March, 1974.

47. Rappaport, I., Boyne, P. J., and Nethery, J.: The particulate graft in tumor surgery, Am. J. Surg. **122**:748, 1971.

48. Reynolds, F. C., Oliver, D. R., and Ramsey, R.: Clinical evaluation of the merthiolate bone bank and homogenous bone grafts, J. Bone Joint Surg. **33-A**:873, 1951.

49. Shira, R. B., and Frank, O. M.: Treatment of nonunion of mandibular fractures by intraoral insertion of homogenous bone chips, J. Oral Surg. **13**:306, 1955.

50. Shulman, L. B.: The transplantation antigenicity of tooth homografts, Oral Surg. **17**:389, 1964.

51. Shulman, L. B.: The current status of allogeneic tooth transplantation, Proceedings of the CIBA Foundation Symposium on Hard Tissue Repair and Remineralization, Amsterdam, 1973, Excerpta Medica.

52. Siffert, R. S.: Delayed bone transplantation, J. Bone Joint Surg. **43-A**:407, 1961.

53. Silverstein, A. M., and Kraner, K. L.: The role of circulating antibody in the rejection of homografts, Transplantation **3**:535, 1965.

54. Staelinga, P. J. W., Tideman, H., Berger, J. S., and deKoomen, H. A.: Interpositional bone graft augmentation of the atrophic mandible, J. Oral Surg. **36**:30-32, January, 1978.

55. Terasaki, P. I., Mandell, M., Van de Water, J., and others: Human blood lymphocyte cytotoxicity reactions with allogenic antisera, Ann. N.Y. Acad. Sci. **120**:332, 1964.

56. Terasaki, P. I., and McClelland, J. D.: Microdroplet assay of human serum cytotoxins, Nature **204**:998, 1964.

57. Valente, L. J., and Shulman, L. B.: Transplantation immunity to a single subcutaneously implanted tooth in mice, International Association for Dental Research, Abstracts of Forty-Fourth General Meeting, Abstract No. 107, March, 1966.

58. Weinreb, M. M., Sharav, Y., and Ickowicz, M.: Behavior and fate of transplanted tooth buds. I. Influence of bone from different sites on tooth bud autografts, Transplantation **5**:379, 1967.

59. Wilson, P. D.: Experiences with a bone bank, Ann. Surg. **126**:932, 1947.

CHAPTER 17

Wounds and injuries of the soft tissues of the facial area

Robert B. Shira

GENERAL CONSIDERATIONS

Trauma to the facial area produces a variety of injuries. These injuries may be simple and limited to the soft tissues, or they may be complex and involve the underlying skeletal structures. Of all injuries, none perhaps is of more concern to the patient than those involving the facial region. All efforts therefore should be directed toward restoration of the injured parts to normal or as near normal as possible. Regardless of the type of wound encountered, early care is of the utmost importance to ensure restoration of normal function and prevent facial disfigurement.

Wounds involving the soft tissues of the facial area are commonplace. In the past, the more severe wounds were encountered as the result of gunshot fire and implements of war. With the advent of the modern automobile, however, a devastating instrument has been placed in the hands of the public, and transportation accidents are occurring with increasing frequency. Injuries resulting from these accidents are severe and complex, and, with the exception of the loss of tissue, they often approximate the type of injury seen in war.

The use of power tools, such as chain saws, which has become popular in recent years, presents another means of inflicting severe soft tissue injuries on the facial areas.

Care of soft tissue injuries of the face is usually performed in the emergency rooms of hospitals by the assigned personnel. The oral surgeon, however, should be capable of rendering treatment for this type of injury. If he or she should be the only one available, the oral surgeon should certainly accept the responsibility for the early correct management of the facial wound. In times of war or civilian catastrophe, training in this field would prove of great value. In this age of thermonuclear warfare, with attack on large population centers an ever-present possibility, casualties would undoubtedly be produced in such catastrophic numbers that care of facial injuries might well be the responsibility of the oral surgeon. Although it is realized that in normal circumstances care of the facial soft tissue injuries might not be delegated to the oral surgeon, he or she should nonetheless be capable of proper management of these wounds should the occasion arise.

Unless the soft tissue injuries are associated with intracranial injuries, fractures of the skull, or other serious injuries, even severe facial wounds are usually not destructive to life. Therefore, initial attention should be directed to any concomitant condition that, if uncorrected, would have serious consequences. It has often been said, "It is better to have an asymmetrical body than a symmetrical corpse." First priority should therefore be given, when indicated, to such lifesaving procedures as establishment and maintenance of a patent airway, arrest of hemorrhage, recognition and treatment of shock, recognition of associated head injuries, and treatment of intra-abdominal or thoracic wounds. These injuries are frequently of such severity that unless they are corrected early, the patient may die. Although facial wounds are important and should be treated as soon as possible, their management cannot take precedence over these lifesaving procedures.

When the general condition of the patient has stabilized and his life is no longer endangered, attention should be directed to the soft tissue wounds of the face. Open wounds in this area should be cleansed and closed as soon as possible, since conclusive evidence shows that early closure of these wounds is desirable. Wounds that are debrided and closed within the first 24 hours do much better, and results from an esthetic, functional, and psychological standpoint far exceed any result possible when treatment is delayed. Early closure seals off the pathways of infection and promotes rapid healing, which keeps scar tissue and contracture at a minimum. It also reduces the need for nursing care, improves the patient's morale, and permits an early return to a satisfactory method of feeding.

CLASSIFICATION OF WOUNDS

Various types of soft tissue wounds are encountered, and a classification is indicated because of the individual management problems associated with various wounds.

Contusion

A contusion is a bruise, usually produced by an impact from a blunt object without breaking the skin (Fig. 17-1). It affects the skin and subcutaneous tissue and usually causes a subcutaneous hemorrhage that is self-limiting in nature. Ecchymosis usually becomes evident in approximately 48 hours.

Abrasion

An abrasion is a wound produced by the rubbing or scraping off of the covering surface (Fig. 17-1). It results from friction, is usually superficial, and produces a raw, bleeding surface.

Laceration

A laceration is a wound resulting from a tear. It is the soft tissue wound most frequently encountered and is usually produced by some sharp object such as metal or glass (Fig. 17-1). It may be shallow or deep and may involve underlying vessels and nerves. When caused by a sharp object leaving a clean-cut wound with sharp mar-

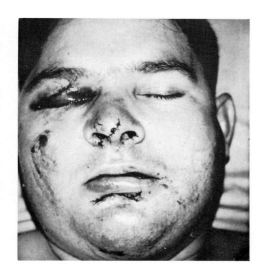

Fig. 17-1. Facial injuries that include a contusion of the right eye, an abrasion of the right cheek, and lacerations of the eyelids, nose, and lower lip. (Walter Reed Army Hospital.)

gins, this type of wound is referred to as an "incised" wound.

Penetrating wound

Penetrating wounds are usually puncture-type wounds produced by a sharp object, such as a knife, ice pick, or nail. They are usually deep and frequently involve other structures, such as the mouth, nose, or maxillary sinus. They may be small or large, depending on the object producing the wound.

Gunshot, missile, and war wounds

These wounds are in reality penetrating wounds but are usually classified separately because of the extensiveness of the wounds and the specialized problems encountered in their management. They are often further classified as penetrating wounds when the missile is retained in the wound, perforating wounds when the missile produces a wound of exit, and avulsive wounds when large portions of the soft or osseous structures are carried away or destroyed. These wounds are produced by gunshot, shrapnel, or other projectiles (Fig. 17-2). They vary greatly in character, depending on the speed, shape, and striking angle of the pro-

jectile. High-velocity bullets usually cause small wounds of entrance and large, ragged wounds of exit. When the bullet strikes bone or teeth, fragmentation of these structures frequently occurs, producing secondary missiles that cause extensive internal trauma. Low-velocity projectiles often become distorted on meeting resistance and cause marked comminution and internal destruction of the wound. Great tissue disorganization with associated fractures of the underlying skeleton and involvement of other facial structures, such as the eyes, nose, oral cavity, and maxillary sinus, are characteristic of these wounds. Shrapnel and blasts produce multiple penetrating wounds with the projectile frequently becoming distorted and scattered throughout the wound. Although marked comminution of bone is seen in this type of wound, much less traumatic loss of the soft and osseous tissue is experienced. Multiple metallic foreign bodies are retained in the wound. Gross contamination is present in all these wounds. Fragments of clothing, dirt, metal, and other debris are often carried deep into the wounds and frequently result in infections of serious proportions.

Burns

Burns often involve the soft tissues of the face. They are caused by contact with flames, hot liquids, hot metals, steam, acids, alkalies, roentgen rays, electricity, sunlight, ultraviolet light, and irritant gases. Burns are classified as *first degree,* which produces an erythema of the skin; *second degree,* which produces vesicle formation; and *third degree,* which causes complete destruction of the epidermis and dermis, extending into or beyond the subcutaneous tissue.

TREATMENT OF WOUNDS
General considerations

When trauma and wounding are inflicted, at least four major phenomena develop that may threaten life unless measures are instituted to control and finally correct the conditions. First, blood is lost, not only to

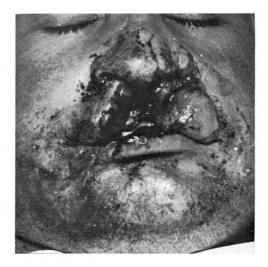

Fig. 17-2. Gunshot wound involving the lips, nose, and oral cavity. (Letterman Army Hospital.)

the exterior, but also into the damaged tissue. Second, tissue is damaged, with derangement of the physiology of the tissue and production of a suitable medium for bacterial growth. Third, the defense against bacteria is broken, which allows the wounds to become contaminated by bacterial invasion of the tissues. Fourth, mechanical defects may develop. These defects may be of major proportion, such as blockage of the airway, hemothorax, pneumothorax, cardiac tamponade, or increased intracranial pressure, or they may be minor problems, such as defects of the soft tissues. These four factors frequently are not limited to the traumatized area alone but may provoke a response in every system of the body. The more severe the injury, the more pronounced will be the systemic response.

Nature has provided the body with an efficient and effective healing response to these major phenomena. Immediately after injury, vasoconstriction, coagulation of the blood, and retraction of blood vessels tend to arrest the local hemorrhage. Damaged, nonvital tissue becomes necrotic and produces a slough that tends to rid the wound of damaged tissue. Wound contamination produces an antibody and leukocytic response that combats the invasion of infectious organisms. Finally, tissue defects may be corrected by proliferation of capillaries, fibroblasts, and epithelium. These natural reparative processes are often sufficient to bring about healing of minor wounds, but in the larger and more complicated wounds, surgical procedures are indicated to complement and assist these natural healing processes. The surgeon's aim should be to aid the body's healing response, and this chapter will deal with the surgical procedures involved in treatment of the specific types of wounds encountered in the facial areas.

Treatment of contusions

Contusions are minor injuries and treatment should be conservative. It consists for the most part of observation, and seldom are definitive measures necessary. Hemorrhage is usually self-limiting as pressure of the extravasated blood builds up within the tissues. The tissue usually remains viable, so necrosis and sloughing are absent. Since the trauma is produced by a blunt force, the skin is usually not broken and contamination and infection of the wound are seldom seen. No tissue defect results from this type of injury, and as the hematoma resorbs, normal contour and function are restored. Because of the hemorrhage in the deeper structures, the contused area first turns blue and later yellow. In this type of wound, nature's reparative processes are usually sufficient to produce complete resolution without surgical intervention. Surgical intervention is indicated only to control hemorrhage that does not stop spontaneously, to evacuate a hematoma that does not resolve, or to suture a superimposed laceration. These complications are rarely encountered.

Treatment of abrasions

Abrasions, being caused by friction, are superficial wounds involving varying amounts of the surface. They are usually painful, since removal of the covering epithelium leaves nerve endings in the subcutaneous tissues exposed. Hemorrhage is no problem because major vessels are not involved, and the involved capillaries retract and are occluded by thrombi. The tissue damage is superficial, and necrosis and sloughing usually do not occur. These wounds occasionally become infected but are so superficial that local therapy is usually sufficient to control the infectious process. If the wound does not extend below the level of the rete pegs of the epithelium, healing without mechanical defect or scarring can be anticipated.

Minimal treatment is indicated for the abraded wound. It should be thoroughly cleansed by mechanical scrubbing with one of the surgical detergent soaps, followed by an antiseptic solution such as benzalkonium (Zephiran). A dressing is usually not required, since an eschar that serves to protect the wound forms rapidly. Epithelization rapidly occurs beneath the eschar, and healing without scar formation is the rule. Occasionally an infection develops under the eschar. When this occurs, the eschar must be removed to permit access to the infected area. Local application of one of the aniline dyes or antibiotic preparations, together with continued mechanical cleansing, is usually sufficient to control the infection. Systemic or parenteral antibiotic therapy is seldom necessary for this type of wound.

Prevention of traumatic tattoo. Abrasions are often produced by traumatic episodes that cause dirt, cinders, or other debris to be ground into the tissue. It is extremely important that these foreign bodies be removed, particularly if they are pigmented. If allowed to remain in the wound, a traumatic tattoo will result that produces an unsightly defect (Fig. 17-3). These particles should be removed by mechanical cleansing. The surrounding area should be cleansed with one of the detergent soaps and then isolated by sterile towels. A local anesthetic solution is then injected and the involved area meticulously scrubbed with a detergent soap on sterile gauze. Frequent

irrigation of the field with sterile saline solution aids in washing the particles from the wound. If the particles are firmly imbedded, it may be necessary to substitute a stiff brush for the gauze, and, frequently a sharp-pointed instrument must be utilized to remove the particles from the tissue. A dental spoon excavator is ideal for this procedure. Recently the use of an electric dermabrader for the removal of large areas of imbedded particles has been recommended. The dermabrader must be held perfectly parallel to the skin while the skin is stretched taut by the assistant to prevent gouging. The procedure is tedious and time-consuming, but the importance of the removal of these particles cannot be overemphasized. The golden opportunity is at the time of original treatment, for if allowed to heal in the wound, their removal at a subsequent time poses a difficult problem.

After this mechanical cleansing, a wound resembling a second-degree burn is produced. This may be left open, but it frequently requires the application of a dressing. Thin mesh gauze applied to the wound and then covered with tincture of benzoin forms a good protective dressing, although petrolatum or scarlet red gauze may also be used.

Treatment of lacerations

Early primary closure. Lacerations constitute the most common of the facial injuries and vary from superficial cuts to deep, complex wounds involving underlying body cavities. Whenever possible, these wounds should be treated within a few hours of the injury, and seldom is a patient so severely injured that early closure of the facial lacerations cannot be accomplished. Even though these wounds may be grossly contaminated, primary closure early within the first 24 hours is preferred to the radical excision of suspected tissue and the open treatment of the resultant wound as recommended for wounds of other parts of the body (Fig. 17-4). Successful closure of facial lacerations requires meticulous atten-

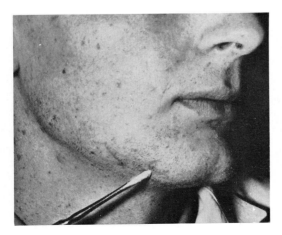

Fig. 17-3. Traumatic tattoo resulting from impregnation of the skin with multiple metallic foreign bodies. (Letterman Army Hospital.)

tion to detail and depends on complete cleansing of the wound, adequate debridement, complete hemostasis, proper closure of the wound, and adequate supportive therapy.

CLEANSING OF THE WOUND. After local or general anesthesia has been obtained, mechanical cleansing of the wound is necessary. The skin about the wound should be scrubbed with a surgical detergent soap, and occasionally ether or one of the other solvents may be needed to remove grease or other foreign substances. The wound is then isolated with sterile towels and scrubbed vigorously. A constant stream of water applied by an Asepto or similar syringe assists in washing the debris from the wound. All areas should be investigated and cleansed, and any foreign bodies encountered should be removed. Great care in the removal of superficial pigmented foreign bodies to prevent a traumatic tattoo is again emphasized. If hematomas are found, they should be re-

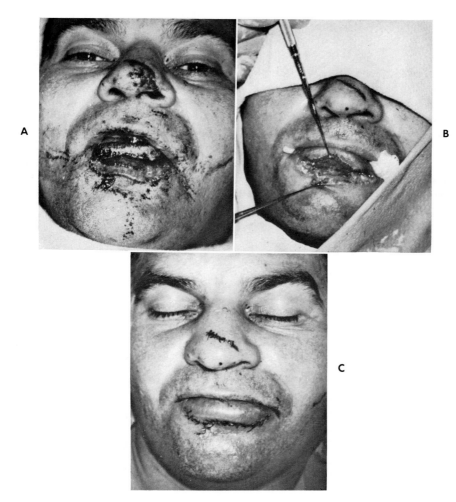

Fig. 17-4. A, Laceration of the lower lip 6 hours after injury. This is an ideal situation for early primary closure. **B,** Wound after cleansing and conservative debridement. **C,** Laceration closed by early primary suture. (Walter Reed Army Hospital.)

moved, since an ideal culture medium for infectious organisms will be produced if they are allowed to remain. Hydrogen peroxide flushed through the wound is of value in eliminating the hematomas (Fig. 17-4, *B*).

DEBRIDEMENT. After the wound has been thoroughly cleansed, the area is redraped, and a conservative debridement is performed. The facial structures are richly supplied with blood and appear to possess a resistance to infection seen in few other tissues. Radical debridement is therefore not indicated. Only the necrotic, obviously nonviable tissue need be removed. It is occasionally difficult to differentiate between viable and nonviable tissue. Bleeding from a cut surface or contracture of a muscle when stimulated is evidence of viability, but when in doubt about viability, conservatism is recommended. Rough, irregular, ragged, or macerated margins should be excised to diminish the ultimate amount of scar formation. Lacerations that have been cut on the oblique require excision of the edges of the skin so that the margins will be perpendicular to the skin surface (Fig. 17-4, *B*).

HEMOSTASIS. Control of hemorrhage in lacerated wounds is essential. Nature provides a degree of hemostasis by vasoconstriction and thrombi formation, but hemorrhage from larger vessels or from the debrided surfaces of the wound must be controlled. Vessels that persist in bleeding are clamped and tied with ligatures. No. 2-0 or 3-0 absorbable or silk ligatures may be used for the ties. Care in grasping the cut ends of vessels to avoid inclusion of excessive amounts of subcutaneous tissue will limit the amount of scar formation. An alternate procedure for smaller bleeding points is to clamp the bleeding point with a hemostat and touch the instrument with the high-frequency coagulation current. Hemostasis must be complete, and the wound should be carefully inspected for frank hemorrhage or seepage of blood. No primary suturing is indicated until complete hemostasis has been secured.

CLOSURE OF THE WOUND. After the wound has been cleansed and debrided and hemostasis has been achieved, the wound is ready for closure. The objective of closure is accurate coaptation of the layers of tissue with elimination of all dead spaces. Lacerations of the face that lie parallel to the lines of skin relaxation may be expected to heal in a favorable fashion with minimal skin closure. If lacerations transect these lines at right angles, immediate Z-plasty may be performed to prevent scar contracture. The

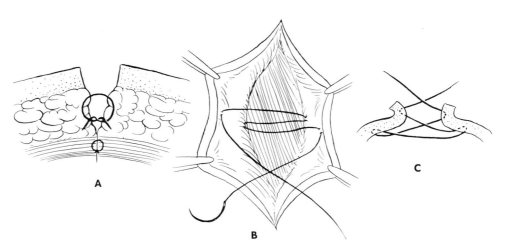

Fig. 17-5, A, Inverted buried sutures for closure of the deeper structures. **B** and **C,** Gillies' near-far far-near relaxing suture, which is valuable in relieving tension on the skin margins.

tissues should be handled gently, by use of tissue hooks rather than forceps whenever possible. If the wound involves the mucosa, this structure should be accurately reapproximated as the first step. An attempt to form a watertight seal of the mucosa by interrupted No. 4-0 or 5-0 nonabsorbable sutures is made. Polyglycolic acid sutures (Dexon), which are made of a slowly re-

sorbable material, may also be used. This is especially advantageous for closure of intraoral lacerations associated with maxillary or mandibular fractures in which removal of sutures would be difficult if not impossible because the patient's mouth is closed by maxillomandibular fixation.

If at all possible, any fractures of the facial bones that may be present should be reduced at this time before completing the closure of the soft tissue. If the soft tissue wounds are closed first, the subsequent manipulative procedures necessary for reduction of the fractures frequently cause a disruption of the soft tissue wound. After the fractures are reduced, deeper muscle and subcutaneous layers are closed by inverted buried interrupted sutures, with care being taken to eliminate all dead spaces (Fig. 17-5). If tension appears to be affecting the wound, the employment of the Gillies[17] near-far, far-near relaxing suture will aid in approximating the subcutaneous tissue and in relieving the tension on the skin (Fig. 17-5). Chromic gut or No. 3-0 silk sutures are utilized for the closure of the deeper layers.

The final step in closure of the subcutaneous tissues is the placement of fine subcuticular sutures just beneath the cutaneous

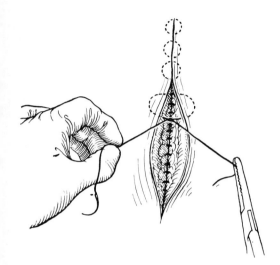

Fig. 17-6. Fine subcuticular sutures beneath the skin, which accurately reapproximate the subcutaneous tissues.

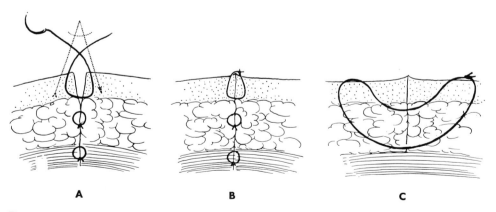

A **B** **C**

Fig. 17-7. A, Interrupted skin sutures are placed after deep layers have been closed. **B,** Eversion of the skin margins should be produced with interrupted skin sutures. **C,** Vertical mattress suture is a useful adjunct in obtaining the proper eversion of the skin margins.

surface (Fig. 17-6). These sutures should accurately reapproximate the subcutaneous tissues and relieve all tension of the skin margins. If any undue tension is encountered, undermining of the skin may be necessary prior to placement of the subcuticular sutures. Plain gut or polyglycolic acid sutures are most commonly used for subcuticular closure. The skin is approximated by No. 4-0 or 5-0 silk or Dermalon interrupted sutures placed in adequate numbers to ensure apposition. Sutures should be placed at equal distance and equal depth on either side of the wound. They should be placed in such a manner that a slight eversion of the skin margins is produced (Fig. 17-7). Interrupted sutures will produce this eversion if properly placed. An occasional vertical mattress suture, however, may be necessary as supplementary support (Fig. 17-7).

Little difficulty is encountered in closing the small or moderately large wounds by this method, particularly if no tissue has been lost. In suturing extensive, complicated lacerations, it may be difficult to determine the proper position of the tissues. In these instances a start should be made at a known point, such as the corner of the mouth, ala of the nose, or the corner of the eye (Fig. 17-8). Each remaining segment is then bisected with a suture until closure is complete. Key surface sutures at these points may be necessary. These may be placed deep into the tissue but should never be placed far from the wound margins, since wide placement is conducive to unsightly scar formation. Fine subcuticular sutures placed between the key sutures will approximate the subcutaneous structures before insertion of the skin sutures. Larger wounds in which no key points are involved may also present difficulties in realignment. Such wounds should be managed by placing a key suture in the center, dividing the wound in half. Each half is then bisected until final closure is accomplished.

Delayed primary closure. For various reasons all lacerated wounds cannot be treated within the initial safe period for primary closure. Such wounds become edematous, indurated, and infected, and early primary closure should not be attempted (Fig. 17-9, *A*). A program of wound preparation should be instigated and followed by a delayed primary closure when conditions are suitable. Chipps and associates[7] have outlined an excellent regimen for the preparation of

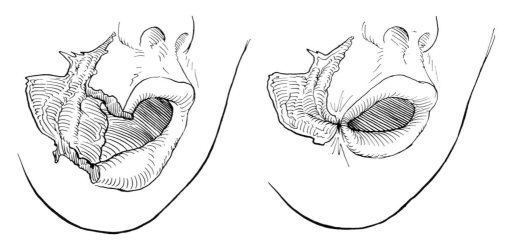

Fig. 17-8. Diagrams that illustrate the principle of starting at a known point, in this instance the corner of the mouth, in suturing large lacerations.

wounds for secondary closure, and their observations stem from vast experience gained at Tokyo Army Hospital during the Korean conflict. The regimen they recommend includes an initial examination and debridement, at which time all obvious devitalized and infected tissues are removed. Concomitant fractures of the facial bones, if present, should then be immobilized. Adequate drainage should be maintained, and an effective and specific antibiotic regimen employed to combat any infection that may be present. Continuous moist dressings applied to the injured tissues assist greatly in preparing the tissues for closure. The wounds should be observed daily, and when necrotic areas are discovered, they should be removed by tissue forceps. Wounds involving the oral cavity should be isolated and oral feeding prohibited to eliminate contamination and fermenting food debris from entering the wound. To accomplish this, feeding by a Levin tube is usually employed. This regimen rapidly controls infection, reduces edema and induration, and renders the wound amenable to delayed primary suture in 5 to 10 days. The wounds are then closed as described under initial primary closure. Success depends on how well the surgeon adheres to the surgical procedures previously described (Fig. 17-9, *B*).

Supportive therapy. The successful treatment of wounds requires consideration of several other factors such as the need for drains, the type of dressing, and the prevention or treatment of various infections.

DRAINS. Superficial lacerations do not require drainage. Deeper wounds, however, particularly those involving the oral cavity, should have a Penrose or rubber dam drain inserted. This allows the escape of serum and tissue fluids and prevents the collection of these substances in deeper structures. Drains may be placed between the sutures or through a stab incision approximating the original wound. Drains should be removed in 2 to 4 days.

DRESSINGS. After suturing, some type of protective dressing is indicated. Small wounds may be covered by fine-mesh gauze, which is then painted with collodion and allowed to dry. Larger wounds require a secure pressure dressing. This dressing should offer tissue support and exert sufficient pressure on the tissue to prevent additional bleeding or the collection of fluid in the subcutaneous areas. A strip of fine-mesh

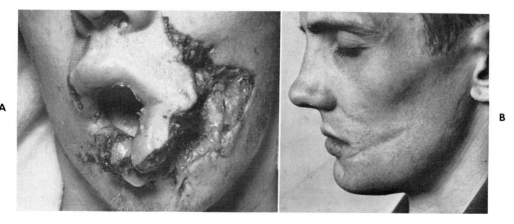

Fig. 17-9. A, Facial laceration as it appeared 11 days after injury. Note the sloughing, edema, and induration. This wound was treated by delayed primary closure. **B,** Six months after delayed primary closure. (Letterman Army Hospital.)

gauze or nylon is usually placed over the sutured wound, and then gauze fluffs, reinforced by elastoplast, are added. Ace bandages, followed by adhesives tape, are applied to exert moderate pressure on the wound. Dressings should be changed in 48 hours. Sutures are removed on the fourth or fifth day, and a collodion dressing is placed over the wound for another 3 or 4 days.

PREVENTION OF INFECTION. All lacerated wounds are contaminated and infected by the time they are seen for treatment. Although this infection is frequently subclinical, efforts should be made to keep the infection at a minimum and to eliminate it as soon as possible. This is accomplished by strict adherence to sterile techniques, thorough cleansing of the tissue, complete hemostasis, conservative but adequate debridement, wound closure that eliminates all dead spaces, and adequate supportive care. This supportive care includes the intelligent utilization of antibiotics or chemotherapy or both. Prophylactic utilization of these substances is indicated in all major wounds as a safeguard against infection.

PROPHYLAXIS AGAINST TETANUS. Because all wounds of the face are contaminated and are often produced by accidents that force dirt and debris into the wound, protection against infection by the *Clostridium tetani* organism must be provided. This is particularly true of laceration, puncture, and gunshot wounds. Tetanus infections are so catastrophic and have such a high mortality rate that if any possibility exists of a wound being contaminated by this organism, active prophylaxis must be provided.

Tetanus is a relatively easy disease to prevent. Active immunization has proved to be both effective in prevention and long lasting. In a large segment of the population, an active immunity against tetanus has been developed as a result of inoculation with alum-precipitated toxoid in three subcutaneous doses of 0.5 ml each. The second dose is given 6 weeks following the first dose and the third dose, 6 to 12 months after

the second dose. Active immunization is effective for a minimum of 1 year, and a repeat booster dose of 0.5 ml of tetanus toxoid given any time within the next 10 years will provide a rapid rise in antitoxin titer.

Tetanus toxoid alone is of little value in those patients in whom no active immunization exists by prior prophylactic inoculation with tetanus toxoid. In these patients passive immunity may be provided using human antitetanus globulin by intramuscular injection of 250 units. Active immunity should then be established immediately by the regimen described previously.

Antibiotics such as penicillin and tetracycline are effective against vegetative tetanus bacilli; however, they have no effect against toxin. The effectiveness of antibiotics for prophylaxis remains unproved, and if used, they should be given for at least 5 days.

FAILURES IN PRIMARY CLOSURE. Whereas the majority of lacerated wounds heal by primary intention without complications, some do break down. Chipps and co-workers[7] report that 30% of facial wounds observed at Tokyo Army Hospital during the Korean conflict failed to heal by primary intention. In an analysis of these cases, they found that six major factors were responsible for this wound breakdown. These were (1) tight closure of the wound without provision for deep tissue drainage, (2) inadequate use of pressure dressings, (3) failure to close the mucosa on the oral surface of the wound, (4) secondary hemorrhage, (5) secondary manipulation of the repaired wound, and (6) inadequate antibiotic therapy. It is obvious that these problems in wound disruption stem primarily from failure to meticulously apply the standard surgical principles of wound treatment. If these principles are strictly adhered to, failure will be kept to a minimum.

For breakdown of small lacerations, conservative management consisting of frequently changed saline-moistened gauze dressings and healing by secondary intention may suffice. In wounds in which breakdown leads to unsightly scar formation or deformation of adjacent tissues, a secondary plastic procedure may be performed but only after complete healing and revascularization have occurred.

Treatment of puncture type of penetrating wounds

Most objects producing wounds to facial areas also produce lacerations, so the isolated puncture wound is rarely seen in this region. When it does occur, the wound of entrance is usually small but may penetrate deeply into the underlying tissue and involve the mouth, nose, or maxillary sinus. This type of wound is dangerous in that it may carry infection deep into the tissue, and the possibility of tetanus infection is always present.

Treatment should be conservative and directed primarily at the control of infection. The wound should be thoroughly irrigated and cleansed under sterile conditions. Hemostasis usually presents no problem because the bleeding stops spontaneously unless larger vessels are involved. Excision of the wound is not usually indicated, since it would require a wide incision to expose and explore the depths of the wound and the resultant scarring would be objectionable. Debridement is not indicated with most wounds of this type, and unless an infection complicates the wound, necrosis and sloughing are rare. Measures to control infection are of primary interest, with particular emphasis being given to prophylaxis against tetanus. The wound should not be closed by primary suture but should be allowed to remain open to heal by granulation. Because of the small wound of entrance, healing usually occurs with little deformity. If an unsightly scar or depression results, it should be managed as a secondary procedure after complete healing and revascularization have taken place.

Treatment of gunshot, missile, and war wounds

Injuries produced by gunshot and other missiles traveling at varying speeds will be considered together, since the resulting wounds present the same problems. These wounds are only occasionally seen in civilian practice, but they become an immediate and major problem in time of war. With the changing pattern of warfare and the possibility of mass casualties resulting from thermonuclear attacks, wounds resulting from missiles and other flying projectiles assume new importance. As seen with lacerations, these wounds vary considerably in extent and character. Many appear hopeless at first sight, but surprising results are usually obtainable by careful surgical technique.

In no other type of facial wound is attention to emergency lifesaving procedures so important. Since these wounds are usually extensive, first attention must be given to the general condition of the patient, and measures to ensure an adequate airway, arrest of hemorrhage, and control of shock must be instigated. The very nature of these wounds produces conditions that tend to interfere with the upper respiratory passages, and if not corrected early, they may lead to disastrous consequences. If any doubt exists as to the ability to maintain a patent airway by conservative methods, no hesitancy should delay the performing of a tracheostomy. Control of hemorrhage is usually not a major problem. Although the facial areas are well supplied with blood vessels, they are mostly small in caliber and well supplied with elastic fibers, and when severed, they retract into bony canals and are occluded by thrombi. The searing action of the missile itself occludes many of the vessels. If hemorrhage becomes a problem, pressure to the bleeding area is usually sufficient to control the bleeding; however, on occasion it may be necessary to clamp and ligate larger vessels. Shock is not a constant finding but is observed in the more severe injuries. When encountered, hemorrhage must be arrested and the blood volume restored as soon as possible to prevent the condition of shock from progressing to its irreversible stage. Surgery can usually be performed as soon as the blood pressure and pulse become stabilized at the desired levels. Neurological disorders must be recognized and carefully evaluated before instigation of treatment. As a rule, treatment of the soft tissue may be started when the vital signs have stabilized.

The method of treatment depends on the problems encountered in each individual case. Gunshot wounds in civilian practice usually receive definitive treatment within a matter of hours, whereas definitive treatment of war wounds may be early or markedly delayed. Regardless of which situation exists, when certain fundamental principles are followed, satisfactory results may be obtained.

Whenever possible, this type of wound should be managed by early primary closure. A general policy of working from the inside out should be followed. Wounds involving the maxillary sinus, palate, and tongue should be sutured first, followed by suturing of the oral mucosa. Associated fractures should then be reduced and im-

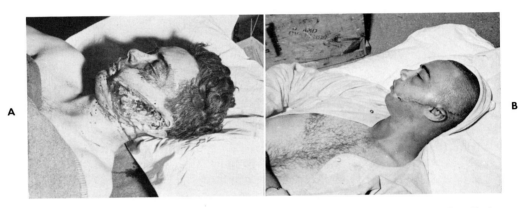

Fig. 17-10. Gunshot wound treated by early primary closure. **A,** Preoperative condition. **B,** Appearance 10 days after operation. (AFIP 55-321-641-47.)

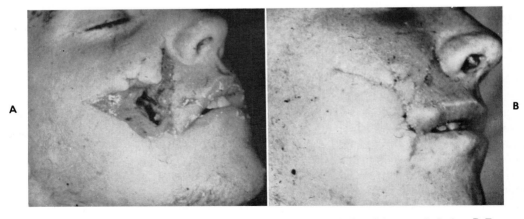

Fig. 17-11. Gunshot wound treated by delayed primary closure. **A,** Condition on admission. **B,** Ten days after operation. (Courtesy Colonel James E. Chipps.)

mobilized, followed by closure of the soft tissue wound (Fig. 17-10).

Unfortunately not all gunshot and missile wounds can be treated early, and many are seen after edema, necrosis, and gross infection are present. Perhaps in no other group of wounds is the delayed primary suturing after a period of wound preparation more effective. By adequate wound cleansing, debridement, utilization of continuous moist dressings, and control of infections, these wounds may be prepared for closure in from 5 to 10 days. The wound is ready for suturing when the edema and

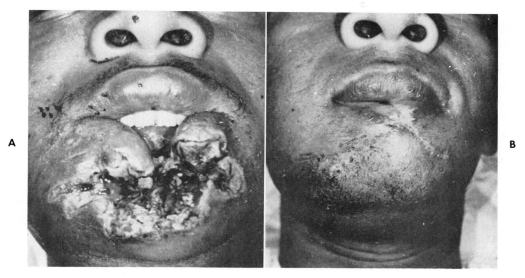

Fig. 17-12. Avulsive wound with moderate loss of soft tissue and bone. An acrylic splint was utilized to stabilize the bony fragments and restore facial contour before the soft tissue was sutured over the defect. **A,** Condition on admission. **B,** Restoration of an acceptable facial contour. (Courtesy Colonel James E. Chipps.)

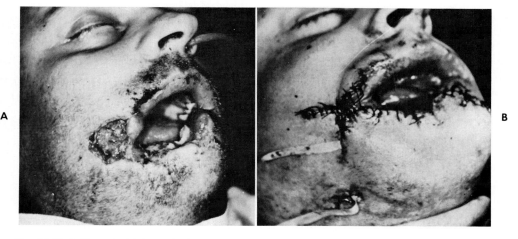

Fig. 17-13. A, Wound with loss of substance at lower lip and corner of mouth. **B,** Suture of mucous membrane to skin. (Courtesy Colonel James E. Chipps.)

inflammation have subsided, when the suppuration has ceased, and when healthy granulation tissue is present. Wound edges containing the granulation tissue are excised and the tissues sutured in layers as described earlier in this chapter (Fig. 17-11).

Not all gunshot and missile wounds can be closed by primary or delayed primary suture. The large avulsive-type wounds, particularly those in which considerable loss of osseous structures has occurred, are not amenable to this procedure. If closed primarily, such wounds may show marked distortion of the remaining tissue and produce unsightly cosmetic defects. However, if the bony fragments can be immobilized in proper position or if an intraoral splint can be utilized to restore normal facial contour, either primary suturing or delayed primary suturing should be utilized if sufficient soft tissue is present. This practice will often produce an acceptable cosmetic result and reduce the number of reconstructive procedures needed later (Fig. 17-12). Avulsive wounds in which it is impossible to restore the normal facial contour by immobilization of fractures or utilization of intraoral splints or wounds with extensive loss of soft tissue must be handled differently. In such instances suturing the skin margins to the oral mucosa (Fig. 17-13) is an acceptable procedure. Reconstructive surgery to restore facial contour can be performed later.

Foreign bodies

Gunshot and missile-type injuries are often complicated by foreign bodies carried into the wound. These foreign bodies range from superficially located debris resulting from explosions and powder blasts to deeply penetrating bullets or metallic fragments of gunfire. They include such objects as pigmented debris, clothing, bullets, and splinters of metal, wood, glass, and stone. Fractured teeth and detached segments of bone may also act as foreign bodies. The question often arises as to the advisability of the removal of these objects. No rule applicable to all conditions can be set forth, but several fundamental principles are worthy of mention. The superficial blast-type of multiple foreign bodies should be removed within the first 24 hours to prevent the development of a traumatic tattoo (Fig. 17-14). Any foreign bodies encountered during the cleansing and debridement of the wound should, of course, be removed. This is particularly true of glass, gravel, wood, teeth, or unattached bone segments, because if they are allowed to remain, infection and delayed healing may result. Metallic bodies present a different problem. Many of these become fragmented and are often so widely scattered throughout the tissue that complete removal is virtually impossible. In evaluating metallic fragments in a wound, the possible deleterious effects of these objects must be weighed against the effect of the surgical procedure necessary for their removal. Many metallic fragments are sterile and will remain in the tissue indefinitely without injurious effect. An old adage often quoted is, "When a bul-

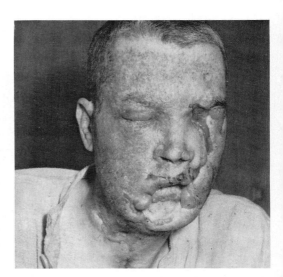

Fig. 17-14. Extensive traumatic tattoo resulting from a shrapnel blast. The metallic fragments are so deeply embedded in the tissue that a permanent tattoo will result. (AFIP B-688-D.)

let ceases to move, it ceases to do damage.'' Although this is not literally true, it is worth remembering. It is considered unwise to perform an extensive surgical procedure to remove these fragments if they are not readily accessible at the time of debridement. It is better to allow them to remain in the tissue, and if any complications develop, removal can be accomplished as a secondary procedure.

Gunshot, blast, and missile wounds are notoriously contaminated, and special precautions are indicated to prevent infection. Antibiotic therapy should be instituted as soon after injury as possible and continued until primary healing is complete. War wounds inflicted in the Korean conflict were for the most part badly contaminated, yet infection was rarely seen by the time the casualties arrived at definitive treatment centers in the United States. This is attributed to the fact that the patients were given antibiotic therapy soon after injury and maintained on this therapy until healing had occurred. If infection did develop, definitive bacteriology and antibiotic sensitivity tests were available to ensure that the proper antibiotic was being used. Tetanus is also an ever-present possibility, and prophylaxis against this infection must be provided. It must also be remembered that tetanus may be a late development in these wounds. Once the organisms are established, they are capable of forming spores that are highly resistant and may remain viable for years. They may lie dormant in the tissues and be activated by some secondary surgical procedure and produce typical tetanus infections. When secondary procedures are necessary on these previously contaminated wounds, it is wise to provide additional protection against this infection.

TREATMENT OF BURNS

The treatment of burns is usually not included in textbooks on oral surgery and rightly so, since the specialist in this field is seldom called on to treat this type of injury.

Because of the current emphasis on mass casualty care, however, and the need for all members of the healing arts to have basic knowledge of the problems that will be encountered in the event of a thermonuclear attack, brief coverage of burns of the facial region is included, with particular emphasis on initial treatment measures.

Burns are perhaps the most severe injuries to which man is exposed, and like so many of the injuries discussed previously, they may vary greatly in extent and severity. Their classification as first, second, and third degree burns depends on the depth of tissue involved. The severity of a burn wound can be estimated from the depth of the wound and the amount of the body surface involved. The deeper the wound and the greater the surface involved, the more severe the burn. Burns, like other wounds, invoke a systemic response that is proportional to the extent of the wound. It has been estimated that a burn of the entire face involves only approximately 3% of the body surface. Thus isolated burns of the face seldom produce a serious systemic reaction. The isolated facial burn, however, is the exception, since facial burns are usually associated with burns on other portions of the body. Collectively these wounds may produce systemic problems of major proportion; therefore, brief consideration of these problems must be given.

The major systemic problem is shock. Immediately after a burn injury a diminution of blood volume occurs as a result of the loss of fluid from the wound and into the interstitial spaces. This results in a hemoconcentration and a loss of colloids and electrolytes. Oligemic (hypovolemic) shock will occur unless the loss of blood volume is corrected. Consequently, therapy to prevent shock is of primary importance and consists of restoration of the normal blood volume, including colloids and electrolytes. The amount of fluid to be replaced is sometimes difficult to determine, and the exact ratio of colloids to electrolytes has not been determined. Use of the hemoglobin determination and hematocrit are of value in replacement therapy, and a workable estimate of replacement needs can usually be determined by knowing the patient's weight and the extent of the burned surface. The estimated need for replacement in the first 24 hours can be derived from the following formula:

> Colloid (blood, plasma, or plasma expander) = Percentage of body burned × Body weight × 0.25
>
> Electrolyte = Percentage of body burned × Body weight × 0.50
>
> Glucose in water = 2,000 ml

Requirements for the second 24 hours are half the amount of colloids and electrolytes estimated for the first 24 hours plus 2,000 ml of glucose in water. By the third day the moderately burned patient can usually be maintained on oral intake of fluids, whereas the severely burned patient will continue to require intravenous therapy, which should consist primarily of electrolyte-free water.

In addition to the loss of fluids and electrolytes, other systemic responses frequently occur. Destruction of red blood cells, certain endocrine abnormalities, as well as aberrations in protein and carbohydrate metabolism are encountered. It is obvious that the systemic involvement is of major concern in the overall treatment of the burned patient.

The burn wound varies with the depth of the injury. First degree burns first become blanched, and then an edema and erythema appear. Small intraepithelial blisters may form. In a few days the surface epithelium may slough, leaving a healthy granulating epithelium. Second degree burns rapidly produce vesicles and blisters that separate the epidermis into layers. Sloughing is more prominent than in first degree burns. Third degree burns produce complete destruction of all layers of the skin. Necrosis deep in the wound is seen, and suppuration is common. Sloughing occurs in approximately 2 weeks, leaving healthy red granulation tissue in the base of the wound.

Therapy

Treatment of the burned patient may be divided into two categories—supportive care and local care of the wound. Only the initial therapeutic measures and first-aid procedures will be considered.

In supportive care the prevention and treatment of shock are of primary importance. With minor burns, this problem is not encountered, but it is of major importance in extensive burns. Control of infection is important, and the aggressive use of prophylactic antibiotics is efficacious in prevention and control of infections. Grossly contaminated burn wounds also call for prophylaxis against tetanus.

Pain is a problem in the burned patient. This is usually controlled within a few days by the local treatment of the wound, but in the early periods, systemic sedation is indicated. This sedation should be administered with caution, particularly to the patient in shock, and doses should be kept to the minimum.

Thorough cleansing of the burned surface is the first consideration in the initial care of first and second degree burns. Bland soap and sterile water gently applied are usually sufficient to cleanse the wound, but occasionally some solvent is necessary to remove oil or grease. The wound is then debrided of all devitalized epithelium, and any vesicles or blisters are removed. Hemorrhage is not a problem in the burn wound, and infection at this initial stage is seldom encountered. Treatment from this point may utilize either the open or closed method. In the former the wound is left open without covering, and within 48 hours, a dry, firm, brownish eschar will form. This eschar protects the underlying wound, and unless infection develops, epithelization will proceed under this protective covering. If cracks in the eschar develop, it should be debrided for a short distance on either side and moistened fine-mesh gauze should be packed into the defects as a precaution against infection. The eschar will eventually fall off, leaving healthy healing tissue exposed.

In the closed method of burn therapy, after the wound has been cleansed and debrided, fine-mesh plain or petrolatum gauze is applied directly to the burned area. A large, occlusive-type dressing is then applied and supported by an elastic bandage reinforced with adhesive tape. This dressing affords protection to the open wound, prevents infection, and relieves pain. It is not necessary to redress the burned areas, except to change the outside bandages, until the wound is healed. If infection becomes a complication, the dressings must be changed, but if the wound has been thoroughly cleansed and the primary dressing is adequate, infection seldom occurs.

Local treatment of third degree burns that involve the full thickness of the skin is essentially the same as for second degree burns. After early cleansing and debridement, a dressing is applied, which is allowed to remain for 10 to 14 days. When the dressing is changed the necrotic, destroyed tissue can be removed with tissue forceps. If the wound becomes suppurative, the dressing will require changing before this time and local as well as parenteral antibiotic therapy should be employed. Third degree wounds should be treated as soon as possible by skin grafting. If no infection is present, grafting is possible when the necrotic tissue is removed. If this wound is allowed to heal by granulation, marked scarring with contracture and deformity will result.

Burns of the face do equally well with either the open or closed method of treatment. The open method is usually employed, but this has the disadvantage of pain during the first 48 hours while the eschar is forming. This pain can be controlled by sedation. Utilization of the closed method is sometimes difficult to apply to facial wounds because of the difficulty in maintaining pressure dressings on the face. If dressing changes become necessary, pain becomes a factor.

First-aid treatment depends a great deal on the extent and seriousness of the wound. For minor burns, which include most of the

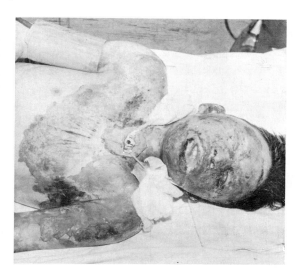

Fig. 17-15. Extensive burn of face that involves the oral cavity and upper respiratory passages. Tracheostomy was necessary to maintain a patent airway. (AFIP 56-8078.)

isolated burns of the face, local care of the wound and relief of pain are usually all that is necessary. Close observation of the patient is essential, and any signs of shock or other systemic reactions call for aggressive therapy. Prophylaxis against infection should be administered as indicated. Patients with severe burns should be hospitalized and replacement therapy started immediately. The burned surfaces may be treated by either the open or closed method, depending on the conditions encountered in each individual case.

One type of burn that presents a serious emergency is the flash or flame burn that involves the upper respiratory passages. Such burns often damage the mucosa of the respiratory tract, and the resultant edema may progress so rapidly that respiratory embarrassment and asphyxia may occur. In such an emergency, tracheostomy may be lifesaving (Fig. 17-15).

Burns in mass casualty care

In the case of mass casualties resulting from thermonuclear attack, burn injuries will undoubtedly constitute a major problem. They will result primarily from exposure to the flash of the explosion or from fires ignited by the explosion. In planning for the types of burn casualties from such an explosion, it has been convenient to divide them into four categories, depending on the magnitude and severity of the injury: self-care burns, moderate burns, severe burns, and overwhelming burns.

Because of the great number of casualties that may occur simultaneously, undoubtedly insufficient personnel will be available to provide complete medical care, and many patients will of necessity have to depend on self-care for survival. It is expected that this group will represent the largest number of burn casualties. Most of these burns will be of the flash variety, which are primarily second degree burns on the exposed surfaces of the body.

Flash burns do well without covering, and the open method of treatment may be the only treatment available. The chief deterrent to this method is pain, and most patients would undoubtedly attempt to cover their wounds. Since sterile dressings may be a critical item, a bland nonirritating ointment applied to the burned surface would afford considerable relief. Fluids should be taken by mouth, and if electrolytes are necessary, the oral fluids can be fortified with the following substances: 3 Gm of salt (NaCl) and 1.5 Gm of soda ($NaHCO_3$) added to a liter of water; this makes a satisfactory electrolyte solution for oral use. Prophylaxis against infection should also be provided.

Persons with moderate burns would require more extensive therapy. They would undoubtedly need some intravenous colloids and electrolytes. During the early period when definitive care is not available, however, they could be managed with oral electrolytes, oral antibiotics, and sedation to control pain. Wounds should be covered by anything available to prevent further contamination.

Severe burns would require aggressive therapy. Patients with severe burns would be unable to tolerate large quantities of fluid by mouth and would be dependent on intravenous therapy. Antibiotics to control infection and sedation for pain should be administered, and, if available, some occlusive type of dressing should be applied to the wound. This type of casualty should be given a high priority for definitive care.

Overwhelming burns would carry a poor prognosis. Even under ideal situations with optimum care administered by trained personnel, the mortality in these cases would be at least 50%. In event of mass casualties, treatment under such adverse conditions would be anything but ideal, and few of the patients with overwhelming burns would be expected to survive. Patients with this type of injury should be made as comfortable as possible and given the lowest priority for definitive treatment.

MISCELLANEOUS WOUNDS
Intraoral wounds

Because of the isolated position of the oral cavity and the protection afforded by the lips and cheeks, wounds of the intraoral soft tissues are relatively rare. The majority of these injuries are part of the complex wounds involving other facial structures and have been considered under other sections of this chapter. Isolated wounds, however, do occur, and they warrant separate attention.

Any type of wound may occur in the oral cavity. Direct blows to the oral mucosa are virtually impossible, so primary contusions seldom occur. Secondary contusions of the oral mucosa, however, are frequently seen as a part of extensive contusions involving the lips or cheeks. In these wounds the mucosa becomes swollen as blood extravasates into the submucosal tissue, and with time the entire area takes on a purplish hue. Treatment of intraoral contusions is not necessary. Infection is no problem, and, as normal reparative processes take place, the blood clot is gradually resorbed, the discoloration fades, and the tissues return to normal in approximately 10 days.

Abrasions are common in the oral cavity.

They may result from any type of trauma that produces a frictional or scraping effect on the mucosa. Characteristic abraded wounds are produced by the irritation of a dental prosthesis, a malposed tooth, or a rough filling. Abraded mucosal surfaces are also caused by habitual lip or cheek chewers or by the occasional accidental self-inflicted bite. These wounds are superficial and require little therapy other than removal of the traumatizing force. Once the irritation has been corrected, the wounds heal rapidly without scar formation. If pain is a factor, the local wound may be covered with tincture of benzoin, which will seal off the nerve endings and afford relief for varying periods of time.

Lacerations are the most common of the isolated intraoral wounds and, for the most part, present little difficulty in management. Lacerations of the oral mucosa are frequent findings in traumatic injuries of the face. This is particularly true of lip lacerations, since the external trauma forces the lip against the sharp incisal edges of the anterior teeth. Accidents caused by the slipping of dental burs or disks during dental procedures or the injudicious use of exodontic instruments are added causative factors for lacerations of the mucosa. If treated early most of these lacerated wounds can be closed by primary suture without debridement. Hemorrhage can usually be controlled by pressure, although it may occasionally be necessary to clamp and tie larger bleeding vessels or active bleeding points. Lacerations limited to the oral mucosa are seldom of sufficient depth to warrant closure of the submucosal tissues as a separate layer, and suturing of the mucosa with No. 4-0 or 5-0 interrupted, nonabsorabable sutures is usually all that is necessary. Deep wounds of the tongue, lip, or floor of the mouth that are occasionally of sufficient magnitude to warrant closure in layers are the exceptions. Mucoperiosteum that has been stripped from the bone should be repositioned and sutured at the earliest opportunity.

A lacerated wound that deserves special mention is the one resulting from tears of the palatal mucosa produced by injuries of the maxilla, which include vertical fractures of the hard palate. These maxillary fragments are occasionally displaced laterally, which may result in a tear of the covering mucosa and produce a communication with the nasal fossa. If these mucosal tears are not sutured early, a nasal-oral fistula may develop that requires a difficult secondary plastic procedure to obtain a closure. If treatment is possible within a few hours after the injury, the maxillary fragments are usually sufficiently mobile to permit the manual molding of the fragments into their proper position, where they can be stabilized with an arch bar. The tears of the palatal mucosa may then be sutured without difficulty. It is obvious that these palatal lacerations must be sutured before intermaxillary immobilization of the fractures. This early primary suturing of the palatal mucosa is a gratifying procedure and, if properly carried out, will prevent the formation of a troublesome fistula.

Intraoral puncture wounds are usually the result of falls or accidents while some hard, pointed object is being held in the mouth. This is a common accident of young children, who frequently run and play with lollipop sticks or similar objects in their mouth. A puncture-type wound results when the sharp object is forcibly driven into the soft tissue. When the soft palate is involved, an actual perforating wound may be produced. Similar puncture wounds of the cheek, tongue, floor of the mouth, or palate are seen as the result of accidental slipping of an elevator during exodontic procedures. Wounds resulting from these injuries are more alarming than dangerous. The puncture wound seldom bleeds profusely, and the tissues usually collapse and obliterate the defect when the penetrating object is withdrawn. The perforations of the soft palate are eliminated by contracture of the muscles around the perforation. Examination to ensure that no part of the perforating object is left in the wound as well as measures to prevent infection are usually the only therapy indicated. Suturing is not necessary. In fact, this is contraindicated, since the wounds should be allowed to heal by granulation. Any accompanying lacerations should, of course, be sutured.

Most burns of the mouth are minor problems and closely simulate first or second degree burns of the skin. They result most frequently from heated instruments or from drugs used during dental procedures that accidently come in contact with the mucosal surfaces. Treatment is almost entirely directed to the local wound, since systemic reaction to such limited burned surfaces is highly improbable. The mucosal surface sloughs early, leaving a raw, denuded submucosal surface. These exposed surfaces are painful, and treatment is directed toward relief of pain and prevention of secondary infection. Systemic sedation is frequently necessary, but considerable relief can be obtained if the burned areas are dried and coated with tincture of benzoin. When large areas of the mucosa are involved, such treatment is not feasible. These patients should be given one of the topical anesthetic solutions such as the viscous type of lidocaine or a 0.25% solution of tetracaine (Pontocaine) to apply to the burned surfaces. A bland, nonirritating diet should be prescribed, since any tart or acid food will aggravate the pain. Secondary infection of the wounds should be prevented. Local application of one of the aniline dyes is helpful, and occasionally systemic antibiotic therapy is indicated. These burns heal rapidly without scarring, and the mucosa returns to normal in approximately 10 days.

Serious burns do occur in the oral cavity. The flash or flame type of burn of the upper respiratory tract may also involve the oral cavity, and the rapidly developing edema of the mucosa may create a real emergency. In such instances, tracheostomy is indicated as a lifesaving procedure, and general supportive therapy should be instigated immediately. The oral burn is usually superficial, and treatment of the local wound should be delayed until the patient's general condition has stabilized. Treatment of the oral wound is essentially the same as previously outlined.

Burns from accidental contact with strong acids and alkalies may be serious. As a rule these substances are swallowed rather than retained in the mouth, and damage to the esophagus and stomach are more common and dangerous than the injuries of the oral cavity. When these substances are retained in the mouth for any appreciable time, however, full-thickness mucosal burns resembling third degree burns of the skin may result. They produce deep necrosis of the tissue that sloughs in from 10 to 14 days, leaving a red, granulating bed. These wounds usually heal by granulation with marked scarring and contracture (Fig. 17-16). When feasible, split-thickness skin grafts should be placed on the granulating surfaces when the slough is removed. This, however, is frequently impossible, and the skin grafting must be done as a secondary procedure. The seriousness

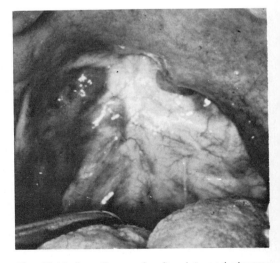

Fig. 17-16. Scar tissue of soft palate and pharynx after accidental swabbing of the throat with phenol. (Walter Reed Army Hospital.)

of these chemical burns may occasionally be minimized by prompt first-aid measures. If they are neutralized with an agent that in itself is not destructive to tissue and then followed by repeated irrigations of the mouth, the depth of the burn may be limited and the resultant scar contraction minimized.

Another oral burn that causes serious consequences is the electric burn. This is seen most frequently in babies who place electric cords in their mouth and chew the cord until a direct short is established. Flash burns occur from the arcing of the electricity, and deeper tissue burns result from the electricity surging through the tissues. Changes ranging from erythema to actual charring may result. In severe electric burns the systemic response is severe and immediate and must be treated vigorouly if the child is to survive. Treatment of the local wound depends on the extent of the injury. Superficial burns heal spontaneously without incident, but deeper burns that destroy considerable tissue heal by granulation with marked distortion of the tissues, which usually requires secondary procedures for correction. In all instances, control of infection is essential.

Severed parotid ducts

Facial lacerations in the region of the parotid gland occasionally sever the parotid duct. This should receive attention at the time of original wound closure to prevent the formation of an external salivary fistula. If both ends of the duct are visible, direct anastomosis of the severed ends is possible. A metal probe or polyethylene catheter is placed into the lumen of the duct, bridging across the severed portion. The duct is then repaired by suture over this probe or catheter, followed by closure of the remaining portions of the external wound. The probe or catheter is removed in approximately 3 days and the flow of saliva stimulated. Once salivary flow has started through the repaired duct, danger of stricture or stoppage of salivary flow is minimal.

Repair of the parotid duct is not always feasible, but a simple alternate procedure produces excellent results. It consists of placing a rubber drain from the mouth into the lacerated region of the cheek through a stab wound in the oral mucosa adjacent to the severed duct. The external wound is then tightly closed, and the saliva is forced to flow along the rubber drain, thus creating a fistulous opening into the mouth. The rubber drain is maintained in position with sutures for 5 or 6 days, and a permanent fistula that functions as a new opening for the parotid secretions is established.

REFERENCES

1. Artz, C. P.: Treatment of burns in atomic disaster, Publication No. 553, Management of Mass Casualties, AMSGS, WRAMC, Washington, D.C.
2. Bethea, H.: The treatment of disfiguring injuries to the exposed part of the face, Surg. Clin. North Am. **33:**109, 1953.
3. Blair, V. P., and Ivy, R. H.: Essentials of oral surgery, ed. 4, St. Louis, 1951, The C. V. Mosby Co.
4. Bradley, J. L.: Primary treatment of maxillofacial injuries, Oral Surg. **9:**371, 1956.
5. Brown, J. B.: The management of compound injuries of the face and jaws, South Med. J. **32:**136, 1939.
6. Brown, J. W.: Characteristic of war wounds of the face and jaws, Army Dent. Bull. **12:**292, 1941.
7. Chipps, J. E., Canham, R. G., and Makel, H. P.: Intermediate treatment of maxillofacial injuries, U.S. Armed Forces Med. J. **4:**951, 1953.
8. Committee on Trauma, American College of Surgeons: Prophylaxis against tetanus. In: The management of fractures and soft tissue injuries, ed. 2, Philadelphia, 1965, W. B. Saunders Co.
9. Department of Army Technical Bulletin: Management of battle casualties, Tech. Bull. Med., p. 147, 1951.
10. Department of Army Technical Bulletin: Early medical management of mass casualties in nuclear warfare, Tech. Bull. Med., p. 246, 1955.
11. Dickinson, J. T., Jaquiss, G. W., and Thompson, J. N.: Soft tissue trauma, Otolaryngol. Clin. North Am. **9:**331, June 1976.
12. Erich, J. B.: Management of fractures of soft tissue injuries about the face, Arch. Otolaryngol. **65:**20, 1957.
13. Erich, J. B., and Austin, L. T.: Traumatic injuries of facial bones, Philadelphia, 1944, W. B. Saunders Co.
14. Ferguson, L. K.: Surgery of the ambulatory patient, ed. 2, Philadelphia, 1947, J. B. Lippincott Co.

15. Fry, W. K., Shepherd, P. R., McLeod, A. C., and Parfitt, G. J.: The dental treatment of maxillo facial injuries, Philadelphia, 1945, J. B. Lippincott Co.

16. Gants, R. T.: Shock in management of mass casualties, Publication No. 569, Management of Mass Casualties, Walter Reed Army Institute of Research, WRAMC, Washington, D.C.

17. Gillies, H. D.: Plastic surgery of the face, London, 1920, Oxford University Press.

18. Harding, R. L.: The early management of facial injuries, Milit. Surgeon 112:434, 1953.

19. Hartgering, J. B., and Hughes, C. W.: Field resuscitation, Publication No. 573, Management of Mass Casualties, Walter Reed Army Institute of Research, WRAMC, Washington, D.C.

20. Hoffmeister, F. S.: Treatment of facial trauma, N.Y. J. Med. 72:373, February 1972.

21. Hughes, C. W.: Debridement, Publication No. 557, Management of Mass Casualties in Nuclear Warfare, Walter Reed Army Institute of Research, WRAMC, Washington, D.C.

22. Ivy, R. H.: Manual of standard practice of plastic and maxillo facial surgery, Philadelphia, 1942, W. B. Saunders Co.

23. Karsner, H. T.: Human pathology, ed. 8, Philadelphia, 1955, J. B. Lippincott Co.

24. Kazanjian, V. H.: Early suturing of wounds of the face, J. Am. Dent. Assoc. 6:628, 1919.

25. Kazanjian, V. H.: An analysis of gunshot injuries to the face, Int. J. Orthod. 6:96, 1920.

26. Kazanjian, V. H., and Converse, J. M.: The surgical treatment of facial injuries, Baltimore, 1949, The Williams & Wilkins Co.

27. Kwapis, B. W.: Early management of maxillofacial war injuries, J. Oral Surg. 12:293, 1954.

28. Loe, F. A., and Gamble, J. W.: Chainsaw injury of the mandibulofacial region, J. Oral Surg. 34:81, January 1976.

29. McIndoe, A. H.: Surgical and dental treatment of fractures of the upper and lower jaws in wartime, Proc. R. Soc. Med. 34:267, 1941.

30. Myers, M. B., and Cherry, G.: Rate of revascularization in primary and disrupted wounds, Surg. Gynecol. Obstet. 132:100, June 1971.

31. Ochsner, A., and DeBakey, M. E., editors: Christopher's minor surgery, ed. 7, Philadelphia, 1955, W. B. Saunders Co.

32. Ordman, L. J., and Gillman, T.: Studies in healing of cutaneous wounds, Arch. Surg. 93:857, 1966.

33. Parfitt, J. G.: The dental treatment of maxillofacial injuries, Philadelphia, 1945, J. B. Lippincott Co.

34. Parker, D. B.: Synopsis of traumatic injuries of the face and jaws, St. Louis, 1942, The C. V. Mosby Co.

35. Robinson, I. B., and Laskin, D. M.: Tetanus of the oral regions, Oral Surg. 10:831, 1957.

36. Rowe, N. L., and Killey, H. C.: Fractures of the facial skeleton, Baltimore, 1955, The Williams & Wilkins Co.

37. Rubin, L. R.: Langer's lines and facial scars, Plast. Reconstr. Surg. 3:147, January 1948.

38. Rush, J. T., and Quarantillo, E. P.: Maxillofacial injuries, Ann. Surg. 135:205, 1952.

39. Sanders, B., Andrews, J., Akers, P., and Lawrence, F.: Management of wound breakdown after primary repair of a facial laceration, J. Oral Surg. 32:531, July 1974.

40. Schultz, L. W.: Burns of the mouth, Am. J. Surg. 83:619, 1952.

41. Smith, F.: Plastic and reconstructive surgery, Philadelphia, 1950, W. B. Saunders Co.

42. Soberberg, B. N.: Facial wounds in Korean casualties, U. S. Armed Forces Med. J. 2:171, 1951.

43. Sparkman, R. S.: Lacerations of parotid duct, Ann. Surg. 131:743, 1950.

44. Stewart, F. W.: The consultant, J. Oral Surg. 26:297, 1968.

45. Sturgis, S. H., and Holland, D. J., Jr.: Observations on 200 fracture cases admitted to the 6th general hospital, Am. J. Orthod. (Oral Surg. Sect.) 32:605, 1946.

46. Thoma, K. H.: Traumatic surgery of the jaws, St. Louis, 1942, The C. V. Mosby Co.

47. Thoma, K. H.: Oral surgery, ed. 5, St. Louis, 1969, The C. V. Mosby Co.

CHAPTER 18

Traumatic injuries of the teeth and alveolar process

Merle L. Hale

TRAUMATIC INJURIES

Traumatic injuries to the teeth and the alveolar process are an all too frequent childhood and teenage accident and a not uncommon adult injury. A traumatically injured tooth is a distressing accident for the patient, and often the final dental restoration leaves much to be desired in appearance as well as in function (Figs. 18-1 and 18-2). However, since the advent of the acid-etch techniques for the bonding of composite resin restorations, there has been a decided improvement in esthetic and functional rebuilding of fractured anterior crowns. Fig. 18-3 illustrates what sometimes can be accomplished in restoring such injuries today.

Review of a long series of accident cases established that, on the basis of frequency, the patient's age must be considered a predisposing cause. The greatest incidence appears to be in children from 7 to 11 years of age (Fig. 18-4). At this period in the development of the anterior teeth the crowns are especially vulnerable because of the large pulp chambers. Also, at this "toothy age," these teeth frequently erupt in positions of isolated prominence in the arch, and they may be exposed to trauma.

Clinical evaluation of the injury

Accidents that produce traumatic injuries to the teeth often are accompanied by hemorrhage, swelling, and laceration of tissue. Such injuries tend to frighten people, and this may complicate the examination procedures. When a small child has been hurt, considerable emotional tension is usually exhibited on the part of both the patient and the parents. By the time this two-

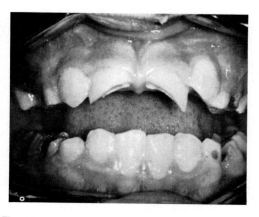

Fig. 18-1. The functional, esthetic, and psychological effects of a dental accident such as is illustrated are distressing and often leave a lifetime mark on the patient.

333

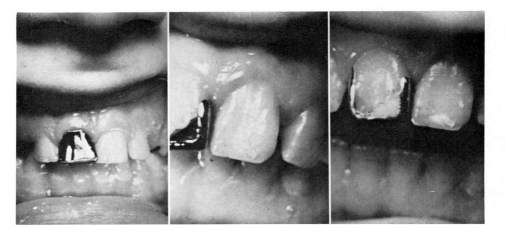

Fig. 18-2. Three case photographs representing dental restorations frequently used in the treatment of traumatic injuries. Permanent disfigurement often follows.

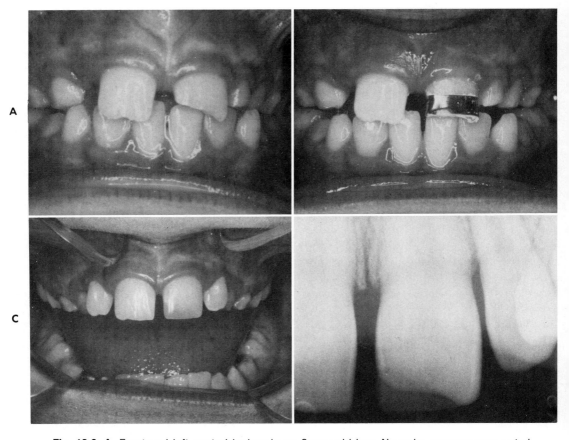

Fig. 18-3. A, Fractured left central incisor in an 8-year-old boy. No pulp exposure was noted clinically. **B,** Incisor treated temporarily until the tooth became more developed and assured a good prognosis. **C,** Incisor restored to good function and esthetics by improved restorative procedure. **D,** Radiograph of incisor at time of reconstruction by the acid-etch technique. (Courtesy of Dr. A. C. Full, University of Iowa.)

some or threesome reaches the dentist, the situation may easily have developed into a difficult problem. To cope with such accidents properly the dentist must conduct himself or herself in a calm and reassuring manner and, in spite of the adverse conditions, must be able to make an accurate diagnosis and decide immediately how to proceed with treatment. It is often expedient to have one of the parents hold a small child while the clinical and radiographic examinations are made. To try to reason with a small child at such times is futile. Gentleness, understanding, and a direct approach to the problem are imperative. In accomplishing the clinical examination, it is necessary to inspect the teeth and alveolar process carefully with a mouth mirror and by digital examination.

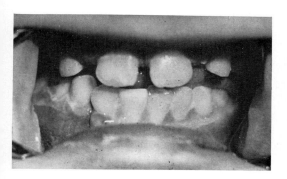

Fig. 18-4. The "toothy age," between 7 and 11 years of age.

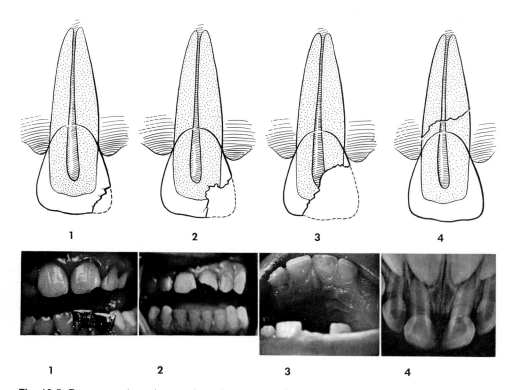

Fig. 18-5. Four cases have been selected, one to typify each of the classifications of injuries to the teeth. *1,* Class I fracture: fracture of the enamel cap only. *2,* Class II fracture: fracture line includes dentine but no pulp exposure. *3,* Class III fracture: fracture of crown with exposed pulp. *4,* Class IV fracture: fracture of root below the cervical line of the crown.

The extent of these dental accidents can be evaluated as follows:

First, the injury to the tooth should be classified (Fig. 18-5).

> Class I fracture: A fracture of only the enamel cap of the crown of the tooth
>
> Class II fracture: An injury extending into the dentine but with no exposure of the pulp
>
> Class III fracture: An extensive injury to the coronal portion of the tooth with a pulp exposure
>
> Class IV fracture: A fracture occurring at or below the cementoenamel junction of the tooth

Second, one should determine clinically if the tooth has been merely loosened or completely displaced from the socket or if it has been forced deeper into the supporting structures. Thus the injured tooth can be classified as *luxated, avulsed,* or *intruded* (Fig. 18-6).

Finally, by digital manipulation, any suspected alveolar fracture should be evaluated. Frequently, during such a procedure minor displacements of the alveolar process, or even slight displacement of teeth, can be detected and sometimes advantageously reduced at once.

Since many of the accident patients have mixed dentitions, it is all the more important that the mouth be charted so that this information will be readily available to aid in later interpreting the radiographs and in planning the necessary supporting treatment.

Radiographic evaluation of the injury

In completing the radiographic examination, it is usually necessary to secure more than one angle or line of exposure to demonstrate fractures. Therefore periapical and occlusal films should be used intraorally. Occasionally extraoral exposures will be required, with both lateral and posteroanterior views. Satisfactory radiographs may help verify clinical impressions and often provide additional findings that

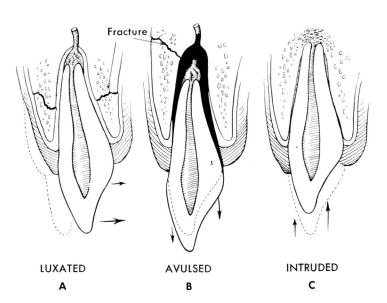

Fracture

LUXATED   AVULSED   INTRUDED

A   B   C

Fig. 18-6. Types of traumatic displacement of a tooth from the socket. **A,** The tooth has been loosened and moved. **B,** The tooth has been displaced from the socket, as represented by the dotted and solid lines. **C,** The tooth has been intruded into the alveolus, as represented by the dotted and solid lines.

are not revealed by the clinical examination alone.

It is necessary to study radiographically the odontogenesis of the apical ends of the teeth receiving the trauma. If radiographs reveal a large, funnel-shaped root canal with an incompletely developed apex, it is logical to assume that the vascular supply to the embryonal tissues in the developing apex will assist repair more speedily than if the root canal and apex are those of a fully developed tooth (Fig. 18-7).

Completing the diagnosis and treatment plan

When clinical and radiographic examinations have been accomplished, sufficient information should be available to permit completion of the diagnosis. At this point, it must be decided whether the injured tooth should be treated as a vital or a nonvital tooth. This diagnostic opinion should be based on knowledge of the following conditions:

1. The stage of development of the root end of the tooth
2. The extent of injury to the tooth itself
3. The condition of the supporting alveolus

Therefore if the injured tooth is not fully developed and has an immature apex, if the coronal injury does not involve the pulp, and if the supporting alveolar fracture will retain itself after reduction or can be readily retained by splinting, then all evidence points toward treating the injured tooth as a vital tooth.

Fully developed teeth with mature apices present a much more difficult diagnostic problem. If a fully developed tooth has only been loosened and not avulsed or impacted, then it should be considered for treatment as a vital tooth, provided nothing more severe than a Class I or II coronal fracture is involved.

If the treatment of the injured tooth as a vital tooth should prove unsuccessful or if it seems to be contraindicated at the time of the examination, it will be necessary to treat it as a nonvital tooth. At the time of this decision a root canal treatment plan may be formulated.

Splinting is usually necessary to retain all displaced teeth in a satisfactory arch position until the supporting structures have healed adequately to retain them. The time factor of the healing period is best evaluated by direct clinical testing of the mobility of the tooth in question.

The basic principle to consider in the treatment of the traumatically loosened or displaced vital tooth is the prognosis for the repositioned tooth. Vascular nourishment of the pulp must be reestablished if possible. If the blood supply to the pulp is lost, the pulp will become necrotic or gangrenous, and this will necessitate early recognition and appropriate treatment. In fully developed teeth the root canal, as revealed by x-ray films, can become narrowed or constricted. It is unlikely that such a tooth, if displaced or impacted, can become revascularized as a vital tooth. If the injured tooth appears not to be fully developed in the radiographic studies, or, if by direct examination of such a displaced tooth, the mesenchymal tissue is found to be present and intact in the cupped-out apex, then repositioning the tooth and retaining it by

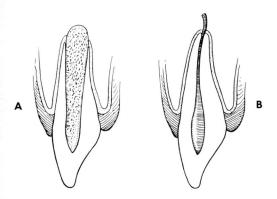

Fig. 18-7. A, Incompletely developed tooth, with embryonal tissues present over the open apical area. **B,** A fully developed tooth. Note the narrowing of the apical end of the root canal and the absence of embryonal tissues.

splinting is justified until sufficient time has lapsed to permit it to prove itself.

Early coronal discoloration alone, especially in teeth having incompletely developed apices, is not sufficient indication for an immediate root canal treatment or extraction. The accumulated extravasated blood in the pulp normally releases hemoglobin, which causes discoloration of the tooth. If, however, the pulp becomes revascularized through the embryonal tissues in the apical area, the injured tooth may recover and continue to be a vital tooth.

In the treatment of a Class I fracture of

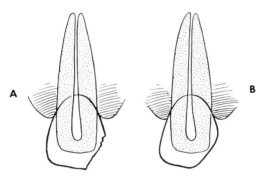

Fig. 18-8. A, An irregular fracture of the crown of a maxillary central incisor tooth. **B,** After treatment with fine abrasives such as sandpaper disks and fine mounted dental stones to remove sharp and irregular enamel rods.

the coronal portion of the tooth, it is usually necessary to reduce irregularities along the fracture line of the crown by the use of abrasive disks or stones (Fig. 18-8). This procedure tends to reduce irritations to the tongue and lips and minimizes the chance of other fracture lines developing under stress along the unprotected enamel rods. This can usually be accomplished at the time of the preliminary examination and often requires no anesthesia.

For the treatment of other than a Class I fracture of the coronal portion of the tooth, the patient will require additional supportive treatment from his dentist. Extended treatment of injuries to a fractured tooth other than emergency treatment, as previously discussed, will not be included here, since this subject is covered in excellent detail in numerous operative and pedodontic texts.

Splinting procedures

Injuries to a tooth alone, without displacement from the socket or a fracture of the alveolus, do not require splinting procedures. However, to stabilize a repositioned tooth with or without an alveolar fracture and to protect the organizing clot at the apex to enhance revascularization of the tooth, a splint is necessary.

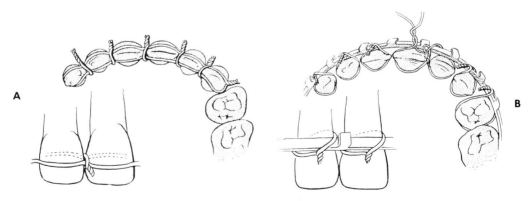

Fig. 18-9. Two techniques that may be used advantageously to stabilize and reposition teeth that have been injured. **A,** Essig type of splinting with 0.018-inch stainless steel fracture wire. **B,** Erich arch bar. This bar is readily contoured and ligated to the arch, and yet by its design it affords good support for intermaxillary traction when needed.

Numerous techniques for this type of stabilization or support have been advocated. As a general rule, the simple, easily managed procedures, such as the application of Erich arch bars or an Essig-type splint, are adequate measures (Fig. 18-9). The primary purpose is to stabilize the repositioned tooth or teeth to minimize traumatic stress on the organizing clot. Sometimes a heavier arch bar or sectional bar is indicated if an impacted alveolar fracture requires slow, elastic traction to secure a functional position. Selected cases may benefit from the use of acid-etched resins as a splinting technique. Usually a section of an arch bar may be incorporated into the resin splint to provide adequate stabilization for such injuries.

Anesthesia

The patient's need dictates the type of anesthesia necessary for the accomplishment of any surgical procedure.

Occasionally, if the patient is seen soon after an injury, minor manipulations and repositioning procedures may be tolerated without any anesthetic agent. However, most of these procedures are painful, and to effectively control the pain and allay the apprehension of the patient, some type of anesthesia is indicated together with preoperative and postoperative sedation.

For the uncooperative and fearful child or adult, it is usually desirable to complete the examination insofar as possible and then to schedule the surgical procedure under general anesthesia. The reassurance to the patient that he will be asleep and not be hurt during the necessary surgery often will aid in quieting him, and this fact alone may permit a more complete preliminary clinical and radiographic evaluation of his injuries.

Postoperative considerations and care

The concept of stages of healing in the repair of bone fractures can be applied in principle to the repair of the displaced tooth, with or without an alveolar fracture.

To the period immediately after the traumatic insult and continuing for approximately 24 to 72 hours, the term *hematoma phase* has been aptly applied. During this period the blood clot is forming and beginning to undergo its earliest organization.

From approximately the third day through the first 3 weeks after injury, the healing progresses and may be described as the *fibrous repair phase*. During this period every precaution should be taken to prevent additional injury to the organizing blood clot by any traumatic movement of the tooth in the socket. During this period, however, gentle, slow repositioning stresses are usually tolerated without impediment to the healing of the supporting tissues.

The fourth through the sixth week usually is considered to be the *final bone-forming phase* in the repair of the supporting tissues. During this period the bone formation is completed, and any undesirable movement or traumatic stress at this time may result in a surgical failure.

It should be remembered that most traumatic wounds of the oral cavity are "open" and, because of the bacteria normally present in the mouth, all such injuries should be treated as infected wounds. The same basic principles in surgical care should be applied here as to any other contaminated wound. Special attention to oral hygiene should be stressed, and systemic antibiotic coverage should be administered as indicated.

An understanding of surgical principles coupled with the proper use of antibiotics should encourage conservative treatment of teeth in the line of an alveolar fracture. Teeth that are determined on the basis of clinical and radiographic findings to have a favorable prognosis should be carefully retained until they have had ample time to prove their status.

REFERENCES
1. Arwill, T.: Histopathologic studies of traumatized teeth, Odont. T. **70:**91, 1962.

2. Baume, L. J.: Physiologic tooth migration and its significance for the development of occlusion, J. Dent. Res. **29:**330, 1950.

3. Clark, Henry B., Jr.: Practical oral surgery, ed. 3, Philadelphia, 1965, Lea & Febiger, pp. 350-404.

4. Ellis, R. G.: The classification and treatment of injuries to the teeth of children, ed. 4, Chicago, 1960, The Year Book Medical Publishers, Inc.

5. Hale, M. L.: Pediatric exodontia, Dent. Clin. North Am., pp. 405-419, July 1966.

6. Korns, R. D.: Incidence of accidental injury to primary anterior teeth (Abstract), J. Dent. Child. **27:**244, 1960.

7. Penick, E. C.: The endodontic managment of root resorption, Oral Surg. **16:**344, 1963.

8. Skieller, V.: The prognosis for young teeth loosened after mechanical injuries, Acta Odontol. Scand. **18:**171, 1960.

CHAPTER 19

Fractures of the jaws

Gustav O. Kruger

GENERAL DISCUSSION
Etiology

Fractures of the jaws occur most often because of automobile collisions, industrial or other accidents, and fights. Since the mandible is a hoop of bone articulating with the skull at its proximal ends by two joints, and since the chin is a prominent feature of the face, the mandible is prone to fracture. The mandible has been compared to an archery bow, which is strongest at its center and weakest at its ends, where it breaks often.

The chin is a convenient feature at which an adversary can aim. It is interesting to note that often the patient will not identify his adversary to the oral surgeon or to the police after a fight. He prefers to gain revenge in like manner later. This philosophy increases the number of jaw fractures, and if the patient has not had 6 months of good healing before the second altercation, he himself may be a candidate for a bone graft to the original site of injury.

A recent survey of 540 fractured jaw cases at District of Columbia General Hospital revealed that physical violence was responsible for 69% of the fractures, accidents for 27% (including automobile accidents, 12%, and sports, 2%), and pathology for 4%. Men experienced 73% of the frac-

tures, whereas women experienced only 27%. Private hospitals in the same area report a preponderance of automobile accidents as the main cause of jaw fractures. Hospitals in industrial cities report a high incidence of industrial accidents.

The automobile has made serious injury to the face and jaws commonplace. Violent forward deceleration causes injury to the head, face, and jaws. When the car stops quickly, the head hits the dashboard, steering wheel, rearview mirror, or the windshield. A middle face fracture can result, in which the maxilla, nose, zygoma, and perhaps the mandible are fractured. The National Safety Council, automobile manufacturers, and other groups have instituted various safety features, including seat and shoulder belts, dashboard padding, rearview mirror of different design, telescoping steering wheel, push-away windshield, dashboard with recessed or absent knobs, and air bags. It seems sensible to insist that children always ride in the back seat, since fewer major facial fractures occur to back-seat riders. The most dangerous seat in the automobile is the front seat next to the driver.

A fracture can occur more easily in a jaw that has been weakened by predisposing factors. Diseases that weaken all bones can

341

be factors. Examples include endocrine disorders such as hyperparathyroidism and postmenopausal osteoporosis, developmental disorders such as osteopetrosis, and systemic disorders such as the reticuloendothelial diseases, Paget's disease, osteomalacia, and Mediterranean anemia. Local disorders such as fibrous dysplasia, tumors, and cysts can be predisposing factors. A patient turning over in bed can experience a pathological fracture if the jaw is weak enough.

Classification

Fractures are classified into various types, depending on the severity of the fracture and whether or not the fracture is simple, compound, or comminuted (Fig. 19-1).

A simple fracture is one in which the overlying integument is intact. The bone has been broken completely, but it is not exposed to air. It may or may not be displaced.

A greenstick fracture is one in which one side of a bone is broken, the other being bent. It is difficult to diagnose sometimes, and it must be differentiated on the roentgenogram from normal anatomical marks and suture lines. It requires treatment, since resorption of the bone ends will occur during the healing process. Functioning of the member and muscular pull can result in a nonunion during healing if the bone ends are not held rigidly in place. However, the time required for healing usually is minimal. This type of fracture is seen often in children, in whom the bone will bend rather than break through.

A compound fracture is one in which an external wound is associated with the break in the bone. Any fracture that is open to the outside air through the skin or mucous membrane is assumed to be infected by outside contaminants. Unfortunately, almost all jaw fractures that occur in the region of the teeth are compounded. The jaw will respond to stress by fracturing through its weakest part. Rather than fracture through the full thickness of the bone at an interdental space, it will separate through a tooth

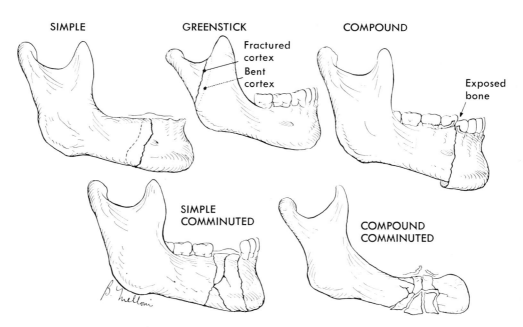

Fig. 19-1. Fracture types.

socket and then extend from the apex of the socket to the inferior border. The periodontal membrane and the thin alveolar mucosa are broken at a point adjacent to the tooth. The edentulous mandible will harbor a simple fracture more frequently. Even though the fracture may be displaced so that a "hump" appears on the ridge, the periosteum and overlying tissues can "give" a little, since the tissues have no close attachment to the teeth.

The oral surgeon is accustomed to dealing with fractures that are compounded into the mouth. Antibiotics have aided in controlling the potential infection. The bones of the jaws appear to have a degree of natural resistance to oral infection. A fracture that is compounded through the outside skin is more difficult to manage, and an osteomyelitis may develop more readily. The orthopedic surgeon finds that compounded fractures of the long bones are much more difficult to manage than simple fractures. This is partly the result of the introduction of plain dirt as well as outside organisms and partly of the fact that the fractured bone ends are more distracted so that one end of the bone can penetrate the skin.

A comminuted fracture is one in which the bone is splintered or crushed. It may be simple (that is, not open to outside contaminants) or compounded. Fractures of the vertical ramus of the mandible are composed sometimes of ten or more fragments, and yet, because of the splinting action of the masticatory muscles, no displacement occurs, and compounding is not present. If comminution occurs in the body of the mandible, the treatment is sometimes revised. Although an open reduction might be done normally (in which the bone is exposed surgically, holes are drilled, and wires are placed to hold the fragments in place), such a procedure would force stripping of the periosteum from the many small bone fragments, and healing would be delayed. A closed procedure may be substituted to ensure viability of the fragments.

Gunshot wounds are usually compound comminuted fractures, and usually bony substance is lost where the missile has traversed.

The District of Columbia General Hospital survey found the following incidence of jaw fractures: simple fractures, 23%; compound fractures, 74%; and comminuted fractures, 3%.

Examination

Every patient who has suffered a head or face injury should be examined for the possibility of a jaw fracture. Not infrequently a leg fracture is treated and facial wounds are sutured only to discover several days or weeks later that a jaw fracture exists. Fractures are more difficult and in some cases impossible to treat satisfactorily at the later date. In most large hospitals every head injury is examined routinely by the oral surgery service while the patient is still in the emergency room.

The general condition of the patient and the presence or absence of more serious injuries are of prime concern. Asphyxia, shock, and hemorrhage are conditions that demand immediate attention. Extensive soft tissue wounds of the face are cared for before or concomitantly with the reduction of bony fractures, except in the few cases in which the fractures can be treated by direct wiring before soft tissue closure is accomplished. However, treatment of minor facial wounds is delayed until intraoral arch bars have been placed, since a beautiful skin closure can be reopened by the stresses imposed by the intraoral procedure.

A history should be written as soon as feasible. If the patient cannot give a good history, the relative, friend, or police officer should be asked for a statement. Relevant details of the accident should be placed in the record. The events that took place between the time of the accident and the time of arrival at the hospital should be recorded. The patient should be questioned regarding loss of consciousness, length of unconscious period if known, vomiting, hemorrhage, and subjective symptoms.

Medications given before arrival at the hospital are recorded.

Questions regarding past illnesses, current medical treatment immediately preceding the accident, drugs being taken, and known drug sensitivity should be asked now. If the patient is uncomfortable, the detailed medical history can be deferred until later. Routine physical examination can be done now or later, according to the judgment of the examiner.

When examining the patient to determine if jaw fracture is present and its location, it is well to look for areas of contusion. This will provide information about the type, direction, and force of the trauma. The contusion sometimes can hide severely depressed fractures by tissue edema.

The teeth should be examined. Displaced fractures in dentulous areas are demonstrated by a depressed or raised fragment and the associated break in the continuity of the occlusal plane, particularly in the mandible (Fig. 19-2). Usually a tear in the mucosa and concomitant bleeding are noted. A characteristic odor is associated with a fractured jaw, which perhaps results from a mixture of blood and stagnant saliva. If no obvious displacement is present, manual examination should be done (Fig. 19-3). The forefingers of each hand are placed on the mandibular teeth with the thumbs below the jaw. Starting with the right forefinger in the retromolar area of the left side and with the left forefinger on the left premolar teeth, an alternate up-and-down motion is made with each hand. The fingers are moved around the arch, keeping them four teeth apart, and the same movement is practiced. Fracture will allow movement between the fingers, and a peculiar grating sound (crepitus) will be heard. Such movement should be kept to a minimum, since it traumatizes the injured site further and allows outside infection to enter.

The anterior border of the vertical ramus and the coronoid process should be palpated within the mouth.

The mandibular condyles should be palpated on the side of the face. The forefingers can be placed in the external auditory meatus with the balls of the fingers turned forward. If the condyles are situated in the glenoid fossae, they can be palpated. Unfractured condyles will leave the fossae when the jaw is opened. This maneuver should be done carefully and sparingly. The patient will experience pain on opening the

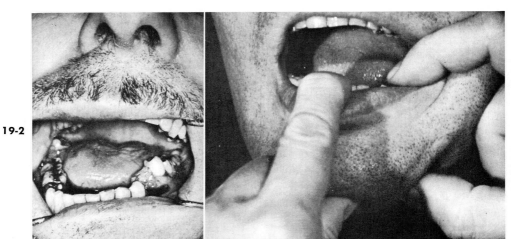

19-2

19-3

Fig. 19-2. The continuity of the occlusal plane disrupted by a fracture.
Fig. 19-3. Clinical examination for fracture of mandible.

jaw and inability to open properly if a fracture is present. The unilateral condylar fracture is suspected in the presence of a shift of the midline toward the affected side on opening. A step sometimes is noted on the posterior or lateral borders of the vertical ramus of the jaw in a low condylar neck fracture if edema has not obscured it.

The maxilla is examined by placing the thumb and forefinger of one hand on the left posterior quadrant and rocking gently from

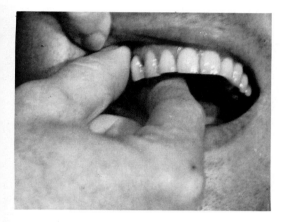

Fig. 19-4. Clinical examination for fracture of maxilla.

side to side, following with the same procedure on the right posterior quadrant and then on the anterior teeth (Fig. 19-4). If a complete fracture is present, the entire maxilla might move. An old fracture or one that has been impacted posteriorly will not move. The latter will be reflected in a malocclusion.

In a unilateral fracture, one half of the maxilla will move. This must be differentiated from an alveolar fracture. The unilateral maxillary fracture usually will have a line of ecchymosis on the palate somewhere near the midline, whereas the alveolar fracture will be confined to the alveolar ridge.

If a maxillary fracture is demonstrated, the facial aspect of the maxilla and the nose should be observed. A pyramidal fracture extending upward in the nasal area may be present. Besides loose bones, the patient usually will have a nosebleed (epistaxis) and black eyes.

All patients with facial injury should be examined for a transverse facial fracture. These fractures are overlooked sometimes because of facial edema and soreness. The examining finger should palpate the infraorbital ridge (Fig. 19-5, *A*). A step in this area indicates a fracture. The normal ridge

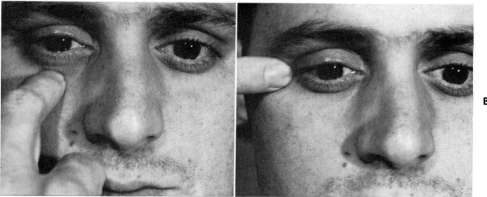

Fig. 19-5. A, Palpation of infraorbital ridge. **B,** Palpation of lateral rim of the orbit for separation of the frontozygomatic suture.

has a roughened area here, which should not be mistaken for a fracture. The lateral aspect of the bony orbit should be palpated next (Fig. 19-5, *B*). Careful examination may reveal a separation of the frontozygomatic suture line. It is found usually if the infraorbital ridge is fractured.

The arch of the zygoma should be palpated. A fracture may be found here even if no other facial or jaw fracture is present. If the infraorbital and lateral orbital areas reveal fractures, the body of the zygoma is detached from the maxilla, and, frequently, one or more posterior fractures are present in the zygomatic arch. Careful palpation may reveal the fracture. A dimple over the course of the zygomatic arch is pathognomonic of a fracture (Fig. 19-6). Overlying edema may make the clinical diagnosis difficult. By standing in front of the patient and pressing a tongue blade from the center of the zygoma to the lateral aspect of the temporal bone on each side, the examiner will note a difference in angulation between the blades that will aid in the diagnosis of a

depressed zygomatic arch (Fig. 19-7). A depressed body of the zygoma may allow a gravitational depression of the orbital contents. The edge of a tongue blade held in front of the pupils of the eyes will incline away from a horizontal plane if one eye is lower than the other.

When a maxillary fracture is suspected, several signs should be looked for before proceeding with manual examination as just described.

1. Bleeding from the ears. This requires differentiation between a middle cranial fossa fracture, a fracture of the mandibular condyle, and even a primary wound in the external auditory canal. A neurosurgical consultation is necessary to help differentiate these conditions. Other neurological signs are present with the cranial fracture. However, the experienced oral surgeon can diagnose the condylar fracture and thereby facilitate the neurological examination. The patient with a suspected or diagnosed cranial fracture is the responsibility of the neurologist or neurosurgeon. Fractures or

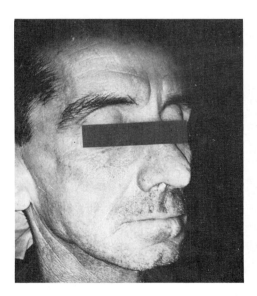

Fig. 19-6. A dimple over the zygomatic arch indicates a depressed fracture.

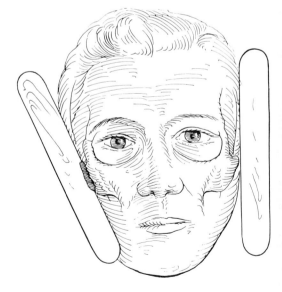

Fig. 19-7. A tongue blade pressed on the zygoma and the temporal bone will incline medially in the presence of a fractured zygomatic arch.

other wounds are treated only when he considers the patient to be out of danger, which in some cases may be a week or two later.

2. Cerebrospinal rhinorrhea. If the cribriform plate of the ethmoid bone is fractured in a complicated maxillary fracture, cerebrospinal fluid will leak out the external nares. Quick diagnosis can be made by placing a handkerchief under the nose for a moment and then allowing the material to dry. Mucus associated with a head cold will starch the handkerchief, whereas cerebrospinal fluid will dry without starching. If doubt exists, test the collected material for glucose. A commercial paper reagent test will identify sugar in normal cerebrospinal fluid; it is not accurate, however, in the presence of significant amounts of blood.

Movement of the maxilla of any type in the presence of cerebrospinal rhinorrhea is dangerous. Infectious organisms can be pushed up into the dura, and a meningitis may result. A few years ago the neurologist insisted that time be allowed for a granulation tissue covering to form over the distracted bone ends so that infection could not enter the meninges when maxillary fracture reduction was attempted. Complete reduction often was not possible by that time. With antibiotics, the reduction is now allowed earlier. Properly reduced bones allow earlier and better soft tissue healing over them with less bridging of voids between distracted bone ends.

3. Neurological signs and symptoms. Lethargy, severe headache, vomiting, positive Babinski reflex, and a dilated and widely fixed pupil or pupils are signposts that point to possible neurological trauma. Neurological consultation should be sought.

Radiographic examination. A patient should be examined radiographically if indications suggest that a fracture exists. Three extraoral are films routinely made: posteroanterior jaw and right and left lateral oblique jaws. The films should be examined immediately with particular attention paid to the bone borders, where most fractures appear.

If a fracture is suspected in the vertical ramus or in the condyle, the oblique lateral view on that side can be remade to concentrate on the suspected area. A lateral temporomandibular radiograph can also be made. If necessary, the x-ray beam can be directed posteriorly through the orbit to a cassette held to one side of the back of the head to obtain a proximolateral view of the condyle head.

In suspected maxillary fractures, a Waters view (nose-chin position taken from a posteroanterior exposure) should be made. If a zygomatic fracture is suspected, a "jughandle" view is made with the tube near the patient's umbilicus and the cassette at the top of the head. Maxillary fractures are difficult to diagnose on the radiograph even by the trained oral surgeon or the radiologist. When a definite conclusion cannot be reached, a lateral skull radiograph should be made. If the frontonasal suture line is opened on the radiograph, the possibility is strong that a maxillary fracture exists. The absence of this sign, however, does not eliminate the possibility of maxillary fracture.[7]

In cases in which a fracture is demonstrated, intraoral radiographs should be made at fracture sites before definitive treatment is given. Extreme trismus or a severly injured patient would preclude this. Intraoral views generally provide excellent definition because of the proximity of bone to the film. They sometimes show fractures that are not seen on the standard views, notably alveolar process, midline maxilla, and symphyseal fractures. The condition of adjacent teeth and detailed information about the fracture can be obtained by this procedure.

The diagnosis of a double fracture at one site, particularly in the mandible, should be made guardedly. A lateral jaw radiograph is not often so made that the fractures of the lateral cortex and the medical cortex superimpose exactly. The two fractured cortical plates may be interpreted mistakenly as two fractures through the body of the bone (Fig. 19-8).

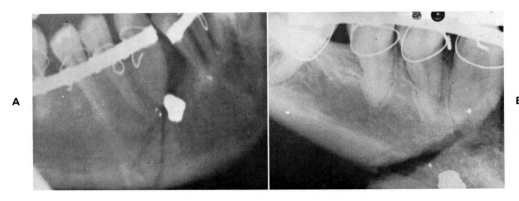

Fig. 19-8. A, Lateral jaw radiograph showing an apparent double fracture. Note that the two radiolucent lines converge at the inferior border. **B,** Intraoral radiograph of the same case, showing that only a single fracture exists. Note metal fragment.

From a medicolegal point of view, a permanent record in the form of radiographs is necessary. In any case in which a fracture might be suspected, it is better to err on the safe side and make the minimum extraoral radiographs, that is, the posteroanterior jaw and right and left lateral oblique jaw films. In children or young adults in whom consideration of the total amount of radiation is a factor, a leaded rubber sheet can be used to cover the gonads and neck.

First aid

The primary consideration is to have a live patient. Accordingly, immediate measures should be taken to assure that his general condition is satisfactory. Specific treatment of fractures in the severely injured patient is given anytime from hours to weeks later.

If the airway is not patent, the fingers should be placed at the base of the tongue and the tongue pulled forward. Dentures, broken-off teeth, and foreign objects should be removed carefully if the finger can reach them. Suction should be employed for secretions and blood. A rubber airway can maintain a patent airway temporarily, or a suture can be placed through the midline of the tongue and tied to the clothing or affixed to the chest wall with adhesive tape. Mandibular fractures may involve the muscular attachment of the tongue with attendant posterior displacement and resultant asphyxia. If serious consideration is given to performing a tracheostomy, it should be done. An emergency tracheostomy may be needed, or, if time and facilities are available, an elective tracheostomy can be done.

However, in a surprisingly large number of cases of temporary airway embarrassment, an intratracheal tube will provide adequate relief until the fracture can be reduced, thus making a tracheostomy unnecessary. Usually, the tube is placed first, and then a tracheostomy is performed only if the tube is found to be inadequate.

Shock is treated by placing the patient in shock position, with the head slightly below the level of the feet. Warm blankets are placed over him. Excessive heat in the form of hot-water bottles is as dangerous as cold. Whole blood is given for definitive treatment of major shock.

Hemorrhage is rarely a complication of jaw fractures unless deep vessels in the soft tissue (for example, maxillary artery, facial vessels, lingual vessels) are involved. Even if the inferior alveolar vessels are severed in the bony canal, the hemorrhage is not severe. Hemorrhage from other wounds, however, demands immediate attention. In most cases the proper pressure point can be held with finger pressure until the vessel can be clamped and tied.

Patients with head injury should not receive morphine, except possibly in case of severe pain. Morphine may complicate further the function of the respiratory center. Tetanus antitoxin is given after a sensitivity test if the skin is broken, provided the patient has not been immunized. If the patient has been previously immunized, then a 1 ml booster dose of tetanus toxoid is given. This is done in the emergency room.

The possibility of spinal cord injury concomitant with cervical fracture or dislocation should be considered. Movement of the head in this instance can cause permanent injury to the spinal cord. Cervical radiographs should be made first if pain is present in the neck or if muscle weakness is present in the extremities.

The best treatment for jaw fractures is immediate intermaxillary fixation. Ideally, the permanent fixation that will be used to treat the fracture should be placed within hours after the injury. In a good many large hospitals the resident is instructed to place intermaxillary fixation immediately after clinical and radiographic examination, regardless of the time of day or night. The patient then is sedated further, given antibiotics and other necessary supportive measures, and ice packs are placed on the face. If these procedures are done soon after admission, the patient is more comfortable. The broken ends of bone are not moving or in malposition, and therefore, the nerve is not traumatized. The organization of the blood clot, which takes place in the first few hours, will not be disrupted by further manipulation in the majority of instances. Intraoral wiring is more difficult to apply the next morning when edema and the trismus associated with reflex spasms of the muscles have occurred. If further treatment is necessary, it is discussed after the immediate measures have been instituted and adequate postoperative radiographs are available for interpretation.

Temporary fixation should be placed if

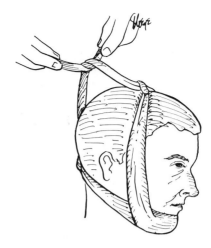

Fig. 19-9. The four-tailed bandage.

definitive fixation is not feasible. Some type of fixation should always be placed to keep the patient comfortable and to keep the fragments in as good a position as possible. A head bandage is the most simple form of fixation. The four-tailed bandage (Fig. 19-9) is one method that can be used. Ivy loops can be placed as temporary measures (p. 364). A method that has been valuable is to string No. 4-0 dress clamps on thin, 28-gauge stainless steel wire. Four of these can be placed in as many minutes, and elastics are stretched between them.

Treatment

The treatment of fractures is directed toward placing the ends of the bone in the proper relation so that they touch and maintaining this position until healing occurs. The term used for positioning the bone is *reduction* of the fracture. The term used for maintaining the position is *fixation*.

Closed reduction. Several methods of reduction are available. The simplest method is closed reduction, that is, manipulation without surgically exposing the bone to view. In closed reduction of long bones, the orthopedic surgeon pulls or manipulates the bone under the intact skin until the fracture is in proper position. The story is told of an old Scottish physician who had a bucket of sand in the corner of his office. A patient suffering a wrist fracture would be directed against his will to pick up the bucket. In so doing, the fractured parts would align themselves perfectly, and a plaster cast was applied.

Most early jaw fractures can be reduced manually. In older fractures in which the bony segments are not freely movable, traction supplied by rubber bands between the jaws exerts a powerful, continuous force that will reduce an obstinate fracture in 15 minutes to 24 hours. The elastic traction overcomes three factors: the active muscular pull that distracts the fragments (the main cause for malposition), the organized connective tissue at the fracture site, and the malposition caused by the direction and force of the trauma. A maxillary fracture often is pushed back by force, and it must be brought forward by manual manipulation or elastic traction. Rarely do the bones require surgical separation except in the case of delayed treatment when a fracture has healed in malposition (malunion).

Open reduction. It is not feasible to reduce all fractures satisfactorily by closed procedures. The often-encountered fracture at the angle of the mandible is difficult to reduce because it is difficult to counter the powerful pull of the masticatory muscles in that area. In the case of the angle fracture, however, open reduction is done more for fixation than for reduction. When the bone is surgically exposed, holes are drilled on either side of the fracture, wire is crossed over the fracture, and the bone ends are brought into good approximation. Besides good fixation, the fracture can be reduced exactly by direct vision. Perfect approximation is not always present after closed procedures. It might be stated in passing, however, that jaw fractures occurring within the dental arch are reduced to a fraction of a millimeter by the action of the dental facets of one arch guiding the other arch into the preexistent occlusion. This is not so likely to be true in fractures in other

parts of the body, where manipulation is necessarily done through large muscle masses. Reduction in these latter instances need not be as critical as in jaw fractures, which must present an exact occlusion.

Another advantage of open reduction, particularly in a late fracture, is the opportunity for the surgeon to clean out the organizing connective tissue and debris between bone ends that would delay healing in the new position if left interposed.

Disadvantages of open reduction are: (1) the surgical procedure removes the natural protective clot at the site, and the limiting periosteum in incised; (2) infection is possible even with extreme aseptic procedures and antibiotics; (3) a surgical procedure is necessary, which increases time in the hospital and other hospital costs; and (4) a skin scar is present.

Fixation. The orthopedic surgeon reduces a simple fracture of the long bones by a closed procedure and then employs a plaster cast for fixation. The oral surgeon frequently combines the two procedures by the use of one apparatus. When the bones of the jaws contain teeth, the occlusion of the teeth can be used to guide the reduction. By placing wires, arch bars, or splints on the teeth and then extending elastic bands or wires from the mandibular to the maxillary arch, the bones are held in proper position through proper and harmonious interdigitation of the teeth. Plaster casts are not necessary or feasible.

The fixation of jaw fractures is approached in graduating steps. Usually intermaxillary fixation by means of wires, arch bars, or splints is the first step. In many cases that is all that is needed. If this is insufficient, however, direct wiring through holes in the bone is done by an open procedure. This is done in addition to the intermaxillary fixation.

Methods other than open reduction and direct bone wiring have been employed to manage the angle fracture. Distal extensions from intraoral splints and external extensions from plaster headcaps to a hole

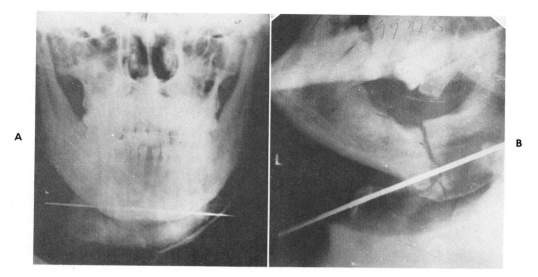

Fig. 19-10. A, Kirschner wire placed across symphysis fracture. **B,** Steinmann pin placed through angle fracture.

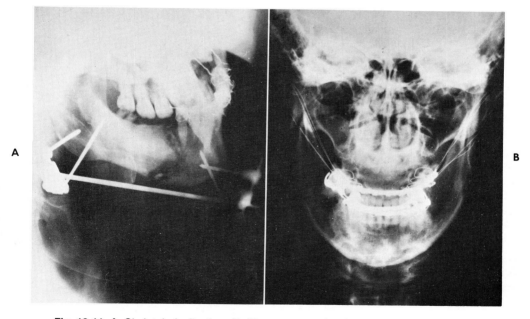

Fig. 19-11. A, Skeletal pin fixation. **B,** Circumzygomatic wire suspension of maxilla.

in the proximal fragments have been discarded by and large. Fixation by medullary pins is used sometimes. The parts are reduced, and a long, sharp, stainless steel pin is drilled into the length of the bone, crossing the fracture line. The pin is used more often in mandibular symphysis fractures and rather infrequently in mandibular angle fractures. (See Fig. 19-10.)

Skeletal pin fixation is used often (Fig. 19-11, *A*). In simplest form, a screw pin, 8 cm long with a diameter of 2 mm, is drilled into the lateral aspect of the jaw through the skin and subcutaneous tissues, through the outer bone cortex, the spongiosa, and just through the inner bone cortex. Another pin is drilled on the same side of the fracture. Two pins are drilled on the other side of the fracture. The pins are attached to each other by a connecting apparatus, and the two connecting units are united across the fracture by a stout metal rod. This is a closed procedure that is simple, but many failures are associated with it. If it is performed by an inexperienced person, the pin will not engage the inner cortex, and the entire assembly will become loose at an inopportune time.

Maxillary fractures must be maintained against the base of the skull. A plaster headcap with extensions has been used for years. Recently, internal wiring has been used more often. Wires are suspended over the intact zygomatic arches or holes are drilled into an unfractured bone superior to the fracture, such as the infraorbital ridge or the bone just above the zygomaticofrontal suture line (Fig. 19-11, *B*). Wires are passed then beneath the skin, and the maxilla thereby is suspended. Since this suspension is not visible, the patient can go about his business during recovery. Less chance exists for movement of the fracture during healing than with the plaster headcap.

It is interesting to note changes in the thinking of the profession over the years regarding open reduction. In the years before World War II, open operations on bones frequently resulted in osteomyelitis. Complicated jaw fractures were treated by all manner of gadgets. Bicycle spokes, fancy castings, and "man-from-Mars" outfits were used. In the years since the beginning of World War II, the popular procedure has been the open reduction. Antibiotics, the introduction of metals tolerated by the tissues, and more predictable results were largely responsible. The gadgets had been uncomfortable to the patient and sometimes inefficient in approximating the bony segments, and the surgeon never knew when one would slip at a crucial moment.

The trend is beginning to regress a bit at present. Largely responsible are the occasional infection of the open wound that is resistant to many antibiotics and the fact that results are not always that much better despite the increased amount of surgery. A tremendous backlog of experience with open procedures can be compared now with conservative procedures. The fractured mandibular condyle is an example. A few years ago almost every fractured condyle was considered for open reduction. Now only a selected few are done. However, many indications exist for open procedures if no other method will give a comparable satisfactory result. Open reduction is still preferable to most of the modern gadgets.

HEALING OF BONE

Healing of bone can be divided into three overlapping phases. *Hemorrhage* occurs first, associated with clot organization and proliferation of blood vessels. This nonspecific phase occurs during the first 10 days. *Callus formation* occurs next. A rough "woven-bone" or primary callus that looks like burlap is formed in the next 10 to 20 days. A secondary callus in which the haversian systems form "in every which way"[12] forms in 20 to 60 days. *Functional reconstruction* of the bone is the third phase. Mechanical forces are important here. The haversian systems are lined up according to stress lines. Excess bone is removed. The shape of the bone is molded to conform with functional usage so that bone may be added to one surface and removed on another side. It takes 2 to 3 years, for example, to completely reform a fracture of the human femur.

Weinmann and Sicher[27] divide the healing of fractures into six stages:

1. Clotting of blood of the hematoma. When a fracture occurs, blood vessels of the bone marrow, the cortex, the perios-

teum, the surrounding muscles, and adjacent soft tissues rupture. The resultant hematoma completely surrounds the fractured ends and extends into the bone marrow as well as into the soft tissues. It coagulates in 6 to 8 hours after the accident.

2. Organization of blood of the hematoma. A meshwork of fibrin is formed in the organizing hematoma. The hematoma contains fragments of periosteum, muscle, fascia, bone, and bone marrow. Most of these fragments are digested and removed from the scene. Inflammatory cells, which are so necessary for the hemorrhagic phase of bone healing, are called forth by this diseased tissue rather than by bacterial organisms. Capillaries invade the clot in 24 to 48 hours. Fibroblasts invade the clot at about the same time.

The proliferation of blood vessels is a characteristic of the early organizing hematoma. A good blood supply is important. The capillary beds in the marrow, cortex, and periosteum become small arteries to supply the area of fracture. As they become more tortuous, a slower flow results in a richer blood supply. At this stage, proliferation of capillaries occurs throughout the hematoma. The hyperemia associated with the slow flow of blood through tortuous vessels is responsible for mesenchymal proliferation. Protein building blocks created by the richer blood supply form the basis for mesenchymal proliferation.

Resorption of bone is a characteristic of an older hematoma. The torrents of blood running through the area of active hyperemia, and not disuse atrophy, cause resorption of bone. When the blood gets into the actual site of fracture where the capillary bed lies (which Johnson[12] likens to a "swamp"), the flow is slowed. This area of passive hyperemia is associated with proliferation of bone. Calcium ion level is increased in this swamp area by the capillary bed.

3. Formation of fibrous callous. The organized hematoma is replaced by granulation tissue ordinarily in 10 days. The granulation tissue removes necrotic tissue primarily by phagocytic activity. As soon as this function is completed, the granulation tissue develops into a loose connective tissue. The end of the hyperemic phase is characterized by a decrease in the number of white cells and partial obliteration of the capillaries. The fibroblasts are now most important. They produce numerous collagenous fibers, which are termed fibrous callus.

4. Formation of primary bony callus. Primary callus forms between 10 and 30 days after fracture. Structurally it has been compared to a crudely woven burlap. The calcium content is so low that primary callus can be cut with a knife. It is for this reason that primary callus cannot be detected on the roentgenogram. It is an early stage that serves only as a mechanical prop for the formation of secondary callus.

Primary callus has been considered in different categories, depending on location and function (Fig. 19-12).

Anchoring callus develops on the outside surface of the bone near the periosteum. It extends some distance away from the fracture. Young connective tissue cells of the fibrous callus differentiate into osteoblasts, which produce this spongy bone.

Sealing callus develops on the inside surface of the bone across the fractured end. It fills the marrow spaces and goes out into the fracture site. It forms from endosteal proliferation.

Bridging callus develops on the outside surface between the anchoring callus on the two fractured ends. This callus is the only one that is primarily cartilaginous. The question has been raised whether true bridging callus forms in the healing of mandibular fracture, since the mandible is one of the bones formed originally in membrane rather than by replacement of cartilage. However, cartilage cells have been identified in such areas of healing in the mandible.

Uniting callus forms between the ends of

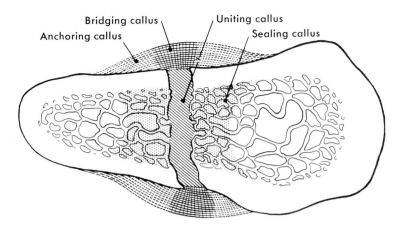

Fig. 19-12. Types of primary callus forming a healing fracture.

bones and between areas of other primary calluses that have formed on the two fractured parts. It does not form until the other types of callus are well developed. It forms by direct ossification. Extensive resorption of the bone ends has occurred by this time. Therefore, rather than merely ossifying the interposed connective tissue at the fracture site, the uniting callus forms in the area of resorption as well. A well-united fracture is the result.

5. Formation of secondary bony callus. Secondary bony callus is mature bone that replaces the immature bone of the primary callus. It is more heavily calcified, and therefore it can be seen on the roentgenogram. It differs from other skeletal bone, however, by the fact that the pseudohaversian systems are not formed in any uniform pattern. It is composed of laminated bone that can withstand active use. Therefore fixation can be removed when secondary callus is seen on the roentgenogram. Formation of secondary callus is a slow process, requiring from 20 to 60 days.

6. Functional reconstruction of the fractured bone. Reconstruction proceeds over months or years to the point where the location of the fracture usually cannot be detected histologically or anatomically. Mechanics is the major factor in this stage.

As a matter of fact, if a bone is not subjected to functional stress, true mature bone will not form. True haversian systems that are oriented by stress factors replace the nonoriented pseudohaversian systems of secondary callus. The secondary callus that is formed in abundance is sculptured to conform with the size of the remainder of the bone. The entire bone is molded by mechanical factors if the healing has not taken place in exact alignment. Steps are reduced on the one side, and deficiencies are filled in on the other side. This process seems to take place in alternative waves of osteoclastic activity and osteoblastic activity.

FRACTURES OF THE MANDIBLE
Causes

Two principal components are involved in fractures of the mandible: the dynamic factor (blow) and the stationary factor (jaw). Common causes for setting in motion the dynamic factors have been discussed at the beginning of the chapter. Physical violence and automobile accidents lead the list in a municipal hospital administering to a preponderance of indigent patients. However, in studies conducted in private hospitals, industrial accidents rate as a close second to automobile accidents. In these hospitals the incidence of physical

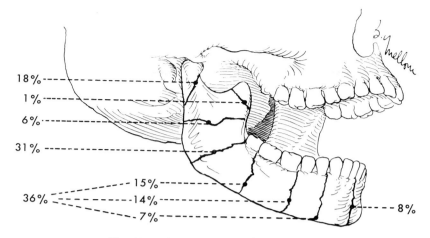

Fig. 19-13. Sites of mandibular fractures.

violence is extremely low, usually about 10%.

The dynamic factor is characterized by the intensity of the blow and its direction. A light blow may cause a greenstick or simple unilateral fracture, whereas a heavy blow with "follow through" may cause a compounded, comminuted fracture with traumatic displacement of the parts. The direction of the blow largely determines the location of the fracture or fractures. A blow to the right of the chin may result in a fracture of the mental foramen region on that side and a fracture of the angle of the mandible on the other side. Force applied to the point of the chin might result in symphysis and bilateral condyle fractures. Severe force may push the condylar fragments out of the glenoid fossa.

The stationary component has to do with the jaw itself. Physiological age is important. A child, with his growing bones, can fall out of a window and experience a greenstick fracture or no fracture at all, whereas an elderly person, whose heavily calcified skull can be compared to a flower pot, can trip over a rug and suffer a complicated fracture.

Mental and physical relaxation prevents fractures associated with muscular tension. A bone that has severe tensions placed on it

by all-out contractions of its attached muscles requires only a slight blow to fracture it. On the other hand, intoxicated persons have fallen from rapidly moving vehicles only to suffer bruises. The muscle masses serve as tissue cushions when relaxed, but the same muscles under tension form strain patterns in the bones.

Vulnerability of the jaw itself varies from one individual to another and from time to time in the same individual. A deeply impacted tooth will make the angle of the jaw vulnerable, as will physiological and pathological conditions such as osteoporosis or a large cyst. Heavier deposition of calcium in the trained athlete will reduce jaw fractures. Jaw fractures in boxers are almost nonexistent because of increased calcification, the use of padded boxing gloves and rubber mouthguards, and a training factor.

Location[10]

In the series quoted previously (p. 341), the following incidence of fracture, by sites, occurred in the mandible (Fig. 19-13).

Angle	31%	Symphysis	8%
Condyle	18%	Cuspid	7%
Molar region	15%	Ramus	6%
Mental region	14%	Coronoid process	1%

The most common bilateral fracture was in the angle-mental regions.

Displacement

The displacement of a fracture of the mandible is a result of the following factors.

Muscle pull. The intricate musculature attached to the mandible for functional movement distracts the fragments when the continuity of the bone is lost (Figs. 19-14 to 19-18). The action of balances between sets of muscles is lost, and each muscle group exerts its own force unopposed by another muscle group. The "sling of the mandible," that is, the masseter and medial pterygoid muscles, displaces the posterior jaw fragment upward, aided by

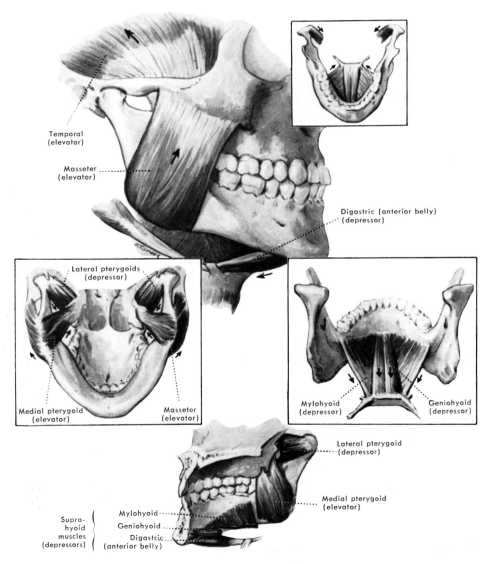

Fig. 19-14. Muscles of the mandible. (From Massler, M., and Schour, I.: Atlas of the mouth; courtesy American Dental Association.)

the temporal muscle. The opposing force, that is, the suprahyoid muscles, displaces the anterior fragment downward. These forces would balance themselves if attached to an intact bone.

The posterior fragment usually is displaced medially, not because of lack of muscular balance as much as because the functional direction of pull is medial. The medial pterygoid muscle is largely re-sponsible. The superior constrictor of the pharynx exerts medial pull from its multi-centric origin on the mylohyoid ridge, pterygomandibular raphe, and hamular process to its insertion on the occipital bone. The lateral pterygoid muscle attached to the condyle will help, and in the case of the condylar fracture, it will tend to displace the condyle medially.

Fragments situated in the anterior por-

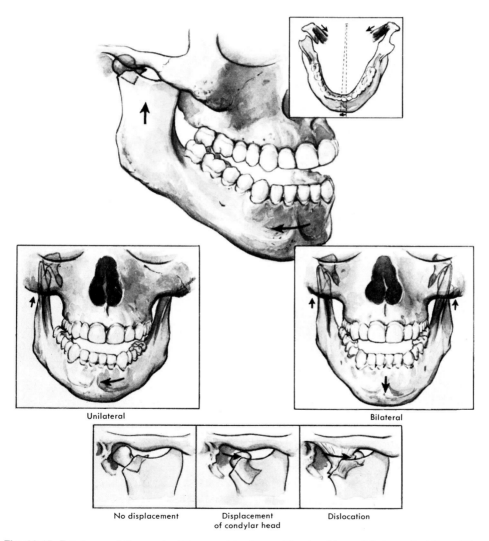

Unilateral   Bilateral

No displacement   Displacement   Dislocation
                        of condylar head

Fig. 19-15. Fractures of the neck of the condyle. (From Massler, M., and Schour, I.: Atlas of the mouth; courtesy American Dental Association.)

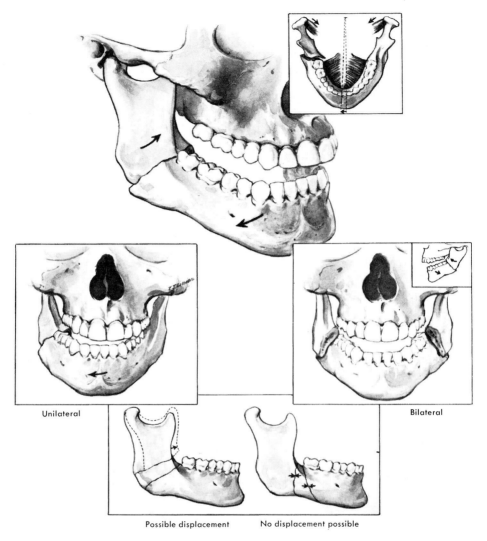

Fig. 19-16. Fractures of the angle of the mandible. (From Massler, M., and Schour, I.: Atlas of the mouth; courtesy American Dental Association.)

tion of the jaw can be displaced medially by the mylohyoid muscle. Symphysis fractures are difficult to fixate because of the bilateral posterior and slight lateral pull exerted by the suprahyoid and digastric muscles.

Direction of line of fracture. Fry and associates[8] classified fractures of the mandible as ''favorable'' and ''unfavorable,'' depending on whether or not the line of fracture was in such direction as to allow

muscular distraction. In the mandibular angle fracture, the posterior fragment will be pulled upward if the fracture extends forward toward the alveolar ridge from a posterior point on the inferior border. This is termed an unfavorable fracture (Fig. 19-19, *A*). However, if the inferior border fracture occurs further anteriorly and the line of fracture extends in a distal direction toward the ridge, a favorable fracture is present (Fig. 19-19, *B*). The long angle of

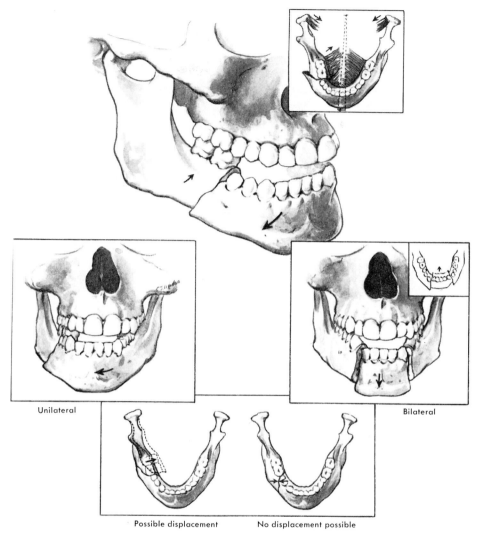

Fig. 19-17. Fractures of the body of the mandible. (From Massler, M., and Schour, I.: Atlas of the mouth; courtesy American Dental Association.)

the anteroinferior portion will lock the posterior fragment mechanically to withstand upward muscular pull.

These distractions are in a horizontal plane, and so the terms horizontal unfavorable and horizontal favorable are used. Most angle fractures are horizontal unfavorable.

Medial displacement can be considered in similar fashion. Oblique fracture lines can form a large buccal cortical fragment that will prevent medial displacement. If the mandible could be viewed directly downward from the upper jaw so that the occlusal surfaces of the teeth are seen in button fashion, a vertical unfavorable fracture line extends from a posterolateral point to an anteromedial point (Fig. 19-20, *A*). No obstruction to medial muscular pull is present. A vertical favorable fracture extends from an anterolateral to a posteromedial point (Fig. 19-20, *B*). Medial muscular dis-

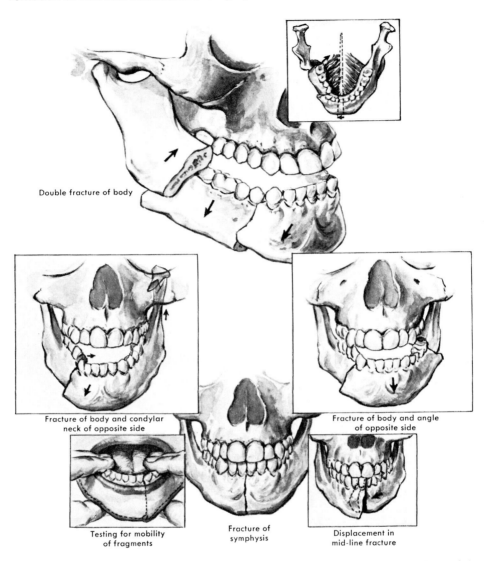

Double fracture of body

Fracture of body and condylar
neck of opposite side

Fracture of body and angle
of opposite side

Testing for mobility
of fragments

Fracture of
symphysis

Displacement in
mid-line fracture

Fig. 19-18. Multiple fractures of the mandible. (From Massler, M., and Schour, I.: Atlas of the mouth; courtesy American Dental Association.)

placement is prevented by the large buccal cortical fragment.

Force. Factors such as the direction of the blow, the amount of force, the number and location of fractures, and the loss of substance as in gunshot wounds are not as important in displacing mandibular fractures as they are in maxillary fractures except insofar as they form the basis for later muscular distraction. Force in itself can displace fractures by forcing the bone ends away, impacting the bone ends, or pushing the condyles out of their sockets, but secondary displacement by muscular pull is stronger and more significant in mandibular fractures.

Force that compounds a fracture or comminutes it serves to complicate the treatment. Events that follow the initial fracture can also complicate it. An initially

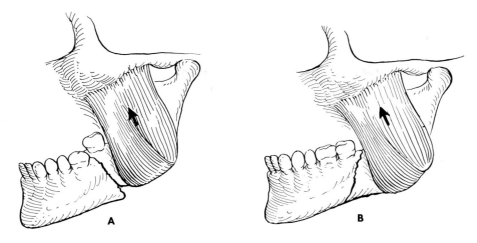

Fig. 19-19. A, Horizontal unfavorable fracture. **B,** Horizontal favorable fracture.

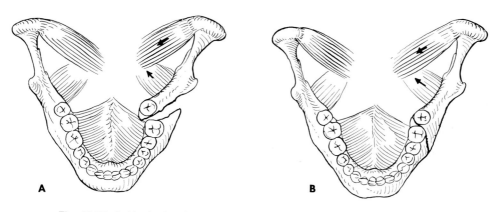

Fig. 19-20. A, Vertical unfavorable fracture. **B,** Vertical favorable fracture.

undisplaced fracture may be displaced by trauma (such as rolling) in the same accident. Placing the patient face down on a stretcher or injudicious and unskilled examination may displace bone segments. Lack of temporary support of the jaw, particularly in the case of a fractured skull, often leads to functional and muscular displacement, which is painful and difficult to treat later.

Signs and symptoms[1]

1. *History of injury* is invariably present, a possible exception being a pathological fracture.

2. *Occlusion indirectly* offers the best index of recently acquired bony deformity.

3. *Abnormal mobility* with bimanual palpation of the mandible is a reliable sign of fracture. By this procedure, separation between mandibular fragments is differentiated from mobility of teeth.

4. *Pain* with movements of the mandible or on palpation of the face often is a significant symptom. When condylar movements are restricted and painful, a condylar fracture should be suspected.

5. *Crepitus* with manipulation or mandibular function is pathognomonic of a fracture. However, this is elicited with

considerable pain to the patient in many cases.

6. *Disability* is manifested by the patient's inability to masticate because of pain or abnormal motility.

7. *Trismus* is seen frequently, especially in fractures through the angle or in the ramus region. This is a reflex spasm mediated through the sensory pathways of the disrupted bone segments.

8. *Laceration* of the gingiva may be seen in the region of the fracture.

9. *Anesthesia* may be noted, especially in the gingiva and lip up to the midline, when the inferior alveolar nerve is injured.

10. *Ecchymosis* of the gingiva or mucosa on the lingual or buccal surfaces may be suggestive of a fracture site.

11. *Salivation and fetor of breath.*

Treatment methods

Treatment of the fracture consists of reduction and fixation. In the case of long bones, this is often done in two stages, particularly if much manipulation is necessary for reduction. In simple mandibular fractures, reduction and fixation are accomplished together. The apparatus that is used to keep the jaws together during healing will often reduce the fracture as well. If multiple-loop wiring is placed, no attempt is made to reduce the fracture until the wiring on each jaw is complete. When the jaws are brought together and intermaxillary elastic traction is placed, the occlusion of the teeth will help to orient the fractured parts into good position. Exceptions occur, of course. Fractures that occur beyond the tooth-bearing portion of the mandible, such as the angle, will not be reduced if initially displaced. Other examples are edentulous jaws and old fractures that are partially healed, which require continuous elastic traction for reduction.

Intermaxillary fixation, that is, fixation obtained by applying wires or elastic bands between the upper and lower jaws to which suitable anchoring devices have been attached, will successfully treat most fractures of the mandible. The main methods for such fixation are wiring, arch bars, and splints.

Wiring

Multiple-loop wiring. The armed services and many civilian institutions use this method almost exclusively. The four posterior quadrants are wired.

PREPARATION. Local anesthesia with sedation or sedation alone is used. General anesthesia is used occasionally when further treatment is necessary after the wiring. Even then it is better to have the interdental wiring completed the day or night before the operation so that the time of the operating room personnel and prolonged general anesthesia are not needlessly required. The wiring is done in a dental chair if possible.

A local anesthetic can be given by two pterygomandibular blocks in the mandible and simple infiltration in the maxilla. Bilateral block anesthesia combined with sedation in a patient who later will be put on his back in bed can be dangerous because of lingual anesthesia. The patient should sit in a chair until the anesthesia has disappeared.

If the contact points of the teeth are not too tight and broad, and if the interdental gingival tissue is not too close to the contact points, no anesthesia is necessary. Sedation alone is adequate if care is taken that the fracture zone is not traumatized by undue movement. Premedication with either meperidine hydrochloride (Demerol), 50 to 100 mg, or pentobarbital sodium (Nembutal), 100 to 200 mg, parenterally is adequate generally. For severe pain or to render the patient almost completely insensible to manipulative pain for 20 minutes, 75 to 100 mg of meperidine hydrochloride can be given intravenously to an average adult. This must be administered slowly over a 2-minute interval.

ARMAMENTARIUM. The materials used for multiple-loop wiring are as follows:

Wire, 26-gauge stainless steel, cut into lengths of 20 cm and placed in a cold-sterilizing solution 20 minutes before use; wire cut on a bevel so that the bevel can act like a needle point if it must go through tissue

Solder, soft No. 20 resin core

Hegar needle holders (two)

Wire cutters

Blunt-nosed crown and bridge pliers

Discoid dental instrument

TECHNIQUE. One end of the wire is placed on the buccal side of the teeth, starting at the midline (stationary wire). The other end goes around the last tooth in the arch (for example, the second molar) and into the mesial interproximal space and emerges under the stationary wire. Then it is bent back above the stationary wire into the same interproximal space. It is delivered to the lingual side and bent around the next tooth (first molar) and into the interproximal space between the molar and the premolar. The wire that goes around each tooth and over and under the stationary wire is called the working wire (Fig. 19-21, *A*).

To make uniform loops on the buccal side, a piece of solder is placed on the buccal surfaces of the teeth over the stationary wire. It can be pressed against the teeth with the finger. The working wire therefore emerges under the stationary wire as well as under the solder, and then it is turned back and passed over the wire and solder to reenter the same interproximal space.

Each time the wire emerges on the buccal side it should be grasped with the needle holder and pulled firmly to reduce slack. The left hand should provide counterpressure on the buccal surfaces of the teeth. The discoid instrument is used to move the wire under the height of contour of the teeth on the lingual side.

When the arch segment has been wired, the working wire and the stationary wire are crossed at the mesial side of the canine or first premolar. They are crossed 1 cm away from the tooth; the needle holder is placed over the cross and twisted clockwise until the wire almost touches the tooth. With the discoid instrument, the wire is pushed beneath the cingulum of the cuspid. The wire is then grasped with the needle holder at the turn nearest the tooth and turned until the tooth surface is contacted. Backward pressure always is placed on the needle holder when wires are tightened.

The solder is cut midway between the last two buccal loops, bent outward, and twisted gently out of the last loop. The wire loop then is given a three-fourths turn in a clockwise direction with the needle holder or pliers. Another cut is made in the solder between the next two loops, and the small distal piece is withdrawn. The loop is tightened with a three-fourths turn. This is continued until all of the solder has been

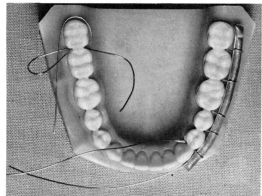
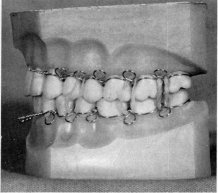

Fig. 19-21. A, Multiple-loop wiring. Note the buccal stationary wire and the lingual working wire that is threaded back and forth through interproximal spaces. **B,** Completed multiple-loop wiring.

removed. Then, starting in the back, each loop is given another half turn. The multiple-loop wiring should be firm by this time (Fig. 19-21, *B*).

The same procedure is followed in the other three quadrants of the mouth. If elastic traction will be used, the loops should be bent away from the occlusal plane so that hooks are formed. If wire will be used between the jaws, the loops are bent toward the occlusal plane.

It is desirable to use elastic traction routinely. This overcomes muscular distraction so that reduction is accomplished more easily, and it serves as a positive force to overcome muscular spasm when the jaw first tires of its forced closed position. If the mouth should have to be entered in the immediate postoperative period for relief of vomiting or the placement of an endotracheal tube for subsequent operation, the removal of the elastic bands is a simple matter. As an emergency procedure, particularly if the patient will be transported later, a wire can be placed on the buccal side under the elastics, bent back on itself over the elastics, and the two ends tied to clothing over the chest. If actual vomiting (not retching) occurs, the patient can jerk the wire and remove the elastic fixation immediately. This procedure is used rarely in civilian hospitals.

Elastic traction is obtained by stretching small or large Angle orthodontic elastics from an upper to a lower wire loop. A 14- or 16-gauge rubber catheter can be cut into bands that provide stronger traction. If the fracture does not position itself properly, elastics can be placed in different directions rather than straight up and down. If the chin fragment is too far forward, several strong elastics can be placed from the lower cuspid region to the upper second bicuspid region. Often the angled elastics can be replaced by straight elastics in one day, thereby eliminating a possibility of overreduction.

Ivy loop wiring. The Ivy loop embraces only two adjacent teeth, and it provides two hooks for elastics. An individual Ivy loop is applied more quickly than multiple-loop wiring, although several Ivy loops are necessary in a dentulous arch. If many teeth are missing, adjacent teeth can be used satisfactorily by this method. If a wire should break, it is simpler to replace a single Ivy loop than it is a multiple-loop wire.

The armamentarium is the same as in multiple-loop wiring. The wire is 26 gauge cut in 15 cm lengths. A loop is formed in the center of the wire around the break of a towel clip and twisted once. These wires can be stored in an emergency room in cold-sterilizing solution.

The two tails of the wire are placed in the embrasure from the buccal to the lingual side (Fig. 19-22, *A*). If difficulty occurs, a

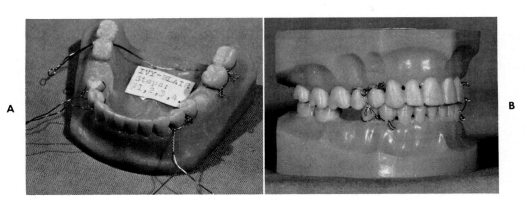

Fig. 19-22. A, Ivy loop wiring. **B,** Completed Ivy loop wiring. Intermaxillary fixation can be obtained by the use of wire or elastics simply by bending the loops down or up.

piece of dental floss can be doubled through the loop. The floss then is carried past the contact point and the wire pulled through the embrasure from the lingual to the buccal side. The floss is removed. One wire tail is carried around the lingual surface of the distal tooth, pushed through the embrasure on the distal side of that tooth, and bent around the buccal surface. It is threaded through the previously formed loop or just under the loop. The other wire tail is carried around the lingual surface of the mesial tooth, passed through the embrasure on the mesial side of that tooth, and meets the first wire. The two wires are crossed and twisted together with the needle holder. The loop is then tightened and bent toward the gingiva. The crossed wires are cut, and a small rosette is made to serve as an additional hook. The rosette is wound clockwise below the greatest circumference of the tooth for two turns and then flattened toward the tooth (Fig. 19-22, *B*). One or two of these Ivy loops are placed in each quadrant. Elastic traction then is placed between the jaws.

Risdon wiring. A wire arch bar tied in the midline is especially indicated for symphysis fractures. A 26-gauge stainless steel wire 25 cm long is passed around the most distal strong tooth so that both arms of the wire extend to the buccal side. The two wires, which are of equal length, then are twisted on each other for their entire length. The

same procedure is followed for the other side of the arch. The two twisted strands are crossed in the midline and twisted around each other (Fig. 19-23, *A*). A rosette is formed. Each tooth in the arch then is ligated individually to the wire arch (Fig. 19-23, *B*). One wire is passed over the arch wire, and the other is passed under the arch wire. After tightening, a small hook is formed with each twisted strand. (Fig. 19-23, *C*). Intermaxillary traction is obtained by stretching elastic bands between the hooks in each arch.

Arch bars

Arch bars are perhaps the ideal method for intermaxillary fixation. Several types of ready-made arch bars are used. The rigid type requires either an impression and a stone cast to which the bar can be adapted carefully by a two-plier technique or a person skilled in the bending of prosthetic bars who has sufficient time to adapt it in the mouth (Fig. 19-24, *A*). A soft type is available that can be bent with the fingers. It must be remembered that teeth lashed to any type of bar can be moved orthodontically if the bar has not been fitted skillfully.

The soft bar can be fitted, using two large needle holders, although wire-bending pliers are better (Fig. 19-24, *B*). In an unfractured maxilla the bending should be

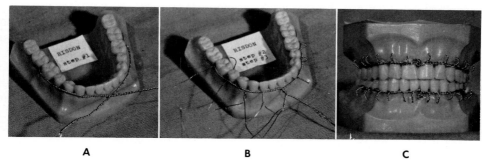

Fig. 19-23. Risdon wiring. **A,** Formation of wire arch bar. **B,** Ligation of separate teeth to wire arch bar. **C,** Completed wiring ready for elastic bands.

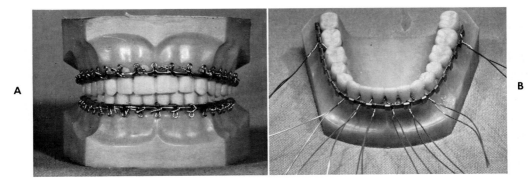

Fig. 19-24. A, Rigid arch bars. **B,** Soft type arch bar. Note that the incisor and canine teeth are wired before the bar is placed, and the bar is then wired to the anterior teeth fixation. The posterior teeth are ligated directly to the bar.

started at the buccal side of the last tooth. The bar is adapted accurately to each tooth. The pliers or needle holder should be kept close together so that previously adapted portions are not bent again. By starting at one end of the bar, progressing past the midline, and finishing at the other end, the bar can be adapted readily and quickly without producing bulges. The bar should be shortened properly and the end filed smooth with a gold file. An overextended bar will cause soft tissue necrosis and severe pain. The midline of the jaw should be marked on the bar during bending so that it will be reseated accurately. As a general rule, the bar should not cross a fracture line except in a greenstick fracture. The bar is cut and adapted to each segment of a fractured jaw.

Wiring the bar to the teeth is relatively simple. Thin 30-gauge wire is used. Before seating the bar, wires are placed on the anterior teeth to seat tightly under the cingulum to resist displacement of the bar to the incisal level. A small loop of wire is placed by "jumping" the contact point or by threading through the two embrasures. The wires are crossed and grasped with a needle holder close to the labial enamel surface. Three fourths of a turn is given to the wire after the wire has been pushed below the cingulum. This is done to each anterior tooth.

The bar then is placed between the open ends of the wires. The midline mark is adjusted, and care is taken that the hooks on the arch bar project upward in the maxilla and downward in the mandible. The individual anterior wire ends are crossed over the bar, grasped, and twisted. The posterior teeth are then ligated individually to the bar. One end of a 7 cm long wire is passed from the buccal side under the bar through one embrasure, circled around the lingual side of the tooth, and then pushed back from the lingual side through the next embrasure to pass over the bar.

The crossed wires are grasped 2 mm away from the bar, and backward pressure is placed on the needle holder before a turn is made. This pressure is maintained during any tightening operation. When the turns approach the bar, the wire is again grasped with the needle holder further away from the bar, and turns are made until the previous turns are reached. The turned strand is cut 7 mm away from the bar while the holder still has the wire in its beaks so that the cut strand will not be lost in the mouth. The strand is grasped close to the bar and given a final turn. The end is turned under the bar so that the lips and cheeks will not be traumatized.

All teeth should be ligated to the bar. This rule has few exceptions.

Perhaps the main failings of the bar technique are improper adaptation of the bar, ligation of an insufficient number of teeth, and inefficient tightening of the wires. Advantages associated with arch bars include less trauma, because of the thin wire, and greater stability in an arch that has many missing teeth, because the edentulous gaps can be spanned by a rigid appliance. If one wire should break during healing, the fixation will not suffer. The hooks on the bar also seem to be less irritating to the soft tissues.

Splints

Splints are used when wiring of the teeth will not provide adequate fixation or when horizontal splinting across a fracture zone is necessary, as well as in some cases in which immobilization of the fractured parts is indicated without closing the mouth by intermaxillary fixation. At one time, splints with distal metal extensions were used to control the posterior fragment in angle fractures, but pain and unsatisfactory results have made it necessary to generally discontinue this procedure.

The acrylic splint is made from an impression so that it covers a minimum of the occlusal surfaces of the teeth and as much of the labial and lingual surfaces of the teeth as do not form an undercut. The gingival margins are not encroached. The lingual surface is continuous. The buccal surface is attached to the lingual portion behind the last molar either by continuous acrylic material or by a wire connector. A vertical cut is made in the midline of the labial flange through a large acrylic button. The splint is placed over the reduced fractured mandible, and the acrylic button is drawn together and held by wire. (See Fig. 19-25, *A*.)

The cast cap silver splint requires impressions of the opposing arches. The lower cast is sawed through the line of fracture. The cast is reassembled in proper occlusion and fixed in this position by pouring a base for the cast. The splint is formed to the gingival margins in 28-gauge sheet wax. Oc-

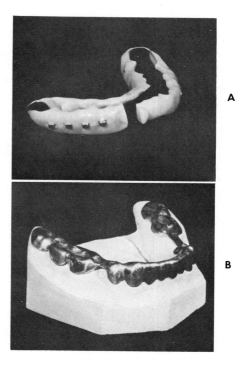

Fig. 19-25. A, Acrylic splint. **B,** Cast cap silver splint.

cusal relations are established in the wax-up by bringing it into proper centric relation with the opposing casts while the wax is soft. The cast is sprued with inlay wax. When the sprues are in place, the wax-up is drawn from the stone cast in an occlusal direction while the wax is warm to eliminate undercuts. The wax-up is mounted in a large crucible former in a single investment technique, with an asbestos liner in the ring. It is cast in coin silver at 1,000° to 1,500° F (538° to 816° C) and finished (Fig. 19-25, *B*).

The splint is cemented to the reduced fractured jaw. If the splint will be needed for weeks rather than months, it is sometimes better to use zinc oxide and eugenol for cementation rather than crown and bridge cement, since these splints are often difficult to remove. The splints can be made of gold, and projections or hooks for intermaxillary fixation can be formed on them. Some gold splints are made in sections for specific purposes.

The splint is generally indicated for the very simple or the very complex case. If an oral surgeon suffered a simple mandibular fracture within the area of dentition, he or she probably would prefer a cast cap silver splint so that the jaws would not be wired shut. In bone graft cases or in delayed union cases, the splints are indicated, since they provide long-term fixation in the presence of function.

Except for these general indications, the use of splints is not great. The acrylic splint has fallen largely into disuse, except for children with deciduous teeth, which are difficult to wire sometimes. The average fracture with good teeth is well on the way to good healing if wired immediately. The splinted patient requires impressions, temporary immobilization, delay of various degrees during construction of the appliance, and then later reduction and cementation. If a tooth should become acutely infected under a splint, a real problem is presented.

Orthodontic fixation is used more often for elective surgery and long-term procedures than for traumatic surgery. It is especially indicated for alveolar fractures.

Circumferential wiring

Circumferential wiring (''wiring around'') usually refers to the procedure of placing wires around a mandibular denture and around the mandible so that the fractured mandible is held firmly into the denture, which serves as a splint. The fracture must be situated within the area covered by the denture base unless secondary procedures for the control of the other segment are contemplated. If the denture is fractured at the time of the accident, it can be repaired satisfactorily sometimes with quick-cure acrylic (Fig. 19-26).

The mouth is rinsed with an antiseptic solution to reduce the bacterial count. The skin is prepared in the usual manner. General or local anesthesia is satisfactory, although skin infiltration is necessary to supplement a local block procedure.

The simplest procedure consists of threading a long, straight skin needle with thin 28-gauge steel wire, which has been sterilized previously. The needle is bent into a slightly concave form with the fingers. It is passed through the floor of the mouth close to the mandible to emerge

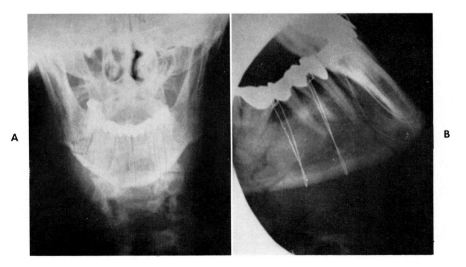

A   **B**

Fig. 19-26. A, Circumferential wiring around cast cap silver splint. The splint was cemented to the teeth. Circumferential wiring pulled the inferior border fragment upward. **B,** Lateral view.

through the skin directly beneath the mandible. The needle is brought out of the skin, turned, and redirected into the same skin puncture hole. It is passed upward on the buccal side of the mandible close to the bone to emerge in the mucobuccal fold. The wires are cut near the needle. The two lingual and the two buccal wires are twisted over the denture, cut short, and formed into a rosette on the buccal side. At least three circumferential wires are placed, one near the distal end of the denture on each side and one at the midline. Occasionally two wires are placed in the anterior region. One side of the denture may have a wire placed anterior and another posterior to the fracture line. (See Fig. 19-27.)

The wires are sawed back and forth several times before tightening, to move them through the tissues to the inferior border of the mandible. Care is taken that a dimple does not persist at the skin wound. The skin around the wound should be released from the subdermal structures after the wires are tightened around the denture. A No. 11 surgical blade is used to release the skin, and a single skin suture is placed.

Several variations in technique are possible. A long, No. 17 hypodermic needle can be used (Fig. 19-28). It is bent to a concave form and passed on the lingual side from the skin through the floor of the mouth. A single 26-gauge wire is introduced into the lumen from the skin side and grasped in the mouth with a hemostat. The needle then is removed. The same needle is introduced intraorally through the buccal fold to emerge through the same skin hole, and the other arm of the wire is threaded through the lumen from the skin side into the mouth.

If the hub of a second needle is cut off so that it can be removed from the wound, it can be introduced from the skin side into the buccal vestibule. The advantage of this method is the introduction of the two needles and the two arms of the wire from the skin surface into the more septic oral cavity, which will enhance the possibility of a noninfected skin wound.

Other variations have to do with the preparation of the denture. Holes for the wires can be drilled in the acrylic buccolingually between the teeth, just above the

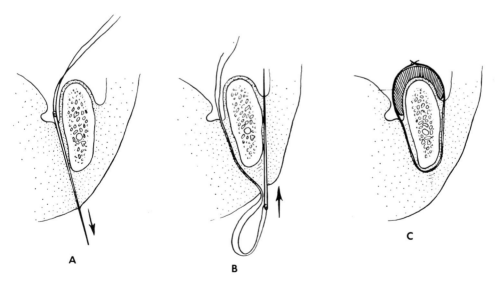

Fig. 19-27. Circumferential wiring technique with straight skin needle. **A,** Penetration of floor of mouth. **B,** Penetration of buccal sulcus. **C,** Wire around denture or splint.

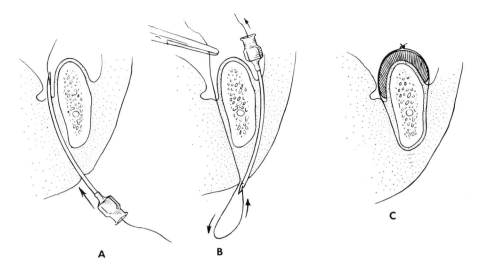

Fig. 19-28. Circumferential wiring technique with hypodermic needle. **A,** Penetration of floor of mouth from skin surface. **B,** Penetration of buccal sulcus from mucosal surface. **C,** Finished wiring.

ridge. Danger of slipping is lessened, and the occlusal surfaces are not separated by the thickness of the wire. These holes also can be used for ligating the maxillary and mandibular dentures together for intermaxillary fixation after reduction, or hooks can be placed on the dentures for this purpose. The anterior teeth of the mandibular denture can be removed to provide better feeding and to eliminate the fulcrum created by the wire when it is tied over the teeth away from the ridge. Edentulous acrylic baseplate splints can be constructed if dentures are not available.

Skeletal pin fixation

Skeletal pin fixation is used in cases in which the management of a fractured bone segment is not satisfactorily accomplished by intermaxillary fixation. Fractures of the mandibular angle can be immobilized by skeletal pin fixation without surgically exposing the fracture. Fragments bridged by a bone graft are immmobilized by skeletal pin fixation. Fractures in edentulous jaws can be treated in similar fashion.

At the time of World War II, skeletal pin fixation became popular for several rea-

sons. The armed services and the British treated simple as well as complicated fractures by this method, without supplementing it with intermaxillary fixation, so that the transported patient who suffered from motion sickness was not endangered by drowning in vomitus, and limited duty was made possible without liquid-diet restrictions. Men practicing in as well as out of the armed services could treat complicated fractures without having training in open procedures.

Skeletal pins can be placed while the patient is under general anesthesia or local block anesthesia supplemented by skin infiltration. It can be done in the dental chair or preferably in the operating room, where greater safety and convenience are possible. Strict asepsis is necessary. The skin must be prepared thoroughly, the field must be draped, and the operating team must be scrubbed and wear gloves and gowns.

After skin preparation, the inferior and superior borders of the mandible are palpated and marked on the skin with a dye such as gentian violet on an applicator stick. The line of fracture is marked, and the general location of the inferior alveolar

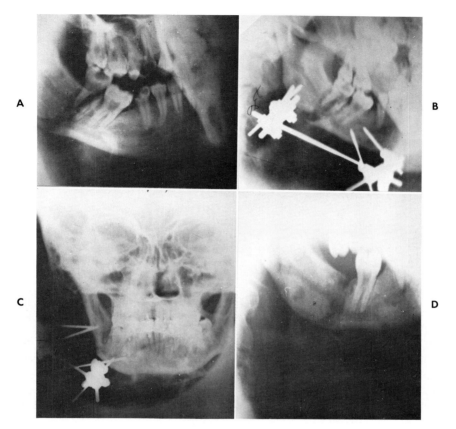

Fig. 19-29. A, Compound fracture extending through molar tooth, complicated by infection. The posterior fragment has been distracted upward by muscular pull. **B,** Skeletal pin fixation in position. **C,** Posteroanterior view. Note intermaxillary wiring. The fractured tooth was removed after this radiograph was made. **D,** Healing 3 months later.

canal is marked after reference to the radiograph. Intermaxillary fixation should be placed beforehand if used. (See Fig. 19-29.)

The pins are positioned usually by an egg-beater-type drill. Two are placed at a 40-degree angle to each other on one side of the fracture, and two are placed similarly on the other side. If each pin is started 20 degrees from the vertical plane, a 40-degree divergence between them will result. The pins should not be placed closer to the fracture line than 1 cm. The skin is tensed directly over the bone. The pin in the drill is placed on the skin and pressed directly down to bone. The drill is rotated slowly under

moderate pressure. The revolving point will be felt to penetrate the outer cortex, transverse the softer spongiosa, and then enter the inner cortex. It should penetrate the entire inner cortex, but it should not be lodged more than 1 or 2 mm in the medial soft tissues. The drill then is removed carefully from the pin. The pin should be tested for stability. If not stable, it has not penetrated the medial cortex and should be rotated deeper with a hand attachment.

Two pins are placed in the anterior fragment parallel to the inferior border. The two pins in the posterior fragment can be placed parallel to the inferior border also, provided that the location of the fracture is not so far

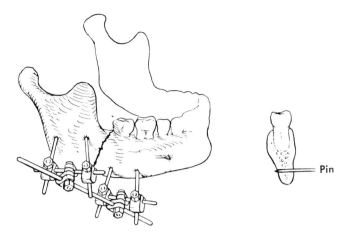

Fig. 19-30. Skeletal pin assembly. Note that the pin traverses both bony cortices.

back that the most posterior pin will be located in the thin bone at the angle of the jaw. If the most posterior pin location is at the angle, it is better to locate the second pin further up on the vertical ramus at the posterior border or in the retromolar area near the anterior border. The pins should be located halfway between the mandibular canal and the inferior border, and care is taken that they do not traverse the facial artery or vein. (See Fig. 19-30.)

A bar assembly is attached to the two anterior pins. A similar assembly is placed on the two posterior pins. A large bar is selected and placed in the attachments on the short bars so that it crosses the fracture. The fracture is manually reduced so that the inferior border is continuous to palpation and the lateral border is continuous. All attachments are then tightened securely with a wrench. A drop of collodion is placed around the pin entrances into the skin. Roentgenograms made in the operating room or later will demonstrate the accuracy of the reduction.

Properly placed pins will remain tight for several months in the absence of infection.

Many variations exist in the design of skeletal pin apparatus. The Thoma bone clamp is useful in cases in which infection

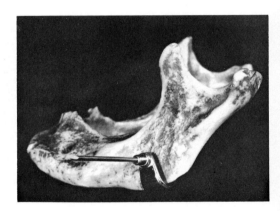

Fig. 19-31. Thoma bone clamp.

makes pins or transosseous wiring uncertain or in long-range treatment cases in which a bone graft is used (Fig. 19-31).

Some operators make use of an electrical drill to place pins rather than the manually operated eggbeater-type drill.

Open reduction

Open reduction with interosseous wiring is a definitive method for anchoring bone segments at the fracture site. Wire is placed through holes on either side of the fracture, reduction is accomplished under direct vision, and immobilization is obtained by tightening the wires. This procedure usually is reserved for fractures that cannot be reduced and immobilized adequately by closed methods. However, fractures that have soft tissue or debris interposed between the fragments and fractures that have healed in malposition are treated by open reduction.

One advantage to this method is direct visualization of the fractured parts, and consequently better reduction is possible. Oblique fractures, particularly those that present a short fracture on one cortical plate and a long one on the other plate (usually the lingual), are reduced with more precision. Complicated fractures are treated in this manner. It should be noted, on the other hand, that a severely comminuted fracture is not treated by open reduction if it can be avoided. The many small fragments may lose their vitality and be sloughed after an open procedure because the surrounding periosteal and soft tissue attachments and the traumatic hematoma and its binding, nutritive, and protective functions have been removed, and infection may be introduced.

Another advantage is firm fixation. Teeth can loosen, wires and appliances can slip, but the bone ends are still held close to each other. If teeth are present, open reduction should be supplemented by intermaxillary fixation for additional stabilization. Experience has shown that direct interosseous wires cannot be relied on for complete immobilization of the fragments if unrestricted use of the jaws is permitted.

Open reduction is done almost always under general anesthesia in the operating room. Intermaxillary wiring should be in place. For that reason, nasoendotracheal anesthesia is indicated. The most common site for open reduction is at the angle of the mandible, and the description will be for that procedure.

Preparation of the site of surgery, draping, and the surgical approach through the skin and soft tissues have been described in Chapter 2. The basic armamentarium is supplemented with the following instru-

ments necessary for interosseous wiring:

2 Periosteotomes, dull and sharp
1 Bone rongeur
1 Mallet, metal, small
3 Chisels
1 Pliers, cutting, wire
4 Forceps, bone, Kocher's
1 Retractor, malleable, narrow
1 Pistol drill, key, and drill points
    Wire, stainless steel, 24 and 30 gauge

Infiltration of the skin with a local anesthetic solution containing 1:50,000 epinephrine or another vasoconstrictor will eliminate clamping and tying the skin blood vessels, resulting in a smoother postoperative skin wound.

The bone is exposed, and the fracture is visualized (see Chapter 2 for technique). The posterior fragment usually will be malplaced in a superior and medial position. Examination should be made of the cortical plates, particularly on the medial side. If the medial cortex is missing for some distance on one fragment, the location of the bur holes will have to be moved back until both cortical plates of that fragment can be traversed by one hole.

A flat ribbon retractor is placed under the medial side of the bone from the inferior border to protect the underlying soft tissue structures. The second assistant holds the superior soft tissue retractor across the face with the right hand and the ribbon retractor at the inferior border of the jaw with the left hand. The first assistant holds a syringe of normal saline solution in the right hand and the suction (if it is used) in the left hand. The operator holds the drill in both hands. Occasionally secondary tissue retraction by the right hand of the first assistant is necessary near the drill bit.

An electrical drill is used more commonly than a mechanical eggbeater-type drill. The first hole should be started on the anterior fragment, near the inferior border, 0.5 cm from the fracture site. The drill point should be sharp. Rotation is started at slow speed until the hole is started, and then the speed may be increased, taking care that burning of the bone does not occur. The operator will feel the penetration of the outer cortex, the spongiosa, and the inner cortex. Saline solution is sprayed on the site during drilling. The drill is removed. Another hole is placed above the first one in the anterior fragment. It should not go through the inferior alveolar canal being slightly below it. Usually it is well to place a 24-gauge wire in this hole immediately after the drill is removed and clamp the two ends with a hemostat outside the wound.

The ribbon retractor is repositioned under the posterior fragment. One hole is placed near the inferior border 0.5 cm from the fracture site. Another hole is placed as high as possible above the first one and still just below the inferior alveolar canal. A wire is placed through this hole and clamped outside the wound.

The medial arm of the wire in the anterosuperior hole (Fig. 19-32, 2) crosses the fracture line and is threaded in the posteroinferior hole (3) from the medial to the lateral cortex (Fig. 19-32, A). It usually is difficult to locate the hole from beneath. Time can be saved by placing a thin 30-gauge wire in the second hole from a lateral to medial direction. This wire is doubled,

and the loop is introduced into the hole first. When recovered with a small curved hemostat from the medial aspect, the medial arm of the original wire is placed through the loop and bent back 3 cm. The thin double wire then is pulled upward (laterally) with care, to thread the original wire through the hole. The two arms of the original wire then are clamped outside the wound.

The medial arm of the wire in the posterosuperior hole (4) is threaded through the anteroinferior hole (1) from a medial to lateral direction, using a similar thin wire loop technique. It is clamped outside the wound.

The bone fragments are grasped with bone-holding or Kocher's forceps, although two No. 150 dental forceps may be employed, and the fracture is reduced by manipulating the fragments. If aberrant soft tissue and other debris are located between the bone fragments, it should be removed at this time. If necessary, major debridement should be done before the wires are placed. The wires are tightened while the assistant holds the bone ends in the reduced position. It is important to place upward traction on the needle holder while twisting the wires. After the wire has been tight-

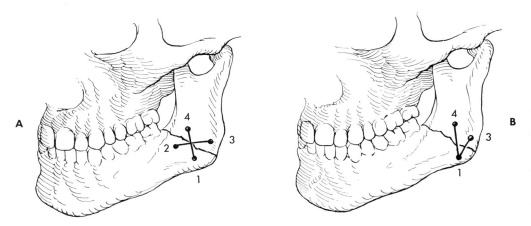

Fig. 19-32. Open reduction and interosseous wiring. **A,** Four-hole technique for mandibular angle fracture. **B,** Three-hole technique.

ened to within 3 mm of the bone surface, a small periosteal elevator is placed on the underside (medial) of the bone and the wire flattened against the bone. The needle holder grasps the strand of wire at the next to last turn, upward traction is made, and the wire is turned down to the bone surface.

The same procedure is followed for the other wire. The first wire is examined for tightness. The bone-holding instruments are removed, and the fracture reduction is inspected. Ordinarily no further manipulation will be necessary. The wire strands are cut off at a length of 0.7 cm, and the ends are turned carefully into the nearest bone holes.

Soft tissue closure is made by layers as described in Chapter 2. No drains are placed unless uncontrollable oozing of blood from deep areas is noted when the platysma muscle layer is being closed. After the skin sutures are placed, a small piece of sterile Teflon is laid over them. Three 10 by 10 cm gauze sponges are placed over the Teflon and held. Drapes are removed together with gloves and operating gowns. Blood and secretions are wiped from the face and neck. Skin areas adjacent to the bandages are painted with compound tincture of benzoin and allowed to dry. Many narrow strips (1 cm) of adhesive tape 20 cm long are placed over the bandages and skin with a fair amount of tension, since a pressure dressing is desired. An operating cap is placed on the head of the patient. A roll of elastic adhesive tape is wrapped around the chin, bandage, and head in modified Barton style. Last, a 10 cm strip of ordinary adhesive tape is placed on the cap over the forehead, and the words "fractured jaw" are written upside down on it. This will remind recovery room personnel that the ordinary practice of holding the chin up to maintain a clear airway must be done with care, if at all.

It is possible to place too much bulk and pressure with the elastic adhesive dressing on the anterior throat instead of under the chin. Immediate respiratory embarrassment will result, necessitating revision.

The endotracheal tube should not be removed until the elastic adhesive dressing is in place. Anesthesia should be continued in sufficient depth until that time so that the patient will not "buck" on the tube. A carefully reduced fracture can be disturbed by "bucking" on the tube, particularly if the fracture is not supported adequately by outside bandaging.

The postoperative orders should be written in the operating room. In most hospitals all preoperative orders are automatically cancelled by an operative procedure.

This basic technique has many variations. Three bone holes are adequate usually (Fig. 19-32, B). This eliminates the need for the anterosuperior hole, with the attendant threading of the wire immediatedly after drilling. All three holes are drilled. The posterosuperior hole (4) is drilled last, and a wire is placed through it. The medial arm of this wire in the posterosuperior hole is threaded into the anterior hole (1). Then one wire is placed from the anterior hole (1) to the posteroinferior hole (3). Two wires therefore are located in one anterior hole. The horizontal (1 to 3) wire is tightened first to impact the bone, and then the oblique wire (1 to 4) is tightened to prevent upward muscle displacement. The first wire is examined for stability, since it often requires another turn.

In the three-hole technique, a figure-of-eight wire in two inferior holes offers advantages in providing downward traction as well as cross fracture traction. As a matter of fact, the technique used most today employs two holes, one on either side of the fracture, connected with a figure-of-eight wire (1 and 3). A figure of eight is made on the inferior border, with the wires crossing near the fracture site. Both ends of the wire can be placed from the lateral side, eliminating the threading from the medial side.

Bone plates are used infrequently in new

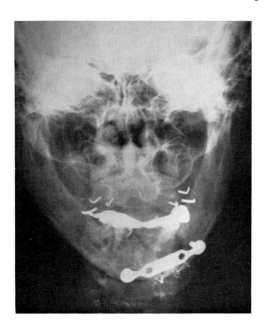

Fig. 19-33. Bone plate used to maintain telescoped comminuted symphyseal fracture. Cast cap splint on mandibular teeth; acrylic splint with metal lugs in edentulous maxilla.

fractures of the jaws (Fig. 19-33). Healing seems to be delayed in comparison with wire techniques that pull the fractured ends together during convalescence. The screws in bone plates hold the bones rigidly. The technique of fastening the plates sometimes will allow a small distraction of the fragments, and the absence of minute functional stresses at the fracture site results in slower healing. Care must be taken that the screws and the plate are made of exactly the same alloy to prevent electrolytic currents from forming, which would cause dissolution of bone around the holes.[14] Even screws cast from the same alloy sometimes cause such currents. In the casting process the metals may have separated somewhat so that the head and point of the same screw are not a uniform alloy.

In comminuted fractures that require open reduction and occasionally in edentulous mandibular fractures that have a strong tendency to override, a metal gutter plate can be placed on the inferior border with screws or wires through bone holes. Ordinary wires without a bone plate will pull an overriding fracture together, but they will not hold an overriding fracture in proper distracted position unless other wires are placed in lateral directions. The principle of the slotted plate used by the orthopedic surgeon in fractures of the long bone is applicable here. Muscular pull across the fracture site is allowed to act to keep the fractured ends together during healing by the sliding of screws in a horizontal slot rather than in a hole in the plate.

The L splint has a right-angle bend across its top surface that is placed in a slot cut through the cortical plate across the fracture zone. Because of its horizontal stability, only two screws are necessary. The L splint is less bulky and more stable than ordinary bone plates.[19]

Treatment of fractures of the mandible
Uncomplicated fractures

A large percentage of mandibular fractures can be treated by simple intermaxillary fixation. The fractures must be located within the dental arch, and at least one sound tooth should be present in the posterior (proximal) fragment. Although specific advantages are inherent in the use of one method over another in a specific fracture, by and large any method of intermaxillary fixation can be used. (See Fig. 19-34.) For example, multiple-loop wiring was used extensively and almost exclusively in the armed services during World War II. The beginning practitioner should be able to manage one method well. Variations can be considered with increased experience.

The question of the removal of a tooth in the line of fracture is managed often by the judgment of the operator. Before the sulfonamides and antibiotics, it was always removed. Most experienced practitioners still will remove this tooth. The following factors influence the decision: the absence

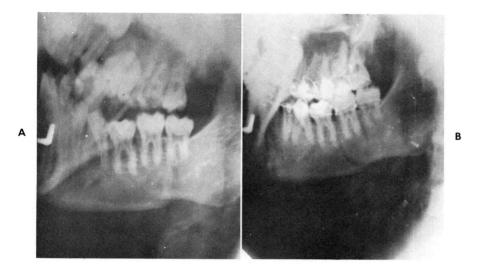

Fig. 19-34. A, Fracture in dentulous region distracted upward. **B,** Satisfactory reduction by simple interdental wiring and intermaxillary fixation.

of fracture or gross injury to the tooth; the absence of caries or large restorations; the absence of periodontitis; the location of the tooth, including esthetics and the possibility of arch collapse; the nature of the fracture; and the probability of adequate response to antibiotic therapy. If serious doubt exists whether or not to extract the tooth, it should be extracted. Persistent chronic infection or an acute abscess occurring later in treatment sometimes will require opening of the fixation to extract the tooth. Delayed union or nonunion can result.

As a matter of fact, infected and grossly carious teeth that are not in the line of fracture should be extracted before placing intermaxillary fixation. This can be done while the patient is under the same anesthesia given for wiring.

Elastic traction is placed to overcome distraction and muscle spasm. With continued changing, elastic traction can be used throughout convalescence. If desired, the elastics can be replaced by intermaxillary wires after 1 week. The wires are easier to keep clean, and they seem to bother the patient less. Recalcitrant pa-

tients who desire a chicken dinner at the end of the third week sometimes require heavy intermaxillary wire fixation supplemented by elastic traction.

Antibiotics are useful for the first week as a prophylactic measure. It is advantageous usually to admit a fracture patient to the hospital. Many patients with simple fractures are treated in the outpatient clinic or office and then allowed to go home, where they are observed. However, a 24- or 48-hour admission will allow the patient to recuperate from his trauma and operation better, his new diet and drug therapy can be introduced to him, and he can be observed more closely.

Complicated fractures

Fractures that cannot be reduced and fixed properly by simple intermaxillary fixation require further measures. Usually the dentulous cases have intermaxillary fixation placed as a starting point.

Mandibular angle. Intermaxillary fixation is placed. The horizontal and vertical favorable fractures require no further treatment. A solid, unfractured tooth in the posterior fragment with an antagonist in the

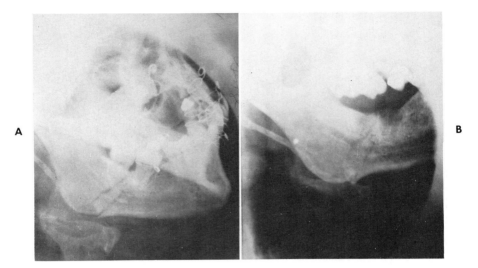

A

B

Fig. 19-35. A, Horizontal unfavorable angle fracture satisfactorily reduced by intermaxillary fixation, aided by the presence of an unfractured third molar in the line of fracture, preventing upward displacement. Note that this tooth is not wired. **B,** Healed fracture. The molar teeth were extracted after healing had occurred.

maxilla will preclude further treatment (Fig. 19-35). Conservatism is necessary in condemning such a tooth for extraction. Many experienced practitioners on occasion have retained such a tooth when one root has been fractured, but as a rule the worry during the convalescent period does not make the procedure worthwhile. The oral surgeon who enjoys life treats the fracture in definitive fashion immediately.

Many methods for controlling the posterior fragment have been advocated. Some have been abandoned, and others are not generally accepted. Skeletal pin fixation and open reduction are the two main alternatives. Individual preference is a strong factor in choice. Skeletal pin fixation is satisfactory if it is placed properly. Pin fixation can be done in the office if necessary. The fact that much external hardware is in evidence during healing and the fact that open reduction takes only about 30 minutes longer to do influence many oral surgeons toward open reduction. Open reduction, despite its drawbacks of the external scar, the loss of the original hema-

toma, the exposure of bone to possible infection, and the operating room procedure involved, still seems to provide more definitive treatment (Figs. 19-36 and 19-37).

Two alternative intraoral methods are illustrated in Fig. 19-37, *C* and *D*. Occasionally a circumferential wire can be placed through a hole in the posterior fragment through an intraoral incision and the wire looped around the inferior border. The angle of the fracture line must be suitable. The other method involves placing two intraoral holes in the buccal cortex of the bone after removal of the third molar. This method is valuable in the case of mandibular fracture associated with removal of an impacted third molar. The wire should lie in a vertical plane rather than a horizontal plane. The technique is especially successful in the horizontal favorable fracture.

Symphysis. Simple wiring often provides satisfactory immobilization. Wiring of the teeth, particularly with the Risdon wiring across the fracture, will reduce the fracture adequately at the alveolar level, but separa-

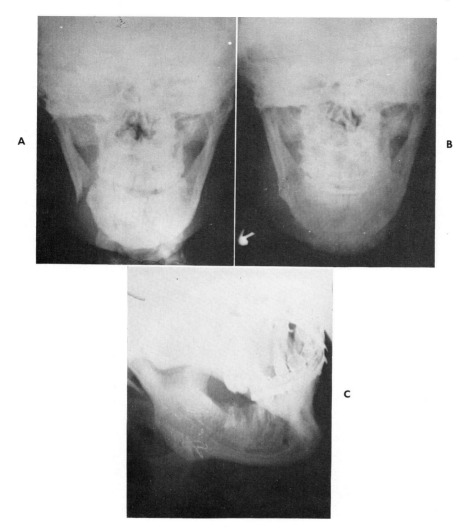

Fig. 19-36. Open reduction, four-hole technique. **A,** Preoperative radiograph. **B,** Postoperative radiograph. **C,** Lateral view showing details of interosseous wiring. The presence of the third molar in this case would not have aided reduction or fixation. The second molar was infected. Both molars were removed.

tion or telescoping may occur at the inferior border. If the wiring is tight and the inferior border separation is minimal, healing will be satisfactory (Fig. 19-38, *A*). However, the principal complication is collapse of the alveolar arch inward, which is difficult to prevent with dental wiring. A simple acrylic splint placed on the lingual aspect of the dental arch before wiring will prevent arch collapse.

Wide separation or other malposition requires further treatment. Skeletal pins can be used. A Kirschner wire or Steinmann pin (Fig. 19-38, *B*) can be driven across the chin by an electrical drill. This is done through the skin surfaces while the fractured ends are held in proper reduction. This is a relatively simple procedure that takes little time.

Open reduction in this region does not

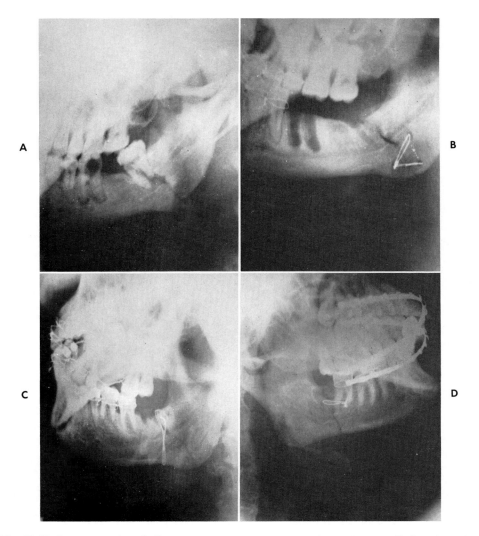

Fig. 19-37. Open reduction. **A,** Three-hole technique, preoperative radiograph. **B,** Postoperative radiograph. **C,** Similar case showing circummandibular wire placed from within the mouth, precluding an operating room procedure. A hole was drilled in the ascending ramus. **D,** Successful use of an intraoral wire through holes placed in the buccal osseous plates after fracture during odontectomy.

encounter large vessels, but the tissue attachments are difficult to raise. Care must be given to locating the linear scar beneath the chin within the skin creases if practicable. More exact reduction and closer fixation are made possible by open reduction. This method is valuable, especially in the grossly telescoped fracture (Fig. 19-39).

In symphysis fractures uncomplicated by

condyle fracture, force of the blow has traumatized the temporomandibular joint, and ankylosis can occur if the jaw is not opened occasionally during the treatment period to free the joint. This maneuver is accomplished better if a lingual acrylic splint stabilizes the symphysis fracture.

Edentulous fracture. Circumferential wiring around a denture or acrylic splint is

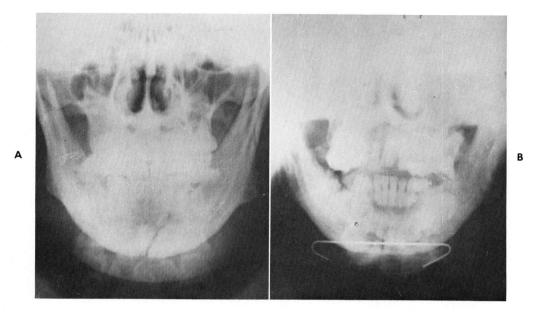

Fig. 19-38. A, Symphysis fracture reduced by multiple-loop intermaxillary wiring. **B,** Steinmann pin through symphysis.

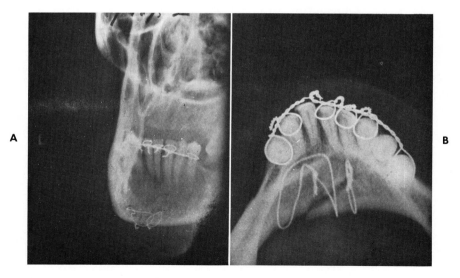

Fig. 19-39. A, Open reduction of symphysis fracture. **B,** Intraoral view to show figure-of-eight wiring to overcome characteristic tendency to telescope in symphysis fractures.

adequate in most cases (Fig. 19-40). All fragments must be covered by the denture base, and they must be held adequately to preclude auxiliary treatment. Fractures occurring distal to the posterior border of the denture, old telescoped fractures, and cases of severe trauma require skeletal pin fixation or open reduction. Some oral surgeons do not place dentures and intermaxillary fixation in edentulous jaws when skeletal pin fixation or open reduction is done, although others feel that all jaw fractures should have intraoral stabilization.

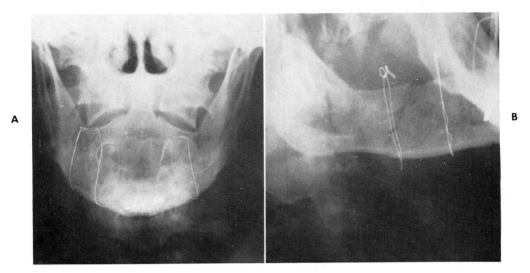

Fig. 19-40. A, Circumferential wiring around acrylic splint in edentulous patient. **B,** Lateral view.

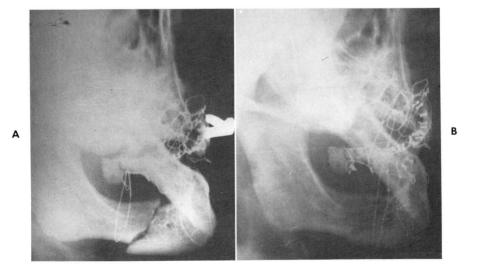

Fig. 19-41. A, Circumferential wire around denture, incorrectly placed. Tightening the wire distracted the posterior fragment upward. **B,** Same case after distal wire was replaced by a wire around the anterior fragment.

In the case of the angle–third molar region fracture that is not distal to the posterior border of the denture, the circummandibular wires should be placed around the anterior fragment. Muscular pull on the posterior fragment will elevate it so that further wires are not necessary in this area (Fig. 19-41).

Keeping the maxillary denture in is often a problem. If the maxillary denture fits well, and particularly if it has one or more minor undercuts, the two dentures connected by intermaxillary fixation may stay in place. Older women with resorbed alveolar ridges will carefully slip the maxilla out of the assembled dentures when the surgeon has gone, turn to the next bed, and start to jabber incessantly. This is an eerie sight with the dentures closed and still moving in unison over fast speech. If the

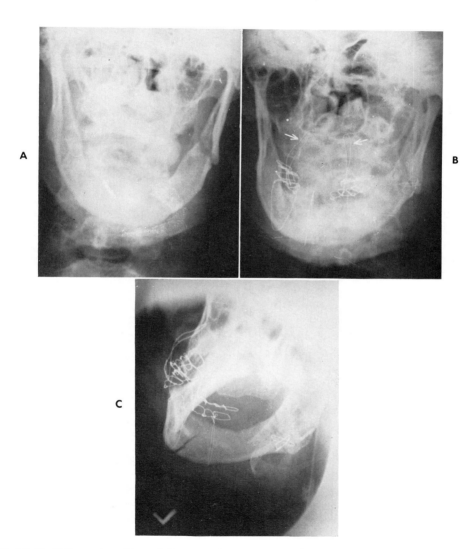

Fig. 19-42. Piriform rim wiring. **A,** Preoperative radiograph. **B,** Circumferential wiring. Piriform rim wiring extends to mandibular denture to aid in immobilizing dentures. **C,** Piriform rim wiring can be seen anteriorly. Note incidental interosseous wiring at angle.

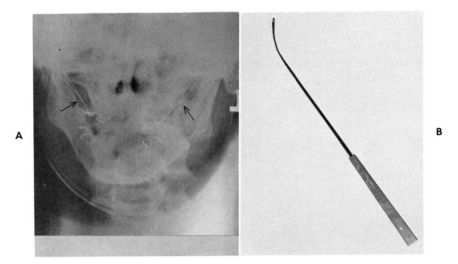

A   B

Fig. 19-43. A, Circumzygomatic and circummandibular wires used to stabilize splints for edentulous fracture fixation. **B,** Instrument for passing circumzygomatic wires (made by Dr. G. E. Morin).

surgeon does not drop in unexpectedly, he or she will find the jaws always fixed in position and will wonder why the fracture heals slowly, if at all.

A head bandage worn continuously is uncomfortable. The cooperative patient can wear an elastic support over the head and chin at night or even during the day. The uncooperative patient will require further stabilization. A simple method consists of direct wiring to the piriform fossa margins (Fig. 19-42).[25] With the patient under local anesthesia or general anesthesia supplemented by infiltration anesthesia, an incision is made high in the labial fold next to the midline of the maxilla. The bone is exposed by blunt dissection. The inferior border of the piriform fossa is followed laterally until the lateral border is reached, where a small hole is placed with a bur. Thirty-gauge wire is placed through the hole and brought out untwisted through the incision. The incision is closed with No. 3-0 catgut. The same procedure is carried out on the other side. The denture is removed from a cold-sterilizing solution and placed in the mouth. The wires are

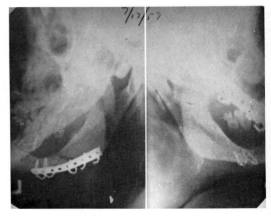

Fig. 19-44. Gutter bone plate used to stabilize triangular segment on inferior border. Note interosseous wiring on other side.

threaded through previously drilled holes in the labial flanges of the denture and tightened moderately. Dental compound is placed over the rosette, and a pressure bandage is placed over the lip.

Pernasal wiring is another method for fixing a denture to the maxilla.[17] A heavy awl is passed just inside the external nares directly through the mucosa and bone of the nasal floor and palate with simple pressure and rotation. A wire is looped through the eye of the awl at its point of emergence on the palatal side. The instrument is withdrawn upward through the palate, but only to a point just beneath the nasal epithelium. It is then guided anteriorly and inferiorly through the labial mucosa into the height of the vestibule. The wire is removed from the eye of the awl, the awl is withdrawn completely, and the two free wire ends (one palatal and the other vestibular) are drawn together around the prosthesis, drawn through a palatal bur hole in the appliance, and tightened on the labial surface.

Circumzygomatic wires are useful also. A long, sharp instrument with a hole near the tip is introduced at the height of the buccal fold just distal to the maxillary first molar region and is pushed upward and posteriorly. A finger on the skin over the zygomatic arch guides the point medial to the arch to emerge on the skin. A wire is threaded into the eye of the instrument, and the instrument is withdrawn into the mouth. The wire is disengaged. The instrument is introduced into the same oral wound and pushed in the same upward direction, this time to pass on the lateral side of the zygomatic arch and emerge through the same skin wound. The other arm of the wire is threaded into the eye of the instrument, and the instrument is withdrawn. The two arms of the wire are sawed back and forth until they contact bone, and they are attached to the maxillary denture flange in the molar region. A similar circumzygomatic wire is placed around the opposite zygomatic arch. The wires can be looped around the mandibular circumferential wires that secure the mandibular denture to the lower jaw (Fig. 19-43).

Open reduction of an edentulous fracture is done best with four holes, using heavy wire. If a triangular segment of bone is found on the inferior border (a not uncommon occurrence in edentulous fractures) and telescoping has occurred, a gut-

ter bone plate on the inferior border will support the segment (Fig. 19-44).

Skeletal pin fixation is excellent. The thinness of the bone makes placement difficult at times. (See Fig. 19-45.)

Multiple fractures

Multiple fractures, in which four or more jaw fractures are present in the same person, occurred in 17% of the fractures in the District of Columbia General Hospital series. When multiple fractures occur in both jaws in the same patient, it is difficult sometimes to find a starting point for treatment. Many fragments at different occlusal levels require the establishment of a baseline, which is usually the mandible. The rule is "bottom up and inside out."[22] After the parts of the mandible have been reduced to a satisfactory plane of occlusion, other segments are fitted to it. If many mandibular segments are present, and if the maxilla is severely fractured so that it cannot be used to establish a plane of occlusion, impressions of the teeth are made and casts are poured. The casts are cut at the fracture lines and reassembled in normal occlusion, and a cast splint that has proper indentations on its superior surface to support the maxillary teeth is made for the mandible.

Multiple fractures that occur solely in the mandible often can be assembled by fixing the teeth of the individual segments to the intact maxillary arch. Wiring or divided arch bars are used. However, many teeth often are lost in this type of fracture. A splint may be used for greater stability, but the splinted mandible in this case is wired to the maxilla to obtain and maintain good occlusion. Oblique fractures and horizontal fractures appearing on the inferior border are treated by circumferential wiring around the splint. Skeletal pins are difficult to place in many small fragments. Open reduction is a last resort. It is definitive treatment, but many small pieces are difficult to wire, and surgical exposure will deprive them of any last vestiges of mechanical and

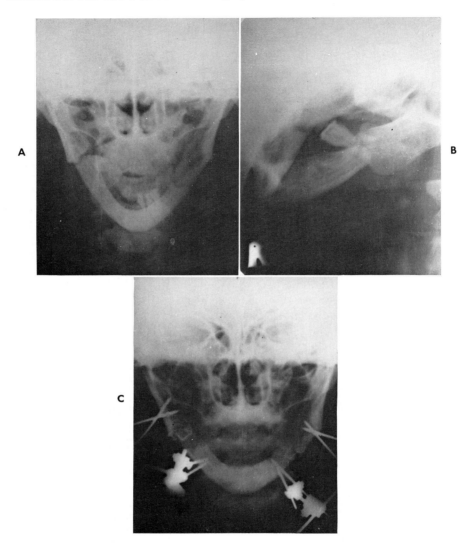

Fig. 19-45. A, Bilateral fracture in edentulous mandible. **B,** Lateral jaw radiograph showing collapse of fragments. **C,** Interosseous wiring supplemented by skeletal pin fixation.

physiological support afforded by the surrounding soft tissues. (See Figs. 19-46 to 19-48.)

Fractures of the coronoid process (2% of the District of Columbia General Hospital series) often are not treated if no displacement has occurred (Fig. 19-49). Tendons of the temporal muscle frequently are inserted low on the ramus, which will prevent displacement. If upward displacement does occur, open reduction can be done

through an intraoral approach. An incision is made on the anterior border of the ramus, and direct wiring utilizing two holes is done. If reduction is not possible and impairment of function is present, the coronoid process is removed.

Condyle

The fractured mandibular condyle has been treated for many years by a closed procedure. Intermaxillary fixation is placed

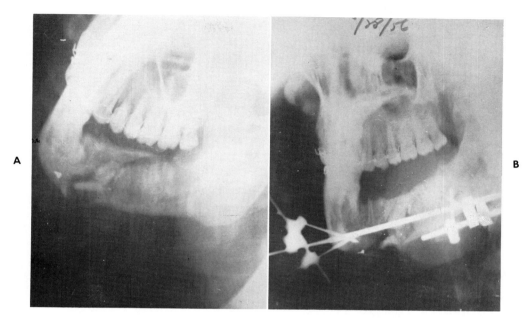

Fig. 19-46. A, Compound comminuted mandibular fracture. **B,** Treatment by skeletal pin fixation.

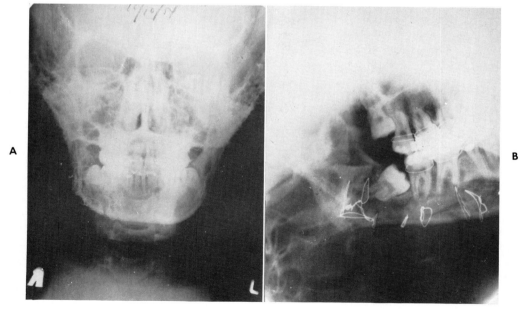

Fig. 19-47. A, Multiple fractures of right mandible treated by interosseous wiring. **B,** Impacted third molar successfully retained for stability.

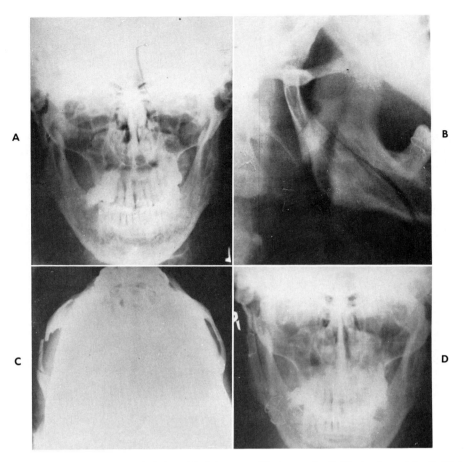

Fig. 19-48. Multiple fractures. A, Infraorbital rim, mandibular angle. B, Neck of condyle. C, Right zygomatic arch. D, Treatment by interosseous wiring through submandibular approach, followed by simple elevation of arch.

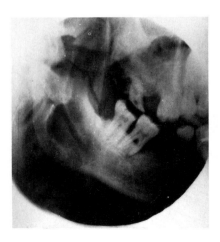

Fig. 19-49. Fracture of coronoid process with minimal displacement.

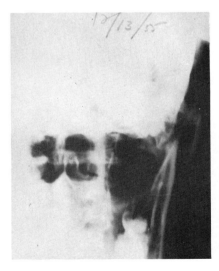

Fig. 19-50. Fracture of condyle with medial displacement.

that immobilizes concomitant fractures and corrects the displacement of the jaws associated with the condyle fracture, that is, a shift of the midline toward the side of the fractured condyle and a slight premature posterior occlusion on that side. The fractured ends of the bone in the condylar region thereby are placed in a somewhat better relationship.

Because of muscular pulls and the stress of the blow, the condylar head often is dislocated forward or tipped medially out of the glenoid fossa (Fig. 19-50). Often the fractured neck of the condyle remains close to the fractured ramus portion. In a subcondylar fracture the fractured segment remains upright in a position lateral to the ramus. Attempts at intraoral as well as extraoral manipulation, the latter including lateral pressure by a sharp instrument through the skin ("ice-pick technique") and various pressure pads on the skin, are usually unsuccessful (Fig. 19-51).

Because of trauma to the joint structures, an ever-present danger exists of ankylosis of the condyle to the glenoid fossa. Healing

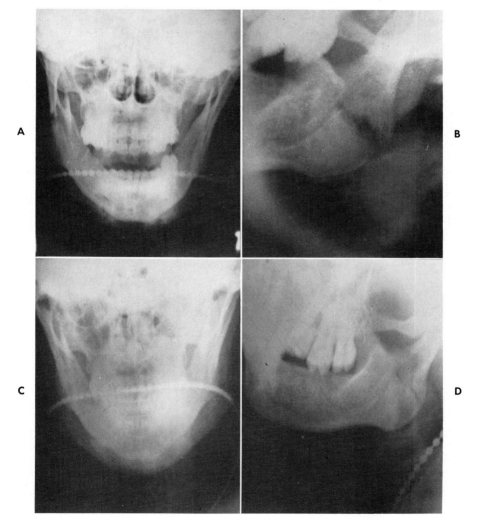

Fig. 19-51. A and **B,** Extracapsular fracture of condyle neck. Preoperative radiographs. **C** and **D,** Postoperative radiographs after "ice-pick" (closed) reduction. Note intermaxillary fixation.

in proper occlusion under intermaxillary immobilization is allowed to progress for 1 week. At that time, with the patient in the dental chair, the jaw is opened carefully once by the operator rather than the patient, care being taken that other fractures do not move, and fixation is again applied. This is done several times in the following weeks.

The effect of this procedure is to ensure motion in the condylar area. Joint surfaces are mobilized so that hemorrhage and edema fluid brought into the joint by trauma are not allowed to organize into a bony ankylosis. The objective is to move the joint without moving the lower fractured bone surfaces, which would lead to nonunion. Such manipulation during healing will create movement in the joint rather than in the fracture zone if it is done carefully, and primary healing of the fractured parts will occur with no ankylosis in the joint.

If the fracture occurs inside the joint capsule, weekly movement of the parts (sometimes more frequently) is especially necessary to prevent ankylosis. In this case, because joint and fracture are together, movement may disrupt the continuity of the fibrous callus in the condylar fracture area. Fibrous tissue rather than bone forms at the junction. The fractured condylar head treated in this manner is nonfunctional. Because of this factor, together with a traumatic hematoma and the damaged synovial membranes, it ankyloses to the base of the skull. The ramus articulates on the edge of the condylar fragment by a fibrous joint. The functioning of the contralateral joint, together with the stability afforded by the fibrous joint, allows satisfactory functioning in good occlusion. The patient can bite as hard on the side of injury as on the other side without experiencing pain.

The head of the condyle that is displaced medially out of the glenoid fossa will ankylose if it touches bone. It is held in place by the soft tissues. Years later it seems to disappear. Fibrous tissue fills the joint cavity.

The occluding dental arches attached to a normal contralateral joint will not allow the ramus to move further upward to form an open bite, whether or not an ankylosed condylar fragment is present in the fossa. Evidence suggests that an attempt is made

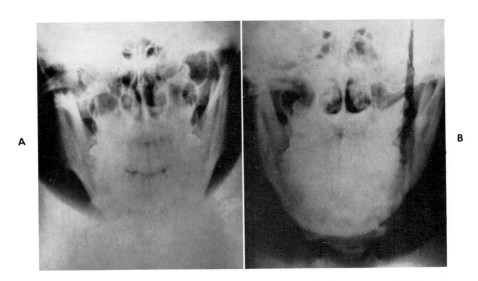

Fig. 19-52. A, Fracture of condyle with medial displacement. **B,** Interosseous fixation after reduction through preauricular exposure.

over the years to re-form the missing condyle from the remaining ramus portion.

Open reduction of condylar fractures has become popular since World War II. The condylar head is placed back in its original position in the glenoid fossa and wired to the ramus. Healing of the fracture takes place by direct bony union, and the healed member functions on the true joint rather than on an artificial fibrous joint.

The surgical procedure for the preauricular approach (Fig. 19-52) is made according to the description given in Chapter 2. Dissection is carried down to the articular capsule. Manual movement of the jaw at this time will demonstrate the joint structure. The capsule is incised horizontally if the fracture is intracapsular or if the condyle has been displaced medially out of the glenoid fossa. This is necessary for access. It is advantageous not to incise the capsule if possible, since the lateral side of the capsule is stronger than the medial side, and the intact capsule stabilizes the condylar head.

A hole is placed in the fragment that lies most superficial. Special retractors such as those designed by Thoma are placed beneath the fragment to protect the maxillary artery. The ramus of the jaw may be pushed upward into the wound to visualize the inferior fragment better and distracted downward to gain access to the superior fragment. A hole is then placed in the other fragment.

The condylar fragment is repositioned carefully in the glenoid fossa. The management of this fragment is a delicate procedure. The fragment is difficult to find if it is displaced deeply to the medial side. It must be placed in its properly oriented position in the fossa with as little damage to surrounding structures as possible. It must be held firmly while the hole is drilled. Any excessive pulling will bring the fragment completely out of the wound.

A wire is placed through the two holes, threading it from the lateral surface of the condylar fragment first and recovering it

from the medial surface to the lateral surface of the inferior fragment by means of a thin wire loop. The wires are twisted over the reduced fracture. It is well to remove the attachment of the lateral pterygoid muscle to prevent redislocation of the condyle. Thoma immobilized the severely displaced condyle that has few if any attachments by means of a catgut suture through holes to the glenoid fossa or by skeletal pin fixation between the condylar head and the eminentia articularis.

The wound is closed in layers, with particular attention to good closure of the articular capsule. A pressure bandage is placed over the wound, and a head bandage made with elastic adhesive tape is placed before the anesthesia is lightened. The endotracheal tube is removed before the patient "bucks" on it.

The submandibular approach is used if the fracture is situated outside of the capsule at the base of the condylar neck (Figs. 19-53 and 19-54). As a matter of fact, this approach is recommended for most cases of open reduction of the condyle. For a description of the surgical approach see Chapter 2. The fracture site can be exposed well with long, narrow-angle Army-Navy retractors. It may be necessary at this stage to administer curare, 60 to 90 units, or succinylcholine hydrochloride, 20 mg, intravenously to provide muscular relaxation.

The same general technique of direct wiring, using two holes, can be employed as described previously. The thin fragments in the condylar neck are usually telescoped. Therefore the ordinary placement of wires will further telescope the fragments rather than hold them distracted in correct position. A small amount of telescoping of the fragments does not seem to affect correct function, particularly in the presence of poor dentition. Lateral contact of the bone ends is important to healing, although the healing is slower. Several methods to overcome telescoping are employed. A figure-of-eight wiring offers some advantage. If one cortex is longer than the other, one hole

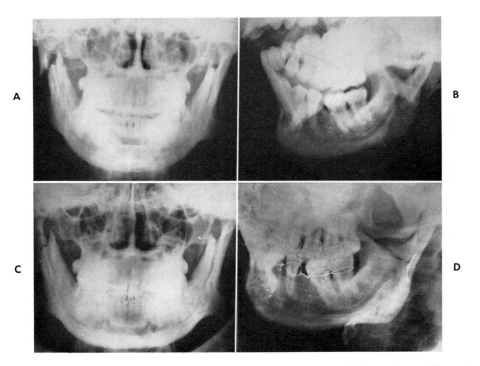

Fig. 19-53. A, Extracapsular condyle fracture with lateral displacement. **B,** Lateral jaw radiograph showing displacement. **C** and **D,** Postoperative radiographs after interosseous wiring.

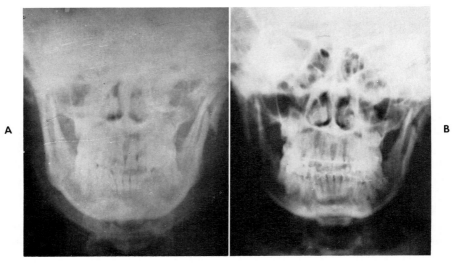

Fig. 19-54. Fracture similar to that shown in Fig. 19-53, with bone contact of fragments, which was successfully treated conservatively. **A,** Preoperative view. **B,** Postoperative view.

is drilled through both fragments and the fragments are wired together. A rounded gutter plate can be placed around the posterior border and wired into place, or a flat, three-pronged plate can be screwed into the lateral surface. The lateral pterygoid muscle attachment often is removed surgically to prevent subsequent dislocation through muscle spasm. Surgical closure of the wound and the immediate postoperative treatment are similar to the procedures described previously.

The Chalmers J. Lyons Club in 1947 reviewed the postoperative results of 120 cases of fractured condyles. They found that fractures treated by closed procedures healed satisfactorily without accurate alignment of the fragments, that ankylosis occurred infrequently, that disturbances to epiphyseal growth did not appear among the younger or skeletally immature patients, and that conservative methods of closed reduction and intermaxillary fixation were simple and effective.

In a 5-year survey of 540 jaw fractures at the District of Columbia General Hospital, 115 cases of condylar fracture were found with a total of 123 condylar fractures (8 being bilateral). Of these, 16 were intracapsular, 64 were extracapsular, and 43 were subcondylar (a total of 107 extracapsular fractures). Thirteen cases were in children. Condyles were fractured in 21% of all cases of jaw fracture. Treatment was as follows: no treatment, 14 cases; conservative treatment, 96 cases; and open reduction, 12 cases. One case of postoperative ankylosis developed in a conservatively treated case.

The general consensus today in the management of the condyle fracture is toward conservative (that is, closed) treatment.[2-4,26] This is particularly true in the unilateral case. No figures are available to indicate the percentage of ankylosis after open reduction of the condyle, which would necessitate later resection of the condyle. This seems to be an infrequent complication. However, function after the open procedure does not seem to be better than that

after the closed procedure, in spite of the rather time-consuming procedure in a hazardous location.

The bilateral case presents a different problem. If proper ramus height is afforded by a nondisplaced condylar fracture on at least one side, open bite may not result. If ramus height is collapsed on both sides, consideration should be given to an open procedure on at least one side. If a low extracapsular fracture occurs on one side, that side should be opened through a submandibular approach. True temporomandibular joint function then will be made possible through direct bone healing on the one side. Both sides can be wired directly if the fractures demand it.

Smith and Robinson[23] presented an interesting case of bilateral joint fracture. The fractures occurred several years apart. Repeated intermaxillary wiring for a total of 3 years and 6 months was followed in each instance by open bite when the wires were removed. When the patient was presented to them, they performed a bilateral joint reconstruction by placing in each glenoid fossa a piece of bone that was designed to ankylose to the fossa and to the ramus. Later the two sides were resected at the graft-ramus junction and preformed metal guide plates were placed to form joint surfaces. Function was excellent.

Observation is continuing on condyle fractures in children (Fig. 19-55). The main growth center of the jaw is located in the condylar region. A study conducted elsewhere was said to show that portions of the growth center in rats extended some distance down the posterior border of the ramus. For this reason, the separation of the growth center from the rest of the jaw is being studied.

The mandibular growth that is associated with the condylar growth center occurs between 1 and 5 years of age in the human. A period of quiescence occurs from 5 to 10 years of age, followed by another period of active mandibular growth from 10 to 15 years of age. This latter growth is asso-

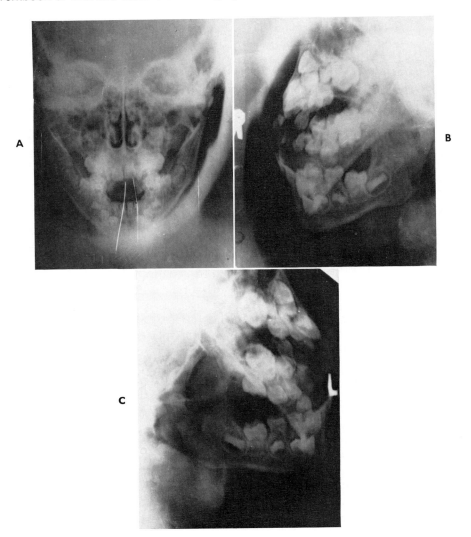

Fig. 19-55. Bilateral intracapsular condylar fractures with medial bowing in a child 6 years of age treated conservatively. **A,** Posteroanterior view. **B,** Right condylar fracture. **C,** Left condylar fracture.

ciated with muscular function more than with the growth center, which is not so important at this age. By this reasoning the most critical period for a condylar fracture would be from 1 to 5 years of age. Perhaps the most critical situation is a fracture-dislocation in a child 2½ years old or less.[18]

Numerous clinicians have presented radiographs showing re-formed rami after closed treatment of condylar fractures. Such reconstruction takes place in conform-

ity with Wolff's law that the shape of the bone conforms to the stresses placed on it during function. The process takes years to accomplish the end result.

Fractured jaws in children

Two considerations are primary in the management of fractured jaws in children. Deciduous teeth are difficult to wire, and growing jaws heal exceedingly fast.

Deciduous teeth have a bell shape. The

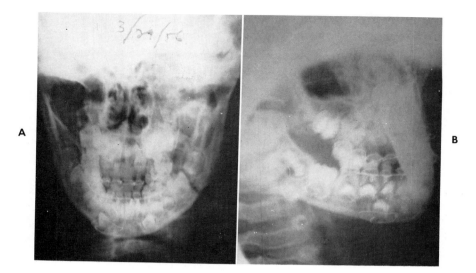

Fig. 19-56. A, Bilateral condylar fracture in a child treated by interdental wiring and intermaxillary fixation. **B,** Note interosseous wiring in canine area with retention of permanent tooth bud.

widest portion of the tooth is at the neck, where the wires are placed. For this reason, many oral surgeons did not attempt to wire deciduous teeth in the past, turning to the use of acrylic splints instead. The splint has the advantages of stability and the elimination of time spent in wiring the patient under general anesthesia. However, often the splint requires the use of circumferential wires. The main disadvantage is the time needed for construction, although if several sizes of preformed acrylic splints are available, one can be selected and adapted with dental compound for immediate insertion. Healing usually is complete in 3 or 4 weeks. If nearly a week is required for impressions and laboratory construction of the splint, the preliminary organization at the fracture site is broken up during reduction and placing of the splint.

The use of a finer wire (28-gauge) makes the wiring of deciduous teeth possible. If the permanent first molar and anterior teeth have erupted, retention is made easier. (See Fig. 19-56.)

Malpositioned angle fractures occurring in children are treated by open reduction. Condyle fractures are treated conserva-

tively in most instances. Intermaxillary fixation is placed while the patient is under general anesthesia or heavy sedation. It is maintained for 2 weeks, and the fracture then is examined. No fixation has been used in isolated instances, with apparently satisfactory results.

Feeding problems

The diet is a high-protein, high-caloric, high-vitamin diet in liquid or semiliquid form. A successful sample diet* containing 2,100 calories is as follows:

Breakfast
    Fruit juice—½ cup
    Cereal—½ cup cooked, thinned with ½ cup milk, sugar to taste
    Milk—1 cup
    Coffee or tea as desired

Midmorning
    Milk shake (4 level tbsp. of protein-vitamin-mineral supplement in 1 cup whole milk)

Lunch
    Meat—6 tbsp. thinned with ½ cup broth or bouillon

---

*Courtesy Dietene Co., Minneapolis, Minn.

Vegetable—¼ cup thinned with ¼ cup vegetable juice

Potato—¼ cup mashed potato thinned with ¼ cup milk

Fruit—¼ cup thinned with ¼ cup fruit juice

Cocoa—1 cup

Coffee or tea as desired

Midafternoon

Milk shake (4 level tbsp. of protein-vitamin-mineral supplement in 1 cup whole milk)

Dinner

Same as lunch, but substitute ½ cup strained cream soup for potato

Bedtime

Milk shake (4 level tbsp. of protein-vitamin-mineral supplement in 1 cup whole milk)

Food selections

Beverages: Milk, cocoa, and milk shakes; fruit and vegetable juices; coffee, tea, etc. only if they do not interfere with schedule

Cereals: Cocoa Wheats, Cream-of-Wheat, Farina, Malt-o-Meal, Cream-of-Rice, corn meal —*thinned with milk*

Fruits: Applesauce, apricot, peach, pear—*strained and thinned with fruit juices*

Fruit juices: Apple, apricot, grape, grapefruit, orange, pineapple, tomato

Meat: Beef, lamb, pork, veal, liver—*strained and thinned with broth or bouillon*

Vegetables: Beets, carrots, wax beans, green beans, peas, asparagus, spinach, mashed squash—*strained and thinned with vegetable juice*

Vegetable juice: Can be the water used in cooking, or liquid from canned vegetables, or commercially prepared vegetable juices

Cream soup: Make with strained vegetable and milk, or use commercial soup thinned with milk

Seasoning: Sugar may be added to tart juices or any seasoning used in any foods to suit your taste

Instructions to patient: Follow the feeding schedule above, selecting foods from the accompanying list. Larger amounts may be taken, but be certain to follow the basic meal plan. For the strained foods you can use prepared baby foods or you can liquefy common table foods in a mechanical blender. Potatoes can be mashed or strained by hand. IMPORTANT: The three protein-vitamin-mineral nourishments ensure nutritional adequacy in this liquid diet and must be taken. Additional liquids and beverages may be taken, provided they do not interfere with feeding schedule.

The patient should be fed six times a day. He is unable to obtain enough nourishment in the ordinary regimen of three meals a day. Perhaps this is associated with the small particle size, which eliminates bulky pieces in the diet.

A calorie chart is important to the fracture patient. He should know how many calories are present in each ounce of the special mixture and how many are in supplementary foods and beverages. He should know also how many calories are necessary to maintain his weight at his present level of activity. The decision then is made whether he should maintain his present weight, gain, or lose weight. Some individuals will lose weight when loss is not indicated, and attention should be given to supplements that will make the diet as attractive as possible. Other persons will gain a tremendous amount of weight, especially with ice cream soda supplements. Some individuals who are over weight will use this situation to lose weight deliberately. This should be encouraged if the amount of loss each week is not too drastic and the patient receives adequate nourishment.

Many modern food advances have a place in this program.[24] Milk and egg powders and protein supplements make nourishment possible without great quantity. The electric food blender makes possible a balanced diet of the same foods that the rest of the family eats rather than the monotonous dairy food diet. The meal is made more palatable by the electric blender because the individual vegetable and meat can be served as separate servings rather than as a nonspecific conglomeration. A soup preceding and a liquid dessert after the meal constitute a normal fare, except for particle size. The importance of meat in the diet is emphasized by faster healing, especially if the meat is not over cooked.

Meats canned for babies are excellent if a food blender is unavailable, although they are expensive.

Intravenous feeding with a supplement of 5% protein hydrolysate and vitamins is the method of choice for the first 24 hours after the treatment of a fracture with intraoral complications or for a severely injured patient. This method keeps food out of the mouth until preliminary healing can take place, and it keeps food out of the stomach. A Levin tube placed into the stomach through the nose will allow feeding into the stomach and still keep food out of the mouth. It is a good method of feeding in the first few days after operation if oral wounds are present.

The patient who has an uncomplicated fractured jaw usually is better off to start with the diet for fractured jaw as soon as possible rather than to be fed intravenously. Ordinary spoon-feeding or a large-bore glass straw is satisfactory. Most patients have one or more teeth missing, and through these spaces the food material can be placed. If no teeth are missing, the food material is brought by means of a straw into the oropharynx through the space existing behind the last molars. When the patient is recuperating well, usually he will want separate blenderized foods by spoon. The larger the entrance space the larger the particle size and the more bulk admissible, which avoids constipation.

An old adage states that as soon as the hospitalized fractured jaw patient complains about his food, he has recovered enough to go home.

Time for repair

Most mandibular fractures heal well enough to allow removal of fixation in 6 weeks. Occasionally the young adult will require only 4 or 4½ weeks. Children require 3 to 4 weeks.

Oral hygiene is difficult to maintain during immobilization. During hospitalization the mouth should be sprayed by means of a 10-pound pressure spray on a dental unit at least once each day. The patient must irrigate the mouth after every meal with saline solution, preferably with a Water Pik. The use of a soft brush is excellent. Failure to keep the mouth clean in a patient who is lying down will permit material to enter the eustacian tubes and allow a middle ear infection to start. The outpatient can have his mouth irrigated with a power spray once or twice each week. Elastics should be changed weekly.

Wires that irritate the lips and cheeks should be turned and the ends protected by dental compound, gutta percha, wax, or quick-cure acrylic.

Pain during healing is not common. For the first few days a satisfactory analgesia level is obtained by giving one 300 mg tablet of aspirin each hour for 4 consecutive hours to obtain a satisfactory level and one tablet every fourth hour to maintain the level. Each day that analgesia is needed, the aspirin level should be built up by taking 1.2 Gm of aspirin in 4 hours and then maintained as just outlined. Some patients may not be able to tolerate this amount of salicylate. However, this method has been found by pharmacologists to be as equally effective as 30 mg of codeine. Because of the possibilities of nausea and addiction, codeine should be used only if absolutely necessary. Then it is ordered in 60 mg doses every 4 hours with salicylates.

At the optimum time for healing, callus formation should be seen on the radiograph. However, the surgeon should be guided by clinical signs of union in determining the length of time immobilization is necessary, since bone healing in the form of secondary callus takes place sometimes before it is demonstrable clearly on the radiograph. The intermaxillary elastics or wires are removed, and the fracture is tested gently with the fingers. If clinical movement occurs, the elastics should be replaced for another week. Reexamination is carried out at weekly intervals until healing has occurred. Even with the best of treatment, some fractures will take several months to heal. In instances in which an unusual delay has occurred, a cast cap splint can be cemented over the fractured member so that the jaws can be opened. Function stimulates healing at this stage. If nonunion is inevitable, all fixation is removed, and the patient is allowed to rest for several months so that the bone ends may round off preparatory to a bone graft. It is not an isolated occurrence to find that the patient has bony union when he returns after moderate functional use of the jaw during the interim.

After removal of the elastics the patient is seen daily for 3 days. If the occlusion and the fracture site remain satisfactory, the wiring or arch bars can be removed at that time. The patient should eat a soft diet for a week, until muscle and joint function have returned. Scaling and polishing of the teeth should be done, and minor occlusion disharmonies should be corrected by grinding.

Complications

Delayed healing in the properly reduced fracture occurs in the presence of inade-quate or loosened fixation, infection, or a fault in the vital reparative effort.

Loosened fixation usually is associated with poorly placed wires. Wires that have not been placed under the cingulum in anterior teeth or those that have not been tightened properly so that they stay under the cingulum will not hold. The multiple-loop wiring technique fails if the strand of wire bridging an edentulous area is not twisted so that it fits the space exactly. For that reason the eyelet wire for double teeth or a thin wire wound twice around a single tooth is preferable in areas of missing teeth. Arch bars should be wired to every tooth in the arch.

The occasional patient who removes his elastics for a small chicken dinner should be strongly advised of the serious consequences. He should be warned that a bone graft is an interesting operation for the oral surgeon and that the patient himself will request such an operation when he tires of a flopping jaw.

Infection caused by bizarre and resistant organisms is becoming more frequent. A

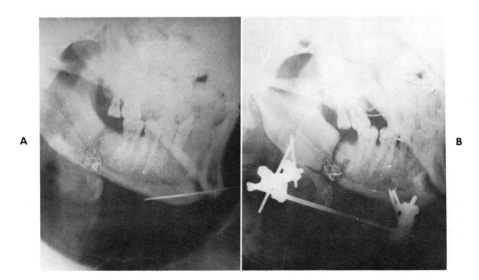

Fig. 19-57. A, Fractures at angle and symphysis treated by interosseous wiring and Kirschner pin. Patient had history of nonunion for earlier wrist fracture. Union occurred at symphysis, but nonunion complicated angle fracture. **B,** Three months later. *Proteus vulgaris* was cultured and found resistant to antibiotics. Skeletal pin fixation. Interosseous wires were later removed and area was debrided before healing occurred.

routine blood culture and organism sensitivity test should be done in all cases of postoperative infection. If pus forms, it should be cultured. Systemic and metabolic disease will cause delayed healing. In some instances the cause for delayed healing is not apparent even after a general medical survey, and healing takes months instead of weeks (Fig. 19-57).

Nonunion is an aftermath of delayed healing if the cause is not corrected. A bone graft is necessary. Sometimes freshening of the area through open reduction is sufficient. A technique for an intraoral approach, freshening, and the placing of homogenous bone chips has been successful.[18]

Malunion is healing in poor position. Poor treatment, an intercurrent accident, or a lack of treatment is responsible. The bone must be refractured and immobilized. However, there is a fine line in judging whether the degree of malposition requires treatment. If the clinical position is satisfactory and the radiograph reveals a small amount of malposition, no treatment may be necessary. Repositioning in this instance is called "treating the x-ray." If facial contours and esthetics are involved as a result of malunion, cartilage or bone onlays have been used successfully.

FRACTURES OF THE MAXILLA

Maxillary fractures are serious injuries because they involve important adjacent structures. The nasal cavity, the maxillary antrum, the orbit, and the brain may be involved primarily by trauma or secondarily by infection. Cranial nerves, major blood vessels, abundantly vascular areas, thin bony walls, multiple muscular attachments, and specialized epithelia characterize this region in which injury can have disastrous consequences.

Causes

Automobile injuries, blows, industrial accidents, and falls can cause such injuries. Rapid deceleration in a fast-moving vehicle can produce a typical middle face fracture known as a "dashboard injury." The force, direction, and location of the blow determine the extent of the fracture. In the District of Columbia General Hospital survey, maxillary fractures represented 6% of all jaw fractures.

Classification—signs and symptoms
Horizontal fracture

The horizontal fracture (Le Fort I) is one in which the body of the maxilla is separated from the base of the skull above the level of the palate and below the attachment of the zygomatic process. The horizontal fracture results in a freely movable upper jaw. It has been called a "floating jaw." An accessory fracture in the midline of the palate may be present, which is represented by a line of ecchymosis. The maxillary fracture can be unilateral, in which case it must be differentiated from an alveolar fracture. The alveolar fracture does not extend to the midline of the palate (Fig. 19-58).

Displacement is dependent on several factors. The force of a severe head-on blow may push the maxilla backward. Muscular pull may do the same. In a low-level fracture, muscular displacement is not a factor. If the fracture is at a higher level, the pterygoid muscle attachments are included in the loose fragment, which is consequently retruded and depressed at the posterior end, resulting in an anterior open bite. Some fractures are depressed all along the line of separation. Many horizontal maxillary fractures are not displaced, and therefore the diagnosis is missed at first examination.

Evidences of trauma may be seen on the teeth, lips, and cheeks. Unless they are severely traumatized, the anterior teeth should be grasped between thumb and forefinger and a forward-backward motion made. The molar teeth on first one side and then the other should be similarly moved. A fractured jaw will move. The distally impacted jaw will not move, but

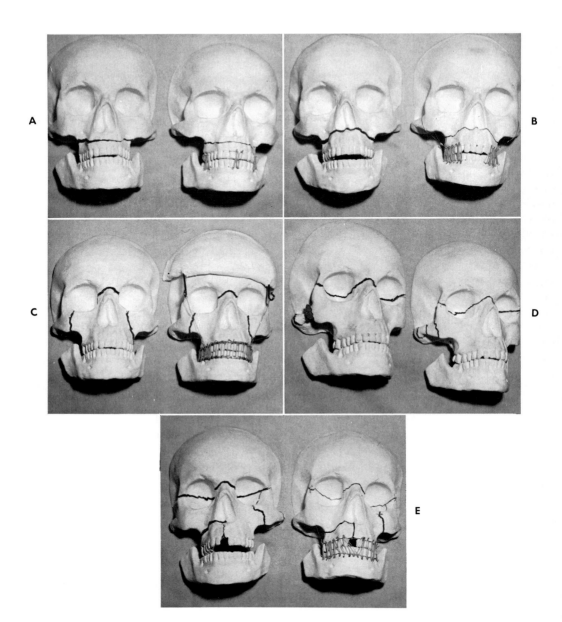

Fig. 19-58. A, Horizontal fracture, low level, treated by intermaxillary fixation. **B,** Horizontal fracture, high level. Note open bite. Treatment by intermaxillary fixation and circumzygomatic wiring. **C,** Pyramidal fracture treated by intermaxillary fixation and suspension from plaster headcap. **D,** Transverse fracture complicated by zygomatic arch collapse. Treatment by interosseous wiring at frontozygomatic sutures, simple elevation of zygomatic arch, and intermaxillary fixation. **E,** Multiple fractures. Note intermaxillary fixation, frontozygomatic wiring connected to maxillary arch bar, and infraorbital rim wiring.

diagnosis can be made from the malocclusion.

Radiographic examination will reveal the fracture on posteroanterior, lateral jaw, and Waters views. Fractures should not be confused with cervical vertebral shadows, nor must intervertebral shadows be diagnosed as fractures.

Pyramidal fracture

The pyramidal fracture (Le Fort II) is one that has vertical fractures through the facial aspects of the maxillae and extends upward to the nasal and ethmoid bones. It usually extends through the maxillary antra. One malar bone may be involved.

The entire middle of the face is swollen, including the nose, lips, and eyes. The patient may have a reddish injection of the eyes, associated with subconjunctival extravasation of blood, in addition to the black eyes. Hemorrhage is present in the nares. If a clear fluid is seen in the nose, cerebrospinal rhinorrhea must be differentiated from mucus associated with a head

cold. An empirical test consists of collecting some of the fluid on a handkerchief or linen cloth. If it starches on drying, it is mucus; if it does not starch, it is cerebrospinal fluid that has escaped through the dura as a result of fracture of the cribriform plate of the ethmoid bone (Fig. 19-59). It is for this reason that clinical examination for suspected upper jaw fractures must be done gently with as little movement as possible. No palpation of the jaw is done in the presence of nasal fluid until cerebrospinal fluid is ruled out. Infected material can be pushed up into the dura if the cribriform plate has been fractured, and a meningitis can follow.

The neurosurgical service should be consulted if positive neurological signs are present or if a fractured skull is suspected. Discreet palpation over the vertex of the skull should be done after a head injury, even if no evidences of skull fracture are noted. Edema masks skull depression that the examining finger often will find. The possibility of a basal skull fracture should not be overlooked in the severely injured patient. More than half of all cranial fractures are complicated by basal skull fractures. A history of unconsciousness is always present, and lesions of the cranial nerves (especially the abducens and facial) are characteristic signs. Battle's sign (ecchymosis in line of the posterior auricular artery in the mastoid area) becomes evident in 24 hours after fracture of the base of the skull. Increased temperature is associated with intracranial damage.

The patient with cerebrospinal rhinorrhea is the responsibility of the neurosurgical service until that service releases him. The neurosurgeon usually will permit temporary bandaging or wiring after a satisfactory antibiotic level is obtained, and definitive treatment is sanctioned often in anticipation of faster healing of the dura on reduction of the bony walls. Only special antibiotics, such as ampicillin, that cross the blood-brain barrier are indicated. Previously no reduction was done until

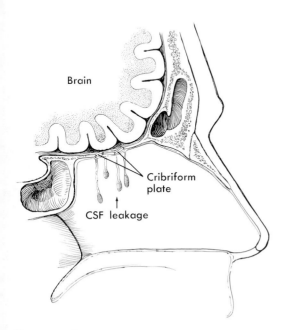

Fig. 19-59. Fracture of cribriform plate of ethmoid with cerebrospinal fluid leakage.

fibrous healing had taken place over the defect, at which time reduction of the fractures was difficult if not impossible to accomplish.

Diagnosis of all types of maxillary fractures is difficult at times. Palpation of bones through massive edema of the facial tissues is inexact. Radiographs are difficult to read. If fracture displacement is present, the radiograph will reveal steps and spaces at cortical borders that can be corroborated clinically. The many structures, including the vertebrae, that are superimposed on the maxilla make radiographic diagnosis difficult in the absence of displacement. The statement has been made that a separation of the frontonasal suture line on the lateral head radiograph usually indicates a maxillary fracture elsewhere, although its absence does not exclude a fracture in the maxilla.[7]

The unconscious or dazed patient should have the facets of the teeth examined carefully to verify the correct occlusion if a suspected maxillary fracture is not confirmed clinically or radiographically.

Transverse fracture

A transverse fracture (Le Fort III) is a high-level fracture that extends across the orbits through the base of the nose and the ethmoid region to the zygomatic arches. The lateral rim of the orbit is separated at the zygomaticofrontal suture line, and the bony orbit is fractured. The zygoma usually is involved either by a fracture of the arch or by a downward and backward displacement of the body of the zygoma.

Because the zygoma is involved, the transverse fracture usually is associated with other fractures. A pyramidal fracture often accompanies the transverse fracture. A unilateral transverse fracture is associated often with a unilateral pyramidal fracture on the other side. Combinations of the basic maxillary fractures are the rule rather than the exception. A severe middle face fracture includes transverse, pyramidal, and horizontal fractures, often in multiple form, zygomatic body and arch fractures, and fractures of associated structures such as the nasal and ethmoid bones.

Transverse fracture cases present a characteristic "dishface" facies because the central portion of the face is dished in. On profile the face appears spooned out in the nasal area because of fracture and posterior dislocation of the maxilla.

Orbital signs are important neurological signs. If one eye is widely dilated and fixed, a 50% probability of death from intracranial damage is present, and if both eyes are involved, the probability of death is 95%.[13] However, the neurosurgeon must differentiate this sign from other conditions such as alcoholism, morphinism, glaucoma, and previous eye operations. Cerebrospinal rhinorrhea, skull-fractures, other neurological signs, and bleeding in the ears should be looked for. Bleeding from the ears usually means a middle cranial fossa fracture. However, trauma to the external ear, scalp wounds, and a condyle fracture must be differentiated.

Palpation should be done as described previously. In all suspected maxillary fractures, the infraorbital rim should be palpated for a bony step, and the lateral orbital rim should be palpated for a separation. If the floor of the orbit is depressed, the eyeball will be lowered, resulting in diplopia. The orbital rims are reasonably easy to visualize on the radiograph, and therefore the presence or absence of a fracture in this region can be diagnosed with certainty. The normally radiolucent frontozygomatic suture line must be differentiated from a traumatic separation.

Treatment
Horizontal fracture

Treatment is directed toward positioning the maxilla in proper relation to the mandible as well as to the base of the skull and immobilizing it there. Since an exact relationship with the mandible is more important, maxillary fractures require intermaxillary fixation. (See Fig. 19-60.)

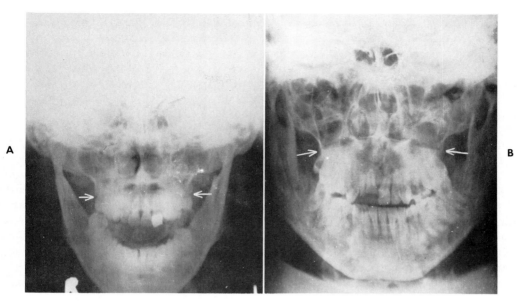

Fig. 19-60. A, Horizontal fracture, low level. **B,** Horizontal fracture, high level.

Concepts of craniomaxillary immobilization have undergone change. Formerly every maxillary fracture was immobilized by wires to a headcap or by internal wires to the nearest superior unfractured bone. These wires often were not tight enough to provide upward traction, or they soon became loose and often were not retightened. Downward positioning of the maxilla was necessary as often as upward positioning. The fractures healed without much effective aid from the craniomaxillary fixation. The intermaxillary fixation provided the effective immobilization. In one series of 116 midfacial fractures only 14% were treated by some form of cranial suspension. The remainder were treated by intermaxillary fixation only.[14]

A simple horizontal maxillary fracture that is not displaced or one that can be positioned manually can be treated with intermaxillary immobilization alone, without craniomaxillary immobilization.

Craniomaxillary fixation is employed in cases of displacement or gross separation to supplement intermaxillary immobilization. The simplest method is that of circum-zygomatic wiring. This pulls the separated upper jaw against the base of the skull, and in the case of open bite, it pulls the downwardly distracted posterior portion upward while the intermaxillary elastics pull the anterior open bite shut.

If the fracture is high and the fragment is displaced backward, considerable intermaxillary traction with the elastic bands directed downward and forward may be necessary for reduction. Occasionally extraoral traction is necessary. A plaster headcap can be used for this. A stationary post or a heavy wire is incorporated into the headcap and suspended in front of the maxilla. Elastic traction is placed from the post to the anterior arch bar. When the jaw has been moved forward, usually in 24 to 48 hours, the post is removed, and intermaxillary fixation is placed.

An old fracture that has started to heal in malposition sometimes can be separated by manual manipulation or elastic traction. If this is unsuccessful, open reduction must be performed by raising mucoperiosteal flaps and separating the bones with thin, broad osteotomes.

A few years ago a plaster headcap was placed on all maxillary fractures to position them against the base of the skull. The plaster headcap has several disadvantages. It looks and feels cumbersome, it is uncomfortable and hot, it tends to move or slide around, and it is time-consuming and messy to construct. Many modifications have been made that eliminate the plaster. Many leather headcaps have been made. The Crawford head frame developed by the Navy has three pins that make contact with the outer table of the skull in tripod fashion.

The plaster headcap is made as follows. The head is shaved to the occiput for men and women. The remainder of the hair of women is piled high on the head. Rubber, 6 mm thick, is taped to the shaved skin over the occipital prominence. A piece of felt 6 mm thick is placed over the forehead and is removed after the plaster is dry, thereby providing space to prevent pressure necrosis and pain. A piece of stockinet 35 cm long is placed over the head to the level of the chin and pulled slightly upward to arrange the hair in an upward direction. A piece of bandage is tied loosely around the stockinet at the top of the head. A small cut is made in the stockinet above the knot, through which the remaining bandage and the knot are pushed. The upper portion of the stockinet is pulled down over the head. This leaves the crown of the head free, surrounded by the bandage, which is used as a purse string to tighten the stockinet. A pencil marks the positions of the ears and eyebrows. A piece of gauze is placed in the center to protect the hair.

Plaster-of-Paris bandage, preferably one impregnated with melamine resin (which is waterproof, porous, lightweight, cool, and stronger), is wetted with water and wrapped around the head over the stockinet to the penciled lines. Two or three layers are placed. A half roll is laid out on a table so that a piece nine layers thick and 22 cm long is formed. This is placed over the back of the head so that it is closely adapted to the region of the mastoid processes. The excess is cut off. A ready-made appliance such as the Erich attachment or a contrivance previously formed of coat hanger wire is placed. Another roll of plaster is placed around the appliance. The lower border of the stockinet is folded up to the penciled line all around to form a smooth border on the cast, and another layer of plaster bandage is placed over it. A wad of dry gauze is bandaged over the mastoid processes by bandaging around the cast. This provides pressure adaptation to this important area for 18 hours while the cast is drying, after which the gauze is removed. The gauze over the hair at the top of the cast is removed.

The headcap can be attached to the maxillary arch bar by two wires passed through the cheek on a straight needle, one on each side lateral to the infraorbital foramen. Today, however, the wires rarely are passed through the cheek. Internal wiring or circumzygomatic wiring has replaced this technique in many cases. The headcap is used mostly as a traction appliance.

The unilateral maxillary fracture is immobilized by intermaxillary fixation. If satisfactory manual reduction cannot be accomplished, elastic traction is placed. A laterally displaced fracture is treated by an elastic band placed across the palate on attachments anchored to the lingual surfaces of the molars. A medially displaced fracture can be pushed outward by a jackscrew placed across the palate or by a bar attached on the labial and buccal surfaces of the arch and bent away from the displaced fragment. Elastic traction between the bar and the attachments placed on the teeth of the fragment pull the fragment laterally. When correct position has been obtained, the apparatus is replaced by a conventional bar and intermaxillary fixation is placed all around or on the contralateral side only.

Pyramidal fracture

Treatment of the pyramidal fracture is directed toward the reduction and fixation

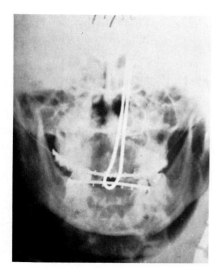

Fig. 19-61. Pyramidal fracture. Bar suspended in front of face from headcap was used to pull backwardly displaced maxilla forward. Note circumzygomatic wires.

of a downward displacement of the maxilla frequently seen in this injury and reduction of concomitant nasal fractures (Fig. 19-61).

Intermaxillary wires or arch bars are placed. Manual or elastic traction usually reduces the fracture, and intermaxillary immobilization is accomplished. The pyrimidal fracture that is severely displaced backward may require manual separation of the lateral portions to disimpact the central pyramidal portion and bring it forward with specially designed forceps. Craniomaxillary fixation then is placed. A head bandage or a headcap may be necessary for extraoral upward traction, particularly in a delayed case, before intermaxillary immobilization is possible. However, internal wiring is used more often. The first intact bone above the fracture is used for suspension on each side. The lateral portion of the infraorbital rim may be used on one side. The lateral margin of the supraorbital rim may be used on one or both sides. Circumzygomatic wiring can be used occasionally, although one or both zygomatic complexes can be involved in this injury.

The nasal fractures are managed by the otolaryngologist or the plastic surgeon.

They are reduced by manipulation and shaping, followed by support. The procedure is accompanied by much hemorrhage, which must be managed effectively in the presence of wired jaws. Some clinicians prefer to wait until the maxillary fracture has healed and then perform a submucous resection to reshape the nose. Others prefer to reduce the nasal fractures immediately after the maxillary fractures are reduced. The immediate reduction is done more frequently.

Transverse fracture

Because the zygoma and possibly the zygomatic arch are fractured, the treatment of the transverse fracture is complicated. The circumzygomatic wire cannot be used except in cases of unilateral transverse fracture, in which it can be used on one side. If internal wiring is used, the maxilla is fixed to the first solid bone above the fractures.

A recent fracture that is not complicated by a skull fracture precluding the use of a headcap can be suspended by means of wires through the cheeks.

If the zygoma is depressed, a small skin incision is made on the face at the antero-inferior border. A small hemostat is used for blunt dissection to the bone. A large Kelly forceps is placed under the zygoma and the zygoma lifted upward and outward. The frontozygomatic suture line and the infraorbital rim are examined for position. The zygoma ordinarily will stay in the reduced position. The wound is closed with a silk mattress skin suture. Some type of craniomaxillary fixation is placed.

If the reduction is not satisfactory or if the zygoma does not stay in place, as determined by examination of the lateral and infraorbital rims, open reduction at one or both of these sites is done.

After the usual preparation, the palpating finger locates the frontozygomatic separation at the lateral rim of the orbit. The eyebrows are never shaved. In addition to the general anesthesia, 1 ml of a local anesthetic containing epinephrine, 1:50,000, is injected into the skin for hemostasis. A skin incision 2 cm long is made under the eyebrow, curving toward the external canthus. It is never carried below the external canthus because the facial nerve branches to the eyelids may be severed. Blunt dissection is carried to bone. A small periosteal elevator is placed medial to the rim to protect the orbital contents. A small hole is drilled in each fragment, preferably directed toward the temporal fossa rather than the orbit,[6] and wires are placed and tightened to immobilize the fracture. At this point, it is well to consider internal wire suspension of the maxilla to eliminate the need for a headcap (Fig. 19-62). A long, 26-gauge wire is threaded through the same superior hole in the frontal bone. Both ends of the wire are attached to a long, straight skin needle or a Morin passer and passed into the wound medial to the zygoma to enter the mouth at the crest of the mucobuccal fold opposite the first molar. The wound is closed. The wire is attached later to the maxillary arch bar.

The same procedure is carried out on the opposite side, or if no orbital fracture is found on that side, a circumzygomatic wire can be placed.

If direct wiring on the lateral rim is not sufficient to reduce the step on the infraorbital rim, the latter also should be wired directly. The same general preparation is done. The palpating finger must press through the edema in these fractures, and the finger should be held in place during the incision. A horizontal incision is made down to bone just inside the bony rim. The periosteal elevator is placed to protect the orbit. Two small holes are made and wired together. The wounds are closed.

Since oral contamination associated with passing wire into the mouth may infect the higher areas, it is best to do the lateral orbital direct wiring first and then the infraorbital wiring if it is necessary. The higher areas are left open, and the infraorbital areas are closed. The suspension wire from the frontal bone then is passed downward on one side so that the assistant recovers the needle in the mouth. A new needle is used on the other side without help from

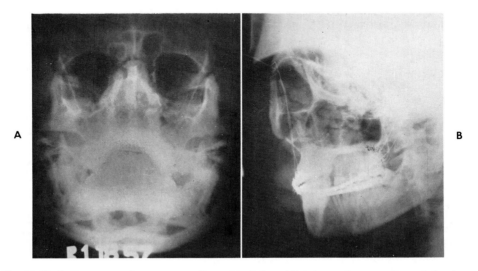

Fig. 19-62. A, Transverse fracture complicated by infraorbital rim and zygomatic arch fractures. **B,** Frontozygomatic wiring. Maxillary suspension by means of wire extending from superior hole in frontozygomatic area, medial to the zygoma, to arch bar.

the assistant who has recovered the needle in the mouth until the second needle needs to be recovered in the mouth. Closure of wounds is accomplished after the assistant has changed gloves. Then the wires are attached to the maxillary arch bars in the mouth in case the mouth has to be opened hurriedly later. If the teeth are few so that the wiring is poor, the wires are attached to the mandibular arch bar or wiring.

Maxillary fixation is maintained for 4 weeks. At that time, maxillary union has usually taken place. Some question exists as to the amount of bony union that actually takes place. The many thin walls may form fibrous unions. At least the thicker pillars of bone heal by direct bony union so that the clinical effect is satisfactory.

The internal suspensory wires are removed while the patient is under sedation or local anesthesia. They are cut from the arch bar or wiring in the mouth, and a needle holder is placed on each end. The two ends are sawed gently back and forth a few times to determine which end of the wire will move more easily. The other end of the wire is cut as high in the mucobuccal fold as possible. The remaining longer end with the needle holder attached is pulled out. Needless to say, the wires should be placed through the tissues without twisting. The intermaxillary wiring is not removed for at least 6 weeks.

Many combinations of the fractures just described are found, and special procedures for treatment are too numerous to be described here. Then, too, the bones may be comminuted. In instances in which intermaxillary fixation is not a suitable adjunct to craniomaxillary fixation, several techniques are useful. One is skeletal pin fixation between the zygoma and the mandible. Another is the use of the Steinmann pin drilled into the bone across the symphysis of the mandible. The pin is allowed to extend beyond the margins of the bone and through the skin. Traction can be accomplished by the attachment of the free margins of the pin to a headcap arm by

elastics or metal attachments. Still another method is the use of a Kirschner pin driven across the maxilla.

Complications

Infection is a possible complication of direct wiring, even under antibiotic therapy.

Malunion or nonunion is not seen often if proper early reduction and fixation are accomplished.[5]

Diplopia may be a complication if the fracture is not reduced soon enough so that proper positioning of the parts is possible. It may result from a depressed orbital floor or an injury to the inferior oblique muscle. In the latter case, cartilage under the eyeball will not correct it.[7]

Persistent periorbital edema is a complication that arises occasionally. It may or may not resolve eventually. No treatment is known. It is speculated that this may be the result of a traumatic blockage of the lymphatic drainage of the area.[7]

Poor occlusion, facial disfigurement, damage to the specialized antrum lining, and an improperly functioning nose are possible complications, but they are less frequent if the fracture can be treated early and adequately.

Dimness of vision infrequently increases day by day. It may lead to blindness. This is caused by a hematoma pressing on the optic nerve. Erich[7] decompresses it by removing a little bone from the lateral wall of the orbit.

ZYGOMA FRACTURES

The zygoma is a heavy bone of the face that is rarely fractured. However, its bony attachments and its arch are frequently fractured, often in conjunction with a fracture of the upper jaw. In a series of 134 zygoma fractures at the District of Columbia General Hospital, the zygomaticotemporal suture line on the arch was fractured most frequently, followed by fractures of the suture line on the infraorbital rim and then by the zygomaticofrontal and zygomaticomaxillary suture lines. Fractures of the zygomatic arch may occur without fracture of the other suture lines. These fractures are usually unilateral and frequently multiple, and they may be comminuted, but because of the thick protective muscle and tissue coverings they are rarely compounded. They are displaced primarily by the blow rather than by muscles forces. As a matter of fact, because of the temporal fascia attachment superiorly and the masseter muscle attachment inferiorly, the fractures rarely are displaced upward or downward. The blow usually pushes the parts inward.

Cause of fracture varies somewhat with habits and circumstances. The municipal hospital series finds the largest number (70%) results from fisticuffs and mayhem, whereas the private hospitals show the largest number to be caused by automobile accidents. Frequently, the municipal hospital history includes the following statement, ''I was standing at the bar, minding my own business, when - - -,'' Because of the difficult sidewise angle associated with sudden blows at a bar, the side of the face approach to the zygoma seems to be more prevalent than the direct punch to the nose, even though the latter is the announced purpose. The municipal hospitals report that 12% result from automobile accidents, 8% from sports, and 6% from falls.

Time of reduction is important. The man at the bar is collected at once by his friends and rushed to the hospital, where his reduction is accomplished immediately. The automobile victim frequently is fractured in many places, including the skull, and sometimes he is in shock. His zygomatic fracture reduction is delayed until more important structures are treated.

It is difficult to treat a zygoma fracture after 5 days. Earlier than that, the bones frequently snap into place with a sound that can be heard over the room, and they stay in place without fixation. After 1 week they can be reduced, but they will not stay in place. After several months it is almost impossible to reduce them, and no attempt

is generally made. Rather, the surrounding structures are treated so that function and esthetics are served.[9]

Diagnosis

The signs of zygomatic fracture are obscured often by edema and lacerations. Swelling of the tissues overlying a depressed fracture can round out the face so that the two sides will be equally full. One unfailing sign of a zygomatic arch fracture, although not always present until edema has subsided, is a dimpling of the skin over the arch. In the presence of moderate edema, any or all of the following signs may be present: flattening of the upper cheek and fullness of the lower cheek, hemorrhage into the sclera of the eye, nasal hemorrhage, antrum hematoma, depressed level of the eye, paresthesia over the cheek, and other middle face fractures. When all four suture lines are fractured around the body, the zygoma is depressed downward. When the arch is deeply depressed, mandibular function may be hindered because of impingement on the coronoid process (Fig. 19-63).

Palpation of the arch, the lateral rim, and the infraorbital rim is necessary. Radiographs include the posteroanterior jaw film to show the orbital rims and the ''jughandle'' view to show the arches. A lateral

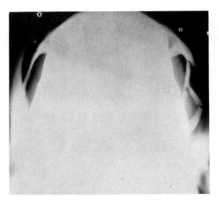

Fig. 19-63. Depressed zygomatic arch impinging on the coronoid process on the right side.

oblique jaw film sometimes will show the body separations better.

Zygomatic fractures can be considered roughly in two categories: fractures of the suture lines surrounding the body of the zygoma and fractures of the arch.

Treatment

The simplest method of treating the depressed body fracture is to make a stab skin incision beneath the bone and lift upward and outward with a Kelly clamp. If this is unsuccessful, an intraoral Caldwell-Luc approach is made into the antrum. The anterior maxillary wall frequently will be found to be comminuted. The gloved finger or a metal urethral sound is used to push the zygoma upward and outward. To support the fragments, the antrum is packed with sterile petrolatum gauze from which most of the petrolatum has been wiped and on which bacitracin ointment has been placed. An inflatable antrum balloon or a Foley catheter can be placed into the antrum to support the reduced parts when it is inflated with air or even water.[11] The edges of the wound are approximated with sutures, but the central portion is left open for removal of the packing materials. The end of the gauze should be brought into the buccal vestibule over a bony edge rather than in the center of a bone void to prevent formation of a persistent oroantral opening. In cases in which the external wall of the antrum is grossly comminuted, nasal antrostomy is made for removal of the gauze. Gross comminution can result in a persistent oral opening if the end of the gauze is brought out in the usual oral opening. Nasal antrostomy is easily accomplished by pushing a small hemostat from the nasal side below the inferior turbinate in the posterior nose. The packing is retained for 2 or 3 weeks, depending on the tolerance of the patient. Further fixation by direct bone wiring at the orbital rim is necessary occasionally.

An eyelet screw is screwed in the body of the zygoma occasionally and attached to elastic traction from a headcap. This is usually a last resort in delayed treatment cases in which manipulation does not succeed or the parts will not stay in place.

The old depressed zygoma can be lifted by means of considerable pull force engendered from an intraoral approach with the help of a large instrument, usually a metal urethral sound.

The simplest method of treating the zygomatic arch fracture is by reduction with a long instrument (for example, a periosteal elevator) through an incision in the mucobuccal fold opposite the second molar (Fig. 19-64). The instrument is passed laterally

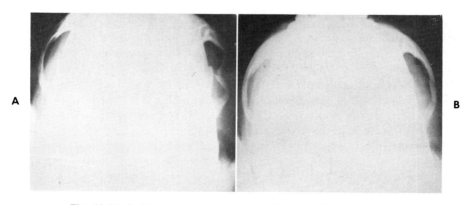

Fig. 19-64. A, Typical depressed zygomatic arch. **B,** Reduction.

and superiorly until it reaches the medial surface of the arch. Lateral pressure is then made, avoiding a lever action on the surface of the maxilla or teeth. The fingers of the other hand are placed on the skin over the arch to guide the reduction. Usually no fixation is required. Some operators feel that continued functioning of the mandible may result in displacement of the fragments by action of the masseter muscle. They place an eyelet wire on the teeth in each posterior quadrant, close the jaws with elastic intermaxillary traction, and maintain closure for 10 to 14 days. Clinical healing takes place in 2 weeks.

If the fracture is older and heavy manipulation can free it, reduction will not be maintained by itself in some cases. A large, semicircular needle can be placed under the arch externally. It is placed through the skin inferior to the arch, behind the arch, and back through the skin on the superior side. The attached wires are placed through the meshes of an ether mask, which has been padded on its edges and placed on the side of the face. Reduction is obtained again, and the wires are tightened around the meshes of the mask. This is maintained in place for 3 days.

The Gillies approach for reduction of the arch is an external procedure. A skin incision in the shaved temporal region is made down to the deep temporal fascia. A special instrument is introduced under this fascia in a downward and forward direction to reach the medial surface of the arch. Lateral pressure is generated for reduction.

After reduction by either method, a round gauze "doughnut" is taped to the side of the head, or a tongue blade is taped vertically over a small roll of gauze bandage that has been taped previously to the side of the temple. This is kept in place for several days until the patient becomes trained not to sleep on that side.

These simple methods are not effective after 9 days at most. Special methods may be successful up to 2 weeks, although 2-month-old fractures have responded to treatment on occasion. Fractures over 2 weeks old are commonly considered untreated fractures and are managed as such.

Complications

The treated zygomatic fracture presents few complications. The antrum may be filled with a hematoma, which usually evacuates itself, but it can become infected. Nerve injuries usually subside. Ocular muscle balance may be impaired because of fracture of the orbital process.

One consideration in any zygoma body fracture is the possibility of orbital fat herniation through a fractured orbital floor into the antrum. Cloudiness on antrum radiographs may represent hematoma, fat herniation, or both, and differentiation is difficult even with laminagrams. The level of the orbit may not be depressed at early examination because an orbital hematoma props it up. When the hematoma disappears later, diplopia and enophthalmos will be noticed. Examination includes a survey of visual fields. Diplopia may be noticed straight away or when the eyes are turned upward and outward. The possibility of entrapment of orbital muscles should be considered at this time.

If orbital fat herniation cannot be ruled out, the antrum is explored through a Caldwell-Luc opening at the time of fracture reduction. If herniation has occurred, the fat is pushed upward, and the antrum is packed with petrolatum gauze. This may be followed by the insertion of a Silastic sheet (or a piece of autogenous bone obtained from the lateral plate of the mandibular ramus[16]) over the fractured orbital floor through an infraorbital incision, although this procedure often is not necessary. If a strong possibility exists that herniation has occurred, the Silastic sheet is placed first to protect the globe from possible injury by sharp bony spicules, followed by the antrum packing if necessary.

The untreated fracture creates a marked flatness of the face. The coronoid process may be impinged on by the depressed fracture so that mouth opening is difficult if not impossible. The coronoid process is removed. The eyball may be depressed downward with its floor. Rarely is an attempt made to correct an old depressed orbital floor, since it cannot be done successfully. Cartilage or bone grafts are placed over the depressed arch and inserted into the orbital floor to prop up the eyeball. Erich[7] advocates a spongiosa paste made from fresh autogenous iliac crest bone for placing in a tunnel over the arch to build it out. It is placed through a temporal incision and molded from the outside. It is firm in 3 days.

Fractures of the facial bones, particularly the zygomatic complex, may on rare occasions be complicated by damage to the contents of the superior orbital fissure, causing the superior orbital fissure syndrome.

The clinical features, following trauma, may be caused by actual disruption of the bony margins of the fissure or by the formation of a hematoma or aneurysm within its boundaries.

Clinically there is ophthalmoplegia, ptosis of the upper lid, proptosis, and a fixed, dilated pupil. The involvement of the third, fourth, and sixth cranial nerves is responsible for the ophthalmoplegia and ptosis. The fixed and dilated pupil is caused by disturbances in the parasympathetic nervous system, and the proptosis is caused by paresis of the extraocular muscles that normally exert a retracing influence on the globe. The syndrome is completed by sensory disturbance over the distribution of the ophthalmic division of the trigeminal nerve.

Prognosis is poor if nerves have been severely damaged or severed. Gradual, complete recovery of motor and sensory function without surgical intervention is the usual case.[20]

REFERENCES

1. Akamine, R. N.: Diagnosis of traumatic injuries of the face and jaws, Oral Surg. **8**:352, 1955.
2. Blevins, C., and Gores, R. J.: Fractures of the mandibular condyloid process: results of conservative treatment in 140 patients, J. Oral Surg. **19**:392, 1961.
3. Boyne, P. J.: Osseous repair and mandibular growth after subcondylar fractures, J. Oral Surg. **25**:300, 1967.
4. Caldwell, J. B.: The consultant, J. Oral Surg. **22**:460, 1964.
5. Crosby, J. F., and Woodward, H. W.: Autogenous bone graft for repair of nonunion of maxillary fracture: report of case, J. Oral Surg. **23**:441, 1965.
6. Crowe, W. W.: Treatment of zygomatic fracture-dislocations, J. Oral Surg. **17**:27, 1959.
7. Erich, J. B.: Unpublished addresses.
8. Fry, W. K., Shepherd, P. R., McLeod, A. C., and Parfitt, G. J.: The dental treatment of maxillofacial injuries, Oxford, 1942, Blackwell Scientific Publications, p. 104ff.
9. Hinds, E. C.: The consultant, J. Oral Surg. **23**:179, 1965.
10. Huelke, D. F., and Burdi, A. R.: Location of mandibular fractures related to teeth and edentulous regions, J. Oral Surg. **22**:396, 1964.
11. Jarabak, J. P.: Use of the Foley catheter in supporting zygomatic fractures, J. Oral Surg. **17**:39, 1959.
12. Johnson, L.: Unpublished address.
13. King, A. B., and Walsh, F. B.: Trauma of the head with particular reference to the ocular signs, Am. J. Ophthalmol. **32**:191, 1949.
14. Kuepper, R. C., and Harrigan, W. F.: Treatment of midfacial fractures at Bellevue Hospital Center, 1955-1976, J. Oral Surg. **35**:420, 1977.
15. Laing, P. G.: The consultant, J. Oral Surg. **23**:86, 1965.
16. Laskin, J. L., and Edwards, D. M.: Immediate reconstruction of an orbital complex fracture with autogenous mandibular bone, J. Oral Surg. **35**:749, 1977.
17. MacIntosh, R. B., and Obwegeser, H. L.: Internal wiring fixation, Oral Surg. **23**:703, 1967.
18. MacLennon, W. D.: Unpublished address.
19. Robinson, M., and Yoon, C.: The 'L' splint for the fractured mandible: a new principle of plating, J. Oral Surg. **21**:395, 1963.
20. Rowe, N. L., and Killey, H. C.: Fractures of the facial skeleton, ed. 2, London, 1956, E. & S. Livingston, pp. 295-287.
21. Shira, R. B., and Frank, O. M.: Treatment of nonunion of mandibular fractures by intraoral insertion of homogenous bone chips, J. Oral Surg. **13**:306, 1955.
22. Small, E. W.: Inside-out and bottom-up: the management of maxillofacial trauma patients, Milit. Med. **136**:553, 1971.
23. Smith, A. E., and Robinson, M.: A new surgical procedure in bilateral reconstruction of condyles, utilizing iliac bone grafts and creation of new

joints by means of non-electrolytic metal. A preliminary report, Plast. Reconstr. Surg. **9:** 393, 1952.

24. Smith, J. F.: Nutritional maintenance of the oral fracture patient, Oral Surg. **19:**705, 1965.

25. Thoma, K. H.: A new method of intermaxillary fixation for jaw fractures in patients wearing artificial dentures, Am. J. Orthod. (Oral Surg. Sect.) **29:**433, 1943.

26. Walker, R. V.: Traumatic mandibular condylar fracture dislocations. Effect on growth in the macaca rhesus monkey, Am. J. Surg. **100:**850, 1960.

27. Weinman, J. P., and Sicher, H.: Bone and bones, fundamentals of bone biology, ed. 2, St. Louis, 1955, The C. V. Mosby Co., pp. 314-330.

CHAPTER 20

The temporomandibular joint

Fred A. Henny

The temporomandibular joint has been the subject of considerable interest and scientific investigation for many years. It is indeed one of the most complex of the facial structures, producing, in its various pathological states, many problems, the correct diagnosis and treatment of which are frequently neither obvious nor easily executed. However, it is now realized that many forms of therapy advocated in the past were basically incorrect, and this is evidence that much has been learned about the joint in recent years. As understanding of the function and pathology of the joint has progressed, so has the management of its many problems. Today the vast majority of temporomandibular joint problems can be corrected with adequate treatment.

ANATOMY

Since a description of the temporomandibular joint is available in standard texts of anatomy, it will not be included in detail here. However, a review of the pertinent points is indicated.

The temporomandibular joint is a ginglymoarthrodial joint differing from most articulations in that the articulating surfaces are covered with avascular fibrous tissue rather than hyaline cartilage. The articular surface consists of a concave articular fossa and a convex articular tubercle. The fossa terminates posteriorly at the posterior articular lip. This ridge prevents the direct impingement of the condyle on the tympanic bone in posterosuperior displacement of the condyloid process. Bony lips also exist at the lateral and medial borders of the articular fossa, the latter being the more prominent. The fossa continues anteriorly to the articular tubercle (eminentia articularis). The tubercle is markedly convex in its anteroposterior direction and slightly concave mediolaterally. The anterior boundary of the tubercle is indistinct.

Condyloid process. The condyle is oval with its long axis extending in a mediolateral direction. It is more convex anteroposteriorly than mediolaterally. The articular surface of the condyle faces upward and forward so that, in a lateral view, the neck of the condyle appears to be bent anteriorly.

Articular disk. The articular disk (meniscus) is positioned between the articular surface of the temporal bone (glenoid fossa) above and the mandibular condyle below, dividing the joint into superior and inferior compartments. The disk is oval and fibrous. It is much thinner in its central portion than along the periphery. The posterior border of the disk exhibits the greatest thickness. The upper surface of the disk is

413

concavoconvex, and the undersurface is concave in its anteroposterior direction. The circumference of the disk is attached to the tendon of the external pteryoid muscle anteriorly; posteriorly the disk continues into a pad of loose neurovascular connective tissue[20] that extends to and fuses with the posterior wall of the articular capsule. The remaining circumference of the disk is attached directly to the capsule.

Capsule. The capsule is a thin, ligamentous structure that extends from the temporal portion of the glenoid fossa above, fuses with the meniscus, and extends below to the condylar neck. The superior portion of the capsule is loose, permitting the anterior gliding movements of normal function, whereas the inferior portion is much tighter where the hinge movements occur.

Synovial membrane. The synovial membrane is a connective tissue membrane that lines the joint cavity and secretes synovial fluid for lubrication of the joint.

Ligaments. The temporomandibular ligament extends from the zygomatic arch inferiorly and posteriorly to the lateral posterior border of the condylar neck. It is the only ligament that gives direct support to the capsule. The sphenomandibular and stylomandibular ligaments are considered accessory ligaments. The former is inserted at the lingula of the mandible and the latter at the angle of the mandible.

Neural and vascular components. Posterior to the articular disk is a loose pad of connective tissue containing many nerves and the blood vessels.[20] The sensory nerves are derived from the auriculotemporal and masseteric branches of the mandibular nerve and are proprioceptive for pain perception. The vascular network consists of arteries arising from the superficial temporal branch of the external carotid artery.

THE PAINFUL TEMPOROMANDIBULAR JOINT

Considerable attention has been devoted to the diagnosis and treatment of the painful temporomandibular joint since Goodfriend[11] published the original work in 1933, followed shortly afterward by the widely read work of Costen[6] in 1934. As a result of these two contributions and continuing study by oral surgeons, prosthodontists, periodontists, orthodontists, and other interested investigators, much knowledge has been accumulated in this challenging field.[1,4,12] Many patients with previously undiagnosed facial or head pain have had the benefit of a concise diagnosis and increasingly effective treatment since that time.

Etiology

Temporomandibular arthralgia is usually attributed to one or a combination of the following factors:

1. Occlusal disharmony
2. Posterosuperior displacement of the condylar head resulting from a decreased vertical maxillary mandibular relation
3. Psychogenic factors producing resultant habits of bruxism and muscle spasm
4. A single act trauma
5. Acute synovitis resulting from acute rheumatic fever
6. Rheumatoid arthritis
7. Osteoarthritis

Many of these factors will be discussed later, so it is not necessary to discuss them in detail here. It is important to note, however, that the role of the decreased maxillary-mandibular relation in the production of joint pain has been greatly minimized in recent years. When it is seen clinically, it is usually either in patients wearing full dentures or in individuals who have been tobacco chewers for many years, so that considerable tooth structure has been lost by occlusal attrition. In either circumstance it is not a frequent cause of difficulty per se, and in patients with full dentures, the deficiency is usually corrected by simple reestablishment of a proper maxillomandibular space. It must be clearly understood that muscles cannot be extended beyond their normal physiological limit. Any contest that is set up between the muscles of mastication on one side and bone, teeth, and gingiva on the other will always be won by the muscles. Instead of setting up such a contest, a precise attempt should be made to adjust the maxillomandibular opening to its normal position. Occlusal disharmony and psychogenic factors are the most common etiological agents and are frequently seen together.

Symptoms

The symptoms arising from dysfunction of the temporomandibular joint are varied. All the various symptoms may occur in one patient, whereas in another only a single symptom may be present. It is therefore of importance that the patient be allowed to describe his symptomatology in detail, and if necessary, the attending clinician may then follow this up with pertinent questions relative to the complaint. The symptoms that are classically present in this syndrome, in the order of their rate of occurrence, are as follows:

1. Pain anterior to the ear, usually unilateral and extending anteriorly into the face; especially marked during use of the jaw
2. Snapping, cracking, or grating sensation in the joint area during mastication
3. Inability to open the mouth normally without pain
4. Pain in the postauricular area
5. Pain in the temporal or cervical areas usually associated with facial pain
6. Inability to close the posterior teeth completely into occlusion on the affected side
7. Rarely pain in the lateral surface of the tongue; usually associated with other more specific joint symptoms

Of these symptoms, the first three are classic and are seen in the vast majority of patients with pain of temporomandibular joint origin. The remainder of these symptoms are usually seen in addition to these three.

Clinical findings

Clinical evaluation is of great importance and must be done with meticulous care. To ensure proper evaluation a routine examination should be developed that is sufficiently inclusive to rule out errors of omission. The clinical signs that are found on examination, in the order of their rate of occurrence, are as follows:

1. Tenderness over the affected temporomandibular joint during normal opening and closing motions. This is best elicited by placing the examining fingers at the posterosuperior aspect of both condyles and expressing pressure anteriorly during their excursion. This finding is consistent and must be present to justify a positive diagnosis of temporomandibular arthralgia. Some discomfort is usually experienced in the normal joint by this diagnostic test, but on the pathological side, the tenderness is greatly accentuated in comparison to the unaffected joint.

2. Deviation of the jaw to the affected side during the normal opening motion. This is a common finding, since muscle spasm frequently accompanies joint dysfunction and, as such, contributes to the pain that ensues. This restricts the motion of the condyle, impairing or completely eliminating the forward gliding motion so that all that remains is a simple hinge action, with the condyle remaining in the fossa. It may also indicate that the joint has degenerated to the point of fibrous ankylosis. It is a significant clinical observation.

3. Crepitation during jaw excursion. Crepitation may be audible, palpable, or both. It is easily discernible with the stethoscope but is usually noted on simple palpation directly over the condylar head during the opening movement.

4. Discrepancy in occlusion. Occlusal discrepancies may be immediately obvious by casual observation or may require careful inspection and study, including the use

of articulated models. The common occlusal discrepancies include the following:

a. Acquired malocclusion. The loss of any tooth or teeth without replacement at an early date is frequently followed by at least a local disruption in occlusal balance by drifting and tipping of the teeth surrounding the edentulous area. This acquired malocclusion disrupts normal occlusal function by producing cusp interference and prematurities of contact that contribute greatly to alteration in joint function and the subsequent development of pain. This alteration, when combined with nervous tension, is the most frequently noted clinical state. Its correction requires treatment that may vary from simple extraction of an extruded maxillary third molar (Fig. 20-1) to extensive occlusal adjustment and so-called equilibration. Such adjustments should be done by someone especially trained and qualified in the correction of occlusal discrepancies.

b. Inherent malocclusion. Many deviations are found from the ideal concept of balanced occlusion. Despite the fact that the teeth may be acceptable cosmetically, either naturally or as a result of orthodontic therapy, cusp interference may be considerable in a dentition in which no teeth have been lost. Here again a nervous tension state is frequently the factor that produces muscle spasm and bruxing habits.

However, purely mechanical factors may also produce joint pain. An example of this is the maxillary third molar that erupts in a posterolateral direction so that it eventually is in the excursion pathway of the anterior border of the ramus of the mandible. This causes deviation of the mandible to miss the third molar during normal chewing movements, which may in turn cause a sufficient alteration in physiology to produce an acutely painful joint. Treatment, of course, consists primarily of extraction of the offending tooth to allow the reestablishment of normal jaw excursion.

c. Improper dental restorations. When dental structures are repaired or replaced, procedures are frequently done without proper consideration for occlusal function. In the vast majority of the population, this is not particularly important. However, in others the end result is either periodontal alveolar bone loss or development of a painful temporomandibular joint. Again, an important contributing factor is nervous tension, with subsequent clenching, clamping, or grinding of the teeth. It is important therefore to check the history of insertion of dental restorations or replacements in relation to the onset of joint pain.

5. Nervous tension. This background factor may not be immediately apparent, but it must be recognized as an active factor in the production of joint pain. Its early

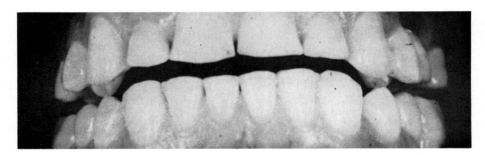

Fig. 20-1. Extruded maxillary third molar that has forced the development of an occlusion of convenience. In centric occlusion the third molar keeps the teeth from coming into proper contact.

recognition as an important factor in a given case may well make the difference between success and failure in treatment. Its importance as an etiological agent can be readily appreciated when it is realized that although great numbers of patients have occlusal disharmonies with cusp interference or even loss of vertical dimension, only a few actually develop joint symptoms. Conversely, those who do suffer with joint pain usually have occlusal disharmonies that are no greater than those of the average population who have no temporomandibular joint problem in any form. The clenching, clamping, and grinding of the teeth are direct results of tension and produce a state of mus-

cle fatigue that in itself may be productive of pain even though the joint may not be involved.

Roentgenographic findings

Proper roentgenographic study should include dental roentgenograms as well as films of the temporomandibular joints (Fig. 20-2). Joint films should be obtained in all cases to classify the type of joint derangement and also to provide a basic record for future reference if the patient develops additional difficulties in the ensuing years. These films should include the normal as well as the painful side to provide proper comparison and should also include both

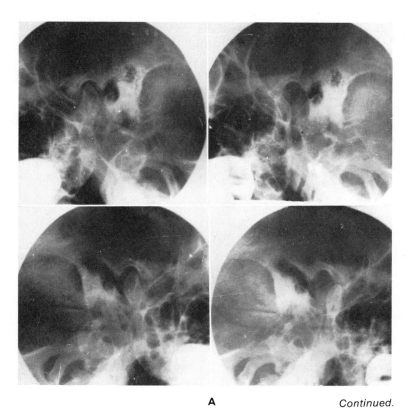

A *Continued.*

Fig. 20-2. A, Normal-appearing temporomandibular joint. Outline of glenoid fossa and of condyle is regular and smooth. Excursion of condyle is normal in degree. No hazing of the joint structures is seen. **B,** Bilateral joint dysfunction. In both the closed views (left) and open views (right) there is lack of regularity of outline, with some evidence of demineralization, opacity of meniscus, and inadequate excursion.

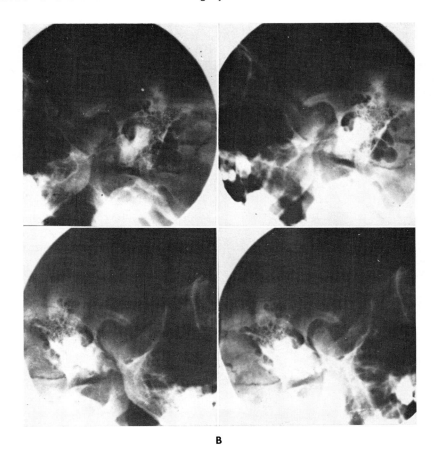

B

Fig. 20-2, cont'd. For legend see p. 417.

open and closed positions to give an indication of jaw function and possible muscle spasm.

Adequate diagnostic roentgenograms are sometimes difficult to secure. Several techniques are available, and one should be selected that gives the most consistently good results in a given operator's hands.[9] When deviations from normal are seen or are questionable, the routine transcranial films should be supplemented by laminograms of the condylar head. Laminograms are not a routine part of study of the typical patient with temporomandibular joint pain. Interpretation of films is also difficult for the inexperienced observer and requires much patience, persistent study, and correlation of clinical and roentgenographic findings. In viewing them it is important to first become oriented to the position of the condyle and glenoid fossa. Often there will be superimposition of other structures over the joint area, further masking the true findings.

The following variations from normal are most frequently noted:

1. Restriction of motion of one or both condyles. This finding is usually unilateral and may indicate either beginning ankylosis or simply muscle spasm. In either event it will immediately verify a clinical impression of joint dysfunction on that side. It is one of the most significant and most frequently seen positive findings.

2. Haziness of the joint space in both the open and closed positions. This is usu-

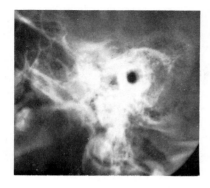

Fig. 20-3. Ankylosis of the temporomandibular joint—condyle no longer identifiable; some indication of outline of the glenoid fossa.

ally indicative of acute inflammation within the joint.

3. Posterosuperior displacement of the condylar head resulting from a decreased vertical dimension. This is difficult to interpret because of variations that may occur in angulation of the films.

4. Erosion or demineralization of the condylar head. This may be a reflection of a generalized metabolic dysfunction, localized osteoarthritis, or may be the result of a localized tumor process. Its presence calls for careful evaluation.

5. Proliferative changes or osteophyte formation, which are portrayed by a diffuse enlargement of the condylar head or by relatively opaque projections from the articular surface into the joint space (Fig. 20-3).

6. Subluxation or luxation of one or both condyles. Relaxation of the supporting ligaments will occasionally allow the condyle to extend anteriorly beyond its normal open position. This may be manifested by true luxation (dislocation) that requires assistance for reduction, or it may be merely an overextended excursion anteriorly that is self-reducing (subluxation).

It should be noted that although many patients have demonstrable roentgenographic changes, others may have persistent pain without demonstable roentgenographic evidence of abnormality.

When this circumstance exists, it is usually the result of an early disease process, or the patient may simply have pain of muscle or myofascial origin without true intra-articular involvement.

Treatment

The treatment of temporomandibular joint arthralgia has varied considerably in the past, but in more recent years a relative unanimity of opinion has existed. At present the treatment program should be considered to be in three progressive stages: conservative supportive and corrective therapy; injection therapy; and mandibular condylotomy.[14]

Conservative supportive and corrective therapy. Every patient who has temporomandibular joint pain should be placed on a specific program that is designed to reduce local inflammatory changes as promptly as possible. Some parts of the program should be continued indefinitely, although others can be discontinued as the patient gradually becomes more comfortable. However, all patients should understand that even though relief is obtained by conservative treatment the joint may again become painful if it is subjected to undue stress. Because of this, they should use the jaw with sensible caution in future years.

PLACING THE JOINT AT REST. This is accomplished in a relative fashion by placing the patient on a regimen consisting of a soft diet and limitation of motion. It is generally unwise to completely eliminate motion by interdental ligation, since this may cause an exacerbation of pain by compression of the condyle against the meniscus and periarticular structures, which are already involved in some degree of inflammation, and will not in itself eliminate bruxism that may be present. Voluntary limitation of motion and subsistence on a soft diet allow the joint structures to rest insofar as possible so that the inflammation and edema that are present may gradually recede. Opening of the jaw should be restricted to whatever opening is possible without production of pain. This reduces the stimulus of pain and therefore tends to reduce the accompanying muscle spasm.

APPLICATION OF HEAT. Muscle relaxation is also aided by the application of heat to the affected area. An electric heating pad is the most practical form to use, although moist packs may also be of considerable benefit. An electric pad can be used with care at night and early morning when muscle spasms are frequently the most bothersome.

ANALGESICS. Buffered acetylsalicylic acid, 0.6 Gm taken four times daily, will do much to eliminate discomfort by its analgesic action, thereby reducing muscle spasm and trismus. It should always be given by prescription with definite directions to maintain the dosage schedule faithfully during the active treatment period. This usually involves approximately 4 to 6 weeks and bears no contraindication unless the patient is allergic to acetylsalicylic acid, symptoms of gastric intolerance occur, or the patient is taking anticoagulants. It is most effective if taken 15 to 20 minutes prior to meals with a full glass of water, with the final daily dose at bedtime.

SEDATIVES AND TRANQUILIZERS. Most patients with a painful temporomandibular arthralgia have considerable nervous tension, which is usually a contributing factor to their problem but on occasion may be secondary to the continuing pain. Mild sedation is therefore in order. Amobarbital (Amytal), 60 mg taken four times daily, is effective and is not depressing. Diazepam (Valium) is an effective tranquilizing agent and induces muscle relaxation as a side benefit. Dosage varies from 2 mg three times daily to 5 mg four times daily in severe cases. It should never be used in association with alcohol, since it has a significant potentiating effect.

REGULAR EXERCISE. Muscle spasm and tension are both relieved considerably by a program of regular daily physical exercise. Out-of-door exercise that is associated with sports is preferred but not entirely necessary. Daily out-of-door walks or bicycling is excellent and is especially effective for the otherwise sedentary individual. The greater portion of patients of this type are women, and as a group they are prone to naturally refrain from physical exercise. However, they should be urged to adopt a well-balanced physical exercise program and to continue it indefinitely. If the patient is especially tense, an evening walk followed by a warm tub bath and the last of the daily dosage of acetylsalicylic acid and amobarbital sodium or diazepam will do

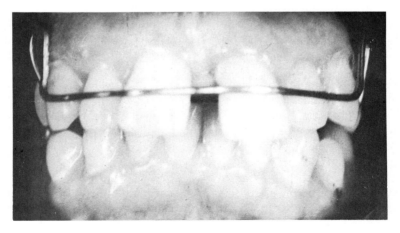

Fig. 20-4. Bite plane in place, allowing contact with the lower incisor teeth only.

much to promote a restful night, free of muscle spasm.

CONSTRUCTION OF A BITE PLANE. A palatal bite plane should be constructed for those patients who exhibit evidences of bruxism. It should be so designed that only the lower anterior teeth can contact the smooth, shiny surface of the plane so that they cannot be locked into occlusion and thereby permit bruxism (Fig. 20-4). The bite plane should not be considered to be primarily a bite-opening splint, but instead, one that will assist the patient in breaking a subconscious habit of clenching and grinding during the sleeping or even the waking hours. It may be necessary for the patient to wear such an appliance continuously for 2 or 3 weeks, but this should be reduced to the night hours as promptly as possible to eliminate the possibility of elongation of the posterior teeth. The bite plane is constructed of clear acrylic, covering approximately the anterior third of the hard palate. The acrylic should be smooth and highly polished. The appliance is held in position by a continuous nonprecious metal wire extending along the labial cervical margins of the maxillary anterior teeth. The appliance should be considered as a temporary splint, since it is used primarily to assist the patient in breaking the bruxing habit. When this has been accomplished, the use of the splint should be gradually discontinued.

OCCLUSAL REHABILITATION. After a conscientious effort by the patient to follow the regimens as outlined above, it is usually possible after 1 or 2 weeks to subject the patient to the indicated occlusal adjustments. The details of this procedure will not be included here. However, the basic objective of occlusal rehabilitation should be the restoration of relatively normal occlusion without premature contacts or cusp interference. This may require extensive occlusal grinding, or it may require a few indicated extractions and restoration of the edentulous areas. The use of carefully articulated models and study of the functioning occlusion are imperative if the objective is to be attained. Ill-fitting restorations that may have been inserted immediately preceding the onset of pain deserve special attention and early correction. Extruded third molar teeth are also of importance, since they may cause a subconscious and spontaneous shift in the occlusion that may be sufficient to set up muscle imbalance and subsequent spasm and joint pain. Occlusal equilibration is a subject unto itself, and the interested student should avail himself of proper postgraduate study to develop a proper concept of its execution.

Injection therapy. Injection therapy consists of two types: hydrocortisone compounds and sclerosing solutions.

HYDROCORTISONE COMPOUNDS. The intra-articular injection of the hydrocortisone compounds has proved to be beneficial in reduction of joint pain throughout the body by reducing the inflammatory process that exists within the joint.[10,16,24] As a result of recent developments, more potent compounds are available. These are prednisolone acetate (Meticortelone acetate) and prednisolone tertiary-butylacetate (Hydeltra-T.B.A.). Rapid and long-acting corticosteroids are combined in betamethasone acetate and betamethasone disodium phosphate (Celestone Soluspan), or the two types may simply be combined by mixing rapid and repository drugs prior to intra-articular injection. With either drug, beneficial effects can usually be obtained by intra-articular injection into the temporomandibular joint. The following indications for injection should be strictly observed:

1. Joint is so painful that occlusal rehabilitation cannot be started.
2. Pain persists despite adequate conservative and supportive therapy.

Hydrocortisone injections should be used only as an occasional adjunct to an overall treatment program. In those cases in which the onset is sudden and no occlusal complication exists, a permanent cure may result. However, in those patients who have a prolonged history, occlusal disharmonies, and an overlying tension state, relief from

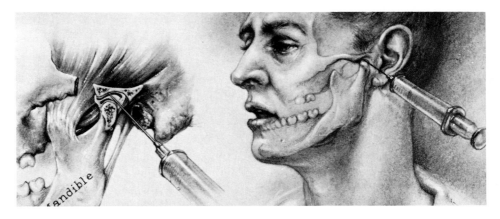

Fig. 20-5. Hydrocortisone injection (25 mg hydrocortisone or 15 mg prednisolone acetate or prednisolone tertiary butylacetate) into the superior compartment of the temporomandibular joint. (From Henny, F. A.: J. Oral Surg. **12:**314, 1954.)

injection alone, without additional supportive and corrective treatment, is usually followed by the prompt recurrence of symptoms in 2 to 4 weeks, when the antiinflammatory action of the drug has disappeared.

Patients in whom roentgenographic evidence indicates extensive proliferative changes within the joint or erosion of the condylar head should, when symptoms persist despite general supportive therapy, be treated surgically. Since both joints are rarely involved simultaneously, the injection is almost invariably given on a single side, although there is no strict contraindication to injecting the drug bilaterally.

The technique of hydrocortisone injection of the joint (Fig. 20-5) is as follows[13]:

1. The injection site must be prepared so that it is surgically clean.

2. The patient's mouth should be opened one third of the normal full distance.

3. When a local anesthestic is used, it is deposited through the sigmoid notch and also into the tissues overlying the joint.

4. With the mouth opened one third of the normal full distance, the hydrocortisone injection is done with a 25-gauge needle. The needle is inserted over the lateral surface of the joint and directed at the glenoid fossa.

5. On contacting the roof of the glenoid fossa, the needle is withdrawn 1 mm, aspiration is done, and the drug is then deposited.

6. The needle is withdrawn, and a small sterile dressing is applied.

Patients who have had such an injection may complain of an increase in symptoms for 24 to 36 hours, but this is almost universally followed by a significant and frequently total reduction in pain and dysfunction. As noted previously, the beneficial results will usually persist for a period of 2 to 4 weeks, which is usually ample to carry out most occlusal adjustments that are required.

SCLEROSING SOLUTIONS. The injection of sclerosing solutions should be restricted to those joints that show demonstrable clinical and roentgenographic evidence of hypermobility (subluxation or luxation). In such a circumstance, relaxation of the capsule and temporomandibular ligament permits the condyle to overextend its anterior excursion. Injection of the sclerosing solution should be restricted to the capsule overlying the upper condylar neck to aid in fibrosis and tightening of that structure. The material used should not be injected into the joint space, such as is done with the hydrocortisone compounds. Usually more than one injection is required, but since a cosiderable local reaction to the injection may occur, it is wise to space them at intervals of 2 to 3 weeks. The patient should understand that a series of as many as four or five injections may be required.

Mandibular condylectomy. Surgical intervention to eliminate temporomandibular joint pain is indicated only when all other more conservative forms of therapy have failed and roentgenographic evidence indicates extensive proliferative changes or erosion of the condylar head.[14,15] Psychoneurotic patients should not be submitted to surgery unless the procedure has been approved by a psychiatrist after adequate evaluation. When surgery is indicated, the procedure of choice is a high condylectomy (condylotomy). This approach to the problem has evolved after the failure of earlier methods, which were associated with a high rate of recurrent pain after surgery for meniscectomy.[8] Selection of patients for surgery must be done with care to be certain that the pain is arising from the joint and not the musculature, since if the latter is true, recurrence of pain postoperatively is the rule. The rationale of the procedure is based on the surgical reduction of the height of the condylar head, thereby relieving the persistent irritation and pressure on the nerve supply to the joint. This tissue has been described by Sicher[20] to be located posterior to the condylar head and to contain "loose connective tissue rich in blood vessels, nerves and nerve endings." It binds the articular disk posteriorly to the capsule. Although one might normally expect unusual shifting of the mandible in the postoperative state to the side operated on, this does not happen (see Fig. 20-8). When deviation does occur, it is usually of a relatively slight degree easily correctable by occlusal adjustment. Preservation of the meniscus is of importance, since it prevents adhesions that would otherwise form between the stump of the resected mandible and the glenoid fossa, the development of which would cause deviation of the jaw to

the affected side. No attempt to restrict motion is necessary in the postoperative state. Instead, the patient should be urged to gradually resume jaw function as promptly as possible.

The recommended condylectomy procedure (Fig. 20-6) is as follows:

1. The hair is shaved for 3 cm above, behind, and in front of the ear.

2. A local anesthetic solution containing epinephrine is infiltrated into the area anterior to the ear and overlying the condyle.

3. An incision is made immediately anterior to the ear, extending from its inferior to its superior attachments and running along the medial surface of the tragus.

4. A skin flap is undermined for approximately 2 cm anterior to the incision. It is sutured forward to the skin to aid in its retraction.

5. Dissection is begun in intimate contact with the ear cartilage. The dissection actually consists of dissecting the attached soft tissues off from the cartilage of the ear and external auditory canal until the zygomatic arch is reached.

6. The condyle is palpated, and the dissection is carried slightly deeper and then forward until the joint capsule is exposed.

7. The capsule is opened through a semilunar incision extending along its posterior and superior borders but avoiding the meniscus, thus exposing the condyle.

8. The condyle is resected 6 to 8 mm below its superior border. This is accomplished rapidly and easily by means of a small, round, tungsten carbide drill.

9. The specimen is removed by limited stripping of attaching fibers of the lateral pterygoid muscle. Most fibers of the lateral pterygoid remain attached above and below the resection site, thus providing good postoperative function.

10. The stump of the condyle remaining is smoothed with bone files, and Gelfoam is placed into the defect to control capillary oozing or brisk venous bleeding that may be present.

11. The capsule is sutured with fine plain

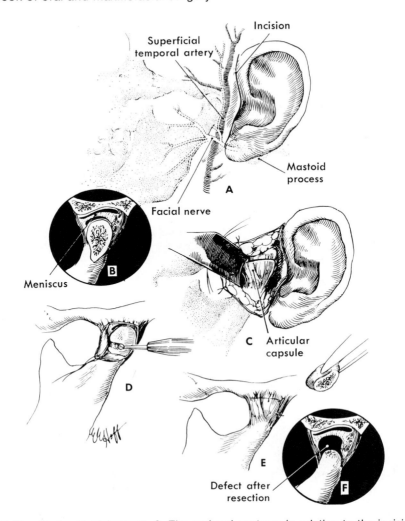

Fig. 20-6. Mandibular condylectomy. **A,** The regional anatomy in relation to the incision and subsequent dissection. It should be noted that by keeping the dissection in contact with the ear cartilage, one can damage neither the vessels nor the nerve. **B,** Cross section of articulation showing relation of meniscus, joint compartments, and neurovascular tissue posterior to the condyle as described by Sicher. **C,** Incision of the capsular ligament. All other overlying tissue has been dissected free and retracted anteriorly. **D,** The condylar head is transected, using a tungsten carbide drill. **E,** Capsule closed with No. 3-0 plain catgut sutures. **F,** Space created by condylar excision. Some rounding off of the resected portions usually occurs. (From Henny, F. A.: J. Oral Surg. **15:**214, 1957.)

catgut. The balance of the wound is closed in the usual fashion.

12. A generous pressure dressing is applied and is left in place for 48 hours.

13. The patient is urged to use the jaw as soon as possible.

14. Because of the spilling of blood into the external auditory canal, it is imperative to irrigate and cleanse the canal postoperatively since clotted blood lying against the drum is highly irritating.

This technique has several advantages. It allows adequate visualization: also, if the soft tissues are dissected off directly from

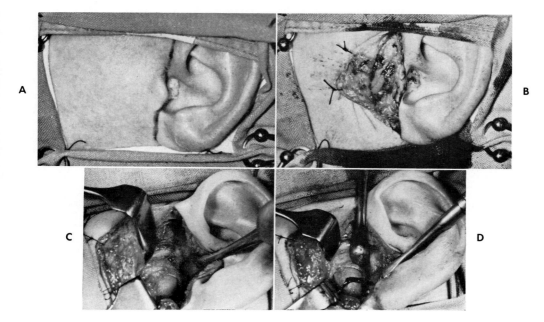

Fig. 20-7. **A,** Outline of preauricular incision. **B,** Skin flap undermined and sutured forward. **C,** Capsule incised and reflected, exposing the condylar head. **D,** Condylar head transected, prior to delivery of specimen.

the ear cartilage as described, it is virtually impossible to damage either the facial nerve or the vessels that richly supply the area (Fig. 20-7).

There has been a tendency in recent years to substitute an alloplastic implant, primarily Silastic or metal, for the resected condylar segment.[5] Although this may be desirable in some surgeons' hands when total condylectomy, including the condylar neck, is done,[21] it has been my experience that insertion of any type of foreign material is not required in the procedure described previously. In the vast majority of cases, the arthritic process is not sufficiently extensive to require resection of more than 6 to 8 mm of the most superior portion of the condylar head. In any event, only the amount required to eliminate the pathologic condition should be excised. If the meniscus is preserved, as it always should be, even though it may require repair by suturing of tears or other perforations, it is by far the best biologically acceptable material

available. Its presence prevents cicatricial adhesions between the condylar stump and the glenoid fossa. It is these adhesions that produce deviation of the mandible to the operated side postoperatively. Thus preservation of the meniscus and early, continued exercise are the key to the return to normal, comfortable function (Fig. 20-8). Since the resection point is relatively high, the inferior belly of the lateral pterygoid muscle remains intact and is a significant asset in the return to normal mandibular function. Preservation of the function of the lateral pterygoid muscle is, of course, impossible to regain when an alloplastic implant is used.

When the entire condyle must be removed or if both condyles must be removed, it has been my experience that jaw dysfunction is almost inevitable without reconstruction of at least one joint. Autogenous and biologically acceptable materials are always preferable. This opinion is shared by others.[2,7,18] My personal exper-

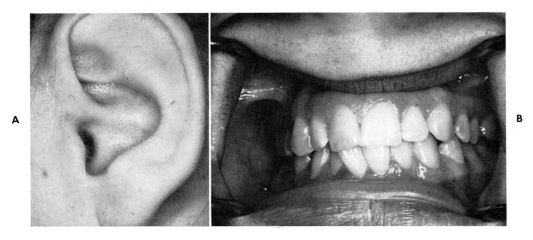

Fig. 20-8. A, Postoperative appearance of surgical area 3 years after operation. **B,** Postoperative occlusion 3 years after condylectomy; note midline.

ience is based on the use of costochondral rib grafts in 14 cases. Some of these grafts also replaced a portion or all of the ascending ramus but others were used to reconstruct the condyle alone or the condyle and neck. When the condylar head only is to be replaced, it can be done through the preauricular incision described above. The graft is morticed into the stump remaining and is held firmly in place with stainless steel wires that perforate the graft and stump and also circumscribe both. If the morticing is well done, the graft is held very firmly in position and will remain there without complication. Costochondral grafts are remarkably adaptable for use in the ramus and temporomandibular joint area.[18] They are especially useful in children with agenesis of the condyle since they can be used early in life when a growth spurt can be anticipated. An increase in the size of the graft in harmony with mandibular growth then occurs, thus eliminating the facial and jaw deformity at a relatively early age and eliminating the need to wait for jaw reconstruction until skeletal maturity is complete.

DISLOCATION

Dislocation (luxation) of the temporomandibular joint occurs with relative frequency when the capsule and the temporomandibular ligament are sufficiently relaxed to allow the condyle to move to a point anterior to the eminentia articularis during the opening motion. Muscle contraction and spasm then lock the condyle into this position so that it is impossible for the patient to close the jaws to their normal occluding position. Dislocation may be unilateral or bilateral and may occur spontaneously after stretching of the mouth to its extreme open position, such as during a yawn or during a routine dental operation. It may also occur when the jaws are forcibly dilated open during general anesthesia.

Treatment

Dislocations can usually be reduced by inducing downward pressure on the posterior teeth and upward pressure on the chin, accompanied by posterior displacement of the entire mandible. It is preferred that the operator stand in front of the patient. Ordinarily reduction is not a difficult procedure. However, muscle spasm may occasionally be sufficiently great to disallow simple manipulation of the condyle back to its normal closed position. In such circumstances it is necessary to induce sufficient muscle relaxation to allow proper reduction of the luxated condyle. This can

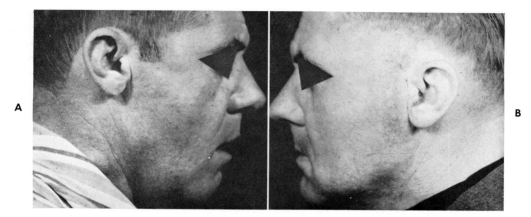

Fig. 20-9. A, Long-standing bilateral dislocation (7 weeks) with repeated unsuccessful attempts at reduction. **B,** Appearance after bilateral open reduction.

be accomplished by the administration of a general anesthetic supplemented, if necessary, by a muscle-relaxing drug. Johnson[17] has reported the successful spontaneous reduction of dislocations of the temporomandibular joint by infiltration of a local anesthetic solution into the musculature surrounding the condyle. This method requires no manipulation, since the muscles become sufficiently flaccid to allow the condyle to drop back into its normal position in the glenoid fossa. It is of interest to mention that Johnson has noted that when the dislocation is bilateral, it is necessary to anesthetize only one side to accomplish spontaneous bilateral reduction.

Occasionally dislocations of long standing may be present without recognition (Fig. 20-9). Frequently, this follows extraction of teeth or tonsillectomy using general anesthesia, the jaw being necessarily forced open. Dislocation may then remain unrecognized if the patient is not examined postoperatively. Frequently, dislocations of long standing require open reduction, since they have usually had the opportunity of developing a new articulation anterior to the eminentia articularis. Open reduction consists of opening into the joint through a preauricular incision as described previously for mandibular condylectomy, expos-

ing the dislocated condyle, and, under deep relaxation medication and direct vision, manipulating the condyle back into the glenoid fossa. I have seen two such cases, one of 13 weeks' duration and the other of 8 weeks' duration. Both were bilateral and resisted all efforts to reduce the dislocation by conservative means. Both patients had normal postoperative courses and have had no additional tendency to dislocate since that time.

When chronic, persistent luxation (dislocation) occurs, surgical intervention may be necessary. In almost every instance of repetitious dislocation, there is abnormal laxity of the supporting ligaments. Several procedures have been advocated by various authors and all report successful results. The procedures vary from simple plication of the loose capsular ligament to removal of the eminentia articularis or ligation of the condylar head to the glenoid fossa. Since I have seen several cases of repetitious dislocation in patients who have lost all of the eminence and have cured them by creating a new eminence by rib grafting, it would appear that excision of the eminence in itself is not responsible for the successful result of the surgery. In fact it would appear that, with success reported from so many varied surgical procedures, the true reason for the success is the postoperative fibrosis produced in the capsular ligament. This in itself produces a functional result that is similar to surgical plication.

Repetitious dislocation may also be caused by hysteria or neuromuscular disease. When hysteria is the cause, it is most frequently seen in young females. The use of routine interdental ligation is usually fruitless since the patient will invariably find a way to break the ligatures loose, given sufficient time to do so. Obviously psychotherapy is imperative and should be carried out without delay. Surgical intervention is *not* indicated and indeed may be strongly contraindicated.

When advanced, incurable neuromuscular disease accompanies repeated dislocation, conservative therapy may be tried, but eventually a complete condylectomy including a generous portion of the condylar neck may be necessary to assist in the nursing and nutritional care of the patient.

ANKYLOSIS

Ankylosis of the temporomandibular joint (Fig. 20-10, *A*) occurs with relative infrequency. Loss of jaw function may vary from partial to complete. Surgical correction of the ankylosis is required in all cases to permit proper rehabilitation of the pa-tient. Whereas ankylosis occurred most commonly as a complication of childhood illnesses some years ago, this has rarely been the case since antibiotic medications have been available to control secondary infections. The commonest cause of ankylosis today is trauma. Fracture of the condyle with involvement of the articular surface, hemorrhage, and subsequent elevation of the periosteum followed by clot organization occasionally produces bony union between the ramus of the mandible and the zygomatic arch. Advanced arthritis may also produce proliferative alterations in the condyle, eventuating in ankylosis.[21]

Surgical correction (arthroplasty) involves exposure of the joint area through the previously described preauricular incision. If the condyle area alone is involved in the ankylosis, it is unnecessary to expose the coronoid process. The osteotomy is usually first extended across the base of the condylar neck. The condyle is then chiseled loose and is removed. In other circumstances, if the condyle has been fractured and displaced medially, it is necessary to perform a 1 cm ostectomy at the superior portion of the ramus. This allows visualization of the medial aspect of the ramus and exposure of the malpositioned condyle, which can then be chiseled from the medial

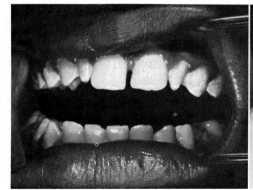 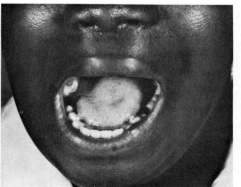

A   B

Fig. 20-10. A, Ankylosis of the right temporomandibular joint (see Fig. 20-3) after fracture of the right condyle. **B,** Jaw excursion after arthroplasty through a preauricular surgical approach and postoperative dilation.

surface of the ramus and removed through the wound.

Two principles are involved in developing a successful arthroplasty:

1. Perform an adequate arthroplasty by removing the displaced condyle if one is present and creating a 1 to 1.5 cm space between the superior margin of the ramus and the zygomatic process.

2. Provide early, vigorous, and sustained postoperative jaw dilation.

An otherwise adequate arthroplasty may fail if the second principle is not carried out with determination. To ensure success it is wise to return the patient to the operating room on the third postoperative day and, under general anesthesia with deep relaxation, forcibly dilate the jaws with a side-action mouth prop. Thereafter, the patient should have forcible daily dilation with the mouth prop for 3 months after surgery. When this program is followed, postoperative results are universally good, and it is unnecessary to interpose any foreign material at the arthroplasty site (Fig. 20-10, *B*). Since the dentition of most patients of this type is usually in poor repair, it is important that the patient be encouraged to complete rehabilitation by undergoing whatever dental procedures may be indicated as soon as practicable.

Metallic condylar prostheses have been used with good results reported by several operators.* Their use appears to be a good procedure when the condyle alone is ankylosed to the glenoid fossa. In our experience with a large number of cases of ankylosis it has been evident that when the ankylosis extends medially to include the coronoid process and the base of the skull, a patient may continue to lay down bone in the area regardless of a metallic implant. In some instances this new bone may completely encompass any alloplastic material that is interposed to create a false joint. We have enjoyed the greatest success by total excision of all new bone from the base of the

skull and reconstruction of the ramus and condyle with a costochondral graft. Early mobility followed by vigorous exercise is, as usual, important to complete recovery.

Micrognathia may be a complication of ankylosis because of the lack of the condylar growth center. Surgical correction of this deformity may also be required to develop an acceptable cosmetic and functional result. Although this is not within the scope of this chapter, it should be stated that a combination of surgery and orthodontics yields good results and usually completes excellent rehabilitation of the patient. Bone onlays over the chin area are only rarely indicated and should not be depended on to mask the jaw deformity, since many of them resorb over a period of time.

---

*See references 5 and 19-21.

REFERENCES

1. Bauer, W. H.: Osteo-arthritis deformans of temporomandibular joint, Am. J. Pathol. **17:**129, 1941.
2. Bear, S. E.: Personal communication.
3. Bellinger, D. H.: Internal derangements of the temporomandibular joint, J. Oral Surg. **10:**47, 1952.
4. Burman, M., and Sinberg, S. E.: Condylar movements in the study of internal derangements of the temporomandibular joint, J. Bone Joint Surg. **28:**351, 1946.
5. Christensen, R. W.: Mandibular joint arthrosis corrected by the insertion of a cast vitallium glenoid fossa prosthesis: a new technique, J. Oral Surg. **17:**712, June 1964.
6. Costen, J. B.: Syndrome of ear and sinus symptoms dependent upon disturbed function of the temporomandibular joint, Ann. Otol. **43:**1, 1934.
7. Dingman, R. O., and Grabb, W. C.: Reconstruction of both mandibular condyles with metatarsal bone grafts, Plast. Reconstr. Surg. **34:**441, November 1964.
8. Dingman, R. O., and Moorman, W. C.: Meniscectomy in treatment of lesions of temporomandibular joint, J. Oral Surg. **9:**214, 1951.
9. Doub, H. P., and Henny, F. A.: Radiological study of the temporomandibular joints, Radiology **60:**666, 1953.
10. Ensign, D. C., and Sigler, J. W.: Intra-articular hydrocortisone in treatment of arthritis; present status, J. Mich. Med. Soc. **51:**1189, 1952.
11. Goodfriend, D. J.: Symptomatology and treatment of abnormalities of mandibular articulation, D. Cosmos **75:**844, 1933.
12. Goodrich, W. A., Jr., and Johnson, W. A.: Roent-

gen ray therapy of the temporomandibular joint, J. Oral Surg. **14:**35, 1956.

13. Henny, F. A.: Intra-articular injection of hydrocortisone into the temporomandibular joint, J. Oral Surg. **12:**314, 1954.

14. Henny, F. A.: Treatment of the painful temporomandibular joint, J. Oral Surg. **15:**214, 1957.

15. Henny, F. A.: Surgical treatment of the painful temporomandibular joint, J. Am. Dent. Assoc. **79:**171, July 1969.

16. Hollander, J. L., Brown, E. M., Jr., Jessar, R. A., and Brown, C. Y.: Hydrocortisone and cortisone injected into arthritic joints; comparative effects of and use of hydrocortisone as local anti-arthritic agent, J.A.M.A. **147:**1629, 1951.

17. Johnson, W. B.: New method for reduction of acute dislocation of the temporomandibular articulations, J. Oral Surg. **16:**501, 1958.

18. MacIntosh, R. B., and Henny, F. A.: A spectrum of application of autogenous costochondral grafts, J. Maxillofac. Surg. **5:**357, December 1977.

19. Robinson, M.: Temporomandibular ankylosis corrected by creating a false stainless steel fossa, J. South. Calif. Dent. Assoc. **28:**186, June 1960.

20. Sicher, H.: Structure and functional basis for disorders of the temporomandibular joint, J. Oral Surg. **13:**275, 1955.

21. Silver, C. M., Motamed, M., and Carlotti, A. E.: Arthroplasty of the temporomandibular joint with use of a vitallium condyle prosthesis, J. Oral Surg. **35:**909, November 1977.

22. Silver, C. M., Simon, S. D., and Litchman, H. M.: Temporomandibular joint disorders, Am. Fam. Physician **3:**90, February 1971.

23. Smith, A. E., and Robinson, M.: A new surgical procedure for the creation of a false temporomandibular joint in cases of ankylosis by means of a non-electrolytic metal, Am. J. Surg. **94:**837, December 1957.

24. Thorn, G. W., and others: Clinical and metabolic changes in Addison's disease following administration of compound E acetate (1-dihydro, 17-hydroxycorticosterone acetate), Trans. Assoc. Am. Physicians **62:**233, 1949.

CHAPTER 21

Cleft lip and cleft palate

James R. Hayward

The congenital deformities of cleft lip (cheiloschisis) and cleft palate (palatoschisis) have been known to afflict man since prehistoric time. Efforts to correct these abnormalities have evolved over the centuries with increasing success as scientific knowledge has advanced. It will be seen that oral clefts involve complex long-range treatment and appear with sufficient frequency to constitute a public health problem. Some form of cleft lip and cleft palate occurs in one out of every 800 live births. Combined clefts of the lip and palate are more frequent than the isolated involvement of either region. With lack of complete knowledge concerning etiology, effective preventive measures are not available to eliminate this deformity. The psychological and socioeconomic handicap of oral clefts may be severe. It is a deformity that can be seen, felt, and heard and constitutes a crippling affliction. Facial deformity with cleft lip involves the structures of the lip and the nose. Further skeletal facial deformity is seen in some forms of cleft palate. The most severe handicap imposed by cleft palate is an impaired mechanism preventing normal speech and swallowing.

The zones involved by common oral clefts are the upper lip, alveolar ridge, hard palate, and soft palate. In a useful classification the normal position of the nasopal-

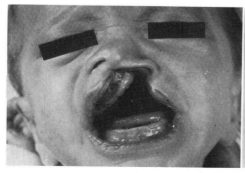
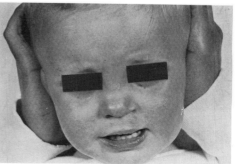

Fig. 21-1. A, Unilateral complete cleft of the lip and palate on the left side. Note the deviation of the premaxilla away from the cleft and the associated deformity of the nasal structures. **B,** Postoperative view of the cleft shown in **A,** patient 2 years of age.

atine canal divides clefts of the lip and alveolar ridge (primary palate) from those of the hard and soft palate (secondary palate). Slightly more than 50% are combined clefts of the lip and palate. About one fourth of this number are bilateral. The isolated clefts of the lip and palate constitute the balance of the varieties seen. Clefts of the lip are more frequent in males, whereas isolated clefts of the palate are more frequent in females. Lip cleft involvement is more frequent on the left side than on the right (Fig. 21-1). These phenomena lack explanation, and the underlying cause of the deformity is incompletely understood. The failure of union of the parts that normally form the lip and palate occurs early in fetal life.

EMBRYOLOGY

The oral cleft problem occurs between the sixth and tenth week of embryo-fetal life. A combination of failure in normal union and inadequate development may affect the soft tissue and bony components of the upper lip, alveolar ridge, and hard and soft palates. The face of the fetus undergoes rapid and extensive changes during the second and third months of development. The embryonic formation of the lip from the nasal frontal and lateral maxillary processes indicates the intimate relation with nasal structures (Fig. 21-2).

During the sixth and seventh weeks the maxillary processes of the first branchial arch grow forward to unite with the lateral nasal processes and continue to unite with the medial nasal processes, forming the upper lip, the nostril floor, and the primary palate. All structures are developing rapidly, and the tongue is ahead in size and differentiation, growing vertically to fill the primitive stomodeal cavity (Fig. 21-3). The palatine shelves expand medially, and as the face broadens and lengthens, the tongue descends. During the eighth to ninth week the palatine shelves further extend medially to contact at the midline and fuse from anterior to posterior for the creation of the palatine partition between nasal and oral cavities (Fig. 21-4). The point of fusion of the future hard palate with the septum is the site for ossification of the future vomer. Normal facial development depends on a harmonious growth of the parts that are undergoing dynamic changes during this critical period. Asynchronous development and failure of mesodermal proliferation to form connective tissue bonds across lines of fusion are cited as embryological variants involved in cleft formation. Without mesodermal bonding, the components of the lip pull apart. Residual epithelial bands have not been penetrated by mesoderm and are left to span some clefts of the lip and alveolar ridge. The effect of teratogenic influences is seen in a variety of clefts of the palate, incomplete or complete and unilat-

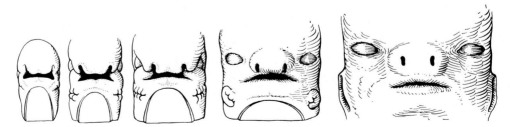

Fig. 21-2. Stages in the embryology of the face. Note that the width between the nostril openings is relatively constant, whereas the remainder of the face expands in development. (Redrawn from Avery, J. K. In Bunting, R. W.: Oral hygiene, ed. 3, Philadelphia, 1957, Lea & Febiger.)

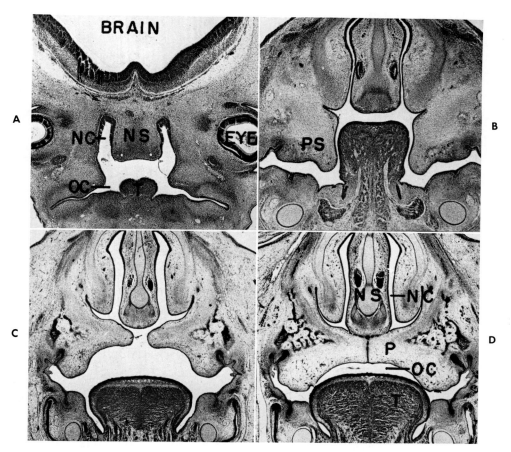

Fig. 21-3. Coronal sections of the developing palate (perpendicular to sagittal). **A,** Six weeks: *NC,* nasal cavity; *NS,* nasal septum; *OC,* oral cavity; *T,* tongue. **B,** Seven weeks: *PS,* palatal shelf. **C,** Eight weeks. **D,** Nine weeks: *P,* palate. (From Avery, J. K. In Bunting, R. W.: Oral hygiene, ed. 3, Philadelphia, 1957, Lea & Febiger.)

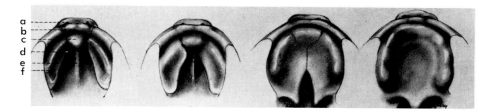

Fig. 21-4. Diagrams of palatal development. Note the fusion of parts and progressive posterior union in stages left to right. *a,* Nasal structures; *b,* prolabium; *c,* premaxilla; *d,* primary palate junction; *e,* alveolar ridge; *f,* palatal shelf. (From Avery, J. K. In Bunting, R. W.: Oral Hygiene, ed. 3, Philadelphia, 1957, Lea & Febiger.)

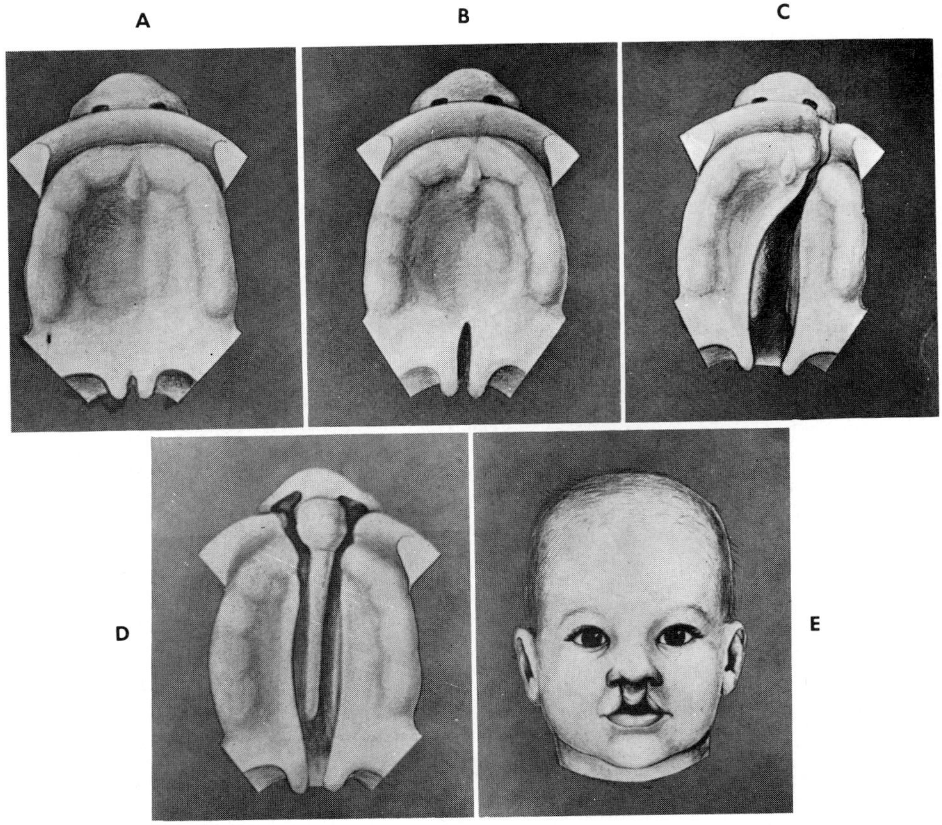

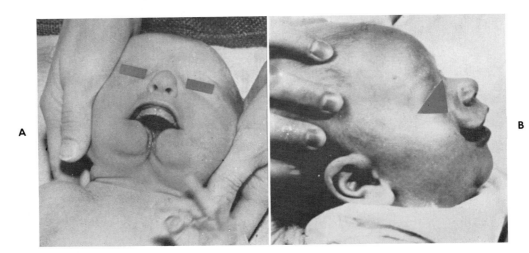

Fig. 21-5. A, Bifid uvula, which may or may not be associated with an occult or submucosal cleft. B, Cleft involving the soft palate only. C, Complete unilateral cleft involving the lip, alveolar ridge, hard palate, and soft palate. D, Bilateral complete cleft of the lip and palate. E, Involvement of structures in the bilateral cleft of the lip.

Fig. 21-6. A, Congenital cleft mandible. B, An oblique facial cleft. C, Complete wide bilateral cleft. D, Deficiency of premaxilla and prolabium. E, Absence of premaxilla and prolabium as well as septum. F, Complete absence of central lip, palate, and nasal structures. G, Absence of primary palatal and central nasal structures. H, Cyclops.

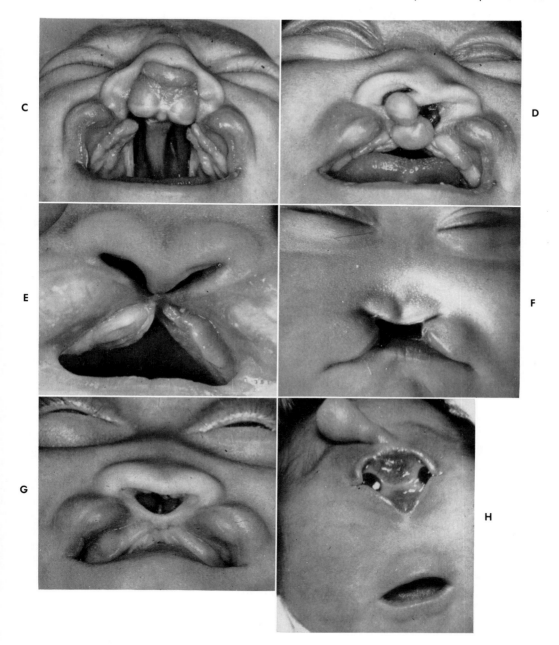

Fig. 21-6, cont'd. For legend see opposite page.

eral or bilateral (Fig. 21-5). Additional rare cleft anomalies may involve other zones of the face (Fig. 21-6, *A* and *B*).

Progressive central deficiencies of the premaxilla and prolabium are seen in the bilateral clefts (Fig. 21-6, *C* to *E*). Further decreases in interorbital distance are seen in arrhinencephalia in degrees progressive to cyclopia (Fig. 21-6, *F* and *H*). The latter are incompatible with life, since midline central nervous system defects and deficiencies are also included. Although severe bilateral clefts of the lip and primary palate include deficiencies in midline structure and decrease in interorbital distance, the opposite appears to be true in some isolated clefts of the secondary palate. Here the interorbital space is increased in varying degrees of hypertelorism with or without epicanthal folds.

ETIOLOGY

Heredity. The genetic basis for oral clefts is significant but not predictable. Hereditary tendency as evidenced by affliction of some known member of the family has been found in 25% to 30% of most reported series throughout the world. Other causative factors obviously must contribute to the production of cleft anomalies. Great variation is seen in the dominant and recessive manifestations of a genetic tendency that fails to conform with common genetic laws. Although the child with an oral cleft is twenty times more likely to have another congenital anomaly than a normal child, no correlation is evident with specific anatomical

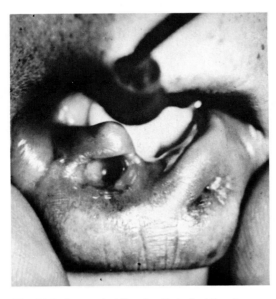

Fig. 21-7. Congenital lip pits. Note that the depression is demonstrated by a stream of compressed air dilating the blind tract.

zones of additional anomaly involvement. Aside from occurrence in certain syndromes of multiple congenital anomalies, oral clefts are related genetically only to congenital lip pits (Fig. 21-7), which appear as depressions in the lower lip associated with accessory salivary glands. The genetic defect for cleft lip and cleft palate is manifest as a lack of potential for mesodermal proliferation across fusion lines after the borders of the component parts are in contact. A fairly common clinical finding of atrophic bands of epithelium across cleft areas and absence of muscle development in the zones of cleft are evidence of mesodermal hypoplasia.

Another theory of cleft production describes an error in transitional shift of embryonic blood supply. Increased maternal age also appears to contribute to embryonal vulnerability to cleft production. The discovery of chromosomal abnormalities as a cause of multiple congenital malformation has directed attention to further genetic background for cleft lip and cleft palate. There seem to be separate genetic disturbances for clefts of the usual type involving the lip or palate or both and those that involve the isolated cleft palate (secondary palate). Several autosomal trisomy syndromes include oral clefts along with other congenital anomalies.

Environmental factors. Environmental factors play a contributory role at the critical time of fusion of lip and palate parts. Animal studies have directed attention to nutritional deficiency as increasing the incidence of oral clefts. Radiation energy, steroid injection, hypoxia, aspirin and many other drugs, amniotic fluid alteration, and other environmental factors have been shown to increase oral cleft incidence. These factors, however, have been demonstrated to increase cleft incidence when susceptible strains of animals with known genetic cleft tendencies were used. They were less significant in their effect when the strain of animal did not have the genetic tendency. Transposition of maternal malnutrition and other environmental theories to explain the appearance of human oral clefts has not brought consistent or supporting correlation. However, one conclusion can be made. The intensity, duration, and time of action appear to be of greater importance than the specific type of environmental factor.

Mechanical obstruction to the approximating margins of component parts often has been cited as contributory to cleft production. The possible role of an obstructing tongue is suggested in the embryology of the parts. Some asynchronous development or fetal position may cause retention of the tongue and the nasal area between the palatine shelves (Fig. 21-3). The isolated cleft palate, which appears more sporadically and often with less genetic predisposition, suggests this mechanical contributory influence of the tongue on the developing oral structures. Adhesion of one cleft palate margin to the mucosa of the floor of the mouth has been reported as the result of fusion when the palate shelf is blocked by the tongue.

At the present time the etiology of oral clefts appears to depend on both genetic and environmental factors that are subtle in their expression, and aside from general principles of maternal health they defy known methods of prevention.

SURGICAL CORRECTION

Surgical procedures for correction of cleft lip and cleft palate are always elective. The goals of surgery require that the child be in an optimum state of health before operation is undertaken.

Cheilorrhaphy

Comprehensive pediatric appraisal must find the infant in optimal physical condition for a cleft lip repair. Operation is usually undertaken at 3 weeks to 3 months of age, when a full-term newborn infant has regained original birth weight or approximates 10 pounds. This allows adequate time for manifestation of other possible congenital anomalies of greater significance than the oral cleft. The first problem of feeding has been overcome by careful instruction, using a soft nipple with enlarged opening or a bulb syringe for formula feeding. Structural defects of cleft lip and palate prevent negative oral pressure required for effective sucking. Since larger than normal amounts of air are swallowed, the infant must be fed slowly while held in a head-elevated position and "burped" frequently.

Surgical anatomy. The cleft of the upper lip entails loss of the important orbicularis oris muscle complex. Without the control of this sphincter group of muscles, the developing parts of the cleft maxilla deviate to accentuate the alveolar ridge cleft when it is seen at the time of birth. In all significant clefts of the lip a nostril defect is present that ranges from mild nostril asymmetry to absence of nostril floor and gross deformation of nasal alar cartilage and septum. Premaxilla and prolabium are found deviated away from the cleft in unilateral cases and found to project anteriorly in bilateral clefts of the lip and palate. This reflects a difference in the dynamics of growth potential in midline structures as compared with lateral structures, a difference that has had over 6 months to be manifest structurally before birth. Thus the premaxilla that is uncontrolled by the lip deviates to accentuate the cleft in unilateral cases and protrudes monstrously in complete bilateral clefts of the lip and primary palate. Blood supply to all structures is excellent. It is of interest to note that in complete bilateral clefts the nerve and blood supplies to premaxilla and prolabium are distributed along midline structures from the maxillary artery and the inner loop of the trigeminal second division.

Surgical goals and techniques. The safety of cleft lip surgery has been greatly enhanced by refinements in modern anesthesia using oral endotracheal intubation techniques.

Surgical correction of cleft lip strives to attain a symmetric, well-contoured lip with preservation of all functional landmarks and

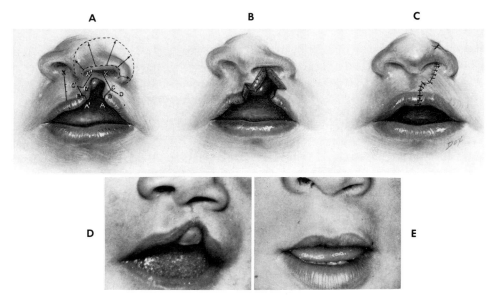

Fig. 21-8. Diagram of the Hagedorn cheilorrhaphy as modified by LeMesurier. **A,** Margin incisions mapped out, using uninvolved side for length guide. **B,** Prepared margins with flap from full side to insert in notch of deficient side. **C,** Closure of margins in three segments (mucosal and muscle closure not shown). **D,** Preoperative incomplete lip cleft. Note the nasal asymmetry and groove into nostril floor. **E,** View 22 months after operation.

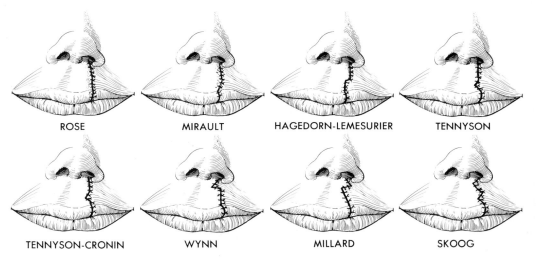

Fig. 21-9. Incision patterns for cleft lip repair. The scar line is broken into segments to achieve greater length in the margins and to offset the contracture of scar tissue into separate planes.

minimal scar tissue in the result. Since cleft margins are composed of atrophic tissues, they must be prepared to provide adequate muscle layers and full-thickness structural definition. Since all scars contract, efforts are made to minimize trauma and sources of inflammation in the procedure and to design the preparation of margins in several planes (Fig. 21-8). This pattern of preparation prevents the linear contracture of a straight-line scar, which would tend to produce a residual notch in the vermilion tissue. All tissue of quality is preserved and utilized in the operation. In unilateral clefts the unaffected side serves as a guide for length and symmetry in the restoration of the lip. The preparation of cleft lip margins to gain length, preserve landmarks, and to compensate for scar contracture has developed numerous patterns that are applicable to variations in types of cleft (Fig. 21-9).

In the past, definitive lip repairs of wide clefts have been postponed to avoid the surgical trauma of extensive tissue undermining in the newborn infant. To establish some control of the orbicularis oris musculature over the deviated and protruded premaxilla, a minimal margin preparation termed "lip adhesion" has been developed. Although inadequate for cosmetic improvement, the muscle control that is established provides action to close the alveolar cleft and greatly simplifies a definitive repair later when the child is approximately 1 year of age. When this more conservative program is followed for wide clefts, there is less undermining of the soft tissues from the anterior maxilla and thus less constricting scar limitation on the future development of the maxilla.

Palatorrhaphy

Surgical anatomy. Palate function is necessary for normal speech and swallowing. The hard palate provides the partition between oral and nasal cavities, whereas the soft palate functions with the pharynx in an important valve action referred to as the velopharyngeal mechanism (Fig. 21-10). In normal speech this valve action is intermittent, rapid, and variable to effect normal sounds and pressures by deflecting the air stream with its sound waves out of the mouth. Without this valve action, speech is hypernasal and deglutition is impaired. It should be recalled that in addition to their action in the elevation and tension of the soft palate, the levator and tensor muscles effect an opening of the auditory tube. This action is demonstrated when middle ear pressures are equalized by swallowing during changes in atmospheric pressure, such as those experienced in rapid changes in altitude. When this mechanism of tube opening is impaired, greater susceptibility to middle ear infections is experienced. The cleft palate anomaly entails this problem and the additional hazard of lymphoid hyperplasia over the auditory tube orifice in the nasopharynx. It can be appreciated that hearing loss from middle ear infections added to a defective mechanism for normal speech complicates and intensifies the handicap of cleft palate.

Copious blood supply is afforded to the palatal tissues by the major and lesser palatine and nasopalatine branches of the maxillary artery. The ascending palatine branch of the facial artery and branches from the ascending pharyngeal artery contribute further sources of blood supply. Nerve supply to the muscles of the palate and pharynx for motor action arise chiefly from the vagal pharyngeal plexus, except for the tensor, which is innervated by the motor branch of the trigeminal nerve, and stylopharyngeus from the glossopharyngeal nerve. Sensory supply for the mucosa in this region arises from the second division of the trigeminal nerve as well as from the ninth and tenth cranial nerve branches of the pharyngeal plexus.

Surgical goals and techniques. The goal of palatorrhaphy is the correction of the embryonal defect to restore palate function for normal speech and swallowing and to accomplish this restoration with minimal disturbance to the growth and development

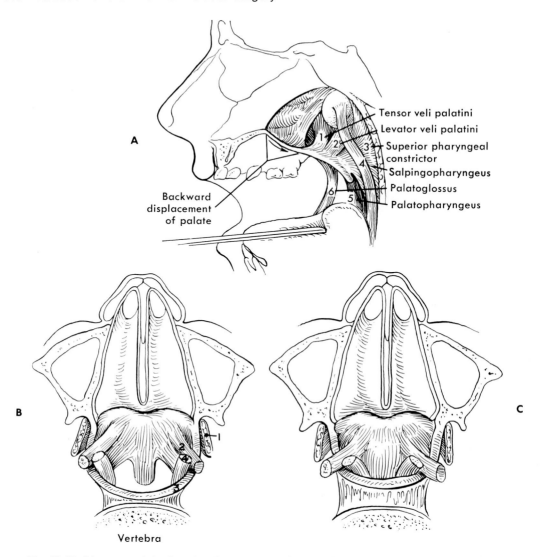

Fig. 21-10. Diagrams of the functional musculature in the velopharyngeal mechanism. **A,** View from sagittal plane to show relations of palate and pharyngeal musculature. **B,** Cross section of soft palate in relaxation, viewed from above. **C,** Muscle position in velopharyngeal closure.

of the maxilla. Cleft palate surgery is always elective, and the child must be free from infection and in optimal physical condition prior to surgery. Because scar tissue defeats the functional goal of a flexible soft palate and, in addition, contracts to deform the developing parts of the maxilla, every effort is made to minimize scar tissue and to establish the functional muscle slings of

the velopharyngeal mechanism. Healthy tissues and minimal surgical trauma are required for the operation. Advances in anesthesia with utilization of nasoendotracheal intubation techniques have added to the safety of the operation.

Since a great variation exists in the degree of deformity as seen in cleft width as well as the quality and quantity of tissues, a

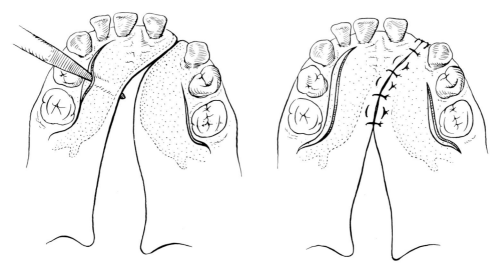

Fig. 21-11. A first-stage palatorrhaphy by the Von Langenbeck method. Elevation of mucoperiosteal flaps mobilized for midline closure. Lateral relaxing incisions heal rapidly.

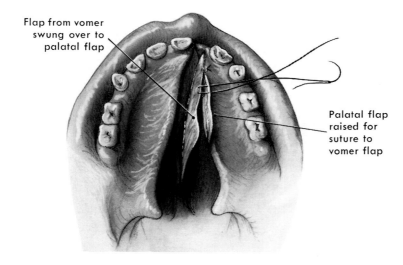

Flap from vomer swung over to palatal flap

Palatal flap raised for suture to vomer flap

Fig. 21-12. Vomer flap for closure of hard-palate cleft.

standard time for best surgical results cannot be stated. However, the majority of cleft palates are corrected surgically in children between the ages of 18 months and 3 years. Surgeons who advocate palatorrhaphy before the child is 9 months of age emphasize the advantage of muscle development in restored functional position for deglutition, early phonation, and auditory tube action. They point out the hygienic advantages of oronasal partition and the psychological benefits of operation at an early age. Advocates of postponement of surgery until after the child is 6 years of age emphasize the need for avoiding surgical disturbance to the developing parts of the maxilla. They also cite technical advantages of larger and more clearly defined muscle

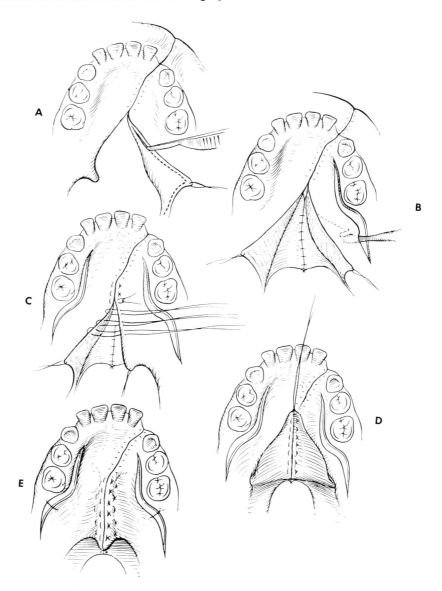

Fig. 21-13. Stages of a second-stage palatorrhaphy (staphylorrhaphy). **A,** Incisions for reflection of nasal mucosa flap. **B,** Broad muscle layer exposed. Nasal mucosal layer closed to form the superior surface. Fracture of hamular processes releases the tendon of the tensor veli palatini muscle. **C,** Vertical mattress sutures close deep muscle and oral mucosa surfaces. **D,** Mucosa closure of posterior uvula seen retracted forward. **E,** Closure completed. Lateral relaxing incisions partially closed.

structures for the operation at a later age. The more widely accepted operation for average clefts of children about 2 years old provides a velopharyngeal mechanism before refined speech habits are acquired, with the added psychological advantage of early repair. Although slight disturbances in maxillary development may be induced by surgery at this age, a correlated and rational utilization of orthodontic therapy may cor-

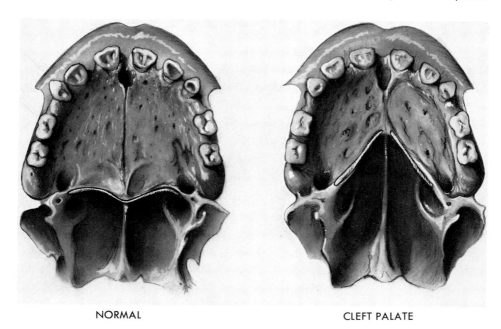

NORMAL

CLEFT PALATE

Fig. 21-14. Diagrams showing the normal attachment of the palatine aponeurosis and the site of attachment in some forms of cleft palate. Note that bone defect brings muscle attachment forward.

rect constriction tendencies in the maxillary arch. In wider clefts the soft palate may be closed without surgical effort to close the hard palate defect. This area is then obturated by a removable acrylic plastic appliance until possible later repair at an older age.

In techniques of palatorrhaphy a bony union of the hard palate area is not accomplished. Cleft margins are prepared and the tissues are mobilized for approximation in the midline. Preservation of the length and function of the soft palate is of fundamental importance. Closure of complete clefts may be divided into two stages, separated by approximately 3 months, in an effort to prevent scar contracture tending to displace the soft palate anteriorly. Techniques for closure of the hard palate are shown in Figs. 21-11 and 21-12. Soft palate closure (staphylorrhaphy) is shown in Fig. 21-13.

Since the work of Passavant and of others in the late nineteenth century, it has been

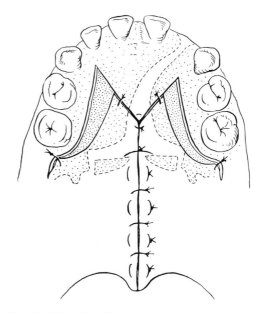

Fig. 21-15. A Wardill "push-back" operation, applicable in cases of complete clefts wherein lengthening is required. Donor sites heal rapidly to cover bone.

known that velopharyngeal function depends on adequate palate length. In addition to adequate length, the muscle vector action must displace the soft palate posteriorly and superiorly. The anterior position of the two halves of the palatine apo-

neurotic attachment found in some clefts is shown in Fig. 21-14. To position the soft palate posteriorly a number of surgical techniques have been devised by Dorrance, Wardill, and others (Figs. 21-15 and 21-16). A superior lining for the extended soft

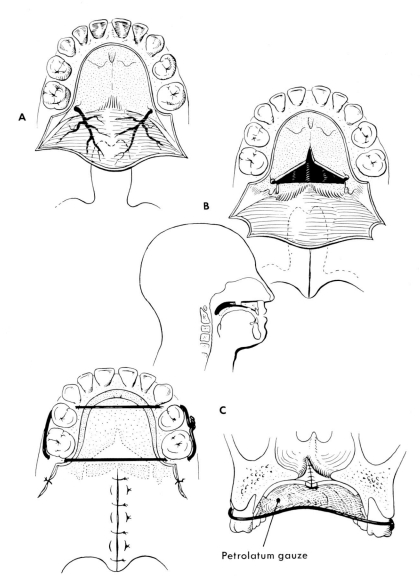

Petrolatum gauze

Fig. 21-16. Dorrance "push-back" operation. **A,** Palate mucoperiosteum reflected. Major palatine arteries preserved. **B,** Section of bone flap (Kemper), allowing muscle attachments to retrude. Sagittal diagram of lengthening procedure. **C,** Soft palate structures and flap repositioned posteriorly with temporary support of gauze pack held with wires during initial healing.

palate, originally advocated by Veau, has been obtained by mobilizing nasal mucosa from islands of palatal tissue pedicled on the major palatine artery and from split-thickness skin grafts. The purpose of this lining is to retain flexibility for soft palate action.

The surgical dissection for set-back lengthening procedures and the "island flap" takes a heavy toll in production of scar constriction of the maxilla. There is strong evidence from research and from long-term observations that extensive dissection of the hard palate tissues should be avoided in young children.

When complete clefts are wide and the hard palate area cannot be closed by a vomer flap, a modified sequence of closure is indicated. The soft palate is closed to establish the velopharyngeal valve, and the hard palate is left open or covered with a removable obturator until the child is 5 or 6 years of age. Maxillary development at this later stage is sufficient to resist major contraction influences from tissue elevation in dissections needed to close the hard palate.

INCOMPLETE CLEFT PALATE

The cleft of the secondary palate alone is often termed "incomplete." However, this group includes some very wide involvements and severe degrees of speech impairment. The aponeurotic muscle attachments seem to be in a more forward position in this type of cleft palate and the palate restored by surgery is apt to be short (Fig. 21-14). The "complete" cleft involves the alveolar ridge (primary palate) as well as the hard and soft palate (secondary palate). It may be unilateral, bilateral, or have varying degrees of completeness at both poles. The relationship with the vomer and the level of the palatine shelves in comparison with the vomer are variable. When the vomer is in good position or attached to one side, it often is utilized in the surgical closure of the hard palate area (Fig. 21-12).

SUBMUCOSAL CLEFT PALATE

In the most minimal variety, the submucosal or occult cleft palate, the muscle slings of the soft palate are not united. No cleft is seen or there is only a bifid uvula with just a web of mucosa spanning the midline area of the soft palate. At a gag reflex the sides of the soft palate will tend to retract and enlarge, but no lifting action of the soft palate occurs. The speech defect in such a case may be as severe as in the type of cleft that is completely observable. In the submucosal cleft a notch may be palpated at the posterior border of the hard palate where the posterior nasal spine is absent. The bifid uvula does not impair muscle action for soft palate and pharyngeal closure, but it may direct an examiner to the detection of a submucosal cleft.

OTHER HABILITATION MEASURES
Presurgical orthopedics

The fact that the premaxilla in complete clefts has been found in distorted positions influenced by intrauterine pressure pointed out the possible benefit of external pressures before surgery. The width of the alveolar cleft may be reduced by pressure tape over a protruding premaxilla. The restoration of the lip musculature by the cheilorrhaphy repair applies this same molding control; however, the posterior maxillary segment on the cleft side may be deviated by this pressure too far medially to produce a so-called "collapsed arch." Prosthetic devices to prevent this collapse or to correct such contractions by expanding the maxillary parts have been used in treatment. In recent years this expansion in early ages has been combined at a few therapy centers with bone grafts to the alveolar cleft. Such grafts are designed to stabilize the arch and to build up a foundation for the nasal alar base. Long-term results await evaluation in respect to growth potentials and later orthodontic possibilities. Limitations of growth and resistance to arch expansion appear probable.

McNeil[11] has shown not only the early presurgical alignment of the maxillary arch by prosthetic devices in infants but has also influenced the level of the palatine shelves and decreased the width of hard palate

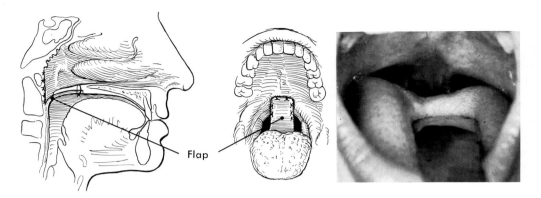

Fig. 21-17. The pharyngeal flap operation to correct velopharyngeal insufficiency (inferior based).

clefts through the influences of prosthetic contact in stimulating growth.

Secondary surgical procedures

The functional potentials of a repaired palate for effective speech can differ from the estimates of morphology that are suggested by the clinical examination. A number of compensatory actions from lateral pharynx contraction and from the existence of adenoid tissue can be involved. Lateral cephalometric radiographs for soft tissue contours and motion picture radiography (cinefluorography) are useful diagnostic aids for estimates of palate function.

If functional soft palate closures have not or cannot be achieved by the methods shown, the procedure known as the pharyngeal flap operation (Fig. 21-17) has been shown to improve velopharyngeal function. Two lateral ports remain between the nasopharynx and the oropharynx. The medial constricting action of the lateral pharyngeal walls produces the intermittent valve action that is desired. Pharyngeal flaps have been based superiorly and inferiorly, but the net result seems to be a combination of holding the soft palate back and up and bringing the posterior of the pharyngeal wall forward. Other pharyngoplasty procedures have been used and materials inserted to advance the posterior pharyngeal wall for this problem of velopharyngeal incompetence.

Short palate structure has motivated some surgeons to add a superiorly based pharyngeal flap to the primary closure of the soft palate. Judgment of these procedures is difficult, since the functional potential of the palate for movement is not always correlated with observations of length. Further guidelines are being developed for decisions as to use of these procedures.

Prosthetic speech aid appliances

Another solution to the problem of velopharyngeal insufficiency may be accomplished with a prosthesis. Occasionally a cleft palate deformity exceeds the possibility of functional repair through surgery. Postoperative cleft palate results may be deficient in functional potential. In such instances satisfactory habilitation has been achieved by the skillful construction of a speech aid appliance (Fig. 21-18).

If a palate is reasonably restored but fails to lift properly to close the velopharyngeal isthmus, a strut can be extended posteriorly from a dental appliance. Often a repaired soft palate is insensitive and may tolerate the contact of such an appliance and its extension without a gag reflex. If the palate is deficient in length, a bulb obturator is added to the posterior lift extension (Fig. 21-19). The posterior bulb extension of the appliance affords a partial closure of the velopharyngeal isthmus on which the pharyngeal musculature may act. The size of the

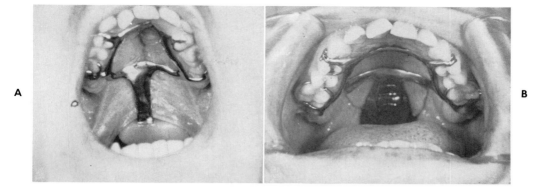

Fig. 21-18. Speech aid appliances for velopharyngeal insufficiency. **A,** Repaired cleft with insufficiency, showing the speech aid bulb extension. **B,** Cleft palate that has not been operated on and is treated with obturator for both hard and soft palate areas.

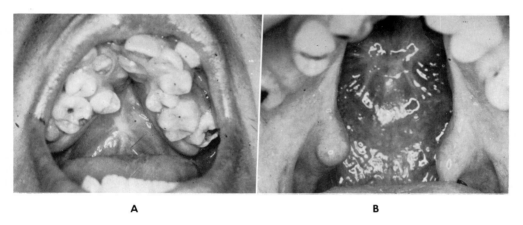

Fig. 21-19. A, Extreme constriction from surgical scar in poorly managed cleft palate. Functional occlusion is lacking, and speech is poor. **B,** Atrophic palate segments where no surgery has been attempted on a wide cleft palate. Anterior arch collapse had been produced by surgical error in amputating the premaxilla and creating a tight lip repair.

bulb can be gradually diminished as more pharyngeal muscle constriction develops for a better velopharyngeal closure. This type of appliance can be used to develop muscle action before a pharyngeal flap operation is carried out. Such an appliance may also be used to supply missing teeth, to cover hard palate defects, and to add support to the upper lip by means of a "plumping" sulcus flange extension. Retention of

the appliance is achieved by anchorage to sound and adequately restored teeth.

Dental care

The importance of preservation of the dentition in the cleft palate patient cannot be overemphasized. Sound teeth are essential to the development of the alveolar process that is deficient in the area of cleft. Teeth are essential to the orthodontic cor-

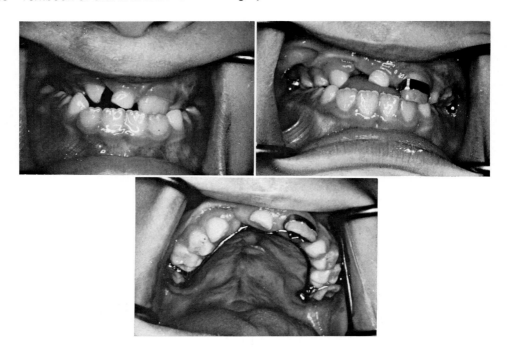

Fig. 21-20. Maxillary collapsed deformity after cleft palate repair and showing orthodontic appliance with "before" and "after" treatment stages. Note the expansion of the maxillary arch.

rection of the position of maxillary segments that show tendency for collapse and underdevelopment (Fig. 21-20). All dentists must be aware of the urgent need for preservation and restoration of the dentition for the cleft palate child.

Repair of residual deformities

Residual deformities of the nose and lip may require additional operations for final results. Residual openings into the nose are hazards for escape of dental impression materials. Labial vestibule openings into the nose are sources of irritation and prevent a peripheral seal for denture appliances. A two-layer flap closure lines both the nasal and oral surfaces with epithelium (Fig. 21-21).

Speech therapy

The most exacting criterion of cleft palate habilitation is the accomplishment of normal speech. The basic significance of speech to personality and socioeconomic achievement is appreciated only when one encounters a speech-handicapped individual. Surgery may be able to provide a palate structurally, but speech training usually is required to accomplish its maximum function. The velopharyngeal closure in speech is not a simple sphincter action, and the refinements of this mechanism are most exacting. In addition to the valve action determinant of nasality in voice quality, many articulatory problems are associated with cleft palate speech. These problems may be complex and require the skill of a competent speech therapist. The status of hypertrophic lymphoid tissue of the adenoids and faucial tonsils often is questioned. Such tissue enlargement may occupy space and compensate for insufficient velopharyngeal closure. A tonsillectomy and adenoidectomy may bring about sudden manifestation of a defective mechanism and marked hypernasality of speech. Lymphoid tissue in these areas undergoes gradual atrophy after puberty, but some workers believe that compensation is more favorable with the lengthened period of atrophy. If diseased adenoids and tonsils are contributing to infections with ear involvement, they must be removed. Careful surgery is required for such procedures to avoid excessive scar tissue, which would further reduce the functional potential of the velopharyngeal mechanism.

The otolaryngologist must manage the chronic serous otitis media problem, which is twice as common in children with cleft palate as in children without cleft palate and which is found in early infancy. Tympanotomy and the placement of temporary plastic tubes will be effective in preserving hearing, so essential in communication and speech development.

Cleft palate team approach

Since the problems of cleft palate habilitation require the services of multiple health care disciplines, centers have evolved to meet these multiple needs. Participants in this effort include the pediatrician, surgeon, pedodontist, orthodontist, prosthodontist, and speech therapist. In addition to the clinical personnel, the social workers and public health nurse contribute much to the function of such cleft palate programs. Special problems may require services of psychologists and a number of medical specialists in individual cases. It is logical that centers for the care of the cleft palate child should develop where these services are available. The diagnosis, treatment planning, active treatment phases, recall observation records, and progress reports are accomplished by conferences and united action of the members of the cleft palate team. The only weakness of the team approach is the danger of an impersonal atmosphere, which can be avoided by good organization and genuine interest in all activities of group members.

It is evident that surgery is only one link in the chain that is vitally necessary to bring

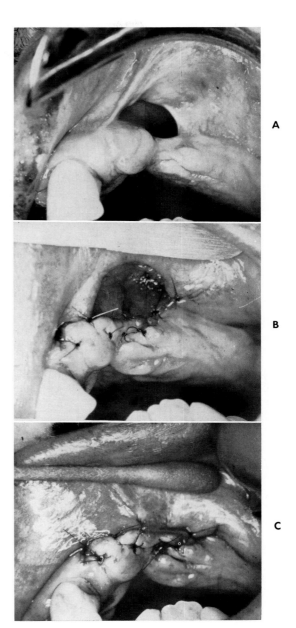

Fig. 21-21. A, The residual oronasal fistula in a middle-aged patient requiring complete denture prosthesis. **B,** Nasal mucosal lining turned down from a flap based on the superior edge of the defect. **C,** Oral mucosal coverage from a mobilized pedicle flap completes the two-layer closure.

the cleft palate child to his rightful place in society.

REFERENCES

1. Braithwaite, F.: Cleft lip and palate repair. In Battle, R. J. V., editor: Clinical surgery (plastic), Washington, 1965, Butterworths.
2. Brauer, R. O., Cronin, T. D., and Reaves, E. L.: Early maxillary orthopedics, orthodontia, and alveolar bone grafting incomplete clefts of the palate, Plast. Reconstr. Surg. **29**:625, 1962.
3. Fogh-Anderson, P.: Inheritance patterns for cleft lip and cleft palate. In Pruzansky, editor: Congenital anomalies of the face and associated structures, Springfield, Ill., 1961, Charles C Thomas, Publisher.
4. Fukuhara, Tatsuo: New method and approach to genetics of cleft lip and palate, J. Dent. Red. **44**(supp.): 1965.
5. Grabb, W. C., Rosenstein, S. W., Bzoch, K. R., and others: Cleft lip and palate; surgical, dental and speech aspects, Boston, 1971, Little, Brown & Co.
6. Graber, T. M.: A congenital cleft palate deformity, J. Am. Dent. Assoc. **48**:375, 1954.
7. Harvold, E.: Cleft lip and palate morphologic studies of the facial skeleton, Am. J. Orthod. **40**:493, 1954.
8. Hayward, J. R., and Avery, J. K.: A variation in cleft palate, J. Oral Surg. **15**:320, 1957.
9. Holdsworth, W. G.: Cleft lip and palate, ed. 3, New York, 1963, Grune & Stratton.
10. Longacre, J. J., and deStefano, G.: The role of the posterior pharyngeal flap in rehabilitation of the patient with cleft palate, Am. J. Surg. **94**:882, 1957.
11. McNeil, C. K.: Oral and facial deformity, London, 1954, Pittman & Sons.
12. Pruzansky, S.: Description, classification and analysis of unoperated clefts of the lip and palate, Am. J. Orthod. **39**:590, 1953.
13. Pruzansky, S.: Factors determining arch forms in clefts of the lip and palate, Am. J. Orthod. **41**:827, 1955.
14. Pruzansky, S.: Pre-surgical orthopedics and bone grafting for infants with cleft lip and palate: a dissent, Cleft Palate J. **1**:164, 1964.
15. Sarnat, D. G.: Palatal and facial growth in macaca rhesus monkeys with surgically produced palatal clefts, Plast. Reconstr. Surg. **22**:29, 1958.
16. Schuchardt, K.: Treatment of patients with clefts of lip, alveolus and palate, Second Hamburg International Symposium, July, 1964, Stuttgart, 1965, Georg Thieme Verlag.
17. Sesgin, M. Z., and Stark, R. B.: The incidence of congenital defects, Plast. Reconstr. Surg. **27**:261, 1961.
18. Steffensen, W. H.: Palate lengthening operations —collective review. Plast. Reconstr. Surg. **10**:380, 1952.
19. Subtelny, J. D.: A review of cleft palate growth studies reported in the past ten years, Plast. Reconstr. Surg. **30**:56, 1962.
20. Swanson, L. T., MacCollum, D. W., and Richardson, S. O.: Evaluation of the dental problems in the cleft palate patient, Am. J. Orthod. **42**:749, 1956.
21. Webster, R. C.: Cleft palate. Part I. (collective review), Oral Surg. **1**:647, 1948.
22. Webster, R. C.: Cleft palate. Part II. Treatment (collective review), Oral Surg. **1**:943, 1948; **2**:99, 485, 1949.
23. Woolfe, C. M., and Broadbent, T. R.: Genetic and non-genetic variables related to cleft lip and palate, Plast. Reconstr. Surg. **32**:65, 1963.

CHAPTER 22

Acquired defects of the hard and soft tissues of the face

Edward C. Hinds

Deformities of the face have been existent since time began, and attempts at correction have been made almost since the dawn of surgery. However, progress in this field has been slow, with few outstanding successes until recent years. Early failures resulted from lack of adequate anesthetics and antibiotics. In addition, religious and moral taboos concerning meddling with human features were also involved.

Four thousand years ago the Hindus were attempting correction of facial deformities and defects by gluing tissues to the affected part. Evidence also indicates that they were utilizing pedicle flaps from the cheek or forehead to repair defects of the nose or lips. Tagliacozzi (1546-1599), who is given much credit for revival of plastic surgery during the Renaissance, wrote extensively on rhinoplasty, using pedicle flaps from the arm. However, he was severely criticized and ridiculed for his plastic operations because of the religious attitudes of the time. Paré and Fallopius are said to have also criticized Tagliacozzi for introducing his operation. Because of this severe criticism from many sources, the rhinoplasty fell into ill repute and did

not become popular again until the early part of the nineteenth century.[79,85]

In Europe, Von Graefe, Dieffenbach, Lisfranc, and Carpue then began the development of modern reconstructive surgery. Since Reverdin's report on transplantation of skin in 1869, a steady improvement has occurred in methods of reconstructive surgery, facilitated to a great extent by the development of modern anesthesia, aseptic technique, and more recently, the use of antibiotics.

According to Peer,[83] König in 1896 was thought to have been the first to use cartilage transplants in man. Ollier studied autogenous bone transplants in animals as early as 1858 but considered such a procedure to be dangerous to humans.[77,78] Macewen[66] performed the first homologous bone graft in 1878. However, bone grafting did not receive any real impetus until World War I.

SOFT TISSUE REPAIR

Defects of the skin may be repaired by transplantation of free segments of skin or by segments with blood supply maintained by pedicle attachment. Free skin grafts may

451

be split thickness or full thickness. Pedicle grafts or flaps usually contain considerable subcutaneous tissue along with the skin and may serve to restore contour defects as well as surface defects.

Free grafts

Free skin grafts find wide usage in lesions of trauma and neoplasia. Glanz[38] states that one advantage of a free skin graft in management of neoplasms of the face is that the wound may be left open during the time that the permanent pathological sections are being made to determine adequacy of therapy. They can then be covered by a delayed skin graft.

Split-thickness grafts can be taken fairly easily and give good assurance of a "take." Disadvantages of split-thickness grafts are their marked tendency to contract, pigmentary changes, and lack of depth for contour problems. Grafts do not take well in infected areas, over exposed cartilage or bone, or in avascular areas. Split-thickness grafts may be used to convert primary traumatic wounds into closed wounds if there is not enough local tissue. They may also be of value in converting secondary wounds into closed wounds such as in the case of burns or trauma (Fig. 22-1).

Full-thickness grafts are much superior to split-thickness grafts as far as matching face color is concerned, and they have less tendency to contract. They may be valuable in various types of lesions of the face, par-ticularly if the tissue loss involves skin only. They have been used successfully in correction of ectropion of the eye and resurfacing of the lip. Perhaps the only disadvantage of the full-thickness graft is the decreased chance of graft survival as compared with the split-thickness graft.

Defects of the oral cavity, nasal cavity, and orbit are best restored by split-thickness grafts. When grafting extensive lesions of the oral cavity, particularly after excision of contractures, the importance of maintaining dilation by means of some type of stent must be realized, and it must be maintained for several weeks to prevent recurrence of the contracture. One of the most difficult problems in surgery is the management of the badly constricted oral cavity resulting from extensive scar tissue.

In repairing an extensive defect of oral mucosa with skin graft, it is best to use a thick, split-thickness graft and to secure it with a stent of gauze or cornish wool saturated in antibiotic solution. This should be left in place 7 to 10 days. These grafts have a marked tendency to shrink; consequently, a generous graft must be used.

The use of skin grafts for extending buccal and labial sulci was originally devised by Esser in 1917, later modified by Waldron, and more recently advocated by Obwegeser.[74] This technique essentially involves the construction of a stent to provide the desired sulcus over which the skin graft is applied so that the raw surface

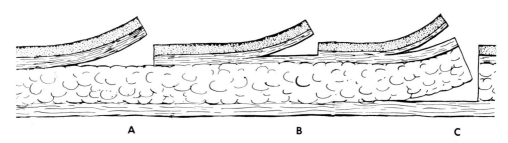

Fig. 22-1. Diagrammatic illustration of free tissue grafts. **A,** Full-thickness skin graft. **B,** Split-thickness skin graft. **C,** Dermal fat graft.

of the graft is adjacent to the raw surface of the newly constructed sulcus. This is secured in place for 7 to 10 days.

Skin grafts applied to a bony surface such as the alveolar ridge will not shrink, but skin grafts applied to soft tissue will manifest marked shrinkage unless counteracted to some extent by an appropriate stent.

Local flaps

Paletta[80] has aptly stated that the simplest repair that closely simulates the tissue being reconstructed should be the method of choice. This objective is probably best achieved by use of the advancement or rotation flap wherever possible.

Flaps may be classified as local and distant. Local flaps utilize contiguous tissue and include the following: advancement (Fig. 22-2), rotation, and transposition. Distant flaps are those carried over an area of normal skin on a pedicle that is later sectioned and returned to the donor site. These may be divided into direct and indirect. The indirect flap may be migrated in steps from a distant area to the face or carried on the arm.

The local flap became popularized by a group of French surgeons shortly after Reverdin's description of the epidermic free graft and is sometimes known as the French flap.[85] The simplest form is probably exemplified by undermining the edges of a wound to facilitate closure. The direct advancement flap is created by undermining the skin of one margin of wound defect and creating parallel incisions at the borders of the undermined area for the purpose of closing the defect.

Although the lip shave (vermilionectomy) in the past has been considered a modification of the advancement flap (Fig. 22-3), in recent years surgeons have performed this procedure without a true advancement in the following manner. The area of altered vermilion tissue to be excised is outlined in an elliptical fashion, beginning anteriorly at the margin of the vermilion. Approximately 5 to 6 mm of vermilion is included in the ellipse near the midline. Posterior and anterior incisions are outlined and brought together near the commissure. Dissection is then carried down to the muscle area, and the entire mucosa and submucosal tissues are excised. The wound is closed directly without undermining the mucosa posteriorly. This allows an ideal closure, without the ecchymosis that occurs when extensive mu-

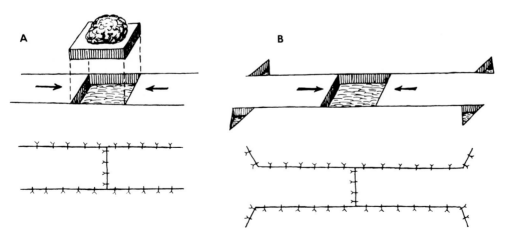

Fig. 22-2. A, Advancement flap. **B,** Modification by removal of triangles of skin at base of flap.

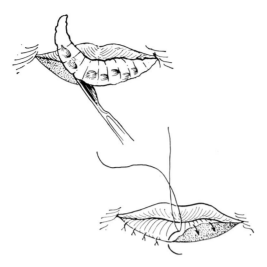

Fig. 22-3. Diagrammatic illustration of lip shave wherein labial mucosa is advanced to form new vermilion after removal of diseased area.

cosal undermining is carried out. The slight decrease in fullness of the lip, if anything, is helpful in protecting the lip from the harmful rays of the sunshine. If one area of the lip is more pathological than the rest, a wedge excision of this area should be done in combination with the lip shave.

A rotation flap is created by incising the donor tissue in semicircular fashion to allow rotation into a defect. The advancement flap and the rotation flap may both be facilitated by either the cut-back or a triangular excision of skin (Fig. 22-2, *B*). A transposition flap is one that is rotated at an angle, jumping an area of normal tissue to reach the defect. Another variety of local flap is the inturned flap in which the margins of a defect are incised, undermined, and turned in to form the back side of the defect if a double lining is required, such as

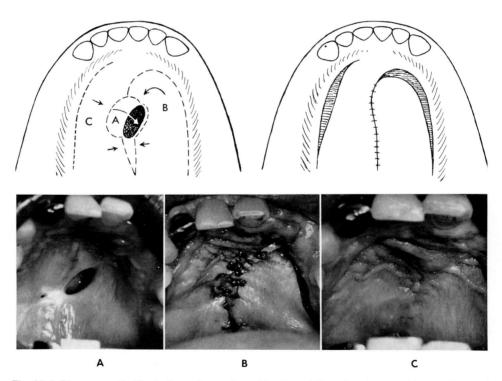

Fig. 22-4. Diagrammatic illustration of use of combination of flaps for closure of traumatic nasal oral fistula: **A,** inturned flap; **B,** rotation flap; **C,** advancement flap. Photographs are of actual case in which the patient was operated on by Dr. William H. Bell and Dr. Robert R. Debes, Jefferson Davis Hospital.

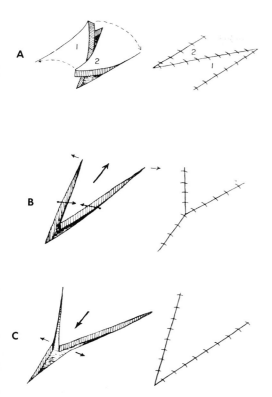

Fig. 22-5. Modification of local flaps. **A,** Z-plasty for breaking up linear scars or for releasing tension of scar band. **B,** V-Y procedure for lengthening localized area. **C,** Y-V procedure for shortening localized area of tissue.

in a nasopalatine fistula or an antral-cutaneous fistula.

Pedicle flaps, in general, have the advantage of possessing subcutaneous tissue as well as skin, thereby providing depth and pliability to the repair. Local flaps have the additional advantages of desirable color and texture as well as simplicity and diminished time requirements. These flaps have wide application, and several variations have been used in closure of oroantral fistulas for many years. Fig. 22-4 demonstrates the use of a combination of local flaps in repairing an oronasal fistula caused by trauma.

Common modifications of the local flap are the Z-plasty and V-Y flap (Fig. 22-5). The Z-plasty is a double rotation flap and may be used as a series of transposition flaps. It is the most effective method for releasing tension on a linear contracture. The rotation of the flaps allows the direction of tension to be changed, with consequent relaxation of the tension of the original axis (Fig. 22-6). It is also applicable if a corner of the mouth or the ala of the nose is depressed or elevated. The V-Y flap is a type of advancement flap that acts as a lengthening procedure when the incision is made in the form of a V and converted into a Y. It acts as a shortening procedure when made in the form of a Y and converted into a V. This may be particularly useful in re-

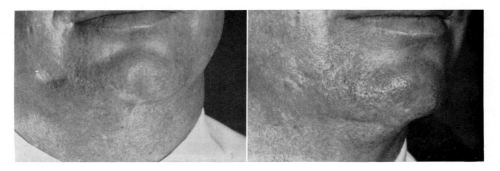

Fig. 22-6. Cicatricial band of segmental area and scar on right side of face corrected by revision and multiple Z-plasty.

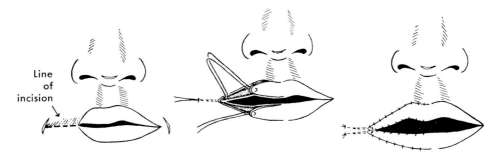

Fig. 22-7. Reconstruction of oral commissure. (Drawn from Kazanjian, V. H., and Roopenian, A.: Am. J. Surg. **88**:884, 1954.)

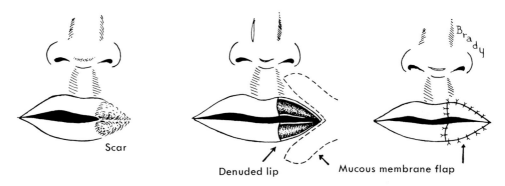

Fig. 22-8. Another method of reconstruction of oral commissure. (Drawn from Kazanjian, V. H., and Roopenian, A.: Am. J. Surg. **88**:884, 1954.)

pairing notch defects of the lips. It may be carried out by mucosal advancement alone or by full-thickness advancement as described by Gillies and Millard.[37]

The commissure of the mouth may be extended by excising a triangular or arrowhead section of skin, cutting through the orbicularis oris, and undermining and advancing the mucosa to form the new lining of the commissure. Palleta[80] described a simple method for reconstruction of the commissure after excision of lesions in this area, using the principle of advancing mucosal flaps.

Two additional methods for reconstructing the commissure of the mouth are described by Kazanjian and Roopenian.[56] The first involves excision of skin, extension of the line of commissure through the muscle, and advancement of adjacent vermilion lip rather than buccal mucosa (Fig. 22-7). The second involves incision of skin, incision of the orbicularis oris and mucosa, and utilization of upper and lower transposition flaps of buccal mucosa for lining the defect of the vermilion (Fig. 22-8).

Full-thickness losses of the lips are best repaired by local flaps and can usually be carried out by one of the following three methods or a variation of one of these:

1. The Abbe or Estlander flap
2. Straight advancement with triangular excision of skin
3. Transposition flap, such as the nasal labial flap

The most common method for repair of

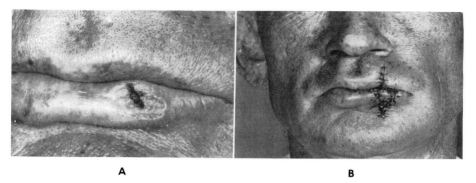

A   B

Fig. 22-9. A, Squamous cell carcinoma of lower left lip. **B,** Wedge excision and primary repair with Abbe-Estlander or rotation flap from upper lip. Pedicle detached and revised 18 days after surgery.

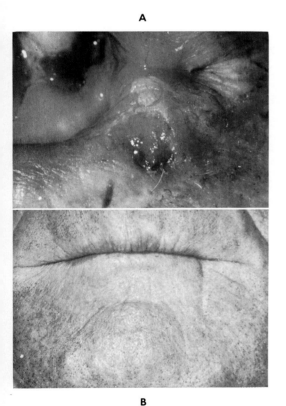

Fig. 22-10. Carcinoma near left commissure of mouth treated by combination V excision and lip shave. **A,** Preoperative photograph. **B,** Postoperative photograph.

full-thickness losses of the lip is probably the rotation flap from one lip to the other. Although rotation flaps from one lip to the other are associated with the names Abbe and Estlander, Pietro Sabattini in 1837 repaired an upper lip defect by rotating a lower lip flap through 180 degrees.[104] Stein in 1847 utilized double adjacent flaps from the upper lip to repair a defect in the midline of the lower lip. Estlander in 1865 first repaired a defect of one lip by a pedicle flap from the other and published his procedure in Germany first in 1872. His technique was characterized by a rotation flap consisting of a single wedge of lip substance and, if necessary, a part of the cheek. The pedicle was located at the angle of the mouth, and the operation, as a rule, was completed in one stage. Abbe in 1898 utilized a rotation flap from the lower lip to the upper lip. (See Fig. 22-9.)

In excising lesions of the lower lip it should be remembered that a V-shaped wedge containing up to one third or more of the lower lip may frequently be repaired by primary suture (Fig. 22-10). Recently a composite V-shaped graft has been transferred from one lip to the other, without use of a pedicle, with success.[30] It does not, however, seem advisable to take this added risk when the disability of the pedicle is minimal. Pedicle flaps of mucosa only from one lip to the other may also be used

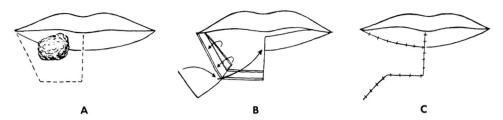

Fig. 22-11. Method of reconstruction of lower lip after wide excision for cancer. **A,** Primary lesion and defect created by excision. **B,** Diagrammatic illustration of method of reconstruction carried out 3 weeks after primary excision. **C,** Closure completed. (Method devised and described by Dr. Richard W. Vincent, New Orleans, La.)

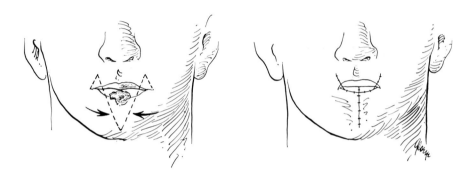

Fig. 22-12. Burow's method of reconstruction of mouth after excision of large lesion of lower lip. (Drawn from Binnie, J. F.: Manual of operative surgery, Philadelphia, 1921, P. B. Blakiston's Son & Co.)

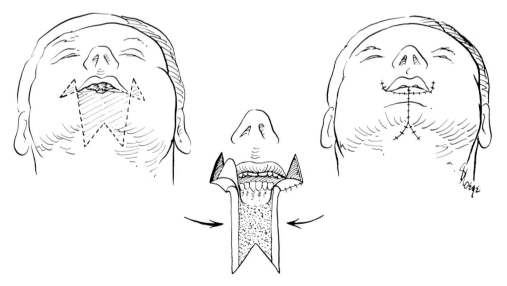

Fig. 22-13. Bernard's method of reconstruction after excision of extensive lesion of lower lip. Triangle of skin removed from upper lip at each lateral margin, saving mucosa for reconstruction of vermilion. (Drawn from Martin, H. E.: Surgery of head and neck tumors, New York, 1957, Hoeber-Harper.)

to advantage. Schneider[91] has described a Z closure of a V excision of the lower lip that gives a more normal-appearing lip.

The literature is somewhat confusing on the origin of the closure of lip defects by excising a triangle of skin and advancing the flaps medially. Burow and Bernard are both mentioned in association with this procedure. The methods of Burow and Bernard were both first published in 1853. Burows' method apparently involved excision of lateral triangles from the upper lip and a V excision of the primary lesion from the lower lip, followed by advancement of the lower flaps to re-create the lower lip (Fig. 22-12). Bernard's procedure involved the formation of lateral cheek flaps mobilized from the mandible, allowing greater excision of the primary lesion, which could be rectangular in outline rather than V shaped[67] (Fig. 22-13).

A great variety of lateral rotation or transposition flaps have been used for closure of lip defects. Bruns, Denonvilliers, and Nealton and Ombrédanne were among the first to describe flaps of this type.[104] The possibilities for use of this principle are almost limitless.

Because of the pliability of the cheek tissue, a large variety of defects can be corrected by rotation, advancement, or transposition flaps. Defects in the anterior portion of the cheek lend themselves to such correction better than defects in the posterior areas. Full-thickness losses of cheek usually require pedicle flaps from a distance for repair.

Distant flaps

Distant flaps are those that are carried over an area of normal skin on a pedicle that is later sectioned and returned to the donor site. It is sometimes difficult to fit all procedures into precise categories. For example, some local flaps, because of their complexity, might best be included in this group rather than in the previous section on rotation of local tissues. Generally speaking, pedicle flaps, or distant flaps, may be

divided into the forehead or scalp flaps, which are supposed to have been developed in ancient India, the open pedicle flap described by Tagliacozzi in Italy, and the tubed pedicle flap developed by Filatov in Russia and Gillies in Great Britain.[85]

A variety of the tube graft is the pillowed or pin-cushioned graft wherein a flap is elevated and turned on itself. Both the tube and the pillowed graft avoid an open wound. The forehead flap, sometimes lined with a free graft, has found wide usage, particularly for extensive repair of the nose. It has also been used for repair of full-thickness defects of the cheek, particularly involving the wall of the antrum. Large flaps from the neck lined with free grafts have also been used for repair of pharyngeal fistulas.

Tubed pedicle flaps seem to have definite advantages over open flaps. Tubing a pedicle flap avoids an open wound, provides better circulation, and may be handled with greater ease, both to the patient and the operator. Pedicle flaps are required for

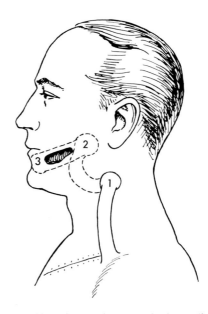

Fig. 22-14. Use of acromiopectoral tube pedicle for repair of full-thickness defect of cheek. Advanced in three stages.

repair if extensive loss of tissue is involved or bone grafting procedures are anticipated and soft tissue covering is not adequate. Of the tube pedicles the thoracoepigastric, the acromiopectoral, and the neck pedicle are used most often (Fig. 22-14).

Although most surgeons have thought that repair of radical loss of the maxilla is best handled by prosthetic appliances, some[27,63] have advocated repair of these defects by means of tubed pedicle flaps. Longacre and Gilby[63] state that a prosthesis for an extensive defect is unsatisfactory, and the efficiency of a prosthesis is inversely proportional to the size of the defect. They have reported reconstruction of extensive palatal defects, utilizing local flaps as well as tubed pedicle flaps. For perforations and defects not exceeding one half of the hard and soft palates, local mucoperiosteal flaps may be utilized. For more extensive losses they have used tubed pedicle flaps from various donor sites such as the arm, the chest, and the neck.

Edgerton and Zovickian[27] also mention difficulties of retention of prostheses. They make use of a cervical tube inserted through an incision beneath the border of the mandible rather than through the mouth. They also use the bulk of the tube to fill out the defect of the zygomatic area where indicated.

Gillies and Millard[37] have used tubed pedicle flaps for repair of traumatic palatal defects as well as cleft palates. In many instances a combination of local and tube flaps is necessary for a satisfactory reconstruction.

CONTOUR REPLACEMENT
Soft tissue

Lacerations of the cheek frequently leave depressed scars, which may be corrected by excision of the scar, undermining of the

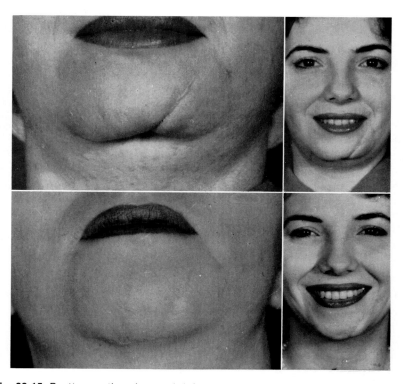

Fig. 22-15. Posttraumatic submental defect corrected by means of dermal fat graft.

skin, and development and imbrication of fat flaps. Free dermal grafts have been used for filling out such soft tissue defects but have definite limits in regard to the amount of correction that can be made. Peer[84] prefers a free graft containing both dermis and fat (Fig. 22-1, C). This is effective in creating a soft, even contour in the cheek and should be inserted with the dermis placed deep in the wound and the fat superficially facing the skin. These grafts almost universally will show a certain amount of shrinkage, and consequently they must be inserted with overcorrection (Fig. 22-15).

Cartilage

Contour loss of the hard structures of the face is usually repaired by substances of a similar texture. Contour defects characterized by loss or displacement of supporting structure may involve the frontal, mental, or malar prominences, the orbital floor or margins, and the external nose and ear. These defects have been corrected by a variety of substances, including viable autogenous tissue as well as a variety of inert materials. Kazanjian and Converse[55] have filled out the prominence of the chin by rotating a fat flap from the neck below the chin, and Gillies and Millard[37] describe the use of a temporal muscle flap for restoration of the malar prominence. These problems are more frequently managed by use of bone or cartilage or an inert material, such as tantalum, Vitallium, or rubber silicone. Good results have been reported with a wide variety of materials, but in some instances this must reflect the amazing tolerance that the tissues sometimes exhibit to any kind of foreign body. A satisfactory implant material by itself will not guarantee success. Meticulous surgical technique must be used, and a satisfactory bed for the implant is necessary as well as adequate skin and subcutaneous tissue covering.

Adequate exposure of the graft bed is essential and requires proper undermining (Fig. 22-16). However, unnecessary extensive undermining is to be condemned. The supraorbital area may be approached through incisions in the eyebrow; the malar

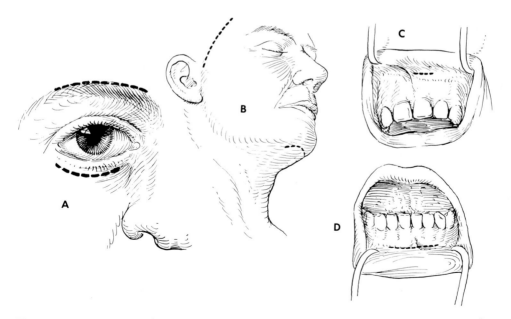

Fig. 22-16. Illustration of routes of approach for implanting filling materials. **A,** Infraorbital and supraorbital. **B,** Temporal and submental. **C,** Intraoral, maxilla. **D,** Intraoral, mandible.

bone may be approached by way of the temporal route, through previous scars, or through an infraorbital incision. The orbital floor is approached by way of the infraorbital route. The chin prominence may be approached either submentally or through the oral vestibule. With either cartilage or bone, the use of preconstructed molds as a pattern for shaping the implant may be of value.

Millard[69] has reported several successful cases of chin implants, utilizing homologous and heterologous cartilage inserted through the oral labial sulcus.

Bone

Bone continues to be popular for correcting contour defects, particularly fresh autogenous bone. As in the case of cartilage, bone grafts have been of three types: autogenous, homogenous, and heterogenous. The physiology of bone growth and bone grafting is one of the most interesting phases of medical science and still a fertile field for new discovery. Excellent historical reviews have been published by Converse and Campbell[21] and by Chase and Herndon.[18]

Opinion overwhelmingly favors iliac bone for grafting procedures. This apparently results from the fact that the large spaces within the substance of the cancellous iliac bone allow early rapid revascularization with survival of many of the graft cells. Abbott and co-workers[1] report new formation of trabeculae, demonstrated microscopically as early as 10 days, with iliac grafts. They state further that tibial cortical bone is low in osteogenic power because of the need for resorption and replacement of the increased amount of dense bone that does not survive. They further state that the same is true of rib grafts, although not to such a great extent, and that split-rib grafts compare more favorably with iliac grafts because of the open spaces presented for revascularization.

Mowlem[72] during World War II began correcting facial defects with chip grafts to facilitate revascularization and survival of graft cells. He found that fixation of these grafts was obtained as early as 10 days, using pressure dressing only.

Iliac bone seems to be much more resistant in the presence of infection. Stuteville[96] and more recently Obwegeser[76] have reported the use of homogenous iliac block graft in the presence of infection. It seems evident that the greater the area of graft recipient bone contact, the more certain and more rapid the regeneration. Adequate fixation is essential, although this does not present such a problem in contour defects as it does in full-thickness defects of the mandible. As with all types of implants adequate soft tissue covering is desired, although ultimate healing in the presence of incomplete soft tissue closure has been reported, particularly with iliac chips.

Iliac grafts for facial defects are implanted by means of similar routes to those used with cartilage in the temporal region, eyebrow, hairline, infraorbital margin, previous scars, and submental area. Ragnell[87] has reported bone implants of the maxillary and nasal areas inserted through an incision in the columella. Adams and associates[2] have applied bone implants to the maxilla through an incision at the alar margin. Converse and Campbell[21] have achieved remarkably good results, inserting iliac grafts to facial defects through the oral cavity.

Block grafts of the ilium are somewhat harder to shape than cartilage. Shaping is done with rongeurs or a Stryker saw. With block grafts a somewhat more extensive dissection is required than with cartilage, and bare bone must be exposed. For this reason Mowlem[72] resorted to chip graft restorations, maintaining that they could be inserted with much less extensive dissection through smaller incisions of access, with easier molding and more rapid consolidation.

It may be advantageous to combine a shaped block graft with iliac chips in filling contours. This will aid both in accuracy of restoration and in early consolidation. The block graft may be placed with the cortex external or with the cortex against the graft bed. More accurate shaping usually can be done if the cortex is left toward the external surface. Usually a moderately firm pressure dressing is all that is necessary for fixation, although direct wiring may be utilized. Where large block grafts are used on a curved surface, it may be necessary to cut or fracture the cortex to allow more accurate bending and shaping of the graft.

Some rather extensive defects of the maxilla have been corrected by bone graft. Gillies and Millard[37] have described replacement of the maxilla by graft from malar prominence to malar prominence. Campbell[16,17] has reported two rather extensive reconstructions of the maxilla. One was made necessary by trauma; the other was an immediate repair at the time of removal of extensive malignant disease. Converse has reported reconstruction of the floor of the orbit and malar bone after extensive excision for neoplastic disease.

Artificial implants

Alloplasts. The use of inert foreign body implants (alloplasts) in surgery continues to be a matter of considerable disagreement. Smith,[94] Kiehn and Grino,[57] and Peer[83] all advised against the use of foreign body replacements. Kiehn and Grino maintained that with slight trauma alloplastic transplants may become infected, absorbed, or extruded and advised use of autogenous tissue transplants whenever possible. In spite of certain apparent objections, there seems to be an increasingly wide usage of such materials, particularly Vitallium and tantalum among the metals, methyl methacrylate, polyethylene, Ivalon, and Teflon among the synthetic resins, and more recently the rubber silicones.

Conley[20] dates the search for a foreign body for implantation purposes back to 1565, when Petronius devised a gold plate for the repair of defects of the cleft palate. Since then many materials have been tried and some, such as ivory and paraffin, dis-

carded because of poor and sometimes harmful results.

In spite of the advantages of cartilage and bone as a filling material, they nevertheless possess certain disadvantages, such as (1) resorption, (2) distortion, (3) difficulty of shaping, and (4) need for additional surgery. For this reason alloplasts continue to be investigated and utilized for purposes of contour reconstruction.

Criteria for a successful alloplastic implant will vary slightly, depending on its function, particularly with regard to texture of the implant. However, in general, a successful implant (1) should not produce a reaction in body tissues, (2) should not produce tumor, and (3) should be easily workable, whether soft or hard, resilient or rigid, according to individual needs.

Metals. Until the work of Venable and Stuck,[100,101] use of metallic implants was characterized by frequent failure. Venable and Stuck showed that corrosion took place through the process of electrolysis in most of the metals then in use. Their investigations revealed three metals that were sufficiently electropassive to be used in surgery: (1) Vitallium, an alloy of cobalt, chromium, and molybdenum; (2) tantalum, a metallic element discovered by Ekeburg in Sweden in 1892; and (3) 18-8-SMO steel, a stainless steel alloy containing 18% chromium, 8% nickel, and 4% molybdenum. Since then these three metals have been used extensively in bone surgery as plates, screws, wires, and trays.

Tantalum and Vitallium have both been used with success for filling in facial defects. Tantalum is strong and, because of its ductility, can be drawn, stamped, or formed in complicated shapes. It may be machined with ordinary steel tools. It has been used in the form of plates for cranioplasty and is easily adapted to defects, although it tends to leave a dead space on the undersurface.

Perforated tantalum plates are readily adapted for correction of facial deformities. Fig. 22-17 shows reconstruction of the infraorbital floor and rim with a perforated

A   B

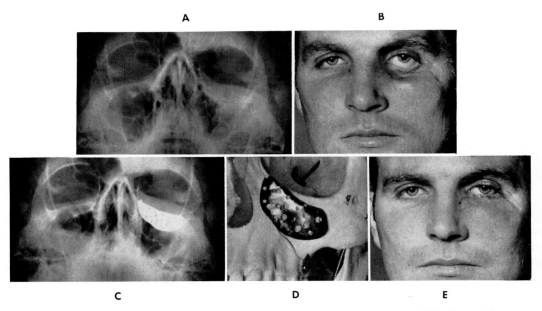

C   D   E

Fig. 22-17. Reconstruction of infraorbital margin utilizing tantalum implant and iliac bone chips. **A,** Preoperative roentgenogram. **B,** Preoperative photograph. **C,** Postoperative roentgenogram. **D,** Contoured tantalum implant adapted to suitable skull. This was the plate used in **C. E,** Postoperative photograph. Note incision beginning at the lateral margin of the nose, carried beneath the margin of the eyelid and laterally along the previous scar to allow reflection of the flap without having the incision lie over the implant.

tantalum plate supported by autogenous iliac bone chips. Construction of such a tantalum plate is carried out as follows.

The bony contours of both orbits are palpated and marked on the skin with indelible pencil for transferring to the plaster model. Vertical and horizontal dimensions of the uninjured orbit are measured and recorded. The impression is made of the patient's face, using hydrocolloid material, and a cast is poured in plaster. From the actual measurements and x-ray films of the facial bones (taken at a 6-foot distance), a skull approximating the patient's dimensions is chosen. Undercuts are eliminated, and a plaster impression is made of that portion of the skull representing the corresponding orbit. The plaster negative is used as a template to restore the orbital margin on the facial cast. The malar portion of the defect is then filled out with Plastiline to correspond to the opposite cheek. From the restored facial cast a stone die and counterdie

are constructed, the die extending at least 1 inch beyond the periphery of the involved area in all directions. A tantalum plate, $1/_{100}$ inch thick, is perforated with a mechanical drill. The plate is outlined from a tin-foil pattern previously adapted to the defect. It is then swaged and adapted over the defect with a wooden mallet. Final adaption is obtained by swaging between the die and counterdie with a hand press.

Similar replacements may be made using preconstructed Vitallium implants; however, technically this may be somewhat more difficult, and adjustment at surgery is impossible.

Beder and co-workers[7,8] have performed extensive studies with titanium, a metal characterized by extreme lightness, a high degree of strength, resistance to corrosion, and low conductivity. These studies indicate that titanium implants are well tolerated by animal tissues. An additional potential advantage of titanium consists of the fact that it is radiolucent and, when buried in the area of facial bones, will allow satisfactory radiographic evaluation of surrounding and underlying tissues. Tantalum and Vitallium both have the disadvantage of being radiopaque, consequently interfering with postoperative x-ray studies.

Synthetic resins. For contour restoration the synthetic resins have probably found much wider usage than metals in recent years. Ingraham and associates[50] published an excellent review of the use of synthetic plastic materials in surgery. Of the synthetic resins only the thermoplastic products have been used in surgical procedures. A thermoplastic resin can be molded without chemical change, for example, by softening under heat and pressure and cooling after molding. Of these synthetic resins, methyl methacrylate, polyethylene, polyvinyl alcohol (Ivalon), and polytetrafluoroethylene (Teflon) have been used successfully. Ingraham, Alexander, and others caution against the use of synthetic resins containing plasticizers and other foreign irritants. They also point out that controlled experimental studies should be carried out before utilizing new plastic materials.

Freeman[33] has reported on 20 clinical cases, using Ivalon sponge for facial reconstruction. He reported four complications, two of which resulted in removal of the sponge. In one instance the sponge survived "a localized infectious process." Freeman noted that the remaining implants, without complications, maintained in a large measure the desired size, position, and fixation but were firmer than desired. He further noted that sufficient time had not elapsed to evaluate the effect of friction, trauma, late scar contracture, and carcinogenic stimulation.

Campbell[17] reports the use of polyethylene in a variety of defects of the facial bones over a period of 4 years with satisfactory results. It has not been necessary to remove any of the implants during this period.

In 1956 Quereau and Souder[86] reported on the use of polytetrafluoroethylene (Teflon) in restoring the floor of the orbit and maxillary contour. They refer to the experiments by LeVeen and Barberio,[60] corroborated by Calnan,[15] indicating that Teflon was the least irritating of the plastics to tissue. The material is white, the surface feels waxy, and the plastic can be whittled and shaped with a sharp knife like soft wood. It is the most chemically inert plastic ever developed. It is stable to temperatures up to 327° C and can be autoclaved. It has a relatively high tensile strength, is flexible, has a memory, and undergoes nearly complete recovery from a deforming load. Nothing will stick to Teflon with any appreciable strength, and water will not wet it.

Rubber silicones. At the present time a rubber silicone (Silastic) is enjoying a high degree of popularity and may prove to be one of the most useful materials yet developed for contour correction. It has several outstanding advantages in that it comes in several different forms and is readily contoured, it can be autoclaved, and it is apparently nonirritating.[73] Of particular interest is an injectable form, which at present is being used experimentally for elimination of wrinkle lines as well as correction of contour deformities (Fig. 22-18).[28,34]

• • •

Unquestionably the use of alloplastic materials must still be considered to be in an experimental stage. However, the eminent surgeon Sir Harold Gillies suggested that one of the plastic materials may eventually take the place of all nonautogenous grafts.[37]

Of particular interest is the current trend to intraoral insertion[54] of the alloplastic implants. Apparently, with improvement in sterile technique, surgical technique, and use of antibiotics, the margin of safety has increased remarkably as far as intraoral procedures are concerned.

Recently Proplast, a microporous implant material consisting of a composite of polytetrafluoroethylene (Teflon) and pyrolytic graphite, has been investigated, both as an

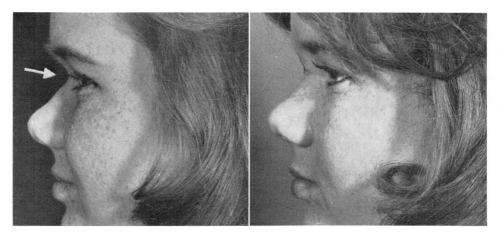

Fig. 22-18. Correction of glabellar defect by means of rubber silicone (Silastic) implant.

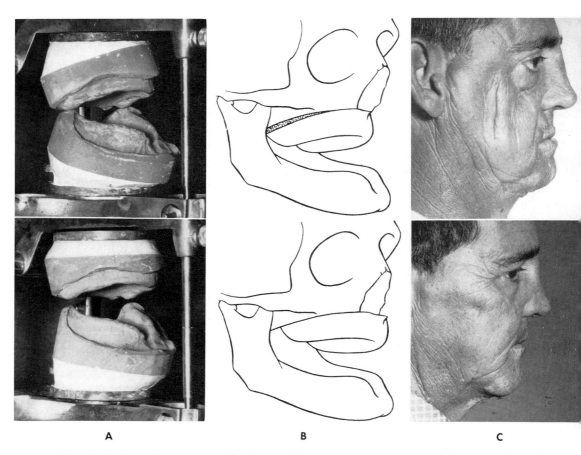

A B C

Fig. 22-19. Repositioning of maxilla 4 years after injury in auto accident. **A,** Preoperative and postoperative study models. **B,** Drawings showing repositioning procedure. **C,** Preoperative and postoperative photographs—patient wearing dentures in postoperative photograph; unable to wear dentures before surgery.

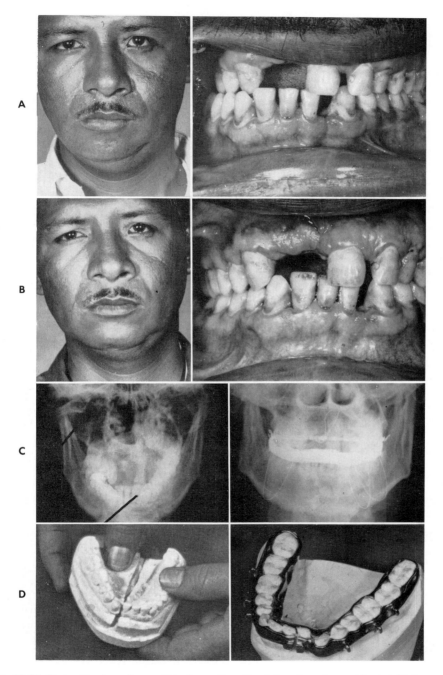

Fig. 22-20. Repositioning of mandible 6 months after injury in auto accident. Initial treatment with headcap and Kirschner wire in malposition. **A,** Preoperative photographs demonstrating crossbite. **B,** Postoperative photographs. **C,** Radiographs showing osteotomy sites and postoperative position. **D,** Correction of crossbite on model. **E,** Construction of splint in corrected position.

implant material and as a stabilizing interface for metal prostheses. Its outstanding qualities are that it allows the tissue cells to grow into its substance, allowing greater stabilization and that it is biocompatible.[46,47] As of this time, it has been used extensively in facial contour corrections, particularly chin implants.

Repositioning procedures

Fractures of the mandible may be corrected by open reduction as late as 6 or 8 weeks after injury. Fractures of middle facial bones usually heal in a shorter time. Even after bony union has taken place, it is possible in certain instances to perform osteotomies and reposition displaced fragments such as is done in treatment of developmental deformities.

Dingman and Natvig[26] have described those procedures that are particularly applicable to the maxillary and mandibular dentition. Impressions may be made and the models cut and repositioned for the fabrication of cast splints where indicated. If feasible, such procedures are preferred to contour corrections or correction by extraction of teeth and construction of prostheses. (See Figs. 22-19 and 22-20.)

RECONSTRUCTION OF THE MANDIBLE

Reconstruction of the mandible presents several problems not found in simple con-tour restorations, particularly in regard to adequate fixation. Mandibular continuity may be lost because of infection, trauma, or neoplastic diseases and may be restored with alloplastic materials or bone grafts.

Alloplasts

The use of alloplastic materials such as Vitallium, stainless steel, and methyl methacrylate has been largely restricted to restoration of continuity after excision of neoplastic disease, particularly with reference to immediate repair. Prostheses used for restoring the continuity of the mandible may be in the form of intramedullary bars or Kirschner wires or in the form of preformed prostheses constructed of methyl methacrylate or Vitallium.

Maintenance of the continuity of the mandible is desirable not only from a cosmetic viewpoint but also to preserve adequate swallowing, speech, and, in some instances, respiration. Losses of the posterior mandible are tolerated much better than losses from the symphysis area. Plates and intramedullary bars may serve the additional function of maintaining the fragments in position until bone grafts can be done, if immediate bone grafting is not indicated (Fig. 22-21).

Full-thickness mandibular segments may be replaced by intramedullary bars or wires, usually of stainless steel. These can be adapted easily to contour. They present

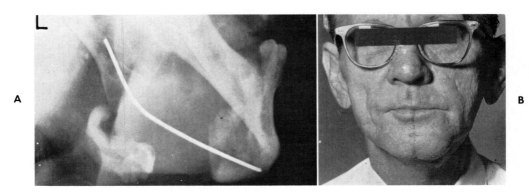

Fig. 22-21. Immediate reconstruction of combined resection of mandible and neck by use of intramedullary bar. **A,** Postoperative roentgenogram. **B,** Photograph showing cosmetic result.

the problem of telescoping, which may be solved by means of threaded pins with flanges or by making L-shaped bends in the pins to prevent further penetration of the marrow cavity. These take up little space and are easily covered with soft tissue. Stainless steel or Vitallium plates, either preconstructed to the individual case or selected from standard kits, may be used. The stainless steel plates are readily adapted to contour. These are secured by means of two screws at each fragment. The screws, ideally, should engage both cortices.

Vitallium replacements of various parts of the mandible may be preconstructed to the individual case, using various-sized mandibles as patterns and the patient's x-ray films and actual measurements for selection of proper size. Such replacements have been used on many occasions in the past, and indeed one author[36] has reported complete replacement of the mandible with such a Vitallium prosthesis functioning without difficulty at least 2 years after surgery. Dewey and Moore[23] have recently reported 13 successful cases wherein varying portions of the mandible were replaced with Vitallium prostheses.

Fig. 22-22 demonstrates an appliance that has remained in place and functioning for 10 years. Matalon[68] has modified Hahn's[41] adjustable Vitallium prosthesis for replacement of segments of mandible lost because of malignant disease. These are cast in ticonium rather than Vitallium, and their chief advantage is their use in more extensive resectioning involving the symphysis area (Fig. 22-23).

Similar replacements may be constructed of methyl methacrylate.[43] These should be

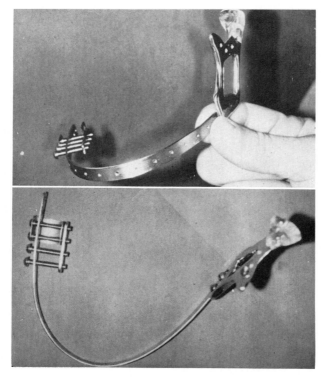

Fig. 22-22. Appliance constructed of acrylic and stainless steel with screw and bolt type of fixation that has been in place and functioning for 10 years. Constructed by Dr. Joe B. Drane and Dr. Duni Miglani, The University of Texas, Dental Branch.

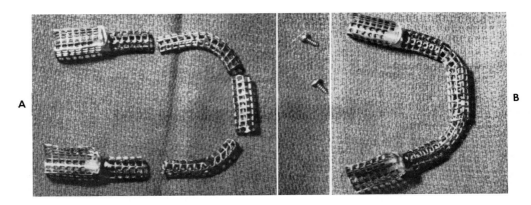

Fig. 22-23. Adjustable cast ticonium prosthesis (Hahn prosthesis modified by Matalon). **A,** Prosthesis dismantled. **B,** Prosthesis assembled.

somewhat smaller than the original mandibular segment to facilitate soft tissue closure. They should be perforated to allow better fixation and fluid drainage and to allow for muscle attachment. Usually direct fixation is all that is necessary, although fixation can be supplemented with other methods such as external pins. Fixation of these prostheses may be facilitated by use of perforated, wedge-shaped attachments at each end that are impacted into the marrow cavity of the mandible.

In all these problems greater difficulty is found in replacement of loss as a result of malignant disease than benign, and it is more difficult to replace the symphysis area than more posterior areas.

It has been my belief that the multiple stresses exerted by the mandible in function would tend to create loosening of most artificial implants, although Freeman[32] noted new bone growth over the screwheads in one implant that had to be removed because of exposure. I have used a Sherman plate as an immediate replacement after excision of a rather large adamantinoma of the body of the mandible. This stayed in place 15 months but had to be removed because of loosening of the screws at the anterior attachment.

Proplast[46,47] may provide a solution to some of these problems. Proplast may be permanently bonded to a metallic prosthesis such as Vitallium. Three cases have been reported in which ankylosis was corrected using ticonium implants with a Proplast interface, which allowed tissue cells and bone to become attached to the prosthesis. In one case in which bilateral ankylosis was corrected and the mandible advanced, the implant has been observed to function satisfactorily for a period of 2 years after surgery.[45] Proplast is also being investigated as a possible means of facilitating long-term fixation of blade vent implants and for alveolar ridge augmentation.[46,47]

Bone

In spite of the recent successes with alloplastic substances, it is desirable to replace lost tissue with tissue of a similar nature, and this is particularly true of the mandible. Hayward and Roffinella[42] have aptly described the peculiar problems associated with reconstruction of the mandible. They describe the mandible as a mobile functioning unit, influenced to considerable degree by the pull of the adjacent muscles and being shaped and constructed in such a manner as to complicate problems of fixation.

An excellent review of bone grafting in defects of the mandible was published by Ivy[50] in 1951. Bardenheuer[5] is credited with being the first to perform an autogenous bone graft of the mandible in 1891. This was in the form of a pedicle flap from the forehead, containing skin, periosteum, and bone. Sykoff[97] in 1900 is believed to have been the first to employ a free bone transplant to the lower jaw. In 1908 Payr[82] reported on the use of free transplants of the tibia and the rib. During World War I, Lindemann[61] and Klapp and Schoeder[58] began to use the iliac crest as the donor site. Klapp also reported on the use of the fourth metatarsal as a transplant to replace the lost ascending ramus and condyle. More recently, Dingman and Grabb[25] have also reported on the use of the metatarsal bone as a replacement for the condyle. Efforts to use this as a growth center graft have not been rewarding.

In spite of the lack of antibiotics and proper metallic fixation of appliances, Ivy[51] reported 76% successful, 7.7% partly successful and 13.5% failures of 103 bone grafting operations of the mandible during and immediately after World War I. Broken down into types of grafts, the figures were as follows: 31 cases of pedicle graft, 87%; 38 cases of osteoperiosteal, 71%; 7 cases of crest ilium, 71%; 17 cases of cortex or tibia, 65%; 6 cases of rib graft, 100%; 3 cases of sliding ramus graft, 2 successful; 1 case of heterologous (ox bone graft), 1 failure. Blocker and Stout,[10] reporting on a large collection of cases from all maxillofacial centers in the United States treating casualties of World War II, reported a total of 1,010 mandibular grafts as follows: 90.7% successful primarily, with an increase to 97% if regrafts are included. Broken down as to types of grafts, they were as follows: 836 from the ilium, 151 from the rib, and 23 from the tibia.

Indications for bone grafting of the mandible. Bone grafts are indicated in cases of nonunion of fractures of the mandible in which freshening of the fractured ends would result in foreshortening of the mandible. Bone grafts may be indicated in cases of extreme atrophy of the mandible. They may be used for filling out contour defects and for full-thickness loss of mandibular segments resulting from infection, trauma, or excision of neoplastic disease.

Watson-Jones[103] has pointed out that variations are possible in healing time of a fracture and that delayed union does not necessarily mean nonunion. Prolonged and proper immobilization may result in union. In the case of the mandible, because of the absence of weight bearing, osseous union may eventually occur even without immobilization if the patient is maintained on a controlled diet.

Types, forms, and techniques of bone grafting of the mandible. All three source types of bone grafts have been used: autogenous, homogenous, and heterogenous. Autogenous bone has been used most widely and is the graft of choice. Preserved homogenous bone has been used both as a block replacement and as chips.

Considerable use has been made of homogeneous bone grafts in repair of nonunion for fractures in which defects are small. Here they seem to exert an osteogenetic effect of definite value. Although full-thickness replacements of mandibular defects with homogenous bone have been reported by Converse and Stuteville, its use in such instances appears to be decidedly inferior to autogenous bone.

Grafts may be used in the following forms: (1) block from tibia, rib, or ilium; (2) osteoperiosteal graft, usually from tibia; (3) chip grafts from ilium; and (4) pedicle grafts from mandible. The osteoperiosteal graft contains all the elements necessary for osteogenesis; it is flexible and easily adjustable to size and shape of defect but is suitable only for small defects. The technique for removal and insertion is simpler than that of any of the other methods. The use of the pedicle graft should also be limited to small defects. Of the block grafts, use of the tibia has for all practicable purposes been discontinued. Most surgeons prefer the ilium; however, the rib still finds favor with some.

Joy[52] has reported on correction of non-union of a mandibular fracture by means of a sliding bone graft from the inferior border of the mandible. This is an efficient method for correction of a limited mandibular defect, avoiding a second operation necessary for obtaining a bone graft from a rib or ilium. Fig. 22-24 demonstrates nonunion of a fracture, which was subsequently treated, utilizing this same principle.[52]

The iliac block graft has several definite advantages. It is largely cancellous, it allows rapid transmission of tissue fluids and nutritive elements, and it provides innumerable pathways for ingrowth of growing cells. It may be readily shaped to meet contour and mortising requirements, and because of its cortical layer and bulk, it may serve to a great extent as its own fixation appliance. Iliac chips have been used extensively in facial reconstruction since Mowlem's[72] report. He was impressed by their resistance to infection and the rapidity with which vascularization and consolidation took place. In addition to contour defects, iliac chips have found considerable use in the management of nonunions and as an added osteogenetic factor in osteoto-

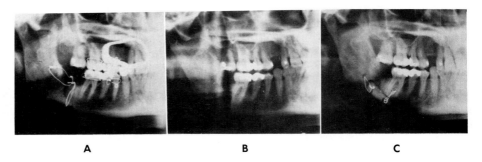

Fig. 22-24. A, Panorex demonstrating fracture in right molar area. **B,** Same patient with subsequent nonunion and flail mandible. **C,** Three months after sliding graft on inferior border of mandible, at which time clinical union had taken place.

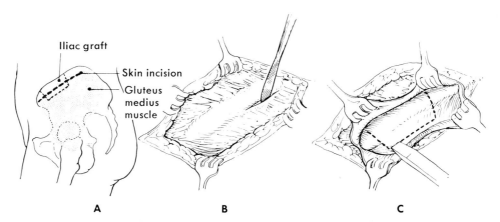

Fig. 22-25. Iliac graft. **A,** Line of incision. **B,** Stripping of muscle and periosteum. **C,** Use of osteotome for outline of graft to be obtained with osteotome.

mies. They are also used to a great extent in combination with larger block grafts for the purpose of filling in minor irregularities and adding to the osteogenetic stimulus. Mowlem's original report described such a technique involving the use of a large cancellous block medially and cancellous chips laterally, the block graft being used to prevent soft tissues from bulging through the mandibular defect and to protect the chips from movement transmitted from the floor of the mouth.

Excellent discussions of the approach to the ilium and the obtaining of the graft are given by Dick[24] and Abbott and associates.[1] The ilium is approached by a transverse skin incision made below the crest to prevent pressure irritation (Fig. 22-25). It is exposed after severing gluteal muscle attachments externally, the external oblique muscle above, and the iliacus medially. Full-thickness grafts may be used, or grafts may be limited to either the outer or the inner plate and medulla.

Chip grafts may be obtained with a gouge after creating a window in the outer cortex, thus leaving the inner cortex undisturbed. I have obtained circular plugs through the outer cortex with an Illif trephine attached to a Stryker saw for repairing nonunions (Fig. 22-26). A circular plug is removed with a No. 7 trephine at the fracture site. The graft is taken with a No. 8 trephine. The outer diameter of the No. 7 trephine

matches the inner diameter of the No. 8. The trephine graft is then wedged into the nonunion defect, providing a precise fit.

Complications after removal of iliac grafts are infrequent, the most common being hematoma formation, which can be prevented to a great extent by careful hemostasis at the time of surgery and the use of fibrin foam or bone wax. However, postoperative pain may be more severe at the iliac site than at the graft site.

Replacement of the angle and entire ascending ramus and placement of large defects of the midline present unusual problems in mandibular bone grafting. Two methods have been used for restoring the angle and ascending ramus. A rib with a portion of its adjacent cartilage may be used, the cartilaginous portion of the graft being placed in the glenoid fossa. The contralateral anterior superior spine and iliac crest may be adapted well to the replacement of this portion of the mandible. However, the chances for resorption in such an extensive graft, attached at one end only, are considerable. There may be some advantage in preserving the condylar fragment when possible to facilitate function and regeneration. In such cases the coronoid process should always be removed because of the harmful muscle pull. In most cases in which a large graft must be prepared, it is advisable to construct a stent of polymethyl methacrylate that will aid in developing the

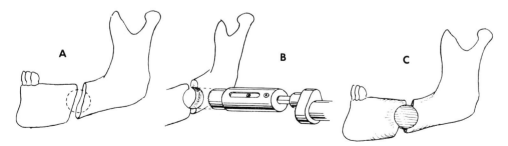

Fig. 22-26. Use of Illif trephine in bone grafting. **A,** Preoperative condition. Site of plug to be removed is diagrammed. **B,** Plug removed from nonunion site with No. 7 trephine. **C,** Graft taken from ilium with No. 8 trephine and inserted into defect. Outer diameter of No. 7 trephine matches inner diameter of No. 8, allowing an accurate fit of graft.

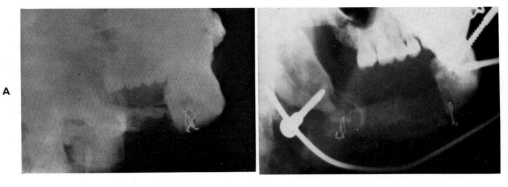

Fig. 22-27. Bone graft. **A,** Fracture of rib graft after atrophy. **B,** Same case, with graft replaced with iliac block, showing fixation by direct wiring and external pins. Graft is intact 11 years after insertion.

graft bed and in obtaining a graft of the proper shape and size.

Description of the surgical approach to the restoration of the angle and ascending ramus is difficult to find in the literature. The object is to develop a plane between the masseter and the medial pterygoid muscle. Kazanjian and Converse[55] utilize three nerves as landmarks in developing this plane. These are the lingual, the inferior alveolar, and the mylohyoid nerves. Because of previous difficulties encountered, Rehrmann[89] made a detailed study of the anatomy of this area and described a method for preparing this area with minimum danger to nerves and vessels. He made use of the stylohyoid muscle and process as landmarks in reaching the glenoid fossa.

The symphysis area may be restored with a split-rib graft or a shaped iliac block. It may be restored by a skewer graft as described by Gillies and Millard[37] consisting of blocks of iliac crest impaled on a Kirschner wire and molded to shape.

Abbott and co-workers,[1] in discussing the merits of cortical and cancellous bone, mentioned the possibility of late fracture in cortical grafts replacing large gaps. Ghormley, in discussing Abbott's paper, stated that cortical grafts, after reaching a stage where they have good circulation, go through a stage of atrophy, during which period some of them may fracture. I have had such an experience with a rib graft (Fig. 22-27). This necessitated replacement with an iliac graft. Because of this problem in large gaps, Abbott has suggested a two-stage procedure wherein cancellous grafts are used initially to establish vascularization, followed by cortical grafts that could then be vascularized throughout their entire length. The necessity for doing this in two stages is not convincing, particularly if one should use split ribs, enclosing cancellous chips for the mandible. The cancellous block, because of its adequate strength, greater bulk, and opportunities for self-splinting, seems more desirable.

Adequate soft tissue covering is of great importance in bone grafting, and, if necessary, grafting should be postponed until soft tissues may be brought in from a distance. Many surgeons advise postponing the graft if the oral cavity is entered during the procedure. In view of the excellent results with iliac crest, the work of Converse on intraoral bone grafts, and the present-day trend toward immediate bone grafting, it would seem that contamination from compounding into the oral cavity should not be cause for postponing the procedure. It may be well to remove teeth near the ends of man-

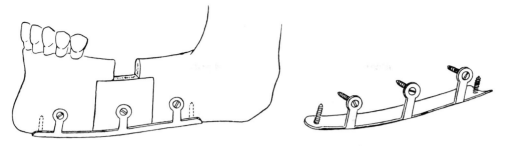

Fig. 22-28. Type of stainless steel splint described by Smith and Robinson.[93]

dibular fragments prior to grafting to avoid cutting through tooth roots when freshening the mandibular stumps.

In spite of the fact that many reports of grafting in the presence of infection have been published, most present-day surgeons believe that it is advisable to eliminate all infection and allow a waiting period of from 2 to 6 months. At the present time, with the use of cancellous iliac bone and antibiotics, it is thought that defects resulting from gunshot wounds and other trauma may be grafted soon after injury, provided adequate soft tissue covering is present. Such early repair facilitates the grafting procedure because of minimal scarring and distortion of fragments. The mandibular stumps should be cut back to an area of good vascularity. Graft and stump should be corticated in areas of contact. The wider the area of contact, the better the chance of "take." Avascular scar tissue should be removed from the muscle bed also.

Fixation. Probably, the most important factor in bone grafting, next to the use of the proper type of graft, is fixation. In mandibular grafts in which teeth are present, intermaxillary fixation is the method of choice. The problems of fixation arise in relation to edentulous fragments and to proximal fragments posterior to the last tooth.

Watson-Jones[103] has pointed out that immobilization serves two significant purposes: (1) control of position of the fragments and (2) protection of growing cells,

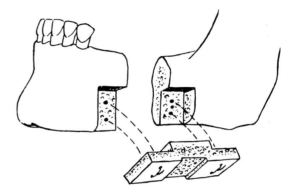

Fig. 22-29. Mortising of iliac block and partial decortication to facilitate revascularization. Fixation by direct wiring.

preventing delayed union and nonunion. Fixation may be obtained by tantalum trays; by stainless steel, tantalum, or Vitallium plates; by external pin fixation; by intramedullary pins; or by a modified gunning splint–type appliance (Fig. 22-28). In addition, direct wiring with 24-gauge stainless steel is advisable and may in itself provide sufficient fixation. A mattress suture should be used. Decortication and mortising at the graft junction will enhance the opportunities for primary union. Mortising may be accomplished by holding the graft in a bone forceps or vise and cutting with a Stryker saw. Decorticating a portion of the body of the graft will aid in revascularization, although some cortex should be maintained for strength (Fig. 22-29).

All these methods have been used with

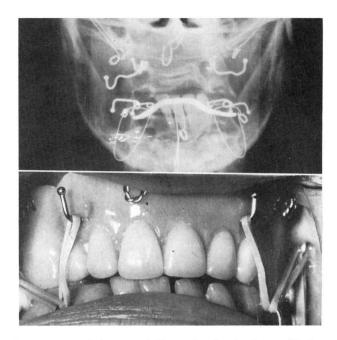

Fig. 22-30. Roentgenogram and photograph illustrating fixation by modified two-piece Gunning splint in which the upper piece is wired directly to the zygomaticomaxillary pillar and the lower is fixed by means of circumferential wires.

success, and it should be emphasized that perhaps more important than method is the exercise of sufficient care in technique. In using the Gunning splint principle, I prefer the two-piece modification shown in Fig. 22-30. Walden and Bromberg[102] have avoided pressure necrosis with this method by constructing the splint larger in all dimensions over the graft area to allow for the pressure of postoperative edema. The upper splint may be wired directly to the alveolar ridge, the piriform fossa, the zygomaticomaxillary pillar, or the infraorbital margin. The lower splint is fixed by means of circumferential wires, and intermaxillary fixation is instituted by means of rubber traction or wires.

The criticism of bone plates is that they hold fragments apart and prevent osteogenesis by compression. This does not seem to be valid from the many reports of successful results. It would seem advisable to use screws that engage both cortical plates.

Branemark and co-workers recently reported 31 cases of mandibular reconstruction utilizing autogenous bone supported by specially constructed titanium splints.[12] My personal preference has been for direct wiring of the graft with fixation augmented by tantalum trays or direct wiring. Fig. 22-31 shows a graft supported by a tantalum tray, inserted when the patient was 5 years old, with subsequent normal and symmetrical development of the mandible over a 7-year period. Intermaxillary fixation, when used, should be maintained for a period of from 8 to 12 weeks. Antibiotics should be used routinely and the patient's general health and nutrition maintained at an optimum level.

Boyne[11,88] advocates use of particulate grafts of marrow and cancellous bone, containing a metal implant mesh device lined with a microporous filter material for bone graft reconstruction of large defects of the mandible.

External pin fixation and intramedullary

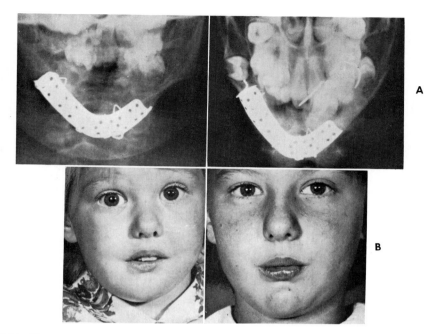

Fig. 22-31. Through-and-through deformity of mandible resulting from excision of atypical fibrous dysplasia corrected by autogenous rib graft fixed with tantalum tray at age 5 years. **A,** Radiographs of patient at 5 and 12 years of age, demonstrating symmetrical facial development over 7-year period. **B,** Photographs of patient at 5 and 12 years of age.

pins may serve both to retain fragments in position at the time of original loss of mandibular structure as well as for immobilization when the graft is performed. Henny[44] has obtained excellent results in such cases with a threaded Steinmann pin containing washers and bolts for additional stabilization.

In recent years there has been a renewed interest in the biphase external pin technique developed by Morris in 1949 and more recently elaborated on by Fleming and Morris.[31] The biphase splint is demonstrated in Fig. 22-32.

• • •

The insertion of alloplastic implants, bone grafting, and other surgical procedures on the mandible and maxilla are being increasingly performed through the oral cavity and oral mucosa rather than the extraoral route with remarkable success for reasons already cited.

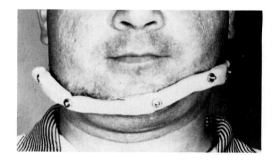

Fig. 22-32. Morris biphase splint.

The factors most commonly associated with graft failure seem to be mobility, infection, and inadequate soft tissue coverage.

Alveolar ridge

Restoration of the edentulous alveolar ridge may be the area of greatest promise for the future as far as reconstruction with autogenous bone is concerned. It is true

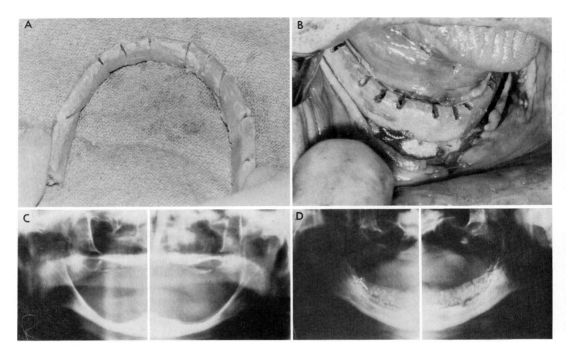

Fig. 22-33. Reconstruction of alveolar ridge with autogenous bone graft (rib). **A,** Rib grooved and contoured. **B,** Rib strut fixed in position. **C,** Preoperative radiographs. **D,** Postoperative radiographs. (Courtesy Dr. William S. Poinsett.)

that such efforts in the past have frequently proved unrewarding, but some authors are reporting successes.

Genest[36] has reported several successful cases using split autogenous ribs and limiting reconstruction to the posterior portion of the alveolar ridge. Obwegeser[75] reports good results utilizing an extensive incision over the alveolar crest, with incision of the periosteum and detachment of the muscles to allow extensive relaxation and advancements of the mucosal flaps. He has used both iliac crest and rib with success. The technique currently preferred has been described by Baker and Connole[4] in a recent issue of *The Journal of Oral Surgery*. An example of this technique is seen in Fig. 22-33.

IMMEDIATE REPAIR OF COMPOUND DEFECTS RESULTING FROM CANCER SURGERY

The trend toward immediate repair of extensive wounds created by removal of malignant tissue, noted on the occasion of the initial publication of this text, not only is surviving but is becoming even more popular, as evidenced by recent articles.* These procedures involve methods previously discussed, including use of free bone grafts, skin grafts, utilization of adjacent pedicle flaps in skin, mucosa, or muscle, and stabilization of mandibular fragments with metallic pins. Such reconstruction done at the time of resection allows optimum exposure as well as prevents contraction of tissues and degeneration of morale. Whether such a philosophy may compromise adequate surgery or hide recurrent disease remains somewhat controversial. Stark[95] has recently reviewed current philosophy with regard to this problem.

---

*See references 3, 19, 35, 48, 62, and 70.

REFERENCES

1. Abbott, L. C., Schottstaedt, E. R., Saunders, J. B. deC. M., and Bost, F. C.: The evaluation of

cortical and cancellous bone as grafting material, J. Bone Joint Surg. 29:381, 1947.

2. Adams, W. M., Adams. L. H., and Jerome, A. P.: Iliac bone graft for correction of maxillary retrusion in cases of cleft palate, J. Int. Coll. Surg. 27:384, sect. 1, 1957.

3. Bakamjian, V., and Littlewood, M.: Cervical skin flaps for intraoral and pharyngeal repair following cancer surgery, Br. J. Plast. Surg. 17:191, 1964.

4. Baker, R. D., and Connole, P. W.: Preprosthetic augmentation grafting—autogenous bone, J. Oral Surg. 35:541, 1977.

5. Bardenheuer: Ver. Dtsch. Ges. Chir. 1:69, 1892.

6. Bauer: Ueber Knochentransplantation, Zbl. Chir. 37:(Beilage 20-21), 1910.

7. Beder, O. E., and Eade, G.: An investigation of tissue tolerance to titanium metal implants in dogs, Surgery 39:470, 1956.

8. Beder, O. E., Eade, G., Stevenson, J. K., Jones, T. W., Ploger, W. J., and Condon, R. E.: Titanium metal in alloplasty, J. Dent. Res. 45:1221, 1966.

9. Bell, W. H.: Personal communication, 1958.

10. Blocker, T. G., and Stout, R. A.: Mandibular reconstruction, World War II, Plast. Reconstr. Surg. 4:153, 1949.

11. Boyne, P. J.: Use of marrow-cancellous osseus grafts in the regeneration of mandibular bone, Proceedings of the Fourth International Congress of Oral Surgery, Amsterdam, 1971.

12. Branemark, P.-I., Lindstrom, J., Hallen, O., Brine, U., Jeppson, P.-H., and Ohman, A.: Reconstruction of the defective mandible, Scand. J. Plast. Reconstr. Surg. 9:116, 1975.

13. Brown, J. B., Fryer, M. P., and Ohlwiler, D. A.: Study and use of synthetic materials such as silicone and Teflon as subcutaneous prosthesis, Plast. Reconstr. Surg. 26:263, 1960.

14. Bush, L. F.: The use of homogenous bone grafts. A preliminary report on the bone bank, J. Bone Joint Surg. 29:620, 1947.

15. Calnan, J.: The use of inert plastic material in reconstructive surgery, Br. J. Plast. Surg. 16:1, 1963.

16. Campbell, H. H.: Reconstruction of left maxilla, Plast. Reconstr. Surg. 3:66, 1948.

17. Campbell, H. H.: Surgery of lesions of the upper face, Am. J. Surg. 87:676, 1954.

18. Chase, S. W., and Herndon, C. H.: The fate of autogenous and homogenous bone grafts, J. Bone Joint Surg. 37-A:809, 1955.

19. Coleman, C. C.: Surgical treatment of extensive cancers of the mouth and pharynx, Ann. Surg. 161:634, 1965.

20. Conley, J. J.: The use of Vitallium prostheses and implants in the reconstruction of the mandibular arch, Plast. Reconstr. Surg. 8:150, 1951.

21. Converse, J. M., and Campbell, R. M.: Bone grafts in surgery of the face, Surg. Clin. North Am. 34:375, 1954.

22. Conway, H., and Goulian, D.: Experiences with an injectable Silastic RTV as a subcutaneous prosthetic material, a preliminary report, Plast. Reconstr. Surg. 32:294, 1963.

23. Dewey, A. R., and Moore, J. W.: Mandibular repair after radical resection, J. Oral Surg. 20:34, 1962.

24. Dick, I. L.: Iliac-bone transplantation. Preliminary observations, J. Bone Joint Surg. 28:1, 1946.

25. Dingman, R. O., and Grabb, W. C.: Reconstruction of both mandibular condyles with metatarsal bone grafts, Plast. Reconstr. Surg. 34:441, 1964.

26. Dingman, R. O., and Natvig, P.: Repair of residual deformities. In Surgery of facial fractures, Philadelphia, 1964, W. B. Saunders Co.

27. Edgerton, M. T., and Zovickian, A.: Reconstruction of major defects of the palate, Plast. Reconstr. Surg. 17:105, 1956.

28. Farrior, F. T.: Synthetics in head and neck surgery, Arch Ophthalmol. 84:82, 1966.

29. Fischer, W. B., and Clayton, I.: Surgical bone grafting with cultured calf bone, Q. Bull. Northwestern Univ. M. School 29:346, 1955.

30. Flanigin, W. S.: Free composite grafts from lower to upper lip, Plast. Reconstr. Surg. 17:376, 1956.

31. Fleming, I. D., and Morris, J. H.: Use of acrylic external splint after mandibular resection, Am. J. Surg. 118:708, November, 1969.

32. Freeman, B. S.: The use of Vitallium plates to maintain function following resection of the mandible, Plast. Reconstr. Surg. 3:73, 1948.

33. Freeman, B. S.: Complications following subcutaneous insertion of plastic sponge, Plast. Reconstr. Surg. 15:149, 1955.

34. Freeman, B. S., Bigelow, E. L., and Braley, S. A.: Experiments with injectable plastic, Am. J. Surg. 112:534, 1966.

35. Gaisford, J. C.: Reconstruction of head and neck deformities, Surg. Clin. North Am. 47:295, 1967.

36. Genest, A.: Vitallium jaw replacement, Am. J. Surg. 92:904, 1956.

37. Gillies, H., and Millard, D. R., Jr.: The principles and art of plastic surgery, vol. 2, Boston, 1957, Little, Brown & Co.

38. Glanz, S.: Skin grafting in reconstructive surgery, Texas J. Med. 52:242, 1956.

39. Gonzales-Ulloa, M., Stevens, E., and Noble, G.: Preliminary report of subcutaneous perfusion of Polysiloxane to improve regional contour, read before the meeting of the American Association of Plastic Surgeons, Chicago, May, 1964.

40. Guillemient, M., Stagnara, P., and Dubost-Perret, T.: Preparation and use of heterogenous bone grafts, J. Bone Joint Surg. 35-B:561, 1953.

41. Hahn, G. W.: Vitallium mesh mandibular prosthesis, J. Prosthet. Dent. 14:777, 1964.

42. Hayward, J. R., and Roffinella, J. P.: Iliac

autoplasty for repair of mandibular defects, J. Oral Surg. **13**:44, 1955.

43. Healy, M. J., Jr., Sudbay, J. L., Niebel, H. H., Hoffman, B. M., and Duval, M. K.: The use of acrylic implants in one stage reconstruction of the mandible, Surg. Gynecol. Obstet. **98**:395, 1954.
44. Henny, F. A.: Personal communication, 1957.
45. Hinds, E. C., Homsy, C. A., and Kent, J. N.: Use of a biocompatible interface for combining tissues and prostheses in oral surgery, Proceedings of the Fourth International Congress of Oral Surgery, Amsterdam, 1971.
46. Homsy, C. A.: Rebuild with Proplast and tissue has a home, Medical World News, Sept. 29, 1972, p. 20.
47. Homsy, C. A., Kent, J. N., and Hinds, E. C.: Materials for oral implantology–biological and functional criteria, J. Am. Dent. Assoc. **86**:817, 1973.
48. Hoopes, J. E., and Edgerton, M. T.: Immediate forehead flap repair in resection for oropharyngeal cancer, Am. J. Surg. **112**:527, 1966.
49. Inclan, A.: The use of preserved bone graft in orthopaedic surgery, J. Bone Joint Surg. **24**:81, 1942.
50. Ingraham, F. D., Alexander, E., Jr., and Matson, D. D.: Synthetic plastic materials in surgery, N. Engl. J.Med. **236**:362, 402, 1947.
51. Ivy, R. H.: Bone grafting for restoration of defects of the mandible, Plast. Reconstr. Surg. **7**: 333, 1951.
52. Joy, E. D., Jr.: Nonunion of a mandibular fracture treated by sliding bone graft: report of case, J. Oral Surg. **25**:356, July, 1967.
53. Judet, J., Judet, R., and Arviset, A.: Banque d'os et heterogreffe, Presse Med. **57**:1007, 1949.
54. Junghans, J. A.: Profile reconstruction with Silastic chin implants, Am. J. Orthod. **53**:217, 1967.
55. Kazanjian, V. H., and Converse, J. M.: The surgical treatment of facial injuries, Baltimore, 1949, The Williams & Wilkins Co.
56. Kazanjian, V. H., and Roopernian, A.: The treatment of lip deformities resulting from electric burns, Am. J. Surg. **88**:884, 1954.
57. Kiehn, C. L., and Grino, A.: Iliac bone grafts replacing tantalum plates for gunshot wounds of skull, Am. J. Surg. **85**:395, 1953.
58. Klapp, R., and Schroeder, H.: Die Unterkieferschussbrüche, Berlin, 1917, Hermann Muesser.
59. Kreuz, F. P., Hyatt, G. W., Turner, T. C., and Bassett, A. L.: The preservation and clinical use of freeze-dried bone, J. Bone Joint Surg. **33-A**: 836, 1951.
60. LeVeen, H. H., and Barberio, J. R.: Tissue reaction to plastic used in surgery with special reference to Teflon, Ann. Surg. **129**:74, 1941.
61. Lindemann, A.: Ueber die Beseitigung der traumatischen Defekta der Gesichtsknochen. In Behandlung der Kieferschussverletzungen, vol. 4, Wiesbaden, 1916, p. 6.
62. Longacre, J. J., deStefano, G. A., Holmstead, K., Leichliter, J. W., and Jolly, P.: The immediate versus the late reconstruction in cancer surgery, Plast. Reconstr. Surg. **28**:549, 1961.
63. Longacre, J. J., and Gilby, R. F.: The problem of reconstruction of extensive severely scarred palatal defects in edentulous patients, Plast. Reconstr. Surg. **14**:357, 1954.
64. Losee, F. L., and Hurley, L. A.: Bone treated with ethylenediamine as a successful foundation material in cross-species bone grafts, Nature (London) **177**:1032, 1956.
65. Losee, F. L., and Hurley, L. A.: Successful cross-species bone grafting accomplished by removal of the donor organic matrix, Naval Medical Research Institute Project NM 004 006.09.01, p. 911, Dec. 5, 1956.
66. Macewen, W.: Observations concerning transplantation of bone, illustrated by a case of inter-human osseous transplantation, whereby over two-thirds of the shaft of a humerus was restored, Proc. R. Soc. **32**:232, 1881.
67. Martin, H. E.: Cheiloplasty for advanced carcinoma of the lip, Surg. Gynecol. Obstet. **14**:914, 1932.
68. Matalon, V.: Personal communication, June, 1967.
69. Millard, D. R.: Chin implants, Plast. Reconstr. Surg. **13**:70, 1954.
70. Millard, D. R., Jr.: A new approach to immediate mandibular repair, Ann. Surg. **160**:306, 1964.
71. Mohnac, A. M.: Surgical correction of maxillomandibular deformities, J. Oral Surg. **23**:393, 1965.
72. Mowlem, A. R.: Cancellous chip bone-grafts, report on 75 cases, Lancet **2**:746, 1944.
73. Mullison, E. G.: Silicones in head and neck surgery, Arch. Otolaryngol. **84**:91, 1966.
74. Obwegeser, H.: Surgical preparation of the maxilla for prosthesis, J. Oral Surg. **22**:127, 1964.
75. Obwegeser, H.: Personal communication, June, 1966.
76. Obwegeser, H.: Simultaneous resection and reconstruction of parts of the mandible via the intraoral route in patients with and without gross infections, Oral Surg. **21**:693, 1966.
77. Ollier, L.: Recherches experimentales sur les greffes osseuses, J. de Physiol. de l'Homme et des Animaux **3**:88, 1860.
78. Ollier, L.: Traite experimental et clinique de la regeneration des os et de la production artificielle du tissu osseux, Paris, 1867, Victor Masson et Fils.
79. Padgett, E. C., and Stephenson, Kathryn L.: Plastic and reconstructive surgery, Springfield, Ill., 1948, Charles C Thomas, Publisher.
80. Paletta, F. X.: Early and later repair of facial

defects following treatment of malignancy, Plast. Reconstr. Surg. **13**:95, 1954.

81. Parkes, M. L.: Chin implants with a newer plastic compound, Arch. Otolaryngol. **75**:429, 1962.

82. Payr, E.: Ueber osteoplastischen Ersatz nach Kieferresektion (Kieferdefekten) durch Rippenstücke mittelst gestielter Brustwandlappen oder freier Transplantation, Zbl. Chir. **35**:1065, 1908.

83. Peer, L. A.: Transplantation of tissues, vol. 1, Baltimore, 1955, The Williams & Wilkins Co.

84. Peer, L. A.: The neglected "free fat graft," its behavior and clinical use, Am. J. Surg. **92**:40, 1956.

85. Pick, J. F.: Surgery of repair, vol. 1, Philadelphia, 1949, J. B. Lippincott Co.

86. Quereau, J. V. D., and Souder, B. F.: Teflon implant to elevate the eye in depressed fracture of the orbit, Arch. Ophthalmol. **55**:685, 1956.

87. Ragnell, A.: A simple method of reconstruction in some cases of dish-face deformity, Plast. Reconstr. Surg. **10**:227, 1949.

88. Rappaport, I., Boyne, P. V., and Nethery, J.: The particulate graft in tumor surgery, Am. J. Surg. **122**:748, 1971.

89. Rehrmann, A.: Autoplastic repair of the ramus mandibulae, avoiding a lesion of the facial nerve and of large blood vessels, Plast. Reconstr. Surg. **17**:452, 1956.

90. Reynolds, F. C., Oliver, D. R., and Ramsey, R.: Clinical evaluation of the merthiolate bone bank and homogenous bone grafts, J. Bone Joint Surg. **33-A**:873, 1951.

91. Schneider, P. J.: V-excision with Z-closure for carcinoma of the lower lip, Plast. Reconstr. Surg. **18**:208, 1956.

92. Sherman, P.: The open method of skin grafting, Am. J. Surg. **94**:869, 1957.

93. Smith, A. E., and Robinson, M.: Individually constructed stainless steel bone onlay splint for immobilization of proximal fragment in fractures of the angle of the mandible, J. Oral Surg. **12**:170, 1954.

94. Smith, F.: Plastic and reconstructive surgery, a manual of management, Philadelphia, 1950, W. B. Saunders Co.

95. Stark, R. B.: Oral cancer: reconstruction and rehabilitation, CA **22**:303, 1972.

96. Stuteville, O. H.: A new concept of treatment of osteomyelitis of the mandible, J. Oral Surg. **8**:301, 1950.

97. Sykoff, W.: Zur Frage der Knochenplastik am Unterkiefer, Zbl. Chir. **35**:881, 1900.

98. Tucker, E. J.: The preservation of living bone in plasma, Surg. Gynecol. Obstet. **96**:739, 1953.

99. Tuffier, T.: Des greffes de cartilage et d'os humain dans les resections articularies, Bull. Mem. Soc. Chir. Paris **37**:278, 1911.

100. Venable, C. S., and Stuck, W. G.: Three years' experience with vitallium in bone surgery, Am. Surg. **114**:309, 1941.

101. Venable, C. S., and Stuck, W. G.: General considerations of metals for buried appliances in surgery, Int. Abstr. Surg. **76**:297, 1943.

102. Walden, R. H., and Bromberg, B. S.: Recent advances in therapy in maxillofacial bony injuries in over 1,000 cases, Am. J. Surg. **93**:508, 1957.

103. Watson-Jones, R.: Fractures and joint injuries, ed. 4, vol. 1, Baltimore, 1955, The Williams & Wilkins Co.

104. Webster, J. P.: Crescentic peri-alar cheek excision for upper lip flap advancement with a short history of upper lip repair, Plast. Reconstr. Surg. **16**:434, 1955.

105. Wilson, P. D.: Experience with a bone bank, Ann. Surg. **126**:932, 1947.

CHAPTER 23

Developmental deformities of the jaws

Jack B. Caldwell
Roy C. Gerhard

Developmental deformities of the jaws are those deformities that present malocclusion of the teeth, malrelation of the jaws, and associated facial disfigurement. They are thought of most often as congenital in origin, but they may also result from other causes.

The surgical correction of these deformities is one of the most challenging and intriguing aspects of oral surgery. Helping persons so afflicted is also one of the most gratifying services that it is possible to render.

Individuals with developmental deformities of the jaws are invariably self-conscious of their abnormal facies and usually have reflected personality problems. Their primary concern is their appearance. However, when correction of these deformities is contemplated, more than esthetic improvement must be considered. Correction of functional deficiencies is even more important, and this factor must be fully considered in treatment planning. In almost every instance personality inadequacies are eliminated automatically after corrective surgery.

For the sake of simplicity, deformities of the jaws will be discussed in their basic forms, namely, prognathism, micrognathia, and apertognathia. It must be understood that many variations do occur and that the primary deformity may be in the maxilla as well as in the mandible, or it may be coexistent in both jaws. A complete knowledge of surgical procedures applicable to the basic deformities should enable the oral surgeon to deal properly with all deformities.

Definition of terms applied to developmental deformities of the jaws is necessary for an understanding of the problem. *Prognathism* is defined as an abnormal projection forward of one or both jaws, whereas *micrognathia* is defined as a smallness of the jaws, especially the underjaw. *Apertognathia,* or open bite, is a condition in which space remains between the maxillary and the mandibular teeth when some teeth are in contact at one or more points. Various other malformations may occur as well, but they are usually variants of these three basic forms. Asymmetries are an example and will be discussed later in the chapter. Hypertrophies and agenesis will also be discussed.

One cannot be fully appreciative of the age in which we live today until one takes the time to read of the experiences of earlier surgeons who dealt with facial deformities. The details of case histories reported by pioneers in this field are truly fascinating to study. It is fortunate, indeed, that men such as Hullihen and Blair had the basic knowledge, imagination, and courage to attempt the surgery that they describe so vividly. Many of the original contributions in this field of corrective surgery are the basis for standard operations today. Refinements in surgical technique, better understanding of physiology and anatomy, and the addition of modern methods of anesthesia and drug therapy have eliminated or minimized the hazards that were so great a few short years ago.

Hullihen[50] can be credited with the first operation for correction of malrelation of the jaws. The patient he described in 1849 was 20 years of age and had been severely burned on the neck and lower part of the face 15 years earlier. The "cicatrix produced a deformity of the most dreadful character. Her head was drawn forward and downward with the chin confined to within an inch of the sternum. The underjaw was bowed slightly downward and elongated, particularly its upper portion, which made it project about one inch and three-eighths beyond the upper jaw."[50] Hullihen studied his patient's problem and resolved it surgically by "sawing out" a V-shaped segment of bone from the upper "elongated portion three-fourths of the way through the jaw" and then completing the section forward horizontally, thus allowing "that portion of the jaw and teeth which before projected and inclined outward" to return to its "proper and original place."

Probably the most important early contributions came from Blair,[14] who was a great philosopher and author as well as a great surgeon. In 1907 Blair wrote: "While surgeons for centuries have expended early talent and energy upon the correction of deformities of almost all kinds, from clubfoot to malrelation of the teeth, both for cosmetic and utilitarian reasons, yet little study or work seems to have been done to alleviate those distressing conditions that arise from excessive asymmetry of the dental arches. Where this deformity was too great to be corrected by orthodontic appliances, the victims have, so far as I can determine, with the exception of a few isolated cases, been compelled to go through life without relief."[14] Furthermore, Blair recognized and classified facial deformities much in accordance with present-day concepts. He stated that ". . . the malrelation consisted either in a disproportionate growth in the length of the body of the lower jaw, in the lack of development of the upper jaw, in a lack of development of the lower jaw, [or] in a bending downward of the lower jaw at or in front of the angle . . . ."[14]

Typical of his optimism was the statement "We have to deal with an upper solid jaw and a lower one that is a hoop of bone *capable of almost any kind of adjustment,* and it is upon the latter that our efforts must be expended."[14] He described ostectomies and osteotomies for correction of prognathism, open bite deformities, and micrognathia. He recognized "three distinct problems: (1) the cutting of the bone, (2) the placing of the jaw in its new position, and (3) holding it there." This classic paper was written 60 years ago but should be prescribed for reading and study today by anyone who contemplates performing surgery for correction of these deformities.

Articles and single case histories describing various operations for correction of these deformities appeared in the literature intermittently thereafter. Among them were many outstanding contributions. The difficulties were many until more recent years, and probably failures went unreported, whereas successful cases were well documented. Much of the difficulty encountered earlier was eliminated with the advent of antibiotics and the increased publicizing of cases and techniques. Refinement of certain techniques has led to their acceptance as standard procedure, the operative details of which will be discussed later.

In Europe the awakening to the possibilities for surgical correction of facial deformities began at the turn of the century. Bruhn[16] of the West German Maxillo-Facial Clinic in Dusseldorf reported in 1927 on the increasing interest in developing new techniques, which was stimulated by the treatment of diseases and wounds of the jaws in Germany during World War I. He stated: "Gradually a new sphere of medical and dental science arose, and soon a new system became possible. Thus a new way was found to remove the deformation of the lower jaw, especially the so-called macrognathy and micrognathy."[16] Unfortunately, this was one of the few significant exchanges of ideas or concepts prior to 1960 between American and European surgeons. The first and most obvious reason for this lack of exchange was the language differences. The translation of foreign scientific literature came as an outgrowth of the ever-widening communications among all nations after World War II. The wars were two-edged swords. They produced the need for the development of new methods of treatment, but they also interrupted the scientific intercourse that serves to embellish the production of scientific knowledge.

Whatever the reason, the significant concepts and procedures developed by European innovators of surgical technique for the correction of facial deformities were not known in the United States until the late 1960s. These outstanding surgeons include Bruhn,[16] Ascher,[2] Perthes[88] (extraoral vertical osteotomy of the mandibular vertical ramus), Immenkamp[51] (modifications of anterior maxillary osteotomy), Wassmund[134] (anterior maxillary osteotomy and Le Forte I osteotomy), Wunderer[136] (anterior maxillary osteotomy, palatal approach), Pichler[90] (mandibular osteotomy), Trauner[127] (mandibular osteotomy at the mandibular angle), Schuchardt (two-stage anterior maxillary osteotomy,[106] posterior maxillary osteotomy, [107] combination surgical-orthodontic horizontal maxillary osteotomy), Köle[58] (augmentation genioplasty, modification of anterior mandibular osteotomy), and Obwegeser (augmentation genioplasty[80] and sagittal osteotomy of the mandibular vertical ramus[82]). These surgeons vigorously applied Blair's observation concerning surgery of the mandible to the development of surgical techniques for the maxilla.

Tessier[121] has made recent significant contributions to maxillofacial surgery. He has improved Gillies original concept of the Le Forte III osteotomy. His newer techniques for surgical positioning of the orbits and the frontal bone are unique and wonderful to behold.

GROWTH AND ORTHODONTICS

Detailed experimental and clinical studies have been made of the growth of the mandible, and it is unnecessary in this chapter to go into a comprehensive review of this subject as it relates to deformities.* Normal growth of the mandible occurs in two ways: (1) appositional at all its borders except the anterior border of the ramus and (2) epiphyseal-like growth of the condyles. No definite etiological factors account for prognathism. Although heredity and endocrines must influence the development of this deformity, it may be a result of hyperactivity of the growth center in the mandibular condyle. Clinically, we have observed that practically all excessive prognathic development of the mandible has occurred someplace in the vertical ramus. This observation is based almost entirely on the preoperative relating of study models. Almost always the dental arches relate to a satisfactory degree, but occlusion may not be ideal.

Conversely, micrognathia is usually a result of an interference in the condylar growth center by systemic or local causes. Trauma at childbirth or during infancy or early childhood is the most commonly ob-

---

*See references 4, 16, 51, 88, and 134.

served etiological factor. Growth interference may be unilateral or bilateral, resulting in asymmetrical or symmetrical deformity.

Prior to surgical correction of jaw deformities the surgeon must establish the fact that the condition is in a static state and that it is not the result of endocrine disturbances such as giantism and acromegaly resulting from pituitary dysfunction. Tumors and ordinary hypertrophy should be recognized in differential diagnosis also.

The most reliable indicator of the cessation of growth of the facial bones is the evaluation of cephalometric roentgenograms. If tracings from three successive cephalometric roentgenograms taken 6 months apart can be superimposed with less than a millimeter of variance, growth can be considered to have ceased.

Whether surgery should be adjunctive to orthodontics or vice versa is debatable. We have seen patients with extreme prognathism who were treated by orthodontics for 3 or 4 years with no benefit or retardation of the progressing deformity. We have also seen patients with prognathism who were treated surgically at an absurdly early age. Developmental deformities must be dealt with at a proper time, and the best interests of the patient are served if the oral surgeon, orthodontist, and speech therapist combine their knowledge on a cooperative basis. Surgical correction and orthodontics should not be undertaken in mandibular prognathism until maturity is reached and maximum growth is attained. Depending on conditions and the operation contemplated, micrognathic mandibles may be corrected surgically at younger ages. Open bite deformities should not be corrected surgically until a speech therapist has controlled tongue thrusting habits. It is sometimes difficult to come to an understanding with younger patients, or more especially the parents, because of the patient's personality problems. If, for psychological reasons, a compromise is agreed to and surgery is undertaken earlier than appropriate, parents must understand that a second opera-

tion may be necessary later. Obviously, a record of this advice should be made.

SELECTION OF AN OPERATIVE PROCEDURE AND PREOPERATIVE PLANNING

No specific operation is applicable to a given jaw deformity. Selection of the most appropriate procedure for correction of the problem is incumbent on the part of the surgeon. Simply because one prefers to operate by way of the extraoral route should not be a reason to exclude all intraoral operations and vice versa; however, if there is a choice, then one should select the operation in which one is most comfortable and able, providing that morbidity is no greater and prognosis is equal. With the wide selection of operations available to us today, maxillary, mandibular, intraoral, extraoral, segmental, and interradicular, it is preposterous to believe that an inappropriate procedure would be selected—that a LeForte I maxillary osteotomy would be done to correct a 4-mm retrusion or simply to log another case or that multiple corticotomy would be offered when conventional orthodontics alone would provide a better result with minimal or no chance for permanent harm to the patient. Anterior maxillary osteotomies have been done when, in fact, the mandible should have been elongated and vice versa, and, occasionally, when the deformity should have been corrected by rhinoplasty alone. As an example, too much dependence is placed on cephalometric analysis when simply *looking* at a facial profile is sometimes more helpful. Illustrations are shown in articles and case presentations at meetings in which it is obvious that the wrong operation was employed for a given problem. This is especially noticeable in the current enthusiasm for maxillary surgery and the resultant questionable outcomes. One must depend on basic principles and especially adhere to the golden rule in selection of operative procedures.

A correct solution is available for each individual deformity problem, but it must be obtained by utilization of every diagnostic adjunct available. Adhering to a fixed preoperative "workup" such as the following will clearly indicate surgical methods adaptable to any case that may present.

Roentgenographic survey. A complete dental roentgenographic survey or Panorex is necessary as a diagnostic procedure prior to surgery to (1) rule out a periapical or periodontal pathological condition, the treatment of which might require mobilization of the jaw after surgery, and (2) aid in the determination of the stability of teeth in the supporting tissue and their ability to withstand the stresses of fixation devices and immobilization.

Study models. Study models of artificial stone are necessary for preoperative studies of occlusal relationship:

1. One set indicating the exact preoperative occlusion is desirable for file, should any question ever arise subsequent to surgery as to the improvement achieved (Fig. 23-1, *A*).

2. One set is needed in cases in which preoperative adjustment of occlusion is indicated. When the lower complement of teeth is moved as a unit at the time of surgery, the new occlusion should be determined and well established preoperatively. Although this preoperative occlusal "equilibration" may or may not be necessary, it is an exceedingly important procedure when indicated. When the study models are occluded into the desired relation, prematurities will be found, but they usually are not excessive, and minor occlusal adjustment will provide normal function. Occasionally orthodontics will be necessary after healing as an adjunctive measure for good functional occlusion.

Preoperative equilibration is accomplished by trimming one inclined plane on a single tooth on the study model at a time. The same degree of adjustment is done in the mouth on the same tooth. Equilibration is thus carried out from one tooth to another until a fairly stable occlusion has been secured on all teeth. Final definitive equilibration is accomplished when the jaws are mobilized after healing is completed. This equilibrated set of study models should be taken to the operating room to be used as a guide to the placement of occlusion when the surgical movement of the jaw is accomplished (Fig. 23-1, *B* and *C*).

Ostectomy or osteotomy in the body of the mandible is rarely necessary; however,

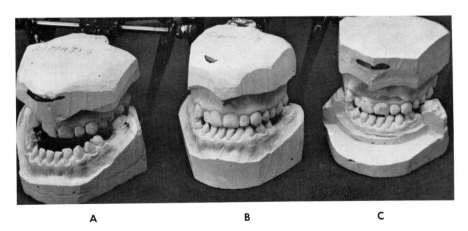

A   B   C

Fig. 23-1. Study models are necessary for permanent record, study of jaw relation and occlusion, determination of operation indicated for correction, and preoperative occlusion equilibration. **A,** Preoperative occlusion. **B,** Osteotomy in vertical ramus. **C,** Ostectomy in horizontal ramus. (U. S. Army photograph; Letterman Army Hospital.)

in the planning of ostectomy for correction of prognatism, measured sections of each side of the ridge are cut out on study models to determine occlusion and jaw relation (Fig. 23-1). When intraoral segmental osteotomy or corticotomy is contemplated, definitive model surgery is essential Fig. 23-2).

All operations on the facial bones involving the dental occlusion must first be accomplished on planning models that are accurate representations of the teeth, the alveolar processes, the adjacent sulci, and the palate. The dental models should be mounted on an articulator in centric jaw relation. The planning of operations on models mounted in the patient's convenience bite is fraught with problems and errors. Planning is most easily and accurately accomplished when the models are mounted on an articulator, which allows for the sectioning and movement of segments of the dental apparatus while the bases remain stationary.

Invaluable information is gained from properly executed model operations. The operation or operations that best suit the needs of the case are determined, the direction and degree of movement of segments is established, and the advisability of the use of orthodontic movement preoperatively or postoperatively is ascertained. Accurate operative guide stents and post-

operative immobilization splints are constructed on the sectioned models.

Cephalometry. *Direct lateral skull roentgenograms (cephalograms),* including the mandible, are essential for preoperative evaluation in all patients regardless of the type of deformity. Cephalometry, primarily utilized in the study of craniofacial growth and orthodontic analysis, is most helpful in the determination of the precise location of jaw deformities and in selection of proper operative sites for surgical correction. The practical application and value of cephalometric techniques are well documented*; however, these studies are adjunctive and must be correlated with clinical observations to arrive at a proper conclusion.

The application of cephalometry to the problems inherent in orthodontic surgery provides information that is indispensible. Oral surgeons recognize that early efforts toward the standardization of measurements of the craniofacial osseous structures made by anthropologists such as Krogman and orthodontists such as Angle, Schwartz, Tweed, Sassouni, Reidel, Downs and Steiner, and the later works of Taylor and Hitchcock provided a means of continuing evaluation of treatment from the preoperative through the postoperative periods.

Portions of each analysis recommended by these investigators have direct application on the evaluation of surgical treatment of developmental deformities. When cephalometric measurements are selected relative to their ability to evaluate the preoperative configuration and postoperative position of the gnathodental complex, numerous measurements useful to the orthodontist are recognized as irrelevant to the surgeon. Thus a method of cephalometric analysis universally applicable to the evaluation of the case treated primarily by surgery has been selected by each surgeon. The most reliable and most universally used is the angle SNA formed at nasion by the intersec-

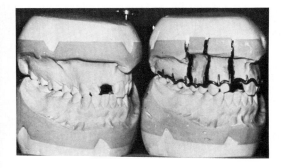

Fig. 23-2. Model surgery to determine degree of movement and feasibility of planned surgical procedure. (Courtesy General Rose Memorial Hospital, Denver.)

*See references 90, 106, 127, and 136.

tion of the line drawn from the midpoint of the sella turcica concavity (S) to nasion (N), or the sella-nasion line, and the line drawn from the subspinale (A), which is the point of greatest concavity of the anterior portion of the maxilla. A second similar angle SNB is formed at nasion by the intersection of the sella-nasion line (SN) and a line from the supramentale (B), which is the point of greatest depression of the anterior portion of the mandible. The angle formed at nasion by the line from subspinale (A) to nasion (N) and the one form supramentale (B) to nasion (N) is called the *ANB difference.* SNA and SNB relate the maxilla and the mandible to the cranial base. The ANB difference relates the anterior maxilla to the anterior mandible. The mean for SNA is 82 degrees and that for SNB is 80 degrees, making the ANB difference 2 degrees. The gonial angle is formed at the angle of the mandible by the interesection of the mandibular plane (line through gonion and gnathion) and a line tangent to the posterior border of the vertical ramus of the mandible, which is tangent at the most posterior point near the angle and the most posterior point of the mandibular condyle. The mean of this angle is 125 degrees. The angles of inclination of the most anterior maxillary and mandibular incisor teeth establish the degree of procumbency or recumbency of each. The inclination of the mandibular incisor is related to the mandibular plane. Normal inclination is 93 degrees. The maxillary incisor is related to the sella-nasion line. Normal value for this measurement is 104 degrees. Schwartz[109] recognized that although skeletal measurements have relevance to the clinician, the soft tissue covering is what the patient, his family, and his associates see. He developed an analysis that combined the measurement of the relationship of bony landmarks with evaluation of the configuration of the soft tissue covering. His analysis used the Frankfort horizontal line as its base. Perpendicular lines to the Frankfort horizontal line were drawn from a point on the skin overlying

nasion, and a second line was drawn from a point on the skin overlying the most inferior point on the infraorbital rim, which was also in line with the pupil of the eye. The infraorbital point was transferred to the cephalometric roentgenogram by fastening a piece of lead shot to the skin in the desired position. Schwartz then classified facial profiles according to the position of the soft tissue chin prominence. He further subdivided the patients classified into those whose palatal plane (this is, anterior nasal spine joined to posterior nasal spine, or ANS-PNS) made an angle of 85 degrees with the soft tissue-nasion line, those with less than 85 degrees at this angle, and those with more than 85 degrees. Within these three groups, he divided his patients into those with average profiles, those with forward profiles, and those with retruded profiles. He believed that the male profile, whatever the classification, should have a more forward position of the chin than the female's. Further improvements on Schwartz's analysis by adding information more relevant to the surgeon are being developed by Obwegeser and Gerhard.[84]

McNeill and co-workers[70] have recently published a cephalometric means of predicting the postoperative profile. They make use of the representation of the soft tissue profile line as reproduced on the roentgenograph by placing radiopaque media on the midline of the face.

The recognition of the basic principles in treatment planning as proposed by Obwegeser[83] indicates the need for more than a practiced eye and the positioning of dental models. He stated that an esthetically pleasing and correctly functioning gnathic apparatus is obtained by the correct positioning of maxillary and mandibular basilar bone, the adjustment of the inclination of the anterior teeth to the basilar bone, and the establishment of the best available dental occlusion.

Recently the scope of possibilities for the surgical correction of facial deformities has expanded greatly. This is partially because

Patient _____ **Georgetown University** Student _____
Birth date _____ **Cephalometric analysis** Instructor _____

		Ref norm								
	Date Taken									
Steiner analysis	SNA	82°								
	SNB	80°								
	ANB	2°								
	SND	76°								
	1 to NA mm	4°								
	1 to NA (angle)	22°								
	1 to NB mm	4°								
	1 to NB (angle)	25°								
	Pogonion to NB mm	Not es-tablished								
	Occ. to SN	14°								
	GO GN to SN	32°								
Down's analysis	Facial angle	87.8°								
	Mand. plane angle	22.9°								
	X axis	59.4°								
	Angle of conventy	+ 0.0°								
	AB plane to facial plane	− 4.6°								
	Cant. of occ. plane	+ 9.3°								
	1 to 1 angle	135°								
	1 to occ. plane	+14.5°								
	1 to mand. plane	91.4°								
	1 to AB plane mm	+ 3.1°								
Holdaway	HNS	73°								
	SNB = HSN (difference)	7°								
	H to nose mm									
	Chin pad mm									
	Upper lid mm									

Ideal

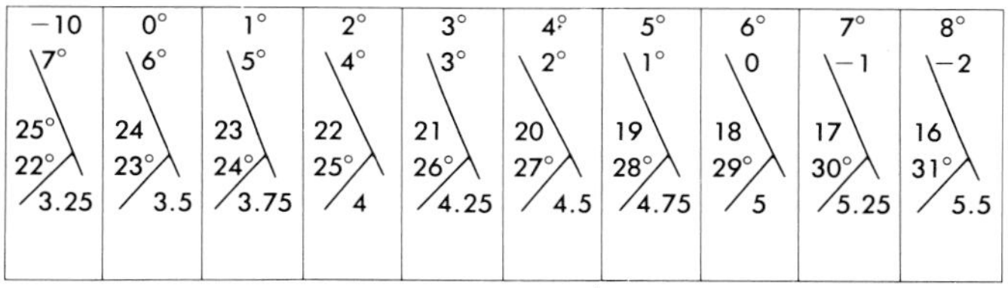

−10	0°	1°	2°	3°	4°	5°	6°	7°	8°	Tracing code
7°	6°	5°	4°	3°	2°	1°	0	−1	−2	
25°	24	23	22	21	20	19	18	17	16	Start—black Progress—blue
22°	23°	24°	25°	26°	27°	28°	29°	30°	31°	Finish—red Ret.—green
3.25	3.5	3.75	4	4.25	4.5	4.75	5	5.25	5.5	1 year—orange

Degrees   Resolved individually

Degrees

PO

Problem

	FMA	FMIA	IMPA
Ideal	25	65	90
Present			
Desired			
Correction factor in degrees			
Correction factor (mm)	1mm/2.5 × 2		
Discrepancy entire arch	mm		
Curve of Spee			
Total arch length needed	mm		
Extraction			
Total net following extraction			

Steiner analysis	+	−
Correcting arch form relocates 1		
Discrepancy		
Expansion		
Relocation 1		
Relocation 6		
Intermaxillary		
Curve of Spee		
Total net		
Extraction		
Total net (mm) following extraction		

	6s	12s
Max. discrepancy mm		
Mand. discrepancy mm		

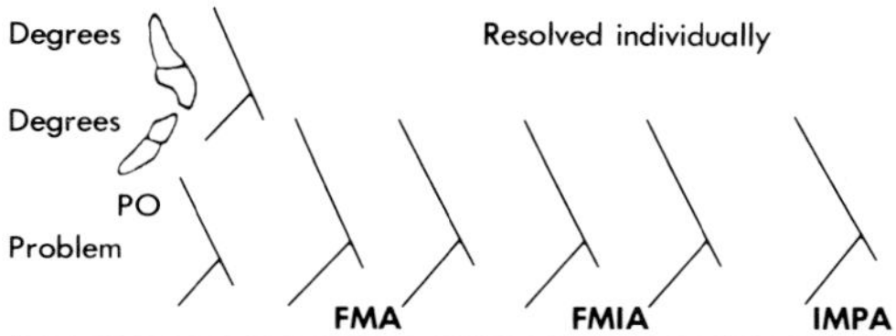

of the increased means of preoperative and postoperative evaluation of surgical procedures. (See form on p. 489.)

Additional extraoral roentgenographic procedure. If a cephalometer is not available, a lateral skull roentgenogram properly made will suffice for evaluation. For this projection a 5-foot target to film distance is recommended, using a technique of 300 milliamperes, 70 kilovolts, and $\frac{1}{10}$-second exposure. The central ray should be directed at absolute right angles to the midsagittal plane through the mandible at the gonial angle (Fig. 23-3). As the exposure is made, the patient should be instructed to take his teeth out of occlusion just enough so that mandibular and maxillary occlusal planes are not superimposed (Fig. 23-3, *C*). One exposure should also be made with the teeth in occlusion so that true degree of retrusion, protrusion, or open bite can be measured.

Preoperative template studies. With the use of tracing paper, the skeletal profile of the mandible and maxilla is traced. Superimposition of one side onto the other makes accurate definition of the occlusal surfaces of the teeth impossible. The occlusal planes can be followed when one roentgenogram has been made with the jaw in rest position. Location of the mandibular and mental foramina and the mandib-

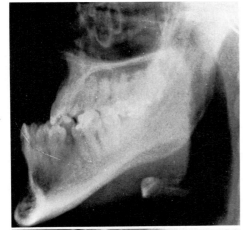
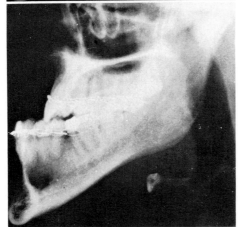
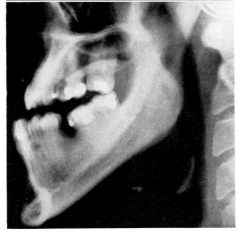

Fig. 23-3. A and **B,** Comparison of cephalogram and direct lateral skull roentgenogram. **A,** Lateral cephalogram. **B,** Direct lateral skull roentgenogram of the same patient, used for diagnostic studies when a cephalometer is not available. The quality of the roentgenogram and its adequacy for this study purpose are equal to the cephalogram. These roentgenograms accurately record actual size of skeletal structures and are valuable adjuncts to treatment planning. **C,** One lateral roentgenogram should be taken with the mandible in rest position so that the mandibular and maxillary occlusal planes are not superimposed. Tracings for study purposes are thus facilitated. (U. S. Army photographs; Letterman Army Hospital.)

ular canal should be recorded on the tracing also (Fig. 23-4, *A*).

This profile tracing is then transferred with carbon paper to thin cardboard (manila letter file holder) (Fig. 23-4, *B,*), and the resulting outline is then cut out, thus producing cardboard templates (Fig. 23-4, *C*).

From these templates, trial sections can be made until a desirable location for osteotomy or ostectomy is found (Fig. 23-4, *D*). The cut sections of the template of the mandible are then fitted back to the tracing in the desired occlusal relation. The section containing the condyle is overlaid in its pre-

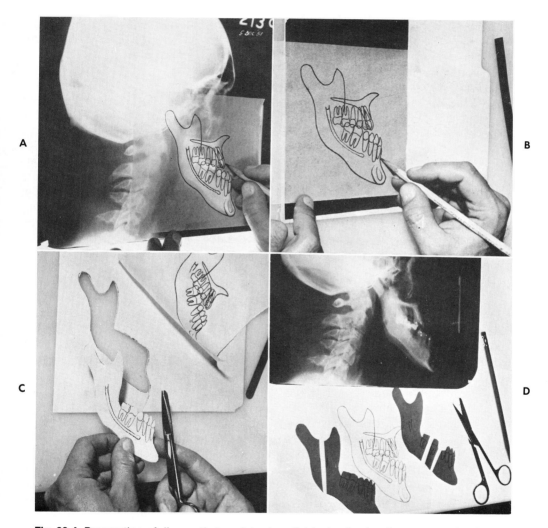

Fig. 23-4. Preparation of diagnostic templates is enlightening in planning an operation for correction of any jaw deformity. **A,** The skeletal profile of the mandible and maxilla is traced onto transparent paper. **B,** The tracing of the mandible is transferred with carbon paper to thin cardboard. **C,** The cardboard "template" is then cut out. **D,** "Trial sections" aid in selecting an operation suitable for correcting the deformity. The roentgenogram and tracings are accurate reproductions of actual size, and measurements are therefore reliable. (U. S. Army photographs; Letterman Army Hospital.)

cise "preoperative" position, whereas the other section is "occluded" and otherwise adapted for the study. This is a helpful and enlightening diagnostic procedure.

Measurements. The amount of protrusion measured in millimeters in prognathic mandibles is not necessarily indicative of the amount of correction necessary. Measurements vary. Occasionally the degree of Class III malocclusion measured in the first molar region will be unequal bilaterally. This measurement cannot be correlated exactly to the incisal edge discrepancy. Therefore, measurements should be standardized in every clinic. In our practice the amount of protrusion is calculated from the incisal edge of lower central incisors to a point lingual to the maxillary incisors where ideal incisal relation is estimated to be.

PREPARATION OF THE PATIENT FOR SURGERY

Routine procedures and miscellaneous preparations. Routine procedures required for any patient undergoing general anesthesia and major surgery should be accomplished the day prior to surgery.

A number of other preparations are considered to be essential in these cases. These are as follows:

1. *Shave and skin preparations.* Most male patient are instructed to shave closely the night before surgery. Those with heavy beards should shave early the morning of surgery. Male patients should shave to the level of the zygomatic arch.

Female patients are instructed to put their hair up in "curlers" or braids the night before surgery so that it can be easily controlled under the drapes.

All patients are ordered to take "lather" showers and shampoos with antiseptic surgical soap the night before surgery. Their instructions are to lather from head to toe out of the shower for 5 minutes (by the clock), rinse, relather for 5 minutes, rinse, and dry.

2. *Antibiotics.* Antibiotics are optional and are ordered only on specific indication or at the discretion and judgment of the surgeon in charge of the case. However, this protection should be routine in all intraoral operations.

3. *Fixation appliances.* Fixation appliances should be placed prior to the day of surgery since most of the corrective surgical procedures are time consuming and anything that can be accomplished ahead of time should be. If orthodontics is to be done adjunctive to surgery, it is good planning to have the necessary appliances in place prior to surgery and utilize them during the period of immobilization.

4. *Oral hygiene.* Prophylaxis should be accomplished if indicated. Any inflammatory condition of the gingiva or oral mucous membranes should be treated and eliminated, especially including pericoronal infections involving erupting third molars and especially prior to intraoral operations.

5. *Mental preparations.* Although the patient will have been psychologically prepared in the preceding weeks of workup as well as advised of the potential morbidity associated with the particular operation planned, there are additional details of the surgery that, if explained on the eve of surgery, will make the immediated postoperative period much smoother for both the patient and the surgeon. In our experience, patients—young or old— appreciate being informed in detail of what to expect. When they first contemplate surgery, they inquire about scarring, length of the operation, number of days hospitalized, how they will eat, and so on—all of which is carefully explained; however, equally important are the answers to questions that they have not thought to ask. Since we have our patients in the office for a final check, placement of fixation appliances, and other preliminaries just prior to admission, we find this to be a convenient time to review hospital routines. Members of the family are with the patient, and this visit is helpful to them also. This review is important since many patients have never been hospitalized and are unfamiliar with the real thing. In addition to information already covered, we tell the patient in terms he can understand:

a. That he will "go to sleep" because of "medicine" given through a "needle in a vein," that the needle will still be in place when he awakens after the operation, and that it will remain overnight and why

b. That a "small tube" will be passed through the nose into the "windpipe" after he is asleep and why and that as a result, he may experience a sore nose and throat for 2 or 3 days after the operation

c. That his head will be fully bandaged when he awakens, with only the face exposed, and that this bandage will be kept in place for 4 or 5 days. (Some patients or parents are concerned by large dressings.)

d. That his jaws will be held together with elastic bands when he awakens, especially that it is important not to fight this restraint, and that the elastics can be removed easily and quickly in case of need

e. That because of the use of modern anesthetic agents and routine administration of other preventative drugs occurrence of postoperative nausea is uncommon

f. That postoperative pain is not great as a rule and, although pain control medicines will be ordered, that requests for them should be on a real need basis, thus further helping to prevent nausea[46]

g. That he will be kept in "overnight recovery" or "intensive care" routinely through the first postoperative day and night and why this precaution is taken

h. That the presence of generalized muscle ache, fatigue, and occasional headache following general anesthesia is common but transitory and why they occur

We have found that communication with patients in anticipation is most helpful to their general well-being. Language they can understand is desirable, with use of technical terms kept to a minimum.

Anesthesia

Choice of an anesthetic is a matter for consideration by both the surgeon and the anesthesiologist. The latter must thoroughly understand the problems related to surgery about the jaws and the need for protection of the airway during the recovery period. The selection of anesthetic agents should take into account the possibility of nausea and related complications that may develop while the jaws are immobilized.

Nasoendotracheal intubation is routine, and the airway is maintained until the patient has reacted from the anesthetic. The stomach is partly emptied by suction at the conclusion of surgery using a nasogastric tube, thus controlling the incidence of vomiting in most cases.

Skin preparation and draping

For extraoral operations the patient should be placed in a supine position on the operating table with his head well extended. After he is intubated and asleep, a Turkish towel is placed under his shoulders, which permits further extension of the head and makes the submandibular area accessible to light and surgery.

The anesthesiologist should be placed at the head of the table to permit direct access to the airway and thus good control of the anesthetic. At the same time the surgical team has ample access to both sides of the patient.

An antiseptic surgical soap is routinely used in preparation of the skin of the operative field. A wide area of skin is lathered for 10 minutes and then blotted dry with a sterile towel. The preparation is started in the immediate area of the incision and circled outward to the perimeter.

Proper draping of the patient for extraoral operations is exeedingly important in maintaining a clean surgical field, preventing postsurgical infection and saving operative time. Step procedure recommended is as follows (Fig. 23-5):

1. A towel and folded sheet arrangement is utilized to drape the head. Both are carried across the table under the patient's head as it is raised by the anesthesiologist or a circulator, care being exercised that the scrubbed area of the face is not contaminated.

2. The head towel is secured under the nasoendotracheal tube with Backhaus towel forceps.

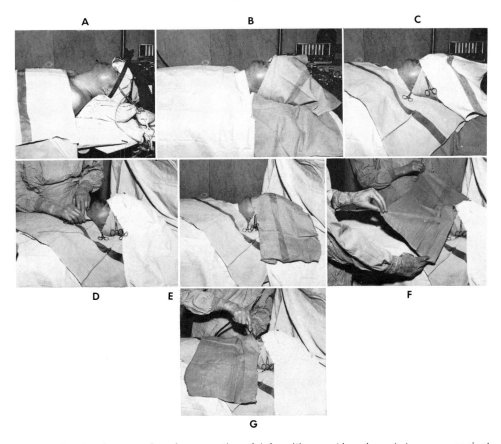

Fig. 23-5. Draping for operations for correction of deformities must be adequate to ensure against contamination. Entering the mouth, turning the patient, and other factors tend to defeat aseptic technique. To cope with these problems and at the same time effect a savings of operative time, draping technique is illustrated. **A,** Position of the patient with the anesthesiologist at the head of the table. **B,** The entire body is covered with sterile sheets, and the head drapes are placed. **C,** The nasoendotracheal tube is covered, and towels are also placed on each side of the face. **D,** A sheet is placed over the patient's head, "draping out" the anesthesiologist. The towel edges at the perimeter of the surgical field are sutured to the skin to prevent shifting of drapes when the patient is repositioned during surgery. **E,** A *"curtain" drape* is sutured across the face, covering the mouth but exposing the chin as well as the surgical field. **F,** The "curtain" drape is adjustable and is a timesaver, permitting access to the mouth with the least possibility of contaminating the sterile surgical field. Before it is turned down to expose the mouth, the surgical area is covered with a sterile towel. **G,** After the mouth has been entered, gloves are changed before reentering the surgical field. (U. S. Army photographs; Letterman Army Hospital.)

3. Another towel is draped over the head towel with the folded edge carried across the upper lip and over the endotracheal tube. It is secured to the head towel on both sides with towel forceps.

4. The entire body is covered with a split sheet extended past the head on both sides.

5. A single towel is then placed on each

side over the patient's neck, with the folded edge about 2 inches below the lower border of the mandible and parallel to it on each side. These two towels are clipped together as they cross at the midline above the sternum as well as to the head towels on each side. All towels are sutured to the skin with No. 4-0 silk at intervals of 1½ inches.

6. A drape sheet is then placed over the

patient's head, secured to the head towels with towel forceps and to IV standards on each side of the table, thus "draping out" the anesthesiologist.

7. One more towel is now placed across the patient's mouth with the folded edge just below the lower lip and the towel draped toward the head, thus "draping out" the mouth. It is also secured on each side with towel forceps and to the skin with sutures at intervals of about 3 cm. It should be sutured to the skin just below the lower lip so that the whole chin is exposed, permitting visualization of areas innervated by the mandibular branch of the facial nerve. Thus as the nerve is stimulated during surgery, it can be identified. This last towel drape is an important one and a timesaver. It protects the extraoral surgical field from oral contamination during surgery and yet provides access to the oral cavity, since it can be turned down over the surgical wound. Thus after occlusion adjustment and fixation of the appliances, the surgeon's gloves are changed, this adjustable "curtain" drape is replaced over the mouth, and surgery is continued.

Suturing the drapes to the skin at the periphery of the surgical field is important, since the patient's head must be moved from side to side during the surgery. Unless so secured the drapes tend to shift and loosen, with contamination sure to occur.

A variation in draping is utilized for intraoral operations. A low-profile anesthesia apparatus permits positioning of the anesthesiologist at the side of the table so that the surgeon may operate from the head of the table if desired. The procedure otherwise is very much the same as already described except that the oral cavity is thoroughly cleansed. The oral pharynx is packed, and the head is flexed somewhat instead of extended as in intraoral operations (Fig. 23-6).

TECHNIQUE OF SOFT TISSUE SURGERY

The standard technique for exposing the inferior border of the mandible through the soft tissue is used (see Chapter 2). However, to ensure success, certain parts of the technique are worthy of emphasis, since the ease with which bone surgery is accomplished is directly dependent on adequate access. This is especially true in access to the ramus.

Location of the incision must be given careful attention to be sure that deeper anatomical structures come to view in proper relation. Positioning of the patient can alter the relation of the incision to the lower border of the mandible as much as an inch. The proposed incision lines should be identified with a marking pen. The patient's head should be centered and not extended so that both sides can be marked symmetrically and the incision lines can be made in proper relation to the lower border of the mandible. Landmarks such as the gonial angle and the mandibular notch are then palpated and dye marks made on the skin, identifying their location. In locating the incision line for surgery to correct prognathism, it must be remembered that an obtuse gonial angle is characteristic and a part of the deformity. Also to be remembered is that when it is corrected, ideally, a more pronounced angle should be developed. This being the case, it is often desirable to have the incision line somewhat lower than normal toward its posterior aspect for a good esthetic result. It should also be kept in mind that with the patient relaxed under anesthesia, the mouth may hang open several centimeters, resulting in a changed relation of skin to border of mandible. Therefore the mandible should be held in a closed, occluded position as incision lines are located.

Incisions for intraoral surgery require the same care in planning and execution. The surgeon must project this thinking toward the closure of the incision before the tissue is incised. Wound margins must be placed so as to not coincide with planned underlying bony cuts. A knowledge of the precise anatomy of any area being treated is mandatory to ensure the most favorable blood supply to flaps generated during the

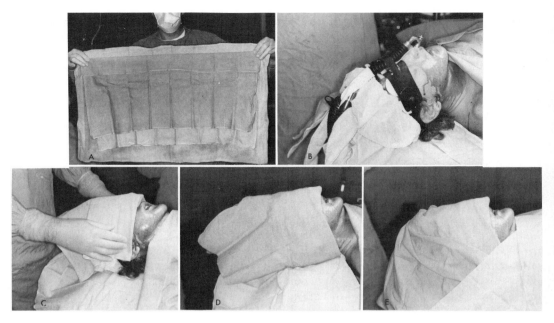

Fig. 23-6. Draping procedure for intraoral operations employing low-profile anesthesia apparatus and with the anesthesiologist positioned at the side of the table. **A,** Three-towel head drape. A bath towel and two draping towels are placed so that the bath towel will lay on the operating table with the two draping towels on it. The towel on which the patient's head will rest is folded and placed so that the edge closest to the patient's shoulders is 3 cm farther away from the shoulders than the towel directly below it. **B,** The anesthesia hose is disconnected and the towels slipped carefully under the patient's head. The hose is reconnected. **C,** A fourth towel is folded on one edge and placed over the anesthesia tubes and the sides of the patient's head. **D,** The topmost towel under the patient's head is brought up, folded over the previously placed head towel, and fastened with a towel clip. **E,** A sheet is draped so that it partially covers the head and closes in the area beneath the operating table. A draping towel is placed on each side of the head and over the chest. Adapter from nasotracheal tube to corrugated connector tube was designed by Lt. Col. Keith J. Marshall, U. S. Army Dental Corps.

surgery. One must always keep in mind the fact that vigorous retraction to provide better observation of the surgical site may displace the soft tissue sufficiently to cause an incision placed over familiar landmarks to be grossly misplaced. Suturing of flap margins to attached gingiva or through the embrasures between teeth is extremely difficult. Gingival tissues are thin and friable. Therefore paragingival incisions, those well into the movable mucosa of the mouth, are preferred to those placed in the gingival sulcus. The surgeon must plan sufficiently ahead to place sutures for closure before splints with wide coverages of soft tissue are wired into position.

PROGNATHISM (MANDIBULAR)

Significant progress in the field of surgery for treatment of prognathism has occurred since the first edition of this textbook. Notable contributions in the literature indicate a marked trend to surgery in the ramus in preference to the body of the mandible for correction of prognathism. Basic operations commonly employed in recent years include (1) subcondylar (or oblique) osteotomy in the ramus (Fig. 23-7, *B*), (2) modification of the earlier horizontal osteotomy* by intraoral sagittal splitting according to Obwe-

---

*See references 17, 43, 55, 75, and 113.

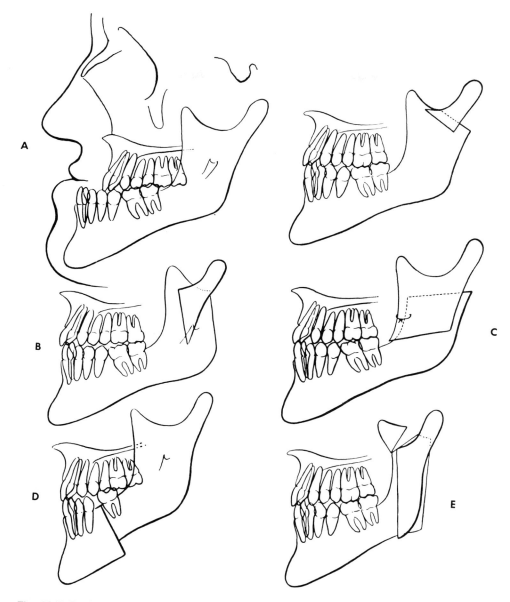

Fig. 23-7. Basic operations employed in correction of prognathism. A 16-mm protrusion of mandible. **A,** Osteotomy through the neck or at the base of the condyle. **B,** Subcondylar (or oblique) osteotomy in the ramus above the angle. **C,** Modified intraoral osteotomy by sagittal splitting. **D,** Ostectomy in the body of the mandible. **E,** Vertical osteotomy in the ramus.

geser (Fig. 23-7, *C*) and its modification by Dal Pont (Fig. 23-24), and (3) vertical osteotomy in the ramus (Fig. 23-7, *E*). Osteotomy through the neck or at the base of the condyle (Fig. 23-7, *A*) and ostectomy in the body of the mandible (Fig. 23-7, *D*) are rarely indicated or utilized. (Osteotomy is the surgical cutting of bone, whereas ostectomy is the excision of a bone or a portion of a bone.) Operations in standard locations will be discussed in detail in the following text. Four of the procedures to be discussed (Fig. 23-7, *A* to *C* and *E*) employ the principle of repositioning the entire body of the mandible. The body of the mandible itself is shortened in the ostectomy (Fig. 23-7, *D*). Osteotomy through the neck of the condyle has never attained general acceptance but is still used by a few oral surgeons. Subcondylar (oblique) osteotomies below the neck of the condyle are quite widely used now. Definition of osteotomy by direction, that is, oblique, vertical, or horizontal, is difficult; for example, an "oblique" subcondylar osteotomy in which the section is carried to a low point on the posterior border of the ascending ramus may well be in a vertical direction. The term *oblique* osteotomy as used in this text originally included all subcondylar osteotomies or those below the condyle head extending from the sigmoid notch to the posterior aspect of the ramus. For the sake of clarity and definition, ramus operations to be described herein will be referred to as (1) osteotomy in the condylar neck, (2) subcondylar osteotomy (oblique and below the neck or base of the condyle), and (3) vertical osteotomy to the gonial angle or anterior to it.

There are few indications for ostectomy in the body of the mandible, since a disparity between the mandibular and maxillary arches is rare. Only 1.5% of our patients required procedures involving ostectomy in the body of the mandible. Hinds[35] found only one out of 20 patients for whom ostectomy in the mandibular body was indicated. Mohnac states "In my series of more than 100 cases, I have rarely found a Class III malocclusion in which the tooth-bearing alveolar region of the mandible was not in proportion with that in the maxilla."[72] Improved surgical techniques and a broader knowledge of operative procedures have also led to greater use of ramus procedures, which are not at all formidable after 25 years of use.

Osteotomy in the condylar neck

Osteotomy in the condylar neck is most commonly accomplished by utilizing the Gigli saw in a "blind" section. It may also be performed through a preauricular incision, a Risdon incision, or by an intraoral approach. The objective is surgical section of the neck of the condyle, creating bilateral surgical fractures, with repositioning of the whole mandible to normal occlusal and jaw relation. In rare instances bony union may not occur or even may not be expected, but a satisfactory functional pseudoarthrosis is hoped for.

History of this condyle site for osteotomy dates back to 1898, when Jaboulay and Berard[52] reported destroying the condyle "piece by piece," "with the aid of gouge tooth-forceps" by way of a preauricular incision. Duformental[34] in 1921 also advocated condylectomy as a means of correcting "a protruded lower jaw." Pettit and Walrath[89] in 1932 were the first to suggest osteotomy through the neck of the condyle. Their "bow back" operation was based on the principle of interposing temporal fascia and the creation of a pseudoarthrosis or flail joint, which had been a standard arthroplastic procedure in treatment of temporomandibular joint ankylosis.

The first refinement to operations in this site came in 1940 when Smith and Johnson[116] suggested the removal of a "parallelepipedonal" section of bone from the region below the sigmoid notch. This was followed by horizontal osteotomy from that point posteriorly below the neck of the condyle to permit posterior repositioning of the mandible. Subsequently, Smith and Robinson[117] reported 57 cases in which the patients were treated successfully by this subsigmoid notch ostectomy.

"Subsigmoid" notch ostectomy and condylotomy suggested by Smith and associates[116,117] offered few advantages over the blind osteotomy in the condylar neck. The method was never popular because of the surgical anatomy involved and the technical difficulties of the operation. In any open surgical procedure through a preauricular incision, the hazards of injury to the facial nerve are almost as great as by the blind Gigli saw method. The delicate excision of a measured section of bone from the sub-sigmoid notch area, as suggested by Smith, is a tedious procedure to contemplate because the depth of the wound is great and retraction of adjacent tissues must be limited.

In 1955 at the Los Angeles meeting of the American Society of Oral Surgeons, Moose suggested osteotomy at the neck of the condyle by an intraoral approach similar to that used for the intraoral sagittal splitting procedure. He recommended establishing an incision line in the bone with drill penetrations, followed by surgical fracture with chisel and mallet. One of us (J.B.C.) assisted with one such operation on a patient with only 7 mm of protrusion. Healing occurred in 6 weeks, and a good result was obtained. Moose[76] reports favorable results using this method in the correction of prognathism in 14 patients. In several other operations he found it impossible to adequately visualize the ascending ramus at a proper height for subcondylar osteotomy and resorted to the "ramus bisection" operation (horizontal osteotomy in the mandibular ramus above the mandibular foramen). This procedure is not recommended because of this experience plus other obvious disadvantages.

Reiter[94,95] was one of the foremost proponents of operations in this region of the condyle and is said to have performed more than 75 such operations, but no published reports are available as to the successful results in his cases. He used a "blind" Gigli saw technique originally suggested by Kostecka[63] for correction of open bite and performed by Schaefer[105] for correction of prognathism. Verne and co-workers,[129] studied 52 cases in which essentially the same techniques were employed. Their published results are impressive.

Technique for blind Gigli saw condylotomy. The technique for blind Gigli saw con-

dylotomy is included for the sake of completeness only. The steps are as follows:

1. An incision approximately 1 cm in length is made through the skin at the posterior border of the ramus, somewhat below the base of the condylar neck, or about halfway between the lobe of the ear and the angle of the mandible.

2. The bone is reached by blunt dissection to prevent injury to the facial nerve or its branches.

3. A curved aneurysm needle is then passed in constant contact with the medial surface of the ramus below the neck of the condyle in an angular direction upward and obliquely forward until it slides out over the sigmoid notch (Fig. 23-8, *2*).

4. As the skin is elevated by the emergence of the needle over the sigmoid notch, another short incision is made to permit exit.

5. At this point the Gigli saw is attached to the needle and carried through the tissues to position for the osteotomy (Fig. 23-8, *3*).

6. It is recommended that "funnellike" cannulas be placed into both wounds with the wire saw passed through them for protection of vital soft tissue components (Fig. 23-8, *3*).

7. With osteotomy completed and the saw removed, one or two sutures are placed in both incisions to close the skin.

8. The mandible is repositioned to the desired occlusal relationship, and intermaxillary fixation is applied to previously placed arch bars.

ADVANTAGES

1. The operation is a simple one to perform.

2. The operating time is short (30 to 60 minutes).

3. It has been done as a clinic or office procedure, although this is not recommended.

4. Instruments required for the operation are available commercially.

5. Fixation appliances need not be elab-

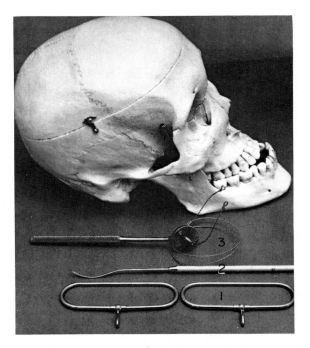

Fig. 23-8. Gigli saw used in oblique subcondyloid osteotomy. *1,* Handles for Gigli saw; *2,* aneurysm needle used to pull wire saw blade into position; *3,* Gigli saw threaded through cannula used in wound to protect soft tissues as section is made with the saw. (U. S. Army photograph; Letterman Army Hospital.)

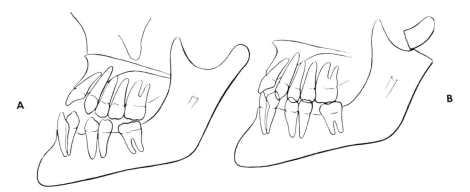

Fig. 23-9. Tracings of cephalograms. **A,** Preoperative. **B,** Postoperative, after correction of 7-mm protrusion by blind Gigli saw osteotomy; a good result was achieved after 7 weeks' immobilization despite poor apposition of bone cut ends.

orate, since immobilization should not require more than 6 to 8 weeks.

6. External scarring is negligible.

7. Teeth need not be sacrificed, and edentulous alveolar ridge area for future denture coverage is not lost.

8. Injury to the mandibular nerve is not likely.

DISADVANTAGES

1. A blind procedure in this area carries the hazards of:

    a. Injury to branches of the facial nerve, with permanent facial paralysis, is a possibility

    b. Deep hemorrhage resulting from severance of the maxillary artery, one of its larger branches, or the posterior facial vein

    c. Injury to the parotid gland or its capsule and formation of a salivary fistula

2. Lack of control of fragments occasionally results in a nonunion with "flail" joint (Fig. 23-9, *B*).

3. Open bite is a distinct possibility that increases with every millimeter of correction beyond 10 to 12 mm. This is caused largely by the strong bipennate temporal

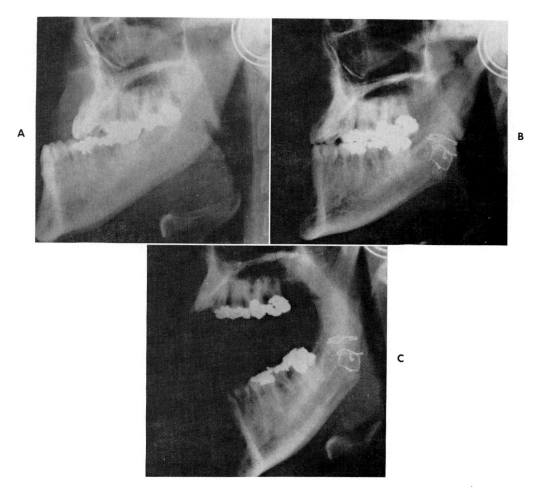

Fig. 23-10. Cephalograms of a patient with extreme prognathism (20 mm), which was corrected by vertical osteotomy in the rami. He was immobilized for 28 days. **A,** Preoperative. **B,** Postoperative. **C,** Functional result. (U. S. Army Photographs; Letterman Army Hospital.)

muscle, which prohibits posterior movement of the coronoid process more than about 10 mm, but also the vertical contracting action of the masseter and medial pterygoid muscles produces a shortening of the vertical ramus resulting in the tendency to open bite anteriorly.

Based on this last disadvantage, the Gigli saw condylotomy operation is not accepted for general use and is not suitable for patients with more than a moderate degree of prognathism. Kaplan and Spring[53] reported seven occurrences of gustatory hyperhidrosis associated with subcondylar osteotomy in 14 patients. They admonish the surgeon to understand and recognize the phenomenon as a relatively frequent complication. It is related to the misdirected regeneration of cut secretory and vasodilator fibers of branches of the auriculotemporal nerve, which results in postoperative sweating and flush of the skin during mastication.

Extraoral vertical osteotomy in the rami

Vertical osteotomy in the rami for correction of prognathism as it is usually accomplished is an extraoral operation through a submandibular approach. The objective is vertical sectioning of the ramus in a line from the lower aspect of the mandibular notch vertically downward over the mandibular foramen or just posterior to it to the lower boder of the mandible at the angle. By decortication of a portion of the distal fragment (ramus, anterior to the vertical section), overlapping of the proximal fragment, and thus creation of a mortised overlay, the whole body of the mandible is repositioned posteriorly to a normal occlusal and jaw relation. It is an operation that is ideally suited to correction of extreme prognathism, which is anything in excess of 10 to 12 mm (Fig. 23-10), and produces excellent results in fully or partially edentulous patients. Details of this operation were described by Caldwell and Letterman[25] in 1954. A follow-up study of the original cases was made in 1965, 10 years

after surgery. Functional and cosmetic results were excellent at that later date.[64] We had used the procedure since 1952 and had operated on eight extreme deformities when the original article reporting three cases was finally published. In 1954[18] this operation was also recommended for selected patients in military facilities since it had been established that healing time was short and need for immobilization did not ordinarily exceed 4 weeks. We have performed this surgery for approximately 650 patients, with generally excellent results. The Walter Reed Army Hospital group while under Shira's[110] direction also operated on a large number of patients using this method with equally successful results.

Technique for extraoral vertical osteotomy in the rami. Certain modifications and improvements have been made in the technical procedure of vertical osteotomy since it was first reported in 1954 (Figs. 23-11 and 23-13).

1. Soft tissue surgery has been described previously. It is done through an incision approximately 3 to 4 cm in length.

2. The lateral aspect of the ramus is exposed to the mandibular notch. Muscle attachments on the medial aspect of the ramus are not disturbed at this time.

3. The prominence overlying the mandibular foramen is identified.

4. A vertical line for bone incision is planned from the lowest point of the mandibular notch to the lower border of the mandible at the angle passing over the prominence of the mandibular foramen or slightly posterior to it. This line may be lightly scribed onto the surface of the bone with a #703 carbide bur before cuts are actually made to be sure the line of osteotomy is correct.

5. Exposure is ample, with the second assistant elevating and protecting the soft tissue with Army-navy retractors and Thompson ramus retractors H135 R and L (Fig. 23-13).

6. A No. 703 taper fissure carbide bur in a straight handpiece powered by a Jordan-

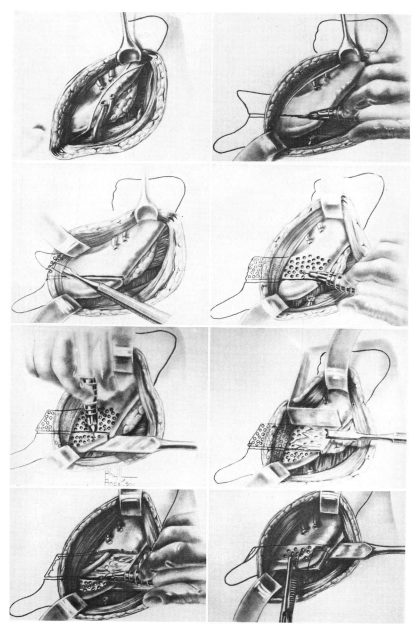

Fig. 23-11. The original vertical osteotomy illustrated here has been simplified over the years. The incision is short—about 3 to 4 cm, the drill holes are not placed in the proximal (condyle) fragment, and decortication is accomplished by a safer more simplified technique. See Fig. 23-77 and related text for details. In minimal prognathism, decortication may not be done at all. Also, the line of vertical osteotomy may vary but usually ends at some point near the angle of the mandible. (Original drawings by Phyll Anderson.) (From Caldwell, J. B., and Letterman, G. S.: J. Oral Surg. **12:**185, 1954.)

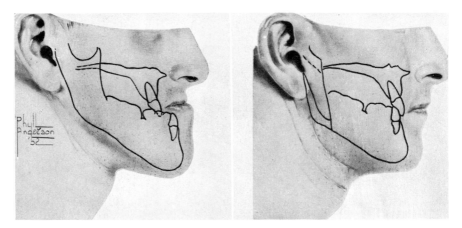

Fig. 23-12. Original vertical osteotomy. (From Caldwell, J. B., and Letterman, G. S.: J. Oral Surg. **12:**185, 1954.)

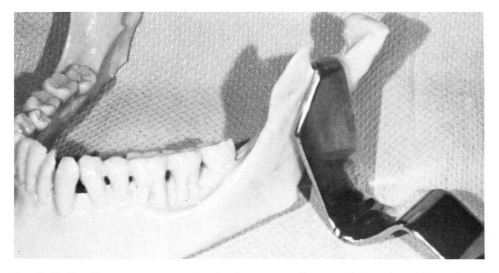

Fig. 23-13. The Thompson ramus retractor hooks over the mandibular (sigmoid) notch and thus serves as a protective device in this critical area, as well as providing much improved visualization of the whole operative site in ramus operations. (Courtesy Medical Illustrations, General Rose Memorial Hospital, Denver.)

Day or Emesco autoclavable explosion-proof engine is used to make the initial vertical cut in the lateral cortical plate. Either of these pulley-driven handpieces provides more torque than is experienced with higher speed air drills, resulting in a more exquisite sense of touch, which permits more intricate and precise cuts in the critical points of osteotomy. Either engine runs at about 18,000 rpm, ample speed for safe, accurate bone cutting.

7. The first assistant maintains a constant flow of water on the bone as cuts are made, aspirating at the same time to prevent soaking the drapes.

8. The initial cut is made carefully over

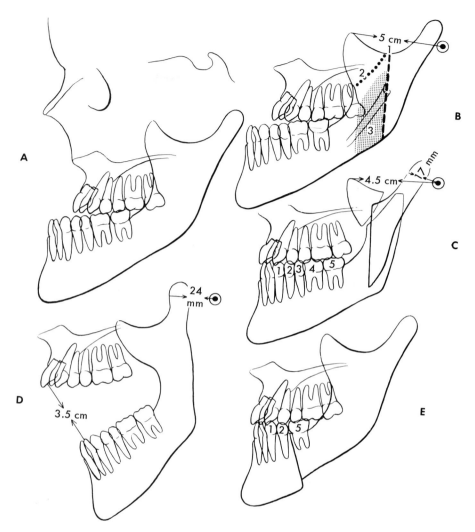

Fig. 23-14. Tracings of cephalogram of patient described in Fig. 23-31. **A,** Preoperative tracing. **B:** *1,* Vertical line of cut; *2,* bur penetrations for coronoidotomy; *3,* shaded area of decortication. **C,** Postoperative tracing from Fig. 23-31, *B,* showing measured distances of coronoid movement as they can best be determined. **D,** Tracing of vertical opening of jaw and condyle excursion. **E,** The hypothetical operation of ostectomy in the body of the mandible applied to this patient (operation actually was vertical osteotomy). Note loss of two teeth and no change in obtuse gonial angle.

the area of the foramen to avoid complete penetration of the lateral cortex, thus avoiding injury to the nerve as it enters the bone (Figs. 23-11, upper right, and 23-14, *B*).

9. The coronoid process is sectioned if indicated. It may be left undisturbed in less

pronounced protrusion, but if a correction of more than 8 to 10 mm is anticipated, coronoidotomy is advisable to obtain unrestricted movement of the jaw posteriorly. In fact the procedure is so simple and completely free of contraindications that it is done almost routinely. (See section on relationship of musculature to surgical correction of jaw deformities.)

10. Sectioning the coronoid is simple. Closely spaced drill penetrations are made obliquely from the sigmoid notch to the anterior border of the ramus using a No. 14 bone drill. The medullary space is usually absent or imperceptible here, so as soon as the high-speed bur no longer meets resistance, penetration through the medial surface has been achieved. The sectioning is then completed by sharp chisel and mallet. Three or four firm, short, sharp blows with the mallet usually suffice. (See Fig. 23-11, left, second from top, and Fig. 23-14, *B, 2.*)

11. If there is special concern about making a straightforward vertical cut between the inferior alveolar foramen and the mandibular notch above, closely spaced drill penetrations can be made with more safety, and this portion of the osteotomy can be completed with a chisel and mallet after the remainder of the osteotomy is completed. The character of bone in this area is the same as in the coronoid process, thin and without medullary space.

12. When *decortication* is indicated, and it most often is, a simplified, safer and faster method has been substituted for that previously described. A second vertical cut is made into the lateral cortical plate approximately parallel to and anterior to the first vertical cut (step 6), with care not to penetrate this cortex especially over the suspected course of the inferior alveolar canal; the two vertical cuts are then connected with several horizontal cuts spaced at about 6 to 8 mm intervals (see Fig. 23-77). These horizontal steps are made with a No. 703 carbide fissure bur, which creates a notching effect that greatly facilitates subsequent decortication. These steps or notches need not be extended above the prominence caused by the inferior alveolar foramen (Fig. 23-14, *B, 3*). Any impingement or interference with bony apposition above this level should be dealt with as described in Fig. 23-16, *E, n.*

13. By use of a sharp, long-beveled, broad, flat chisel (Stout's No. 3 chisel is ideal) with the bevel down, the notched steps of cortex are fractured off without fear of injury to the inferior alveolar nerve and vessels. These cortical segments chip off cleanly, exposing the medullary spaces, and even the neurovascular bundle is usually visualized and its course identified. Having the bevel down allows for better protection for the nerve as the cortical segments are chipped off. It is helpful if the location of the neurovascular bundle is known when the vertical section is completed or when a hole is drilled to provide for transosseous wiring.

14. At this point, while the first side is still intact, one may wish to turn the patient to the other side and repeat steps 1 through 13. The operation on the second side is then completed as follows:

15. A sharp Molt No. 4 curet is used to initiate elevation of the periosteum and anterior attachment of the medial pterygoid muscle, starting at the inferior border.

16. Once the elevation is started, a broad, blunt periosteal elevator is used to push off soft tissue to an approximate level of the lower margin of the mandibular foramen. *Troublesome bleeding may be caused if sharp elevation is used or if these medial attachments are raised too far. A No. 9 Molt periosteotome is recommended.*

17. With a broad, protecting elevator in position on the medial aspect of the vertical cut, the incision through the bone is completed from the area of the inferior alveolar nerve to the lower border through the medial cortex of the ramus. Use of water and suction during all bur cuts in bone permits clear vision of structures encountered and protects the bone from injury.

18. The vertical section above the nerve is completed in the same manner or with a No. 3 chisel and mallet, fracturing through the drill holes to the mandibular notch. Occasionally the No. 702 bur can be used to facilitate the completion of the osteotomy at this level.

19. If the vertical sectioning is incomplete in a critical area, such as immediately

around the neurovascular bundle at the foramen, a Lane periosteotome may be inserted into the vertical cut and, with gentle manipulation, the thin remnants of uncut bone will usually fracture. In older patients or when the ramus is very thin, one must be careful to avoid fracture of the proximal fragment at the level of the foramen.

20. The proximal segment is rotated slightly to permit visualization of the medial surface. Periosteum and the medial pterygoid muscle attachments are elevated posteriorly but only enough to permit direct bone-to-bone onlay without soft tissue impingement. (See discussion on p. 509.)

21. Irregularities along the vertical cut, especially on the medial side of the proximal fragment, are planed away with a chisel or No. 703 bur until acceptable adaption of the medial surface of the proximal (posterior) fragment can be anticipated when it is lapped onto the distal (anterior) decorticated surface.

22. At this point the patient's head is turned back to the first side and steps 15 through 22 are repeated unless these were completed initially.

23. Both wounds are now covered, and the "curtain" drape is turned down over the surgical fields, exposing the mouth. *On oral*

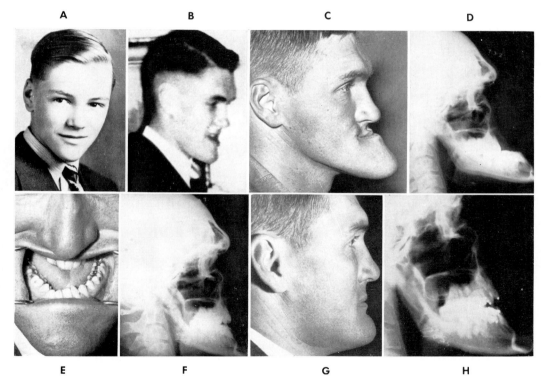

Fig. 23-15. A, When the patient was 14 years old there was only slight suggestion of chin prominence. **B,** Pronounced prognathism was present at age 20 but was minimal when compared to that at age 33. **C,** When he was 33 years old, with extreme prognathism, the patient was 6 feet 8 inches tall and weighed 265 pounds. **D,** From this preoperative cephalogram a required 32-mm correction was confirmed. **E,** The mandible completely encircled the maxilla without any occlusion prior to surgery. **F,** Postoperative cephalogram. **G,** Profile of patient after *modified vertical osteotomy.* **H,** Appearance 4½ years postoperatively. Genioplasty was offered for cosmetic benefit, but the patient was satisfied to have good masticatory function. (Courtesy General Rose Memorial Hospital, Denver.)

examination and when the jaw relation is inspected, the mandible should be hanging posteriorly in a completely free and unrestricted relationship and it should be possible to relate the teeth into a predetermined occlusion without forceful effort. If this is not the case, coronoidotomy is indicated. If impingement is present in the mandibular notch (subsigmoid) area or the sphenomandibular ligament is restricting movement, corrective measures should be taken.

24. The jaw is manipulated until desired occlusion is secured and intermaxillary elastic ligatures are generously placed.

Firm fixation is necessary to prevent displacement as transosseous wiring of the osteotomy is accomplished.

25. The curtain drape is replaced to its previous position, instruments used in the mouth are discarded, gloves are changed, and the surgical field is reentered.

26. The posterior fragment is lapped onto the decorticated area anterior to the vertical osteotomy in a relationship visualized on the templates preoperatively. Both parts are held in the desired relation, and small holes are placed strategically for wiring. *The posterior fragment (proximal or condyloid part) should lap onto the decorti-*

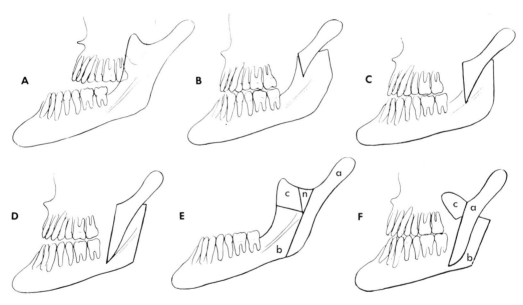

Fig. 23-16. A, From a preoperative cephalogram of patient in Fig. 23-15, *D,* tracings and numerous cardboard templates were made. **B,** Relationships if condylotomy had been the surgical method employed (Reiter, Verne). Obviously the ramus would have been retruded excessively, resulting in functional impairment of the jaw, and the *coronoid process cannot be retruded 32 mm.* **C,** Relationships if subcondylar (oblique) osteotomy had been employed (Hines, Robinson). The same problems are evident as in **B** with condylotomy. **D,** Vertical osteotomy (Caldwell, Letterman) required *modification* as shown in cutouts **E** and **F. E,** The lines of *modified vertical* osteotomy as planned. The vertical cut was made more nearly parallel to the posterior border of the ramus. A V-shaped segment below the mandibular (sigmoid) notch, labeled *n,* was sectioned free and depressed medially, permitting complete freedom of movement of the mandible posteriorly and eliminating interference in overlapping of the proximal portion (segment *a*) onto the distal part (segment *b*). Good mortising is frequently interfered with in the area of segment *n.* At the same time this V-shaped segment, *n,* resulted in a decreased anteroposterior dimension and eliminated any chance of impingement posteriorly as in **B** and **C** above. *Coronoidotomy* was essential in this case, as it is in all surgery for extreme prognathism.

cated part freely and without binding or bowing. If it does not, recheck step 22. It may be necessary to excise portions of medial cortex at points of impingement; the posterior fragment may be rotated outward somewhat to accomplish this. Occasionally the thin portion of ramus below the mandibular notch, above the mandibular foramen, requires sectioning. It need not be removed, simply depressed medially. See Figs. 23-15 and 23-16, E and F.

27. The parts are not wired as securely as previously, since two undesirable sequelae can occur. The condyle may be distracted or rotated, which later may result in poorer occlusion than should have been expected, or there may be chronic temporomandibular joint pain. Usually a drill hole is made just anterior to the decorticated area, and a single, 0.016-inch stainless steel wire is threaded through and carried circumferentially around the stump of the proximal fragment. Usually the wire is not twisted tightly but only enough to assure reasonably good approximation of the parts. An exception is when the operation is used to correct apertognathia (Fig. 23-77). In *all* cases one must always check to be sure that the condyle head is well seated in the glenoid fossa before the wire is tightened and the wounds are closed. The complication of operative condyle dislocation occurred in one of our cases, and reoperation was necessary 3 weeks later (Fig. 23-17, *A* and *B*).

28. The tendinous attachments of the masseter and medial pterygoid muscles are picked up and closed together. The masseter muscle, which may have been entirely elevated, and the pterygoid muscle, partially or often completely elevated, are readily reapposed in their normal anatomical position. Their relationship to the bone that was moved may be changed, but reattachment in harmonious functional position occurs.

29. Closure of soft tissue is completed according to the prescribed technique. Careful attention is given to reapposition of tissues in proper anatomical relation to ensure a good cosmetic and functional result. It is especially important to close the platysma muscle accurately prior to the subcutaneous layer.

30. Pressure dressings are avoided. Gauze toppers are placed on the wound and held firmly with Kerlix gauze applied according to the Barton method.

Discussion. The necessity for sectioning the coronoid process has been a point of controversy. Our attitude toward the inelasticity of the temporal muscle explains why we consider this essential for the per-

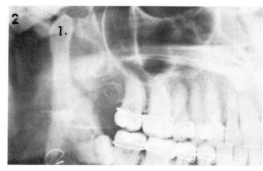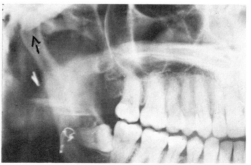

Fig. 23-17. A, The condyle head *(1)* is completely dislocated and anterior to the glenoid fossa *(2)* and articular eminence. Note teeth are in proper occlusion, and the right condyle was in normal relation. This was an operative complication noticed 3 weeks after vertical osteotomy for prognathism. **B,** The patient was readmitted, and the condyle dislocation was reduced surgically. (Courtesy Medical Illustrations, General Rose Memorial Hospital, Denver.)

fect results obtained in correction of moderate to severe prognathism. If one remembers that the central tendinous attachment of the temporal muscle extends for a considerable distance downward along the anterior border of the ramus and also broadly over the medial surface of the coronoid process, the effect of this sectioning should be clear; it is that of a hinge. As the body and anterior portion of the ramus are repositioned in the posterior direction, the coronoid process swings forward, with its tip remaining to a large degree in its original position. Its base anteriorly, still attached below and medially by the tendon of the temporal, is the joint of the hinge. The strong fibers of this tendon's attachment act much the same as the old-fashioned leather barn door hinge. Finally, bony union of the coronoid occurs as illustrated (Fig. 23-14, C and D).

Another point deserving clarification is application of the technique of vertical osteotomy in slight to moderate degrees of prognathism. Results have been equally good in all patients who have been operated on, but the technical details of the operation are more difficult in patients requiring less than 10 to 12 mm of correction than in more severe cases. There are two reasons for this: (1) decortication of a more narrow area anterior to the vertical line is more tedious than the broader area needed in extreme cases and the nerve is usually deeper, probably because the ramus may be thicker (mediolaterally) than in the longer, more obtuse rami and (2) the overlapping and mortising procedure. The proximal (posterior portion) of the ramus does not overlap as readily, and this fragment tends to "bow out." This usually can be overcome by partial decortication of its medial surface and other "fitting" bone adjustments as mortising is accomplished, following step 21 of the technique. For these reasons our operating time in minimal prognathisms is sometimes longer than in more extreme cases; however, as technique and operative skills have improved, our operating time never exceeds 3½ hours and frequently is

less than 2½ hours, including coronoidotomy, decortication, and transosseous wiring. For these reasons we favor *vertical osteotomy* in more *extreme prognathic* surgery and *subcondylar osteotomy* in *less severe cases*.

Bell and Kennedy[11] emphasize the importance of preserving as much soft tissue attachment to the proximal fragment as possible since the bone is entirely dependent on this source for nourishment and revascularization. In their reseach on adult rhesus monkeys, they found that when the proximal segment was not pedicled to soft tissue, there was a tendency to intraosseous necrosis, vascular ischemia, and delayed healing. Similar studies of *pedicled* vertical ramus osteotomies showed early osseous union and minimal osteonecrosis or vascular ischemia. One of their conclusions was that "osteonecrosis and sequestration of the relatively ischemic distal tip of the proximal segment might be obviated by sectioning the ramus more obliquely and thereby shortening the proximal segment or by excising the distal end of the proximal condylar segment."[11] Their research is convincing, and the theory is sound. Their conclusions, however, are not entirely corroborated in practical application. In practice, neither making a "more oblique section" nor "excising the distal end" is practical in all cases. To the contrary, it is essential in certain situations for this proximal segment to be made extremely long (Figs. 23-15 and 23-16 and Fig. 23-75). Other examples of the survival of bone when there are long extensions completely denuded (not pedicled) are illustrated in Figs. 23-51 (L and C osteotomies) and 23-58 (Z osteotomy). In practice, we have literally scores of cases in which extremely long extensions of bone were denuded as described previously, and in not one case have we observed resorption beyond that expected in normal remodeling. Perhaps the reason for this record is that we *decorticate* and *approximate the fragments* in a high percentage of cases.

In application of the "vertical osteoto-

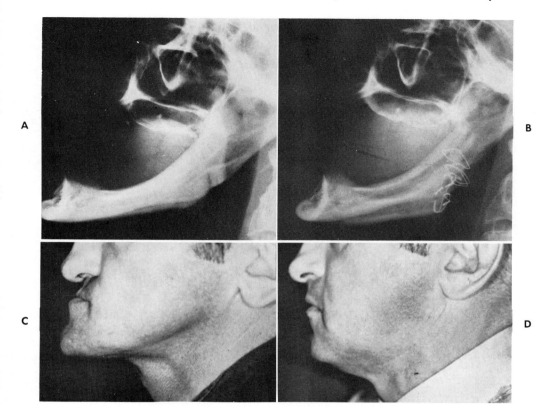

Fig. 23-18. Cephalograms of a completely edentulous patient who had a moderate degree of prognathism. He was treated by vertical osteotomy without benefit of fixation appliances. Dentures were initiated 3 weeks postoperatively and inserted 2 weeks later. **A** and **C,** Preoperative. **B** and **D,** Postoperative. (U. S. Army photographs; Letterman Army Hospital.)

my" technique for edentulous patients, careful preparation of the template from the cephalogram and measurements of its relationship are adapted arbitrarily in the osteotomy. Positive, firm, intraosseous wiring of the sectioned parts usually provides adequate fixation and intraoral "Gunning" splints are not essential.[24] Shira[111] uses preoperatively fabricated and arbitrarily related splints, the lower of which he has secured by circumferential wiring to the mandible. Either procedure is satisfactory, and healing is such that dentures can be initiated 3 to 4 weeks after surgery (Fig. 23-18).

ADVANTAGES

1. Although almost universally suitable for correction of all cases of prognathism

that we have observed over a 25-year period, the procedure is especially applicable in cases of severe prognatism. It produces ideal results in patients requiring 10 mm or more of correction.

2. Clinically union occurs in 3 to 4 weeks, and relapse or nonunion has not occurred.

3. Simple fixation appliances suffice, eliminating a need for orthodontic banding, elaborate splinting, or arch bars. (We use Stout's or multiple-loop intradental wiring in the majority of cases.)

4. As a result of advantages 2 and 3, teeth are not extruded or damaged by protracted stress.

5. Standard, commercially available instruments are used entirely.

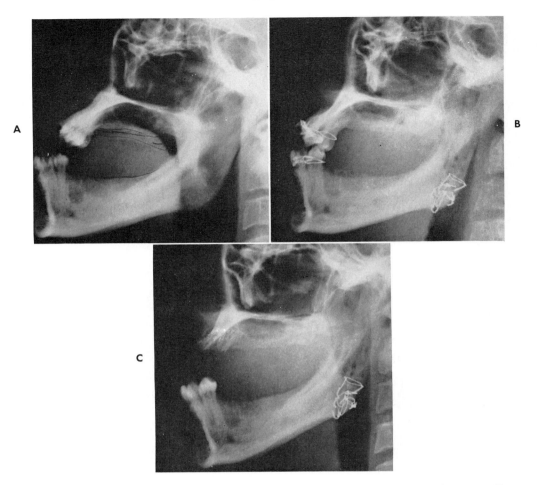

Fig. 23-19. Cephalograms of a partially edentulous patient with moderate prognathism treated by vertical osteotomy. **A,** Preoperative. **B,** Postoperative. Immobilization using Ivy loop wiring was maintained for 21 days postoperatively. **C,** Later the patient's remaining maxillary teeth were removed, and a complete upper denture and partial lower denture were furnished. (U. S. Army photographs; Letterman Army Hospital.)

6. Injury to the inferior alveolar and facial nerves can be completely avoided.

7. The body of the mandible is not shortened anteroposteriorly, and no teeth need be sacrificed as in ostectomy.

8. In addition to preservation of the alveolar ridge, the vertical dimension is positively assured in partially or completely edentulous patients, and dentures can be provided at an early date (initiated within 3 to 4 weeks) (Figs. 23-18 and 23-19).

9. Normal temporomandibular joint relation is also assured, and no joint malfunctional sequelae should occur in patients treated by this method (Fig. 23-14, *D*).

10. In addition to excellent functional results, there is a cosmetic benefit in every instance. The characteristic obtuse angle deformity is corrected at the same time a good profile is achieved. Also, since early bony union is positively assured, no "open

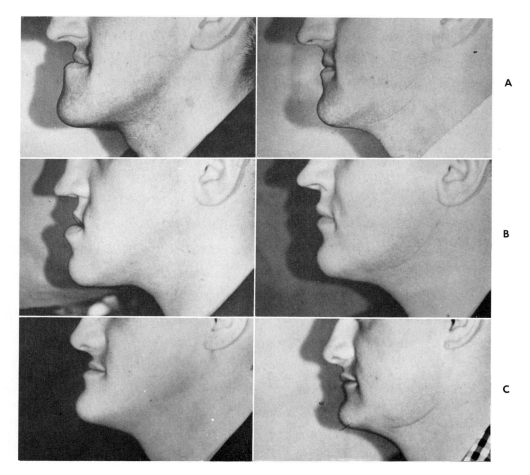

Fig. 23-20. Three patients, all with 15 mm or more of prognathism treated by vertical osteotomy in the rami, have good profiles and normal-appearing gonial angles. None was immobilized in excess of 4 weeks; all functioned normally 6 weeks after operation and were stable 1 year later. These were among the earlier cases treated, and incisions were unnecessarily long. Adequate exposure can be obtained through a 3 to 4 cm incision. **A,** Two months postoperative. **B,** Two months postoperative. **C,** Six weeks postoperative. (U. S. Army photographs; Letterman Army Hospital.)

bite deformity'' occurs. Examples of normal facial contours achieved by vertical osteotomy in the rami are illustrated in Fig. 23-20.

DISADVANTAGES

1. Operating time, which is ordinarily 2½ to 3½ hours, is not considered excessive or a disadvantage.

2. External scarring is minimal but is objected to by some patients; however, the incision line is indiscernible after 6 months in most patients. Those who, from history, tend to form keloids may be treated prophylactically at the time of surgery by local injection of steroids.

Extraoral subcondylar osteotomy (oblique)

Subcondylar osteotomy for correction of mandibular prognathism was reported by Robinson[96,98] and Hinds[44,45] from independent endeavors. Both writers described open procedures with the line of osteotomy almost identically placed in the ramus (Fig. 23-7, *B*). Robinson used a nasal saw to perform the osteotomy; Hinds made drill holes, used a No. 8 round bur to cut a connecting groove along the line of holes, and then completed the osteotomy with an osteotome. Both operated through short incisions (2-5 to 4 cm), and neither saw a need for transosseous wiring. Robinson referred to his operation as *vertical subcondylotomy*, and Hinds referred to his as *subcondylar osteotomy*. Thoma[124] referred to the same prodedure as *oblique osteotomy*. He believed it to be the ideal method by which most Class III occlusal problems could be solved. All these osteotomies were in essentially the same location anatomically, and all were reminiscent of the "vertical osteotomy" of Caldwell and Letterman,[25] the difference being that the line of bone incision was somewhat posterior to the mandibular foramen, no decortication or mortising was done, less hazard existing to the mandibular nerve, and the entire procedure was greatly simplified. Subcondylar osteotomy (oblique) is an acceptable operation for correction of mandibular prognathism, especially when protrusion is not extreme. It is a more desirable procedure than vertical osteotomy in minimal cases (less than 10 or 12 mm correction). It is definitely not the operation of choice in extreme cases (Figs. 23-15 and 23-16), and therefore preoperative appraisal must *never* be neglected. Subcondylar osteotomy must not be utilized simply because it is technically easy. Its use must be limited to cases in which it is indicated. The need for simplified, standard subcondylar technique was recognized by Robinson, Hinds, Thoma, Kruger, and many others.

Technique for extraoral subcondylar osteotomy (oblique). Extraoral subcondylar osteotomy (oblique) follows the same general technique described for vertical osteotomy except for a few modifications.

1. The incision may vary in length from 2.5 to 4 cm.

2. The line of osteotomy is scribed from

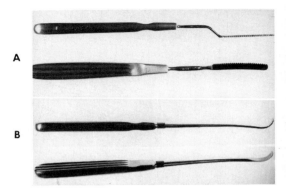

Fig. 23-21. A, Nasal saws are preferred by many surgeons for performing oblique or vertical subcondylar osteotomy in the rami. **B,** A deeply hooked side-cutting periosteal elevator (Obwegeser), essential for elevation of periosteum and muscle attachments in performance of intraoral sagittal osteotomy and necessary to permit unrestricted movement of the sectioned jaw either anteriorly or posteriorly. (Courtesy General Rose Memorial Hospital, Denver.)

the lowest point in the mandibular notch obliquely (it may be a vertical line, depending on the obtuse angle of the mandible) downward to a point on the posterior border of the ramus, 1 to 2 cm above the angle of the mandible (Fig. 23-7, *B*).

3. The osteotomy may be accomplished using a nasal saw (Fig. 23-21, *A*) or a No. 703 carbide taper fissure bur. In either case, care must be exercised to avoid injury to soft tissues on the medial surface of the ramus. However, injury to the inferior alveolar nerve or vessels is not expected, since the line of osteotomy is posterior to the mandibular foramen.

4. Musculature and periosteal covering must be elevated sufficiently to permit lateral placement of the proximal (posterior) fragment and unrestricted movement of the distal (body) fragment posteriorly to a satisfactory degree.

5. Decortication of the lateral surface just anterior to the line of osteotomy is usually not contemplated, but, if it is desirable to obtain better bone apposition of the parts, it may be accomplished as previously described on p. 506. Need for this

step in the procedure should be predetermined in the planning phase (p. 490). Decortication, if needed, is more easily done before the sectioning has been completed.

6. Transosseous wiring may or may not be used, but wire ligatures should not be applied as a means of overcoming a tendency of the proximal fragment to "bow out" or displace posteriorly. If either situation exits, the meticulous surgeon will correct it to a necessary degree by decortication as indicated.

7. The rule governing coronoidotomy applies in subcondylar osteotomy also. If posterior movement of the jaw is limited, regardless of the measurement of correction, the coronoid process should be cut free from the distal (body) fragment. If it is contemplated, this step is also easier to accomplish before the sectioning is completed.

8. The teeth are placed in occlusion as already described (vertical osteotomy). However, immobilization should be accomplished by use of well-adapted arch bars or splints for 6 to 8 weeks to ensure against unnecessary injury to the teeth (extrusion), which may occur if ordinary intradental wiring is used for this period of time.

Advantages and disadvantages are similar to those enumerated for vertical osteotomy, with the following exceptions:

1. Longer immobilization period required (6 to 8 weeks as compared with about 4 to 5 weeks for clinical healing in vertical osteotomy)
2. Probably more suitable for minimal to moderate deformities
3. Shorter operating time (1½ to 3 hours as opposed to 2½ to 3½ hours for vertical osteotomy)

Intraoral subcondylar osteotomy (oblique)

In 1968, Winstanley[135] described an intraoral technique for subcondylar osteotomy using surgical burs in a straight handpiece and approaching the ramus from the lateral aspect. The major disadvantage of the procedure was the need for excessive elevation and retraction of soft tissues for access to the lateral surface of the ramus. Hebert, Kent, and Hinds,[42] in 1970, reported using the Stryker oscillating saw and a 6-mm right-angle blade, which allowed for better visibility by way of the intraoral approach and also accomplished the osteotomy with much less soft tissue elevation. Since these first efforts, Massey[68] and others have reported refinements in the procedure and good results in 14 patients operated on. They established certain criteria for "mandibular divergence angles" that made possible the selection of patients on which the procedure would be acceptable. Others,[1,39] reporting their experience with this intraoral operation, have endorsed it but describe varied morbidity.

After intraoral vertical (oblique) osteotomy in 125 cases, Walker[130] has standardized his technique sufficiently that morbidity is minimal, and he also endorses the procedure. In our discussions, he emphasizes the importance of strict adherence to prescribed technique, use of prescribed instruments only, and good visualization. In his series of cases there has been less than 1% paresthesia, and *all* prognathic cases that he has admitted have been treated by this procedure, with the greatest correction being about 16 mm. All cases were immobilized for 8 weeks. We must endorse the operation based on reports available, but with reservation. As with any new operation, it is wise to observe the procedure before undertaking it. We prefer to correct prognathic problems by way of extraoral operations; however, patients with a history of keloid formation and those who will not accept a skin incision may be offered this operation or the sagittal splitting procedure, but they must be fully informed of possible undesirable sequelae.

Technique for intraoral subcondylar osteotomy (oblique). Intraoral subcondylar osteotomy (oblique) is undertaken in essentially the same manner as described on p. 520 for intraoral sagittal osteotomy. Fixation appliances (orthodontic or arch bars) are placed prior to the operation. The oral pharynx is

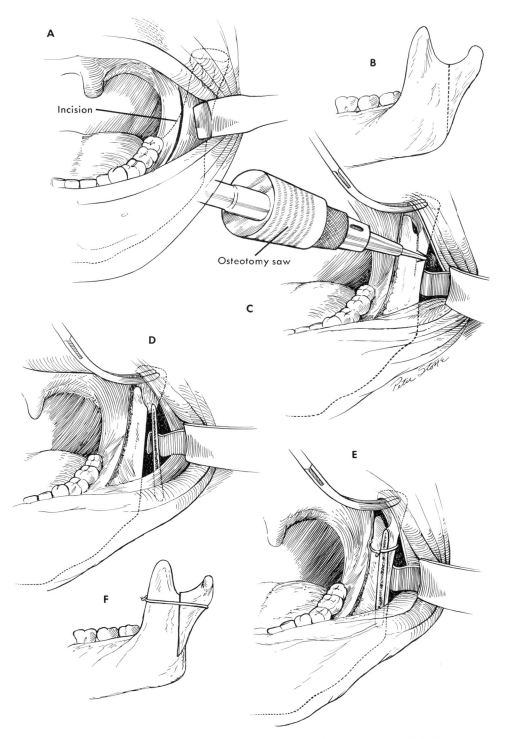

Fig. 23-22. Technique for intraoral subcondylar osteotomy (oblique). (After Hall, Chase, and Pryor.)

packed in the routine manner. The muco-periosteal incision is made firmly onto the external oblique line from about the level of the inferior alveolar foramen to the area of the first molar. The mucoperiosteal tissues are elevated superiorly and held firmly in the retracted position with Obwegeser's V coronoid retractor. The periosteal and overlying soft tissues are elevated broadly from the lateral surface of the ramus from the level of the mandibular (sigmoid) notch to the lower border of the mandible. As soon as adequate access is available, the LeVasseur-Merrill* intraoral retractor fitted with a fiberoptic light is introduced to provide visualization necessary to accomplish the osteotomy. The mandibular (sigmoid) notch, posterior border of the ramus, angle of the mandible, and convexity of bone over the mandibular foramen are positively located. With these landmarks well in mind, the osteotomy is accomplished using the Stryker gas-powered saw fitted with an 11-mm blade offset at a 20-degree angle.† The cut is made from the lowest point in the mandibular (sigmoid) notch obliquely down toward the angle or slightly above it and posterior to the mandibular foramen (Fig. 23-22). Coronoidotomy and circumramus wiring are optional depending on the surgeon's judgment of the individual case, keeping in mind the tendency of the condyle to "sag" from the glenoid fossa. Wiring is technically difficult and adds considerably to the operating time but may be essential for a good result. Routine supportive care used in all intraoral operations is necessary, including steroids to control edema, antibiotic prophylaxis to prevent infection, and vacuum drains to prevent hematoma formation.

In addition to the usual immediate postoperative swelling and lip abrasions, there may be long-term sequelae that may be of some concern. Hypoesthesia or anesthesia

---

*Available from Walter Lorenz, N. Y.
†Available from Walter Lorenz, N. Y., or Stryker Corp., Kalamazoo, Mich.

over the distribution of the mandibular nerve has been common; necrosis of the tip of the proximal segment has been reported on occasion; condyle displacement (sag) and, secondarily, occlusion relapse and anterior open bite may occur.

Horizontal osteotomy in the rami

Blair[14] first proposed horizontal osteotomy in his original article on developmental deformities in 1907. In the past many surgeons were proponents of the method, but there is never an indication for the operation today. As originally conceived this procedure appeared to be simple and consisted of passing a long, curved Blair needle or a Gigli saw guide through a short skin incision at the posterior border of the ramus, introducing the Gigli saw to the medial surface of the ramus above the foramen, and making the section. The hazards were numerous, including possible (1) injury to the branches of the facial nerve, (2) hemorrhage resulting from severance of the maxillary artery, (3) severence of the inferior alveolar nerve, which may not regenerate, resulting in permanent anesthesia to the teeth and lower lip of the injured side, and (4) injury to the parotid gland or its capsule, with formation of salivary fistula.

Because of these potential hazards, "blind" horizontal osteotomy has been discarded as an acceptable operation, and the only reason for reference to it is for its historical value. Many of today's accepted orthognathic procedures have evolved from practices and techniques of an earlier era. Perhaps the widely used intraoral sagittal osteotomy is an evolution from Blair's horizontal osteotomy of 70 years ago. One of the first modifications of the blind Gigli saw procedure was offered by Hensel[43] in his appraisal of deformities of the mandible in 1937. Based on photognathostatic studies, he specifically located the ramus osteotomy on an oblique line from high on the coronoid process downward and posteriorly to the posterior border of the ramus, passing through a central safe area midway

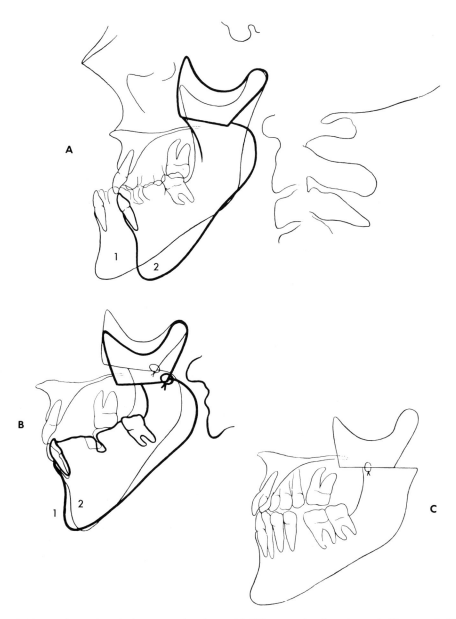

Fig. 23-23. Tracings of cephalograms of patient with 15-mm protrusion shown in **D,** corrected by extraoral horizontal sliding osteotomy with direct wiring posteriorly. **A:** *1,* Preoperative tracing **(D);** *2,* final postoperative tracing 7 months after surgery **(F).** The tip of the coronoid process has been distracted superiorly 15 mm, and the point of the mandible (menton) has been retruded 23 mm, whereas the incisal edges of the lower anterior teeth have been retruded only 13 mm. **B:** *1,* Tracings made from cephalogram 1 month postoperatively; *2,* tracing 3 months postoperatively when union was present clinically and immobilization was discontinued. **C,** Theoretical results possible by intraoral osteotomy, with transosseous wiring anteriorly preventing the open bite tendency and resisting the distracting force of the temporal muscle.

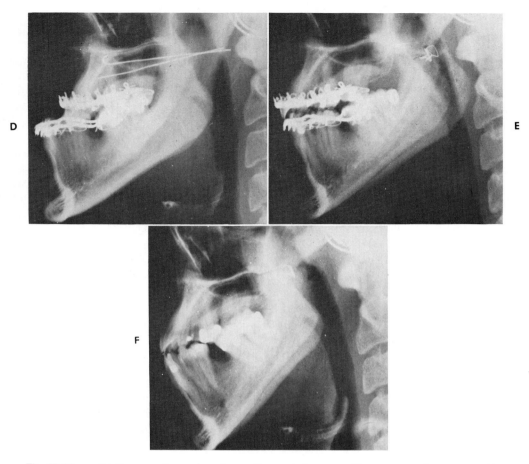

Fig. 23-23, cont'd. Preoperative and postoperative cephalograms; 15-mm protrusion corrected by horizontal sliding osteotomy. **D,** Preoperative. **E,** One month postoperatively. **F,** Follow-up, 7 months postoperatively. The anterior open bite tendency and the tendency of the vertical ramus to shorten are overwhelming because of the power of the masticator and depressor muscles, and, therefore, horizontal osteotomy is not recommended as an acceptable operation by any approach. It is illustrated here to demonstrate the power of the muscles involved with orthognathic surgery in the mandible. (U. S. Army photographs; Letterman Army Hospital.)

between the sigmoid notch and the mandibular foramen. He advocated a direct surgical approach to ensure a correct line of osteotomy.

Moose[75] in 1945 proposed an intraoral direct visualization osteotomy, which he performed with an orthopedic, power-driven, short-stroke, cross-cut saw (designed by Dr. E. A. Cayo of San Antonio, Texas). By utilizing the intraoral route the hazards of blind osteotomy were lessened. Moose also endorsed a hand saw suggested by Sloan[114] in 1951. Sloan suggested wiring the sectioned parts in apposition by looping a strand of stainless steel wire over the sigmoid notch and tying the proximal fragment down to the anterior border of the distal fragment of the ramus through a drill hole previously placed. Skaloud[113] also recommended this method of fixation, although he performed the osteotomy using a Gigli saw. The result, of course, was vertical collapse and foreshortening of the ramus.

In 1941 Kazanjian[55] advocated horizontal

osteotomy above the mandibular foramen by an extraoral Risdon submandibular approach and accomplished the section using a surgical bur. Later, in 1951, he recommended an incision through the bone on an angle using a sharp osteotome. He believed that "beveling in this fashion allowed for a greater area of contact of the cut ends, promoting early consolidation."[55] This may have been the initial conception of the Obwegeser[79]-Dal Pont[31] sagittal splitting procedure (see section on intraoral sagittal osteotomy following).

The disadvantages of horizontal osteotomies in the ramus were numerous and included a tendency to (1) open bite anteriorly produced by the power of the major masticator muscles and the counter action of the depressor muscles, (2) nonunion induced by minimal bone opposition and the displacing action of the musculature, and (3) the need for excessively long periods of immobilization resulting in secondary damage to the teeth (Fig. 23-23).

Intraoral sagittal osteotomy

Intraoral operations for correction of a wide variety of facial and jaw deformities are often indicated and desirable. Obwegeser[79] described a method of splitting the vertical ramus of the mandible sagittally. He surgically modified conditions he had noted in some traumatic fractures of the vertical ramus. His method added many improvements to earlier operations proposed by Moose, Schuchardt, and Kazanjian. Dal Pont[31] later added modifications that Obwegeser endorsed as definite improvements of the original procedure. Dal Pont's modifications ensured a broader bony contact surface and an esthetic improvement of the gonial angle. Bell and Schendel[12] have recommended an additional modification of the sagittal ramus split operation (Obwegeser-Dal Pont) that eliminates the wide detachment of periosteum and masseter and medial pterygoid muscle attachments to reduce the amount of vascular ischemia induced in the proximal fragment of the mandible when operated on by the original method. Their animal studies, beautifully illustrated, leave no doubt that the reduced elevation of tissues contiguous to the mandible results in a richer blood supply to the osteotomized bone postoperatively, thus reducing materially the incidence of complications and degree of morbidity.

Technique for intraoral sagittal osteotomy. The procedure suggested by Obwegeser and modified by Dal Pont is as follows (Figs. 23-24 to 23-26).

1. An intraoral incision over the anterior border of the vertical ramus of the mandible and the external oblique line is made through mucosa and periosteum from 1 cm. above the depths of the curve on the anterior border to the area lateral to the second bicuspid tooth. Care is taken to prevent excessive lateral retraction of buccal tissues, which would cause difficulties in final closure. Specially designed Obwegeser retractors of the Army-Navy type but with longer retracting arms provide the best retraction at this point.

2. The periosteum lateral to the mandible is elevated with a sharp broad-bladed elevator to the inferior border and posteriorly to the posterior border of the vertical ramus. A long-bladed Obwegeser retractor is inserted well into the space between periosteum and bone to retract the lateral flap.

3. Medial tissues superior to the mandibular foramen on the medial side of the vertical ramus are also elevated with a broad-bladed elevator. Care must be exercised to avoid damaging the inferior alveolar nerve, artery, and vein. For this reason, dissection is carried superiorly initially to the sigmoid notch. When this landmark has been located, dissection is carried posteriorly and slightly inferiorly to the posterior border of the vertical ramus.

4. When sufficient periosteum has been elevated medially, a channel retractor of the type recommended by Obwegeser is inserted with care to protect the inferior

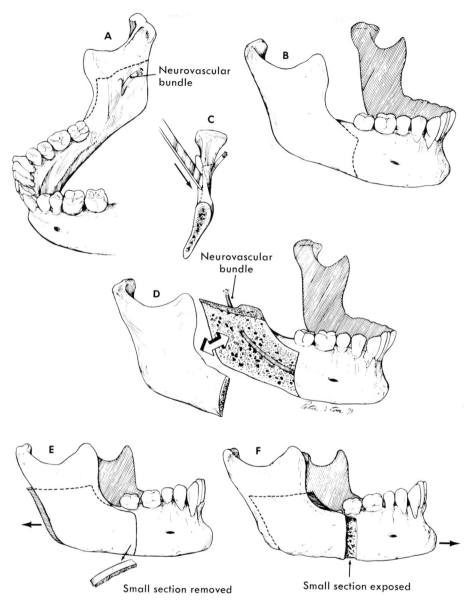

Fig. 23-24. Technique for mandibular sagittal osteotomy. This procedure requires precision in all its aspects. **A,** The medial horizontal bony incision is made from anterior border to posterior border halfway through the mediolateral thickness of the vertical ramus. **B,** The vertical bony incision is carried to the anterior limits of the external oblique ridge. The lateral bony incision is made at right angles to the inferior border of the horizontal mandibular ramus to bleeding bone. **C,** The ramus is split with an osteotome. **D,** The split ramus is separated so that the inferior alveolar neurovascular bundle may be dissected from the proximal fragment. **E,** After correction of a Class III (Angle) malocclusion, a small section of lateral bone is removed to afford good bony approximation of the segments. **F,** After correction of a Class II (Angle) malocclusion, a section of medullary bone is exposed as a result of the lengthening of the horizontal ramus.

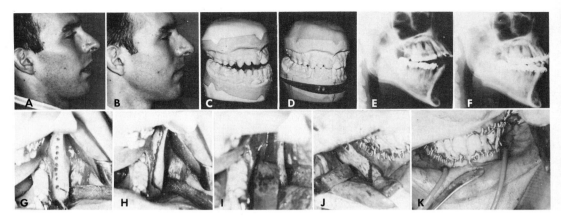

Fig. 23-25. The apertognathia of skeletal origin exhibited by this patient was treated surgically with a sagittal osteotomy of the vertical ramus of the mandible. This method is believed to provide the largest quantity of bone in apposition postoperatively. Relapse is countered by freeing all possible muscle attachments from the osteotomized segments. **A,** Preoperative profile. **B,** Postoperative profile. **C,** Preoperative model. **D,** Postoperative model. **E,** Preoperative cephalometric roentgenogram. **F,** Postoperative cephalometric roentgenogram. **G,** Exposure of operative site showing lateral bony incision and bur holes for sagittal incision on anterior border of ramus. **H,** Completed sagittal bony incision. **I,** Split segments showing exposed neurovascular bundle. **J,** Distal segment immobilized and upper border transosseous wire placed. **K,** Suction catheters in wound.

alveolar neurovascular bundle. Excessive medial retraction at this point can cause damage to the nerve and vessels as they are stretched over the sharp edges of the mandibular foramen. The technique for insertion of the channel retractor follows closely that for the elevation of the periosteum; it is inserted toward the sigmoid notch, then slightly inferiorly toward the posterior border of the vertical ramus.

5. The periosteum lateral to the mandible is now elevated from an area between the sigmoid notch and the second bicuspid tooth. The remaining tissues adherent to the posterior and inferior borders of the mandible are elevated by the properly curved, side-cutting periosteal elevator suggested by Obwegeser (Fig. 23-21, *B*). Complete elevation of these tissues is essential to the successful accomplishment of the operation.

6. The medial bony incision is accomplished by first gaining better vision of the area by making a shallow groove at the anterior end of the proposed bur cut with a Hall No. 1377-07 bur. A horizontal cut with a Hall No. 1373-15 bur is made at a level inferior enough to engage the thicker portion of the ramus in this area and superior enough to avoid the inferior alveolar neurovascular bundle. This cut is made from posterior border to anterior border to a depth of one half the mediolateral thickness of the ramus in this area. The use of an extra light source such as that provided by the Viconex system adds immeasurably to the operator's assurance of adequate visualization of the operative field.

7. The placement of the bony incision on the lateral cortical plate is now made in the area recommended by Dal Pont in his modification of Obwegeser's original operation. The anatomical configuration of the mandible lateral to the molar teeth is the key to the placement of the lateral cut. Indeed, the breadth of the area between the molar teeth and the external oblique line is the indicator whether sagittal osteotomy is surgically feasible. The lateral bony incision is made perpendicular to the in-

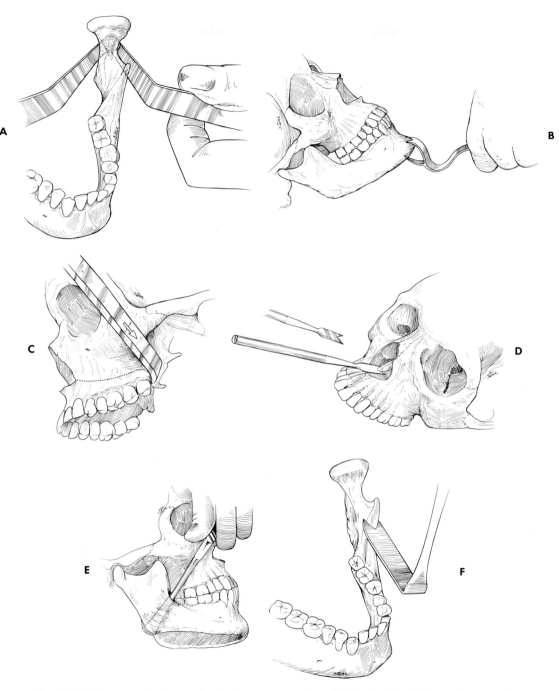

Fig. 23-26. Obwegeser instruments. **A,** Channel retractors. **B,** Chin holder. **C,** Curved pterygoid chisel. **D,** Nasal septum chisel. **E,** Curved periosteal elevator. **F,** Ramus hook-type tissue retractor.

ferior border of the mandible, down to bleeding bone, from the external oblique line to the true inferior border. The more anterior the cut, the easier the splitting procedure becomes.

8. The medial and lateral cuts are now connected along the anterior border of the ramus with a No. 700 bur. The narrow cut prepares the area for a true splitting action by the osteotomes.

9. The mandible is now split by the use of broad, thick osteotomes to which a sharp staccato blow with the surgical mallet is applied. The osteotome must be directed parallel to the lateral cortex of the ramus. Further splitting is accomplished by twisting and prying with one or two Obwegeser osteotomes at the same time. The orthopedic chisels in common use, although large enough, do not have handles that facilitate the necessary twisting action.

10. The contents of the mandibular canal are usually visualized at this time. Care must be taken to ensure that they are not adhering to the proximal fragment. The preceding steps are repeated on the other side.

11. The throat pack is now removed and the teeth fixed in the prearranged occlusion with intermaxillary fixation. The proximal fragment is now positioned and its proper length established in the case of the prognathism operation or merely properly positioned in the case of the retrognathism operation. A so-called upper border wire is placed posterior to the second molar tooth area bilaterally, with care taken that the mandibular condyle is in the glenoid fossa.

12. A suction catheter is placed lateral to the mandible along the entire length of exposed bone and brought out of the wound through a stab incision in the buccal sulcus anterior to the distal extent of the operative incision. The wound is then closed with a running horizontal mattress suture. *No pressure dressings are used.* Antibiotics and steroids such as dexamethasone (Decadron) are prescribed routinely.

Ostectomy in the body of the mandible

There is rarely an indication for *ostectomy* in the body of the mandible for correction of prognathism. When performed, it consists of the excision of a measured section of the body of the mandible to establish normal relation of the anterior teeth and correct protrusion of the lower jaw. It may be performed by an intraoral approach, an extraoral approach, or a combination of both in one or two stages.

Blair[14] described this operation first in 1907. He used a hand saw for removal of bone in the bicuspid or molar region. In 1912 Harsha[40] reported a case in which he had corrected prognathism by excision of a rhomboid section of bone from the third molar area. The section removed was wider above than at the lower border of the mandible in an effort to increase the angle from the obtuse deformity, which is characteristically observed in prognathism. He used "bone-cutting forceps and rongeurs" to accomplish the excision of bone and then placed "wire sutures to maintain apposition of bone during healing." New and Erich[78] in 1941 favored ostectomy in the bicuspid or first molar regions and preferred to accomplish the surgery by an open method "in which the mandible is exposed both externally and from within the mouth." Excision of bone was accomplished by a combination of a motor-driven circular saw, chisel, Gigli saw, and rongeurs in an effort to preserve the continuity of the mandibular nerve. In 1948 Dingman[33] made a comprehensive review of the literature on prognathism and also made a detailed appraisal of various methods utilized for its surgical correction. He had previously described in 1944 a two-stage method of ostectomy in which he overcame the disadvantage of compounding the extraoral surgical wound intraorally and at the same time avoided injury to the mandibular nerve.[32] These articles were classics and served to popularize ostectomy in treatment of prognathism.

Ostectomy, or the Dingman two-stage operation, as it is frequently referred to, was probably the most widely used of all the methods in the late 1940s and early 1950s. Thoma[125] recommended intraoral ostectomy utilizing bone drills and osteotomes. Ramus osteotomies, except horizontal, are indicated in almost 100% of prognathic mandible corrections in preference to *ostectomy* in the body by any method. *Osteotomy* in the body is indicated in certain cases, especially *asymmetrical prognathism*.

Technique for ostectomy in the body of the mandible. When correction of prognathism by ostectomy is indicated, it may be accomplished at one operation or in two stages (Figs. 23-27 to 23-29). In our opinion the two-stage approach is rarely indicated. Complete ostectomy in a single operation is much more desirable. In operations such as this that are open and directly communicate to the oral cavity, antibiotic prophylaxis starting the day prior to surgery is indicated.

1. The patient is specially prepared for the initial part of the operation by thorough washing of the face with surgical soap and scrupulous cleansing of the oral cavity. Draping is standard for operations in the mouth.

2. Incisions are made into the interdental papillae adjacent to the site of the ostectomy and also through the mucoperiosteum at the crest of the edentulous ridge if a tooth has been removed previously.

3. An incision should be carried obliquely anteriorly and downward into the buccal vestibule, one or two teeth anteriorly to the site of ostectomy.

4. Since no such oblique incision should be made on the lingual aspect of the mandible, it is usually necessary to incise papillae as far forward as the cuspid or lateral incisor to permit detachment of the lingual periosteum without tearing.

5. The mucoperiosteal flap on the buccal aspect intraorally is then elevated from the bone. Caution is exercised to protect the mental nerve. For flap retraction intraorally, a smaller periosteotome (Molt No. 9) is preferred, and therefore both the No. 2 and No. 4 Molt curets are used for periosteal detachment and elevation.

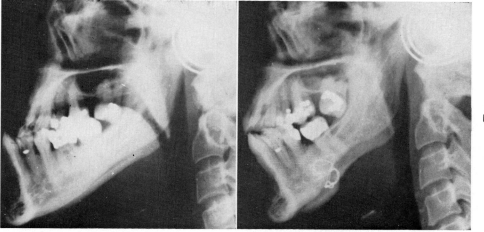

A **B**

Fig. 23-27. Lateral cephalograms of a patient with 10 mm of protrusion corrected by ostectomy in two stages. **A**, Preoperative. **B**, Postoperative. (U. S. Army photographs; Letterman Army Hospital.)

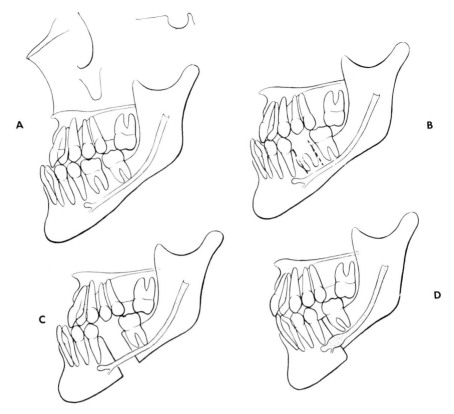

Fig. 23-28. Tracings of cephalogram in Fig. 23-27. **A,** The gonial angle was not markedly obtuse in the preoperative tracing, a satisfactory case for this operation. **B,** Intraoral first stage of bone incisions. **C,** Uninterrupted continuity of inferior alveolar nerve after second-stage ostectomy. **D,** Tracing of cephalogram 9 months postoperatively. Clinical union was present after 10 weeks of fixation by splinting of the teeth. This was an acceptable result of ostectomy, usually observed in patients with no more than 10 to 12 mm of correction necessary.

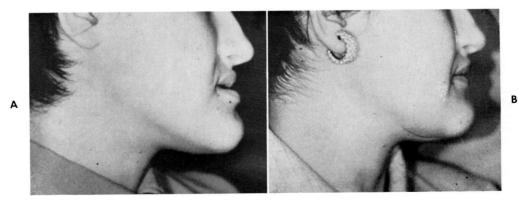

Fig. 23-29. A 20-year-old woman with only 8 mm of protrusion that was corrected by two-stage ostectomy in the body of the mandible, with excellent functional and esthetic results. **A,** Preoperative. **B,** Postoperative. (U. S. Army photographs; Letterman Army Hospital.)

6. The lingual flap is raised in a similar manner down to the mylohyoid muscle. It need not be detached at this time.

7. For precise bone incision, a caliper or measured metal template is used to guide the bone cuts.

8. Vertical cuts across the alveolar ridge are accomplished with a No. 703 fissure bur in an 18,000 rpm engine and handpiece to a safe level above the course of the mandibular nerve. They are extended as low as possible into both buccal and lingual cortices, and the alveolar portion of bone is removed by rongeur and chisel and mallet. The inferior alveolar nerve may or may not be seen at this time.

(If the operation is to be completed in one stage, the intraoral wounds are covered with moist gauze sponges but not closed. If a delayed "second stage" is planned, the following steps 9, 10, and 11 are carried out.)

9. The soft tissue flaps are closed as each side is completed, and the wounds are permitted to heal for 3 to 5 weeks before the second stage of ostectomy is undertaken.

10. During this interim period between the two surgical procedures, the fixation appliances (splints or orthodontic appliances) are prepared and inserted.

11. Local anesthesia may be utilized for all preparatory work, including the first surgical stage. The patient need not be hospitalized unless a specific, unusual reason makes this necessary.

12. The skin of the face and neck is again prepared by washing with soap and draped for the extraoral surgery, and the versatile curtain draping technique is used, since the mouth must be entered later in the operation.

13. The soft tissue dissection extraorally is carried out as previously described.

14. When the lower border of the mandible is reached, the periosteum is incised sharply, and then, using a Lane periosteotome in the left hand for retraction of soft tissue, the surgeon elevates the periosteum sharply with a Molt No. 4 curet.

15. The mental foramen will come to view quickly on the lateral aspect of the mandible, and elevation of the periosteum is carried superiorly beyond it, with caution being exercised to protect the mental nerve. Blunt spreading of soft tissues around the nerve with a curved mosquito forceps will gain relaxation of the flap as it is elevated and prevent damage to the nerve. The cuts in the lateral cortex will be visualized for orientation of the final phase of ostectomy.

16. Periosteum on the medial aspect is elevated in the same manner and with no more difficulty until the attachments of the mylohyoid muscle come into view.

17. Both the lateral and medial surfaces of the bone should be exposed for a distance of 4 to 5 cm for adequate access for bone excision without injury to soft structures.

18. A No. 703 carbide bur is used to complete the previously made bur cuts down to the lower border of the mandible. These cuts on the lateral aspect of the mandible are made through cortical bone only. The shape of the bone segment outlined by the bur cuts has been determined by previous careful measurement. For those who are more comfortable using a Stryker saw the vertical cuts can be done using a reciprocating blade.

19. When both vertical cuts through the cortex are completed, they are connected anteroposteriorly at the lower border of the mandible with the No. 703 carbide bur. (All bone cutting with the bur should be irrigated with sterile saline solution to prevent thermal damage to bone.)

20. A broad, flat-bladed periosteotome is now placed into the anteroposterior connecting cut at the lower border of the mandible and turned, thus elevating off the lateral cortex.

21. The mandibular nerve is exposed and identified by removal of cancellous bone with curets.

22. The medullary bone is removed in this manner until the dense substance of

the lingual cortex is reached. The cortical plates anterior and posterior to the cuts are undermined slightly by scooping out more medullary bone to create space into which the nerve and vessels may coil when the ends of the bone are approximated.

23. The inferior alveolar neurovascular bundle is protected with a blunt retractor (Molt No. 9), and the soft tissues lingual to the mandible are guarded with a broad Lane periosteal elevator.

24. Assuming that transosseous wiring is planned, drill holes to accommodate it are made at this time using a No. 14 bone drill in the handpiece.

25. With protection afforded as in step 12, the ostectomy is completed through the lingual cortex using the No. 703 carbide bur at 18,000 rpm under saline irrigation. As this plate of bone is removed, the mylohyoid muscle attachments must be sharply dissected free to avoid tearing.

26. Lingual ostectomy on the first side may be left incomplete until the second side is finished to afford stability of the jaw as the surgery progresses.

27. When the lingual ostectomies are completed, the transosseous wires are placed in both sides, but they should not be tightened completely at this time, merely enough to hold the parts in approximate relation with some movement still possible.

28. The mouth is now entered. Intraoral soft tissue flaps are replaced and sutured. Previously placed fixation appliances are secured and intermaxillary immobilization is accomplished with the teeth in the desired new occlusal relationship.

29. Gloves are changed, and the extraoral wound is again entered.

30. If the ostectomy was properly planned and executed, the bone ends should now be in close apposition. The wire sutures are twisted down tightly to add to the stability of the mandible during healing.

31. The wound is closed in anatomical layers as previously described, but a small rubber dam drain should be placed from deep in the wound to the outside. Since we routinely keep our dressings on for 4 days, the drain is not removed until the fourth day, when the sutures are also removed.

Technique for intraoral ostectomy. The intraoral ostectomy suggested by Thoma[125] requires more extensive reflection of buccal and lingual mucoperiosteal flaps intraorally. In fact, the buccal exposure must be to the lower border of the mandible, a procedure difficult to achieve and still protect the mental nerve. The operation should be done with the patient under general anesthesia, because complete relaxation is essential. Its application is somewhat limited, and patients with large mouths and pliable, tractable tissues are most suitable for it.

The excision of bone is achieved in the same manner as described previously, using No. 703 carbide burs in a handpiece driven by an 18,000 rpm engine, with removal of the lateral cortex, exposure and identification of the mandibular nerve, and then excision of the medial or lingual cortex. Thoma preferred long-shanked Henihan drills in a contra-angle handpiece, since they are long enough to penetrate both cortices of the bone. It is more difficult to control the progress of the bone incision with a contra-angle handpiece, and, furthermore, one can never be positive as to the exact location of the nerve until it can be uncovered laterally. It has also been difficult to perform the cuts in the precise direction desired, even when the facial muscles are completely relaxed. Completing the ostectomy from an extraoral approach is therefore preferred, unless the patient is absolutely and unalterably opposed to an external scar.

Advantages of ostectomy. The advantages are few:

1. Dissection through the soft tissue to the lower border of the mandible at the midportion of the body can be accomplished quickly, and adequate access to the site of ostectomy is acquired without difficulty.

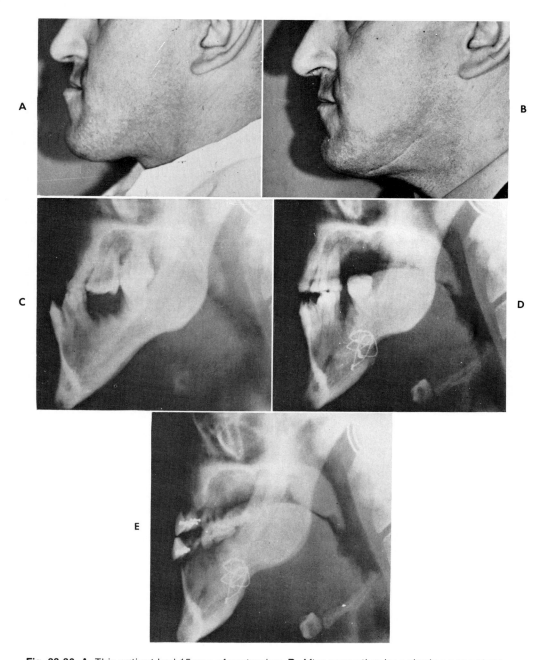

Fig. 23-30. A, This patient had 15 mm of protrusion. **B,** After correction by a single or one-stage ostectomy in the body of the mandible there appears to be a disproportionate vertical length of his face compared to the short anteroposterior length. Although he has a good postoperative profile, he does not have a desirable correction of the gonial angle. **C,** Preoperative cephalogram. Moderately advanced periodontal disease was present, indicating complete extractions and dentures after surgical correction of prognathism. **D,** Postoperative cephalogram showing downward tilt of anterior portion of mandible caused by action of depressor group of muscles, permitted by unstable periodontally involved teeth, despite interdental splints and intramaxillary immobilization. **E,** Poor skeletal profile with pronounced obtuse gonial angle present in final cephalogram. These poor results are commonplace after ostectomy in extreme prognathism. (U. S. Army photographs; Letterman Army Hospital.)

2. Excision of bone can be done without injury to the mandibular nerve, and if the nerve is damaged, it tends to recover.

3. Immobilization of the sectioned bone is possible when stable teeth are available in both fragments and the parts are secured by intraoral splinting or orthodontic appliances augmented by transosseous wire ligatures.

4. An acceptable cosmetic result can be achieved in slight to moderate cases of prognathism (Figs. 23-28, *D,* and 23-29).

Disadvantages of ostectomy. Following are the disadvantages to be considered:

1. Although a good profile can be produced in every case, a good cosmetic result is not attained in moderate to extreme cases of protrusion for the simple reason that the obtuse angle of the mandible is not corrected by the surgery. The excision of bone in the body merely shortens the length of the bone, and the obtuse gonial angle deformity is often accentuated (Figs. 23-30 and 23-31).

2. If it becomes necessary to remove more than one tooth, the sacrifice of functional surfaces is too great to contemplate this method, thus contraindicating the procedure in moderate to extreme prognathism. When two teeth on each side are sacrificed, the difference in the transverse distance between the two second molars

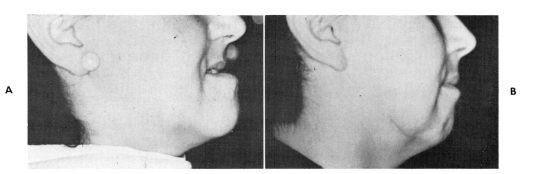

Fig. 23-31. A, Another patient (prognathism measuring 13 mm) was treated by ostectomy in the body of the mandible. **B,** The complication of nonunion occurred on one side; the angle of the mandible was not improved; scarring was conspicuous because of "bunching" or "folding" of soft tissues when the mandible was shortened. (U. S. Army photographs; Letterman Army Hospital.)

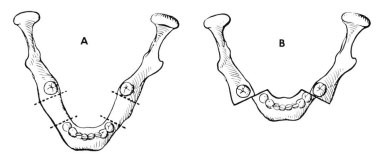

Fig. 23-32. A, Removal of a large segment of bone from the body of the mandible (ostectomy) results in imperfect bone end apposition, **B,** or excessive medial rotation of the proximal (ramus) fragments.

and the two first bicuspids is excessive, and the degree of medial rotation of the proximal fragments is unduly great (Fig. 23-32). Also one must consider the decrease in area available to the prosthodontist if the patient subsequently becomes edentulous.

3. Nonunion, although not a common occurrence, is a complication to be considered. The potential is in direct proportion to the degree of bone end approximation and postoperative immobilization, not to speak of the possibility of contamination from the oral cavity and possible postoperative infection. If, through miscalculation in bone excision, the bone ends are not in direct apposition, nonunion may occur. If as much as 2 to 3 mm of space exists, nonunion is sure to result. Absolute immobilization of the parts is also essential if union is to be assured.

4. Firm clinical union cannot be expected in much less than 8 weeks in the most favorable cases and may not be attained for up to 3 months or more.

5. It is cited as an advantage by advocates of ostectomy that the muscles of mastication are not interfered with; however, no mention is made of the action of the depressor muscles and their continual action tending to produce open bite. If this does not occur, there is the tendency of the anterior teeth to be extruded because of this muscle action. Preoperative tongue thrust

habits may add to these complications (Fig. 23-30).

6. External scarring is an objection unless ostectomy is done intraorally. This should not be objectionable if the incision is well below the lower border of the mandible and closure is carefully accomplished. However, occasionally resulting from an excessive bulk of soft tissue, an irregular scar with "folding" is observed (Fig. 23-31).

Asymmetrical mandibular prognathism

Asymmetrical mandibular prognathism is nothing more than a greater protrusion of the mandible on one side than the other, which results in *deviation* to the side of lesser growth. Hinds and Kent[46] refer to this deformity as a "horizontal asymmetry," which is a good description since there is no condylar or mandibular hypertrophy. The deformity is manifest (1) in the occlusion in which there may be unilateral or bilateral cross bite, a greater Class III discrepancy on one side, and shift at the midline to the side of lesser growth and (2) in the appearance when the prognathic look is not as dominant as the asymmetry of the lower one third of the face in a front view (Figs. 23-33 to 23-35).

Study of models will usually indicate that rotation to the side of greatest growth will produce a normal occlusion; thus, oper-

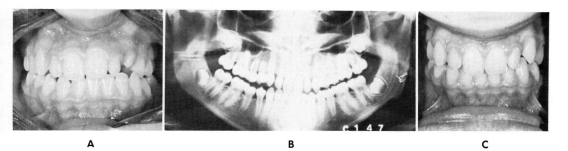

A	**B**	**C**

Fig. 23-33. A, The patient was a 14-year-old girl with marked deviation of occlusion to the left. **B,** Unilateral vertical osteotomy in the right ramus permitted rotation of occlusion to the right, resulting in bilateral Class I occlusion and normal midline, **C.** (Courtesy General Rose Memorial Hospital, Denver.)

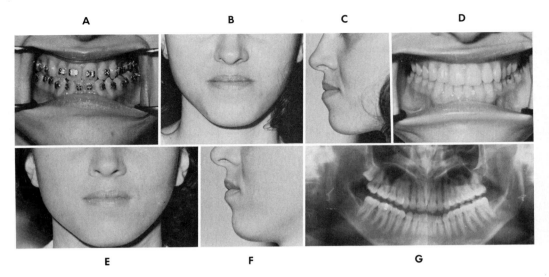

Fig. 23-34. A, The patient was a 24-year-old girl with bilateral Class III malocclusion and deviation to the left side. **B,** There was associated facial asymmetry. **C,** Prognathism was slight. **D,** Postoperative adjunctive orthodontics was minimal to achieve nearly perfect occlusion. **E,** Symmetry was restored to the face. **F,** Her profile was normal, and scarring was undetectable. **G,** Bilateral vertical ramus osteotomies were done—simple subcondylar on the right and decortication with lapping on the left—to accommodate the rotation to normal Class I occlusion. (Courtesy General Rose Memorial Hospital, Denver.)

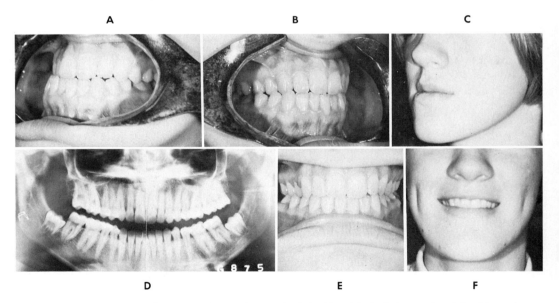

Fig. 23-35. A, There is Class III malocclusion on the left side with deviation to the right side and cross bite to the first molar occlusion, **B.** The molars are in normal Class I occlusion. **C,** There is marked asymmetry with a definite prognathic appearance. **D,** The treatment was by vertical osteotomy in the left ramus with decortication, lapping, wiring, and coronoidotomy and *osteotomy* in the body of the mandible between the second bicuspid and first molar on the right side. This panogram was made 2 months postoperatively and showed good bone healing. **E,** Normal Class I occlusion was achieved, and her face was symmetrical, **F.** (Courtesy General Rose Memorial Hospital, Denver.)

ations used for correction of ordinary prognathism are suitable for correction of most of these problems.

When there is Class I first molar relation on one side and Class III on the other, *unilateral vertical osteotomy* and rotation to that side of greatest growth will usually suffice (Fig. 23-33). Because of the rotation, the proximal fragment will overlap without lateral bowing and decortication is not needed. Osseous wiring is recommended. Also as a result of the rotation, a slight torque occurs in the temporomandibular joint on the unoperated Class I side. The joint adapts to the change, and patients as a rule have no subjective complaints. When there is extreme asymmetry (8 to 12 mm of deviation), it is better to perform a simple vertical or oblique osteotomy on the second side, with osseous wiring optional, and thus eliminate the risk of undesirable joint sequelae. If there is Class III occlusion on both sides, but more on one than the other, it is obvious that bilateral osteotomies are indicated and that decortication will probably be appropriate on the side of lesser correction (Fig. 23-34). This is associated with the lateral swing of the distal (body) fragment at the site of osteotomy in the ramus as rotation to normal occlusion is achieved. If this decortication and morticing is not done, the proximal fragment will "bow out" laterally to an undesirable degree.

When there is *normal Class I occlusion without cross bite* on one side but Class III malocclusion on the other side, plus deviation, vertical or oblique osteotomy in the ramus is indicated on the Class III side while osteotomy or ostectomy should be done in the body of the mandible on the other side at the point where discrepancy in occlusion occurs (Fig. 23-35). This body osteotomy follows the same general technique described on p. 525 for ostectomy except that a tooth need not be extracted and the operation is not staged. The vertical cut on the lateral (buccal) surface is made with a Stryker reciprocating saw or a No. 701 taper fissure bur but is made through the cortical bone only. The vertical osteotomy is begun intraorally, using the No. 701 bur to positively locate the cut in the alveolar part exactly between the teeth—again avoiding penetration into medullary space. Cortical bone on the medial surface is sectioned with a No. 703 bur, and it may be necessary to excise as much as 6 or 7 mm of this bone to permit the rotation that is necessary. Orthodontic appliances or a cast splint are recommended for fixation of this body osteotomy, since union of bone in this area takes about 8 weeks and firm immobilization is essential.

Supportive and postoperative care

The details of supportive and postoperative care must be governed by the extent of surgery and the requirement of the individual patient.

With the mandible immobilized by intermaxillary elastic ligatures, it is routine practice to pass a nasogastric tube through the unused nostril to the stomach so that it can be partially emptied by suction on completion of surgery. This does much to eliminate nausea, and if vomiting does occur, it is of such minimal proportion that no hazard to the airway develops.

If the patient is not reacting from the anesthetic when ready for transfer from the operating room to the recovery room, he should be placed on the litter or his bed *on his side* to ensure dependent drainage of fluid from the mouth. While in the recovery room he should be moved from one side to the other occasionally until he has completely reacted. It is also wise to impress on the patient that when he awakens from anesthesia his jaw will be fixed closed so that he will not fight against the appliances or become panicky. From this time on emergency instruments, such as scissors, wire cutters, and a tracheostomy set, should be immediately available at the bedside to permit immediate access to the oral pharynx in case of airway obstruction.

Fluid requirements must be met. When the patient has been deprived of fluids for several hours prior to surgery, the daily requirements must be furnished by intravenous infusion during the day of surgery. The type of replacement must be calculated individually. If an excessive blood loss has occurred, part of the replacement may be in the form of whole blood. If the patient has lost fluids through the skin (perspiring), part of the replacement may be in the form of saline infusion. The bulk of fluid replacement, however, is usually in the form of 5% glucose in distilled water or Ringer's lactate solution.

Patients undergoing this type of surgery may require antibiotics to protect against infection, but this is a matter of judgment in each case. Intraoral operations demand antibiotic protection.

Pain can be controlled by administration of appropriate opiates or analgesics.

Decreased postoperative edema has been noted when proper drainage and steroids have been employed.

Ordinarily if the patient has not voided within 6 to 8 hours after returning to the recovery ward, catheterization is indicated.

If normal bowel movements have not occurred by the third day, an enema should be ordered.

Early ambulation hastens recovery. The patient is permitted bathroom privileges on the first postoperative day, and activity is encouraged thereafter. Most patients are discharged on the third or fourth postoperative day.

The initial dressings are left in place until the fourth or fifth postoperative day at which time all sutures are removed, but the skin is immobilized with collodion gauze strips for another week or more.

Relationship of musculature to surgical correction of jaw deformities

In appraisal of various surgical methods of correction, authorities on the subject invariably consider the effect that musculature has on the healing of the jaw and the influence that this musculature may exert in causing relapse or a tendency to reversion of the part to its former malrelation.

In the past, if the cosmetic objective was achieved, the result was considered to be satisfactory even when function was impaired or bony union had not occurred. This philosophy is no longer tenable. Complete repair and good function must always be expected as well as improved appearance.

The complexities of this matter of muscle balance, abnormal stresses, and imbalance resulting from surgery vary with the extent of repositioning and the operations performed in surgical correction. The compensatory powers of the musculature are often adequate to reestablish normal function after corrective surgery, although the direction and functional length of muscles are changed. However, certain limitations to the adaptability of the musculature must be recognized and due cognizance taken when a method of surgical correction is selected.

Foremost of the muscles that potentially mitigate against good results is the temporal. It is bipennate muscle, which, according to Batson, "accounts for the *short length of the muscle fibers* and for the strong pull that this muscle exerts."[7] Batson's description of the muscle and its attachments, action, and function explains certain difficulties encountered in surgical correction of jaw deformities, especially prognathism. He states that "from anatomic evidence the temporal muscle is capable of lifting the coronoid process some fifteen millimeters and retracting it seven or eight millimeters."

The strength of the temporal muscle was noticed especially after horizontal osteotomies above the mandibular foramen when the coronoid process tended to rotate superiorly (Fig. 23-23). The tendency is present after intraoral sagittal osteotomy, but good opposition of bone and transosseous wiring prevents a problem.

Clinically we have observed that the temporal muscle places a definite restriction on the posterior repositioning of the mandible in operations in which the coronoid process is carried back with the body of the mandible (osteotomy in the condylar neck, subcondylar or oblique osteotomy and vertical osteotomy in the ramus). This places a definite limit on the amount of correction that may be successfully achieved by blind osteotomy through the neck of the condyle. We are positive of this restriction imposed by the temporal muscle, because in vertical osteotomy by the open surgical method, we have been unable to obtain adequate posterior movement in certain instances after the vertical section has been completed until the coronoid process with its muscle attachments has been sectioned free. About 1 cm seems to be the limit of repositioning freely obtainable without coronoid section.

The lateral pterygoid muscle is probably least affected of all the muscles of mastication in any of the operations for correction of prognathism. It probably also has the least effect or interference with the re-established positions of the mandible. It may tend to distract the head of the condyle after osteotomy through the condylar neck, and nonunion may result.

The medial pterygoid and masseter muscles, because of their overpowering strength, possess a great potential to cause overriding of cut bone ends after horizontal (sliding) osteotomy above the mandibular foramen, and direct transosseous wiring is unreliable to counteract the tendency. This plus the action of the hyoid depressor group of muscles creates a forceful muscle action, with the posterior teeth acting as a fulcrum, and accounts for the tendency to open bite in the anterior part of the mouth. According to Reiter[94,95] open bite does not occur in condyle osteotomy as a result of these same factors because of the counteracting action of the temporal muscle. However, bilateral traumatic fracture-dislocations of the condyles that are untreated surgically have posed many plaguing problems of open bite. On this basis it seems that the entire musculature would also operate to produce

open bite complications after osteotomy in the condylar neck.

The effect on the action and function of the medial pterygoid and the masseter muscles after vertical osteotomy in the ramus is negligible. This is because the masseter muscle is elevated intact from its mandibular attachments and the medial pterygoid is partially elevated. After the sectioning of the bone is completed and the parts repositioned, the muscle attachments are returned to essentially their original relationship, and their detached stumps are sutured together under the lower border of the newly established gonial angle. Thus healing and reattachment may occur in normal functional position as a result of shifting the location for the muscle insertions.

The depressor or suprahyoid musculature functions in harmony with the principal muscles of mastication and also the infrahyoid muscles. This group action common to muscles throughout the body may be disrupted after traumatic injury or surgical ostectomy. Interruption in unity of the body of the mandible bilaterally is followed by a tendency to distraction of the anterior segment (distal fragment) inferiorly. Thus, in addition to the part played by these muscles in contributing to the open bite tendency after osteotomy in the ramus, they also exert considerable influence toward separation of the bone ends after ostectomy in the body of the mandible and open bite anteriorly. Although not great, this effect is present and must be combated by proper fixation appliances.

The complex musculature of the tongue is another factor worthy of comment. This powerful group of muscles, by virtue of uninhibited or uncorrected "habit," is a potent factor in the tendency of the mandible to return to a preoperative protrusive or open bite relationship. Added to the actions of the depressor group, the tongue musculature has considerable displacing effect after osteotomy or ostectomy. This plus the action of the major

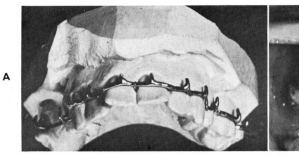
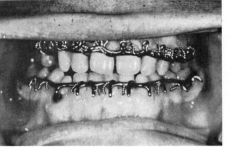

A   B

Fig. 23-36. A, Individually fabricated arch bar. Fourteen-gauge half-round clasp wire is adapted to a stone model, and 18-gauge round wire lugs are soldered or welded onto it. **B,** Mandibular individually made or custom-made arch bar. Maxillary arch bar of the commercial type. Arch bars should be adapted to stone models unless they are made of malleable metal and are readily adaptable. Otherwise they are likely to cause tooth movement or extrusion when not perfectly adapted. (U. S. Army photographs; Letterman Army Hospital.)

muscles of mastication may constitute the total force needed to overcome fixation appliances after any corrective jaw surgery. Direct transosseous wiring cannot be relied on under these conditions either. The combined force of all these muscles places a tremendous stress on the teeth bearing the fixation appliances, and over long periods of immobilization, even though this musculature may relax from trismus and compensate to a degree to new relations and length, there is undoubtedly a great potential for irreversible damage to the teeth and supporting structures. Examples of poor results for these reasons are seen in Figs. 23-23, 23-30, and 23-31. If a tendency to relapse is observed after correction of any deformities, especially in cases of apertognathia, partial glossectomy may be indicated after mobilization of the mandible.

In addition to unfavorable thrusting habits the tremendous bulk of the tongue in patients with extreme protrusion has been a matter of considerable concern. Conceivably it could result in mechanical obstruction of the oral pharynx, since the tongue, in its entirety, is also repositioned posteriorly when the mandible is retruded to desired occlusal relationship. Added to these mechanical factors is the potential of

edema. Ample precautionary postoperative observation is necessary.

Fixation appliances and immobilization

Arch bars (Fig. 23-36) or custom-made cast labial splints (Fig. 23-37) are indicated for fixation of the mandible after any corrective surgery in which immobilization is expected to extend beyond 4 weeks. They should be well adapted to afford protection to the teeth against movement or extrusion over protracted periods of immobilization.

Since it is technically difficult to remove a section of bone with absolute accuracy of measurement (as in ostectomy in segmental operations), some type of adjustable appliance should be planned. Many surgeons obtain orthodontic banding for this reason even if orthodontic treatment is not contemplated, and this may be the most practical and dependable appliance.

The simple expediency of Ivy loop or multiple-loop wiring should not be utilized except when fixation is needed for only a short period of 3 to 5 weeks. This type of fixation is utilized in vertical osteotomy, since the desired occlusion can be established with greater accuracy (Fig. 23-38).

Robinson[96] is a strong advocate of the use of an intermaxillary splint (clear acrylic

A
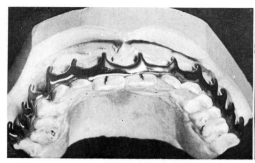
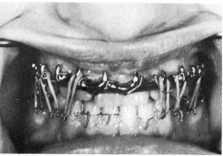
B

Fig. 23-37. **A,** Cast labial splints are more reliable than arch bars, especially when immobilization is expected to be necessary for a long time (more than 8 to 10 weeks). **B,** This appliance actually splints and protects the teeth against stresses of intermaxillary fixation. (U. S. Army photographs; Letterman Army Hospital.)

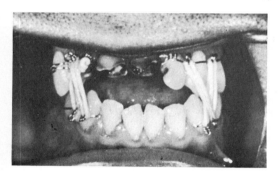

Fig. 23-38. Simple Ivy loop or multiple-loop wiring is often adequate for immobilization after vertical osteotomy in prognathism. This example of wiring used on the few remaining anterior teeth is typical of the simplicity of fixation in this particular operation. (U. S. Army photograph; Letterman Army Hospital.)

"wafer") interposed between the teeth at the time of surgery to ensure postoperative occlusion. Use of such a splint is highly desirable when many teeth are missing and a relation cannot otherwise be positively assured (Fig. 23-39). Routine use of the intermaxillary splint is not desirable or recommended, especially if good jaw relation and reasonably good occlusion are anticipated.

It has been noted already that edentulous patients with prognathism can be treated by vertical osteotomy in the ramus without benefit of intraoral splinting or immobilization, provided that firm transosseous wiring is inserted. No doubt dentures or Gunning-type splints wired to place give added stabilization and ensure correct jaw relation during healing.

Discussion

As previously stated, no single operation is universally applicable to all deformities of prognathism. Before undertaking the surgical correction of these deformities, the problem must be evaluated thoroughly by all adjunctive diagnostic means available. Preoperative planning and selection of a proper technique for correction of any given case of prognathism cannot overemphasized. When several acceptable techniques are available, the surgeon should select the method most suited to the problem. Size of individuals is variable, and it is possible that a small woman with 1 cm of protrusion of the mandible would be considered as having prognathism, whereas a large man needing 1 cm of correction might be considered as slightly prognathic. As an average, vertical osteotomy is recommended in cases requiring correction in excess of 1.5 cm.

Modification of any standard operation is

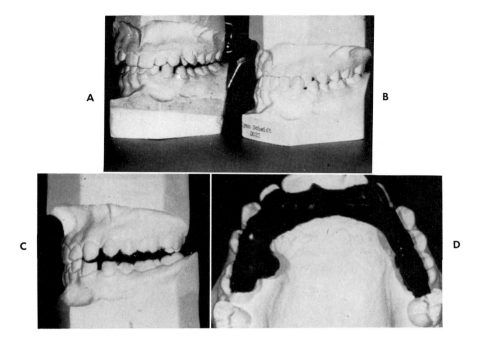

Fig. 23-39. A, A clear acrylic "wafer" interposed between the teeth at time of surgery should be used when the jaw and occlusion are insecure in the new position or if it is desirable to block the teeth from extrusion or other shifting during the period of immobilization. **B,** Study casts show lack of occlusion in bicuspid and molar areas. **C,** Study casts with interposed "wafer" to prevent extrusion of teeth that will be moved by controlled orthodontic management later. **D,** When many missing teeth make a stabilized occlusion doubtful at the time of surgery, a modified Gunning-type splint should be planned to guide the repositioning and ensure proper jaw relation through the healing period. (Courtesy General Rose Memorial Hospital, Denver.)

often needed. For example we have varied the vertical technique that we reported in 1954 many times since then, and in 1963 the most severe prognathism in our experience was treated by a modified vertical operation.[19] The patient was a 33-year-old man whose prognathism measured 32 mm. No occlusion of teeth was present because of the gross size of the mandible and its complete encirclement of the maxilla (Fig. 23-15). It was evident that correction of the problem could only be achieved in the ramus. Osteotomy at the base of the condylar neck, subcondylar (oblique) osteotomy, and vertical osteotomy were considered, but none of these procedures appeared to be acceptable (Fig. 23-16, *B* to *D*). A modified vertical operation was planned and used with good results (Fig.

23-16, *E* and *F*). Decortication, coronoidotomy, and transosseous wiring were necessary to achieve the correction. It was also necessary to obtain access through a fairly generous submandibular incision and to elevate all involved musculature to permit unrestricted posterior repositioning of the mandible. It must be concluded then that simplified techniques have a place in corrective jaw surgery, but that more difficult technical procedures must be mastered also.

Another lesson of importance is that no infallible rule exists regarding the correct age to operate on prognathic patients. The patient illustrated in Figs. 23-15 and 23-16 grew 2 inches in height from age 20 to 28, and he is certain that his mandible grew more after age 20 than during his teen-age years. He was a rare exception and should not influence criteria for surgical scheduling. However, all prognathic patients should be advised of this possibility, and most physcially mature teenage patients should have their surgery deferred and be measured cephalometrically for at least 1 year before surgery is provided. We generally believe that prognathic deformity attains its maximum when full body growh and development is attained. In boys this is usually age 16 to 18 and in girls about 2 years earlier. Psychological problems and poor social adjustment often justify consideration for surgery earlier.

MANDIBULAR HYPERTROPHY (UNILATERAL MACROGNATHIA)

Mandibular hypertrophy is a rare overgrowth of the mandible, occurring on one side only. There is associated hyperplasia of the condyle head, and the condylar neck is elongated. The deformity is characterized by extreme facial asymmetry caused by the gross enlargement of the affected side, which produces a shift of the midline to the unaffected side. Since the maxilla grows in accommodation, there is a slanted plane of occlusion, being lower on the affected side. Hinds and Kent[46] have provided a comprehensive classification of facial asymmetries, dividing these into two main categories: (1) unilateral facial overdevelopment and (2) unilateral facial underdevelopment, which will be discussed later. The condition to be discussed here is one of the more extreme types of unilateral overdevelopment. In differential diagnosis, benign tumors such as osteoma and chondroma should be ruled out.

Treatment of mandibular hypertrophy is complex, especially if the maxilla has become involved and must be subjected to surgery also. When the diagnosis is made early and interceptive condylectomy accomplished at an appropriate point in the development, maxillary osteotomy may be obviated. In fully developed hypertrophy, the maxilla must be raised, and this should be the first stage of treatment (see section on horizontal maxillary osteotomy for discussion of technique). Surgery on the mandible should follow in one operation, with condylectomy and ostectomy of the lower mandibular body on the affected side by an extended Risdon approach. Subcondylar (oblique) osteotomy in the ramus on the unaffected side may be necessary because it will permit freedom of rotation over to the affected side and up to the previously raised maxilla without putting the joint on the unaffected side into a torque relation.[28] Preauricular approach to the condyle and intraoral degloving approach to the hypertrophied body have been suggested, but we do not favor either in treatment of this particular problem for technical reasons.[46] The preauricular approach is anatomically limited, making removal of a mass the size of these hyperplastic condyles extremely difficult. Also, since contouring the lower border of the mandible can be done more accurately and with less morbidity from an extraoral view, both it and the condylectomy can be done through the one opening. Among our objections, the most serious drawback to wide intraoral incision and radical "degloving" is that perioral musculature is frequently so severely damaged that facial expression is permanently impaired and thus a second deformity is created.[21]

A brief review of procedure and technique is outlined and illustrated with three case histories showing the variables of the problem.

Case 1. A 36-year-old woman was referred by her dentist for evaluation and possible treatment of gross mandibular hypertrophy. The left side of her face was enlarged, and the midline was distorted to the unaffected side (Fig. 23-40, *A*). A flattening of the affected side with bowing out of the ramus on the unaffected side was characteristic. Viewed obliquely toward the affected side, mandibular protrusion and the overdeveloped lower border were obvious. There was a 3 cm disparity between the lower borders of the mandible as measured on the lateral cephalo-

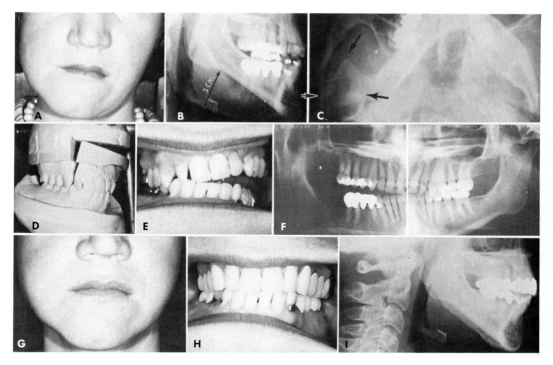

Fig. 23-40. A, Gross mandibular hypertrophy in a 36-year-old woman showing protrusion and gross downward overgrowth of mandibular body. **B,** Lateral cephalogram shows a 3-cm disparity between the lower borders of the manbible. **C,** Massive condylar hyperplasia is demonstrated in the submentovertex projection. **D,** Sectioned upper model in preparation for maxillary osteotomy and an interocclusal splint. **E,** Space between the posterior teeth after maxillary osteotomy and before mandibular surgery, which was corrected by temporary lower prostheses until mandibular surgery could be accomplished. **F,** Interocclusal space and normal maxillary plane of occlusion after maxillary osteotomy. Note enlarged condyle and elongated condylar neck on left side. **G,** Postoperative symmetry has been achieved, protrusion has been eliminated, and lower mandibular contour is normal. **H,** Restored dentition and normal occlusal plane. **I,** Bilaterally equal lower borders on a final postoperative cephalogram. The mandibular canal parallels the newly formed lower border, and a new articular condylar head has formed. (Courtesy General Rose Memorial Hospital, Denver.)

gram (Fig. 23-40, *B*). The massive size of the condyle hyperplasia is demonstrated best in a submental vertex projection (Fig. 23-40, *C*).

Workup should include face bow transfer and mounting of study models on an articulator so that a correct maxillary plane of occlusion can be established (Fig. 23-40, *D*). From this laboratory procedure an intraocclusal splint is prepared for insertion when the maxillary osteotomy is accomplished. It is fixed between the posterior teeth on the affected side, and intermaxillary fixation is secured on both sides. In addition, a suspension wire is run from the zygomatic arch to further secure the maxilla in its raised position.

Treatment included maxillary surgery as well as the final mandibular procedure. The maxillary surgery in this case was in two stages, the palatal procedure preceding the second procedure by 19 days. Anesthesia was induced with methohexital (Brevital) and halothane (Fluothane) for both procedures. There was appreciable blood loss during the second procedure, but the patient did not receive a tranfusion then. However, because of the unexpected development of anemia, she did receive a tranfusion on the first postoperative day and had an allergic reaction to transfusion. Six days after the operation the patient became jaundiced, and 4 days later hepatitis was positively diagnosed. This complication occurred too soon to be attributed to the whole blood transfusion, and twice-used halothane was considered to be the cause. Because of this problem, the mandibular surgery was postponed indefinitely and a semipermanent removable prosthesis was provided for an interim functional occulsion in the interocclusal space (Fig. 23-40, *E*). The normal maxillary occlusal plane was maintained through this waiting period. A Panorex film shows the intermaxillary space, well-healed maxillary osteotomy, aerated maxillary sinuses, and elongated hyperplastic left condyle (Fig. 23-40, *F*). Normally the final mandibular operation would be scheduled 6 or 8 weeks after the maxillary surgery. In this case it was deferred 8 months.

The mandibular procedure that we prefer and that was used in this case is as follows:

1. A submandibular approach to the condyle area is accomplished in the usual way through a fairly long incision.

2. When the mandibular (sigmoid) notch is identified, a Thompson ramus retractor is installed, and the periosteum is further elevated, exposing the joint and as much of the condyle as possible. Strong distraction of the ramus using a bone-holding forceps clamped to the angle facilitates access. The condyle is freed as completely as possible prior to osteotomy.

3. A straightforward bur cut is made through the neck of the condyle beginning at the sigmoid notch and extending horizontally to the posterior border. If the situation warrants, the osteotomy can be completed with a chisel, but undesirable vertical splitting may result in a jagged uneven stump.

4. When the horizontal osteotomy at the neck is completed, the mandible is again distracted downward and a Kocher forceps is clamped onto the neck of the condyle. Rotation of the condyle permits access and visualization of the medial surface and further freeing of the condyle by blunt dissection. It is better to detach the lateral pterygoid muscle in this manner than to simply tear the condyle free from it, although there is a certain amount of disengagement by tearing in any condylectomy.

5. Once the condyle is removed, the depth of the wound is packed with hot, moist, gauze compresses.

6. Ostectomy of the hypertrophied lower mandibular body is then begun by scribing on the lateral surface a design for the cut using a No. 703 carbide bur. It should not necessarily paral-lel the lower border, since the contour in hypertrophy is usually abnormal. It is important to carefully estimate the distance of the mandibular canal from the lower border and to try to stay just below this level.

7. If there is doubt about the location and level of the canal, decortication of the lateral cortex can be carried out and the course of the canal identified.

8. Usually the ostectomy is accomplished in a straightforward way, but the cut through to the medial cortex is completed with a smaller size bur (No. 702 or No. 701).

9. Since the hypertrophied side is usually flattened and deficient in lateral contour, even after condylectomy permits a swing to the affected side, the excised bone from the lower border may be saved and onlaid onto the lateral surface just above the newly created lower border. A plumping effect can thus be achieved.

10. If there is any restricting influence from the unaffected side a subcondylar (oblique) osteotomy should be done on that side at this time. Since this is usually necessary, access should be planned for in preparation and draping. The unaffected side should be draped in view anyway so that it is available for comparison as the ostectomy is designed and accomplished.

11. The jaw is immobilized for about 3 weeks, and then light intermaxillary elastic ligatures are maintained for another 2 to 3 weeks to guide occlusion and help develop a new and functional joint at the site of condylectomy.

Symmetry has been achieved in this case (Fig. 23-40, *G*). The protrusion has been eliminated, and the contour of the mandible on the affected side is normal postoperatively. The line of the incision crosses the crease lines in the skin, but this was necessary for good access to the bone surgery. The patient had complete rehabilitation of her dentition and now has an excellent functional occlusion with a normal plane (Fig. 23-40, *H*). The lower border of the mandible is equal bilaterally as viewed in a postoperative cephalogram (Fig. 23-40, *E*). On the postoperative Panorex film the mandibular canal runs parallel and immediately adjacent to the lower border on the operated side. The patient had no nerve damage. A new functional articular surface has formed at the site of condylectomy, and the patient can open her mouth to a normal degree with minimal deviation.

Case 2. A 55-year-old woman was referred by her dentist for correction of gross mandibular

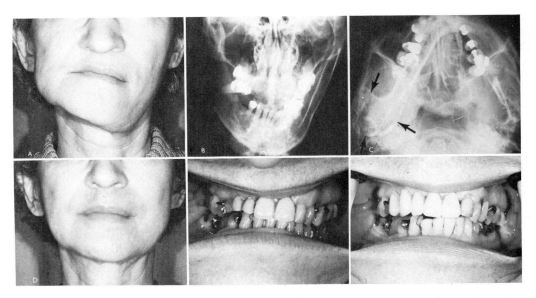

Fig. 23-41. A, Asymmetry typical of mandibular hypertrophy—grossly enlarged, elongated, and flattened affected side with the midline swinging to right unaffected side, which flares outward. There is a slight protrusion of lower jaw and gross overgrowth downward. **B,** Posteroanterior x-ray film shows grossly enlarged condyle and elongated neck, a long, flat ramus and body on the affected left side, and deviated midline. **C,** Arrows point to grossly hyperplastic condyle on submentovertex x-ray film. **D,** Postoperative facial symmetry. **E,** Preoperative view shows only slight slanting of the occlusal plane and poor dentition. **F,** Postoperative view shows acceptable plane of occlusion but more restorative dentistry needed. (Courtesy General Rose Memorial Hospital, Denver.)

hypertrophy. The left side of her face was enlarged, and the midline was distorted to the unaffected side. There was the characteristic flatness of the affected side and the bowing out of the unaffected side (Fig. 23-41, *A*). The long circular extent of the hypertrophied mandible was pronounced, and there was a slight protrusion. The maxillary plane of occlusion was slanted down to the affected side, but only modestly, and the dentition was generally poor. The posteroanterior skull x-ray film exhibited exactly what would be expected after examining the patient: (1) a grossly enlarged condyle with an elongated neck and (2) a long, flat ramus and body on the affected left side, deviated midline, and rotated unaffected right mandible (Fig. 23-41, *B*). The typical grossly enlarged left condyle is again well visualized in the submental vertex projection (Fig. 23-41, *C*). The treatment plan in this case did not include maxillary osteotomy, since the plane of occlusion was not that far off (Fig. 23-41, *E*), and it was expected that a good functional occlusion could be provided by dental prosthesis and rehabilitation. Surgery to correct

her deformity therefore was accomplished in one operation. It included condylectomy of the hyperplastic left condyle, ostectomy of the hypertrophic lower portion of the left mandibular body, and free augmentation graft to the lateral surface using the excised lower border. Subcondylar (oblique) osteotomy was also done in the ramus of the right or unaffected side. The patient's postoperative appearance was symmetrical (Fig. 23-41, *D*), her profile was normal, and the plane of occlusion was acceptable (Fig. 23-41, *F*).

Case 3. A 23-year-old man was referred with the identical facial characteristics and roentgenographic findings as those seen in Cases 1 and 2 (Fig. 23-42, *A*). The only difference was seen clinically in his occlusion. He had an open bite on the right side with a slanted mandibular occlusal plane and early cross bite on the left. The maxilla was level and had not, as yet, tended to accommodate by growth downward on the affected side (Fig. 23-42, *B*). Treatment included removal of the hyperplastic right condyle and excision of the hypertrophic lower border of the

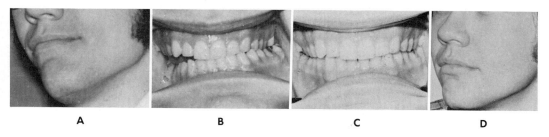

Fig. 23-42. A, A 23-year-old man with the typical asymmetrical face characteristic of mandibular hypertrophy. Radiographs showed hyperplasia of the right condyle and an increase in the vertical height of the body of the mandible. **B,** The maxillary occlusal plane was level while the mandibular plane was slanted as a result of canting of the mandible, which resulted in unilateral open bite on the right side. **C,** The open bite was corrected by removal of the hyperplastic right condyle. **D,** Vertical shortening from condylectomy plus excision of the lower border of the right mandibular body produced a symmetrical face. (Courtesy General Rose Memorial Hospital, Denver.)

mandibular body—all through a submandibular incision. Preoperative plans included simple vertical osteotomy in the left ramus, but this was not done since perfect occlusion occurred after the condyle was removed (Fig. 23-42, *C*). Immobilization was by intramaxillary multiple loop wiring for 3½ weeks, after which function was encouraged and light "guide elastics" were used on the normal left side only to aid in establishment of a new articulation in the area of the temporomandibular joint. This light elastic guidance was continued for 5 additional weeks. Normal function developed as well as normal facial symmetry (Fig. 23-42, *D* and *E*).

The treatment of these rarely seen and difficult problems is interesting. The results are more certain and gratifying than those obtained in the other extreme asymmetrical condition of agenesis described later. Perhaps as more of these unusual deformities are treated and reported, more knowledge will be available and better service can be provided.

MICROGNATHIA AND RETROGNATHIA

A distinction should be made between *micrognathia* and *retrognathia*. Micrognathia is defined as abnormal smallness of the jaw, especially the lower jaw, whereas retrognathia simply implies a retruded position (Angle's Class II) of the mandible without diminution. Another term deserving

definition is *microgenia,* or abnormal smallness of the chin. Surgical correction of the micrognathic mandible has always been a more difficult undertaking than correction of prognathic deformities. Two principle reasons account for the difficulty: (1) bony substance in which to perform osteotomy is minimal. and (2) availability of investing soft tissue to cover the surgically elongated jaw may also be less than adequate or desirable.

An ideal surgical technique for correction of mandibular micrognathism should provide (1) improved acceptable occlusion of the teeth into Angle's Class I relation, (2) cosmetic benefits, including mental prominence and pronounced gonial angle, (3) psychological benefits, (4) improved phonetics, and (5) technical feasibility including (a) adequate bone contact at site of osteotomy to ensure bony union, (b) minimal or no injury to important anatomical structures such as contents of mandibular canal, (c) surgical repair and closure assuring no permanent disruption of function, and (d) reasonable operating time.

Innumerable operations have been suggested for the correction of this deformity. Blair,[14] in his article published in 1907, advocated oblique section of the ramus at the level of the mandibular foramen. In 1909 he reported two cases treated in that manner.[15] In 1928 Limberg[66] reviewed the literature on this subject. At that time a number of methods had already been advocated for osteotomy and forward repositioning of the mandible in micrognathia. He proposed a "step" operation in the body of the mandible, with the addition of a rib graft. He credited Pehr Gadd (1906) with the original conception of the principle of step sliding osteotomy in the body of the mandible, which was commonly employed in correction of micrognathia or retrognathia. In 1936 Kazanjian[54] described an L-shaped sliding osteotomy that is suitable for correction of the deformity also. This and the step procedure were the principal operations used up until the mid 1950s. If teeth are present in the ridge posterior to the proposed location for osteotomy, the L-shaped incision in the bone was preferred, since bony contact could be assured. Obwegeser[79] suggested vertical (sagittal) splitting of the posterior body of the mandible anteroposteriorly through the lower portion of the ramus and gonial angle. Caldwell and Amaral[22] and Robinson [97] modified the vertical ramus osteotomy used in prognathic cases and added iliac bone to permit advancement of the mandible. This mortised inlaid onlay of autogenous bone provides desirable additional substance. The procedure is indicated in selected cases and will be discussed in further detail. Thoma[124] suggested using a rib graft instead of illiac bone. When more prominence at the gonial angle is desirable, he recommended securing the rib with attached cartilage from the costochondral junction, since projecting cartilage at the gonial angle will not resorb as does bone. Robinson and Lytle[100] reported 14 micrognathic patients surgically corrected by the same vertical (or oblique) section in the ramus, but bone was not added. Wire sutures were inserted to ensure bone contact and union. This is similar to the procedure that Limberg[65] reported in 1925 for correction of open bite deformity. In view of the newer vertical L or C osteotomy, this simple vertical osteotomy of Robinson's is not recommended because of the minimal

bony contact, loss of gonial angle, tendency to distract the condyle head, and regression. In 1968 Caldwell, Hayward, and Lister[23] presented a new approach to this difficult problem and with their methods have eliminated to a great extent many shortcomings and technical difficulties encountered heretofore in the previously accepted standard operations. Details of the surgical technique will be described later in the text. This technique more nearly satisfies criteria for an ideal surgical approach for correction of either micrognathia or retrognathia. In 1973, however, Hayes[41] reported modification of this procedure by "sagittal separation in the inferior region of the body of the mandible." We agree that sagittal osteotomy as he suggests "produces better bone contact than the 'C' osteotomy and is technically easier than the intra-oral sagittal procedure." We have adapted this modification to our techniques and recommended its general acceptance. Details are included later in the text.

Preparation for surgery

Planning of surgery for the correction of micrognathia must be meticulous and detailed. The workup should follow the outline found on pp. 485-492. The cardboard templates are made from cephalometric roentgenograms (Figs. 23-44, 23-51, and 23-57).

Since the body of the mandible in micrognathia is smaller than normal, when osteotomy is contemplated in this area, it must be determined that a sufficient bulk of bone exists to afford ample apposition of bone and union. The mandibular notch anterior to the gonial angle is often accentuated, and it is the vertical dimension from this area to the apices of the molar teeth above that may limit use of L or C osteotomy. This vertical dimension can be determined by use of cephalograms and the Panorex x-ray film; however, there is no way to accurately measure the *mediolateral thickness* of the mandible, and for that reason, sagittal splitting as suggested by Hayes[41] may be im-

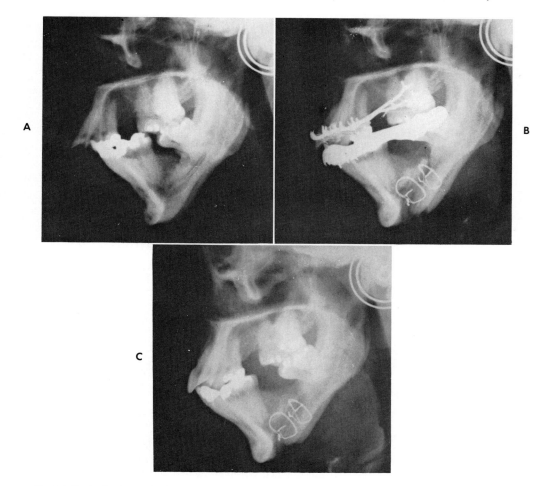

Fig. 23-43. A, Cephalogram of patient with micrognathia, requiring 11 mm of forward movement. **B,** Corrected by step sliding osteotomy and addition of autogenous bone chips, with fixation by sectional screw lock splints. Splinting was supplemented by intermaxillary fixation for 1 month. **C,** After 3 months of intradental splint fixation, union had occurred. (U. S. Army photographs; Letterman Army Hospital.)

possible because of the thinness of bone at the planned location for osteotomy. When splitting is in the preoperative plan, but on exposure, the bone is found to be so thin that splitting may result in unplanned fracture, the standard L osteotomy may be resorted to as an alternative.

There is infrequently an indication for step or "sliding L" osteotomies in the body of the mandible (Fig. 23-44); however, the need may arise in rare cases. Apposition of bone along the horizontal cut can be as-

sured as the mandible is moved forward in step or L osteotomies in the body of the mandible if no teeth are located posterior to the vertical incision in the alveolar ridge. However, if teeth in the proximal (posterior) portion occlude with maxillary teeth, an appreciable space may result between the cut fragments (Fig. 23-44, *B*). Plans for a step operation should be discarded if it is evident that bony contact between the cut sections will be inadequate for union to occur. Addition of autogenous bone chips

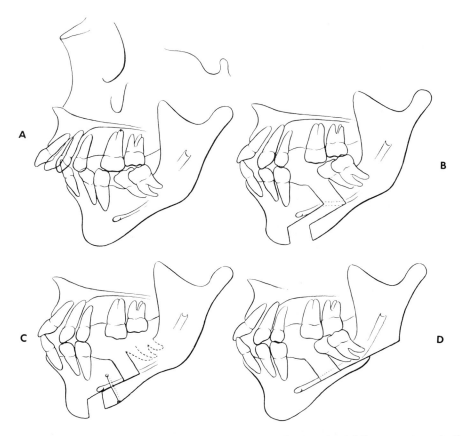

Fig. 23-44. The value of tracings of lateral cephalograms in planning sliding osteotomy in the body of the mandible is illustrated (case shown in Fig. 23-40). **A,** The lack of adequate medullary space between the apices of the teeth and the relatively thick lower cortical border make section without injury to the neurovascular bundle technically impossible. **B,** The deformity was corrected by step sliding osteotomy in an effort to protect the contents of the canal, but voids thus created had to be filled with bone chips to assure union (see Fig. 23-43, *B*). **C,** Had there not been teeth in the proximal (posterior) fragment, contact on the horizontal plane could have been attained, but fixation of one part to the other would have been by transosseous wiring only. **D,** The cosmetic result would be poor, with practically no gonial angle in this L osteotomy. In either operation, stretching of the neurovascular bundle will result in hypoesthesia or prolonged anesthesia even though it remains intact.

from the ilium affords one solution; however, selection of another operation is better.

If the lower third of the face is exceptionally tiny, ramus osteotomy with addition of iliac bone or rib should be considered. If the bulk of the bone seems to be adequate, the L or C osteotomy in the rami is no doubt the method of choice, especially if sagittal splitting of the body portion can be a part of the plan.

Technique for step sliding osteotomy. It has been suggested that this operation be done in two stages on the premise that there is less likelihood of creating a compound wound into the oral cavity and that chances for injury to the mandibular nerve are minimized.[33] This is a suggestion worthy of consideration, even though it is exceedingly difficult to avoid injury to the mandibular nerve. Also, because periosteum is inelastic, it is inconceivable that the man-

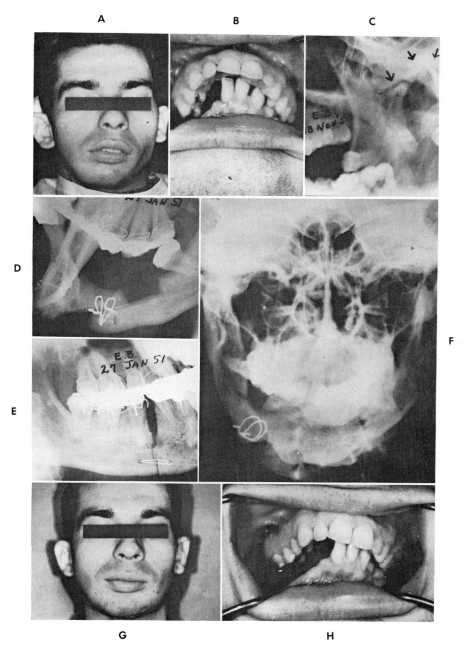

Fig. 23-45. A, Unilateral facial deformity caused by osteomyelitis, with loss of much of the right ramus and mandible when the patient was 6 years of age. **B,** Class II malocclusion resulting. **C,** Pseudoarthrosis of right temporomandibular joint (false joint indicated by lowest arrow, glenoid fossa above and posteriorly). **D,** Right mandible lengthened by step sliding osteotomy. **E,** Left mandible sectioned to permit "swinging" advancement of right side. **F,** Union of bone with bilateral symmetry. **G,** Unaffected left side of face was contoured with a cartilage onlay implanted for final facial symmetry. **H,** Improved occlusion and jaw relation, making replacement of missing teeth possible. (L or C osteotomy in the ramus with or without sagittal splitting would also be acceptable.) (U. S. Army photographs; Letterman Army Hospital.)

dible can be elongated in this step sliding osteotomy without interrupting the continuity of the oral soft tissues at some point, either by frank laceration or detachment of gingival margins. It is recommended that step sliding osteotomy be performed in one operation, following essentially the same technique as described for ostectomy in correction of mandibular prognathism (p. 525). Exceptions to that technique and other considerations include the following:

1. As a rule the whole procedure can be accomplished by an extraoral submandibular approach; however, preparation of skin and draping should include the oral cavity and curtain draping, since splinting and intermaxillary immobilization must be attended to when the osteotomies are completed.

2. The incision must be of sufficient length to permit access without undue trauma to the soft tissues; however, if deeper tissues and periosteum are opened sufficiently to allow for instrument ma-

nipulation, the skin incision may be kept to 4 or 5 cm in length.

3. The Stryker reciprocating saw and a No. 702 carbide fissure bur are used to make the vertical cuts.

4. A horizontal cut is then carried posteriorly, paralleling the plane of occlusion. The Stryker oscillating saw with a 3-mm blade or burs are employed for this purpose. If the inferior alveolar nerve is cut or otherwise injured it usually regenerates.

5. Final separation of the bone through the cuts may be facilitated with a thin, flat chisel and mallet or simply by placing the edge of a Lane periosteal elevator into cuts and prying the bone apart gently. Frequently, incompletely severed areas can be freed in this manner.

6. At this point the mouth is entered and the teeth are fixed into occlusion, which has been previously determined. It is essential that splints or orthodontic appliances be planned. The connections that have been

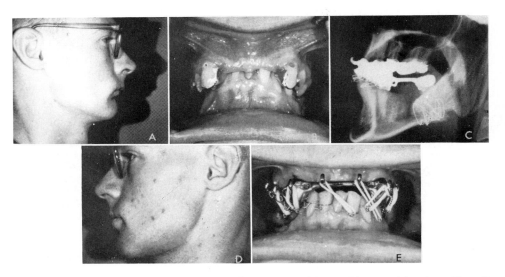

Fig. 23-46. A, Young man with retrognathia. **B,** Nonrestorable dentition resulting from Class II malocclusion with complete lingual version of all mandibular posterior teeth on the right side. **C,** Postoperative profile roentgenogram shows step sliding osteotomy and prominence of gonial angle retained. **D,** Stronger appearance of jaw and face with improved lower lip relation. **E,** Improved occlusion permitted dental rehabilitation. (Courtesy General Rose Memorial Hospital, Denver.)

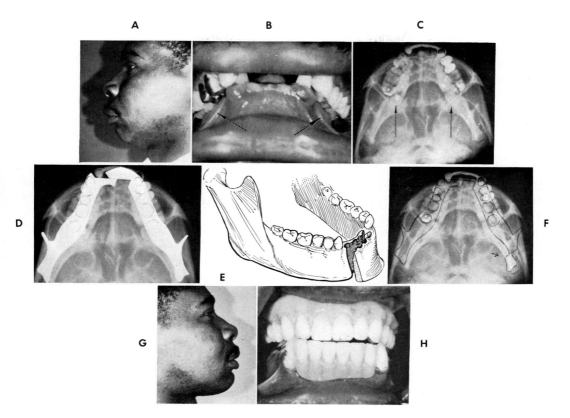

Fig. 23-47. A, The profile view of a patient who appears to have a receding lower jaw gives a *false* impression. **B,** Anteroposteriorly the teeth are in Class I relation, but buccolingually there is *no* occlusion—the whole lower arch closes into the palate of the maxilla. **C,** A submentovertex roentgenogram clearly shows the mandibular teeth in lingual version to the maxillary teeth. **D,** A paper cutout traced from the roentgenogram was "step" cut to show how expansion of the mandible could be obtained to establish proper occlusal relation in the posterior teeth. However, if the whole body of the mandible is moved laterally on each side, the *condyle* also moves laterally from the glenoid fossa. **E,** By an extraoral submental approach, the step expansion of the mandibular symphysis was done by osteotomy through the labial cortex in one lateral incisor area, across the midline, and out through the lingual cortex in the other lateral incisor area. The lower four incisor teeth had been removed to allow for the procedure. There was no problem maintaining the symphysis in the expanded relation using a cast metal lingual splint, but there was a tendency to relapse posteriorly with collapse medially as healing progressed. **F,** A line tracing on the roentgenogram shows that the problem in **D** was overcome by subcondylar oblique osteotomy bilaterally (arrow). **G,** The final result was excellent cosmetically. **H,** A full upper denture was furnished to replace the upper natural teeth, since the lingual alveolar bone support was entirely destroyed by trauma from the relation of the lower teeth preoperatively. Six lower incisors were needed to replace the four lower natural teeth that had been sacrificed to allow for symphysis expansion. To ensure lateral expansion of the mandible posteriorly, it may be necessary to do coronoidotomies, and detach sphenomandibular ligaments at the lingula bilaterally as well as subcondylar (oblique) osteotomies.

arranged are placed to stabilize the sectioned dental arch.

7. The intraoral instruments are discarded, gloves are changed, the curtain drapes are readjusted to expose the surgical field, and the paralleled edges of the horizontal cuts are wired together.

8. Closure and dressings are as previously described. The technique is illustrated in Figs. 23-43, 23-44, *B* and *C,* and 23-45.

Horizontal L sliding osteotomy (Fig. 23-44, *D*). Horizontal L sliding osteotomy is a variation of the step operation that has just been described, and it is performed in essentially the same manner. However, if this design is ever indicated it is better to discontinue the horizontal cut anterior to the angle and complete the osteotomy with a vertical step that will leave the prominence of the gonial angle for a better esthetic result (Fig. 23-46).

The principle of step operations to secure elongation of the mandible may also be utilized to correct other abnormalities in jaw relationship. For example, the patient illustrated in Fig. 23-47 had a Class I jaw relation, but with no occlusion of teeth. The entire mandibular arch was in lingual version to the maxillary arch, with contact of buccal surfaces of the lower teeth to lingual surfaces of the upper teeth. At one time the patient had gross anterior maxillary protrusion, but when we first saw the patient, an effort had been made to correct this cosmetic problem with a six-tooth anterior bridge. The step operation was used in this case to *widen* the mandible (Fig. 23-47, *E*).

Vertical osteotomy in the rami with bone grafting

In 1954 Caldwell and Letterman[25] predicted that modification of vertical osteotomy as it is utilized in correction of prognathism would also make possible correction of micrognathia. In 1960 the technique was completely described.[22] The principles of vertical section in the ramus, coronoidotomy, and decortication are applicable in this operation. The objectives are (1) separation of the ramus vertically from the mandibular notch to the lower border of the mandible at the angle in a line over or just posterior to the mandibular foramen (Fig. 23-48, *B*), (2) angular section of the coronoid process from the mandibular notch obliquely downward and forward to the anterior border to permit forward repositioning of the distal fragment (body and anterior ramus) without interference (Fig. 23-48, *B*), (3) decortication of the lateral cortex over a broad area of the lower aspect of the ramus as a recipient area for bone graft (Fig. 23-48, *D* and *E*), (4) movement forward of the distal (body of the mandible) fragment to the desired occlusal relation (Fig. 23-48, *B* and *F*), (5) interposition between the fragments and onlay into the decorticated area of a measured full-thickness block section of bone from the crest of the ilium (Fig. 23-48, *G* to *I*).

Technique for vertical osteotomy in the rami with bone grafting. The basic approach is similar to that for prognathism.

1. The patient is prepared and draped in the manner already described. In addition, the pubic area is shaved the day before, and the iliac donor site is prepared and draped for the removal of the bone for grafting.

2. The lateral aspect of the ramus is exposed in the manner already described, and the prominence of the mandibular foramen is identified.

3. A vertical cut is made from the mandibular notch to the lower border of the mandible as described for vertical osteotomy in prognathism, and the coronoid process is also detached in the same manner.

4. The course of the mandibular canal from the foramen downward and anteriorly is extimated and so marked with a surgical marking pen.

5. Multiple drill penetrations are made into the lateral cortex from the mandibular foramen and the estimated level of the mandibular canal to the lower border of the mandible. They are extended from the pos-

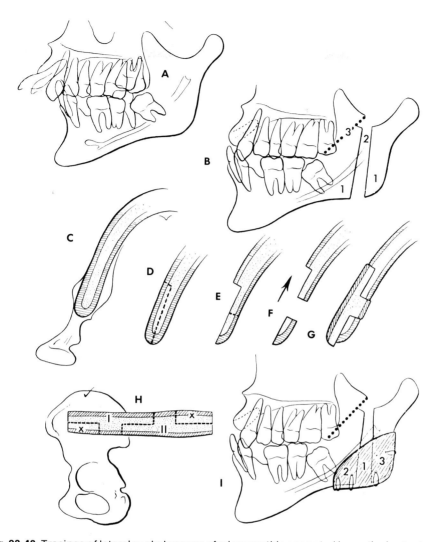

Fig. 23-48. Tracings of lateral cephalograms of micrognathia corrected by *vertical osteotomy* with bone graft. **A,** Protrusion of maxillary anterior teeth and retrusion of the mandible. One centimeter of discrepancy in incisal relation corrected by removal of maxillary anterior teeth and moderate alveolectomy and 1 cm of discrepancy corrected by movement of the whole mandible forward. **B,** Technique of procedure: *1,* areas decorticated on lateral aspect of ramus; *2,* vertical section of ramus over mandibular foramen; *3,* oblique section of coronoid process to permit it to remain in proper relation with temporal muscle as mandible is moved forward. **C,** Mandible viewed from below; lined areas represent lower border and lateral and medial cortices. **D,** Heavy broken line indicates extent of decortication on lateral aspect of ramus as viewed from below. **E,** Lateral cortex removed and vertical section made (dark dotted line). **F,** Body of mandible moved anteriorly the desired distance. **G,** Bone graft from ilium onlaid onto decorticated lateral aspect of ramus with full-thickness graft filling void created by forward movement of mandible. **H,** Iliac graft viewed from the crest of ilium showing method of sectioning graft for both sides of mandible: *I,* graft for left side; *II,* graft for right side; *X,* shaved-off medullary bone for use as filler chips. **I,** Bone graft wired into place: *1,* full-thickness graft in void; *2* and *3,* split thickness of ilium onlaid over decorticated surfaces.

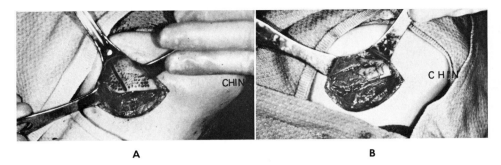

Fig. 23-49. **A,** Exposure of the ramus, the vertical cut for vertical osteotomy and drill holes for bone grafting. **B,** Onlay of bone graft over lateral surface of ramus for correction of micrognathia after decortication was completed. (U. S. Army photograph; Letterman Army Hospital.)

terior border to a point approximately 2 cm anterior to the vertical cut in the ramus (Fig. 23-49, *A*).

6. The lateral cortex is removed from this broad area with the flat, long-beveled Stout No. 3 chisel, creating a flat surface onto which the bone graft will subsequently be fitted. Care should be taken not to injure the inferior alveolar nerve during the decortication, but it should be identified so that it can be avoided when the vertical section is completed.

7. The wound is packed, the patient's head turned, and the procedure just described repeated on the other side.

8. By this time the surgical team that is to obtain the graft should be started.

9. The procedure on the second side is completed except for fitting and placement of the graft.

10. The vertical sections are completed on both sides, following the technique described for the treatment of prognathism.

11. It will be found that the mandible and anterior portion of the ramus are easily repositioned anteriorly. The mouth is entered, and intermaxillary elastic ligatures are placed to fix the teeth into desired occlusion. Arch bars wired to all teeth should be utilized because heavy traction must be placed to ensure maintenance of teeth in proper occlusion during the manipulation necessary to inlay the bone graft.

12. The length of the section of bone needed can be measured with accuracy by calculating the replacement as graphically illustrated in Fig. 23-48, *H* and *I*. It can be cut accurately, also, if an assistant holds it securely on a wood block while the surgeon sections it to the desired size with the Stryker oscillating saw. The full-thickness portion of the graft must be tapered to a lesser width to fit superiorly, since the void to be filled is less superiorly than at the lower border (Fig. 23-48, *I*). The full thickness of the graft with both cortices remaining serves to maintain the elongation of the mandible, and union of the well-mortised graft occurs in about 8 weeks.

13. Once fitted into the voids, the graft is wired onto the decorticated bed with fine, stainless steel wire sutures (0.016 inch) (Fig. 23-49, *B*).

14. Scraps of medullary bone that have been saved during trimming of the graft are added in the void above the block inlay and in any other spaces not filled or in close contact (Fig. 23-48, H, areas marked X).

15. Closure and postoperative care are the same as previously described.

Discussion. There are two objections to this procedure that cannot be circumvented. First, it is a long operation, requiring 4 to 5 hours. However, with the patient adequately supported during and after the surgery, the course is ordinarily uneventful. The second objection concerns use of the ilium for the donor site. Patients always

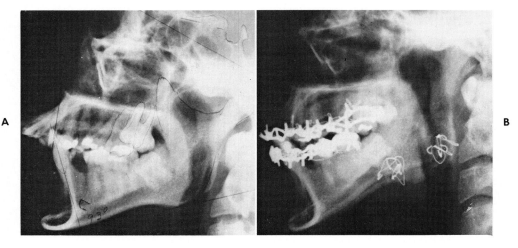

Fig. 23-50. Lateral skull roentgenograms from which tracings (Fig. 23-48) were made. **A,** Preoperative. **B,** Postoperative. (U. S. Army photographs; Letterman Army Hospital.)

complain much more about the hip than the jaw. "Bank" bone is not believed to have the potential for a "take" that autogenous grafts have.

Results in cases of micrognathia treated by this method have been so successful that the principal disadvantages just mentioned can be accepted. By comparison to other methods, the operation has the following advantages:

1. It is adaptable to the usual cases of micrognathia.

2. As much as 1 to 2 cm of advancement can be secured.

3. The small size and bulk of the body of the mandible are not contraindications.

4. Firm clinical union is rapid, requiring about 8 to 10 weeks.

5. The cosmetic result is excellent because the angle of the mandible is maintained or improved at the same time the body is advanced to provide a good profile.

6. The operation can be done without injury to important nerves (that is, mandibular and facial).

7. Elaborate splints are not needed. Orthodontic appliances or ordinary arch bars will suffice for fixation during the period of immobilization (Fig. 23-50).

An acceptable substitution for this iliac bone graft procedure is one described by Thoma.[124] A rib graft does not provide the bulk of bone substance obtained by onlaying with a block from the ilium; however, it is easier to obtain and is less disabling for the patient. The surgical technique is the same as described for placement of iliac bone. Edges of the rib graft are perforated with a drill to afford medullary bone contact when it is interposed between the proximal and distal parts to obliterate the space created as the distal (body portion) is advanced.

Vertical L, L modified, or C sliding osteotomy (without bone grafting)

When there is no need for the addition of bulk in correction of retrognathia (micrognathia is not a factor) but simply an advancement of the mandible to Class I relation is desired, the vertical L sliding osteotomy (or modified) is an excellent procedure and one to be considered.[23] (See Fig. 23-51.)

1. This operation is accomplished by an extraoral submandibular approach, using curtain draping to permit access to the oral cavity for intermaxillary immobilization.

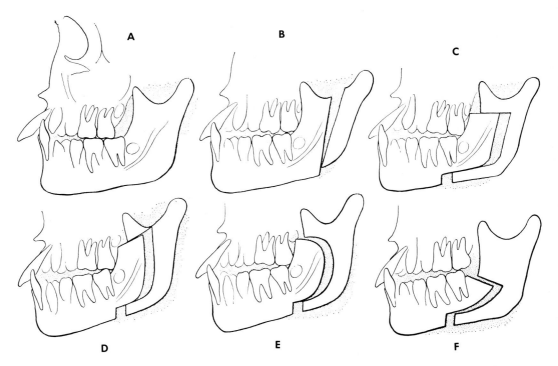

Fig. 23-51. A, Tracing from a lateral cephalogram, which shows the retruded mandible and Class II occlusion of the teeth (note relation of first molars). **B,** Vertical (or oblique subcondylar) osteotomy in ramus permits advancement of the mandible, but does not allow for much bony contact at site of osteotomy and also reduces prominence of the gonial angle. **C,** The inverted L of Pichler and Trauner with a horizontal cut made between the base of the coronoid process and the mandibular foramen and then vertically downward parallel to the posterior border of the ramus and rounding anteriorly as in **D. D,** L osteotomy with line of bone incision made from the mandibular notch "vertically" downward parallel to the posterior border of the ramus and then curved with the angle anteriorly, parallel to the lower border of the mandible as far as necessary to permit the planned advancement of the mandible and then downward through the lower border. Thus a "hockey stick" shape is given to the proximal fragment, and as the mandible is advanced, sliding contact is maintained along the horizontal line of osteotomy at the lower border. Coronoidotomy must be done also. **E,** Another modification of the cut according to Lister is a circular cut in the form of a C. The effect obtained in **C** to **E** is essentially the same. **F,** Osteotomy suggested by Hayward is paralleled to the arc of movement of the mandibular anterior teeth, resulting in maximum bony contact as the bone is advanced after osteotomy. The operation is done in two stages—one intraoral and one extraoral.

2. The incision should be about 5 to 6 cm in length to ensure adequate access to the whole lateral surface of the ramus and several centimeters of the lower border of the mandible anterior to the angle.

3. The outline of osteotomy should be scribed on the lateral surface of the bone as preplanned from tracings of a lateral cephalogram (Fig. 23-51). This line of osteotomy may be vertical down from the mandibular notch (Fig. 23-51, *D*) or horizontal from the anterior border of the ramus above the mandibular foramen and then vertically down, to within about 1.5 cm of the angle of the mandible (Fig. 23-51, *C*). The *line of cut is then curved anteriorly* and may be extended in this direction as far as necessary to allow for necessary "sliding" advancement of the jaw and to maintain bone apposition on the horizontal plane at the

lower border of the mandible. A third line of osteotomy may be in the shape of a C circling around the mandibular foramen from the anterior border of the ramus to the angle of the mandible and then anteriorly, as already described. Lister used this C cut (Fig. 23-51, *E*).[23]

4. If a straight vertical cut from the mandibular notch is planned, coronoidotomy should be accomplished to eliminate interference of the temporal muscle with the forward placement of the mandible.

5. Osteotomy is accomplished as usual, with much care exercised in the parts of the cut above the mandibular foramen, since "guarding" on the medial surface is technically not feasible. We depend on 18,000 rpm, sharp bone drills and the sense of feel to ascertain lack of resistance as penetration of the medial cortex occurs. Points of incomplete osteotomy are severed using short, sharp taps with a broad-bladed, sharp chisel and mallet.

6. From about the height of the mandibular foramen on down parallel to the posterior border of the ramus and anteriorly parallel to the lower border, the osteotomy can be accomplished rapidly, since medial soft tissue may be guarded with a broad, flat Lane periosteotome. A No. 702 or 703 carbide fissure bur in the Jordan-Day engine is used to take advantage of the side cutting effect. As the cut is extended anteriorly parallel to the lower border, it is first scribed into the lateral cortex using one of the larger burs, and then the osteotomy is completed through the medial cortex with a No. 701 carbide bur. This results in minimal bone excision and reduces chance of injury to the neurovascular bundle.

7. When osteotomies are completed on both sides, the mouth is entered, and the new occlusion relation is fixed by heavy intermaxillary elastics. A clear acrylic "wafer" occlusal guide plate is more routinely used in retrognathic cases.

8. After a change of gloves the curtain drape is readjusted, and the surgical field is reentered. Freedom of the proximal frag-

ment (posterior ramus and condyle part) is ensured from muscle binding. Bone approximation is checked along the horizontal cut above the lower border. At least one wire suture is placed on each side to ensure proper bone fragment control.

9. Closure of soft tissue follows a standard technique.

An addendum is necessary here. The patient shown in Fig. 23-52 and previously reported on[23] has since been followed up. Her first operation was in March, 1965, at age 14. Orthodontics had been planned in conjunction but was not accomplished. Regression occurred. A protrusion habit developed in a subconscious effort to compensate for the regression. When seen with this result in November 1969, 4½ years postoperatively, the patient was satisfied and rejected a suggestion for reoperation. She had *acquired* a normal Class I relation of the jaw but without posterior occlusion. No doubt the condyle resided well forward of its normal position in the glenoid fossa most of the time. By 1972 the patient, then 20 years old, had developed an acute temporomandibular joint arthritis produced by her protrusion habit and abnormal joint relation. She accepted surgery to overcome the problem. Fig. 23-53 illustrates the course in this case. Much has been learned from this case as summarized in the following:

1. It is reiterated that vertical L sliding osteotomy or a modified version is an excellent operation for the correction of retrognathia.

2. In micrognathic conditions, autogenous bone grafting should be considered and is recommended.

3. Best results can be expected when treatment is carried out with orthodontic support.

4. Overcorrection should always be attempted, since there is a strong tendency for regression to some degree.

5. The condyle head must not be distracted from the glenoid fossa during surgery when the distal (mandibular body)

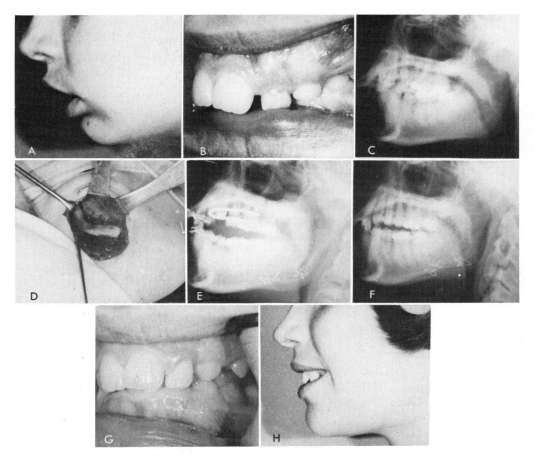

Fig. 23-52. A, This 14-year-old girl was a shy introvert, no doubt influenced by her retruded lower jaw. **B,** She had a typical Class II malocclusion. **C,** The overbite and overjet are demonstrated in a profile roentgenogram. The lower incisors related high onto the palatal mucosa. **D,** Bilateral L osteotomies were accomplished—one side according to Fig. 23-51, *C,* and one as seen in Fig. 23-51, *D.* Photograph after osteotomy, but before advancement of the mandible and wiring. **E,** A "wafer" was placed to ensure desired occlusion and to prevent extrusion or other injury to these young teeth during the 6 weeks of immobilization. **F,** There was improvement in the posterior occlusion during the first year postoperatively as the permanent teeth erupted to the normal occlusal plane. **G,** Although an overbite still existed 1 year after surgery, her occlusion was orthodontically correctable. **H,** She had a remarkable improvement in personality and appearance. (Courtesy General Rose Memorial Hospital, Denver.)

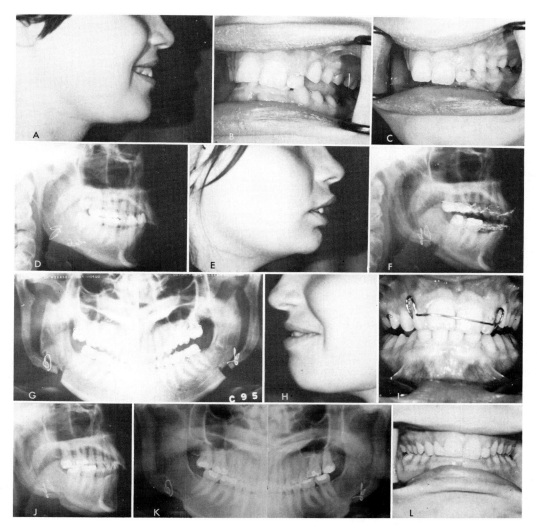

Fig. 23-53. Four and one-half years after L osteotomy for retrognathia, the patient shown in Fig. 23-52 returned for follow-up examination. **A,** At first glance she had a pleasing profile. **B,** Examination of occlusion revealed an open bite posteriorly. **C,** With difficulty she could close to a normal centric relation—precisely what she had prior to surgery 4½ years previously; in the closed position her profile was better than seen in Fig. 23-52, *A,* but not pleasing. **D,** Cephalogram of her in normal centric relation. **E,** Her appearance on return in 1972. She suffered with acute arthritis in both temporomandibular joints as a result of habitual protrusion of the jaw and malrelation of the condyle heads; the occlusion was unchanged. L osteotomy was repeated in May 1972. **F,** Cephalogram. **G,** Panorex film (note *direction* of transosseous wire placement). **H,** Profile is satisfactory (overcorrected). **I,** Occlusion is retained with incisal guide until occlusion posteriorly can be restored with orthodontics or onlays. **J,** Class I jaw relation in centric (cephalogram). **K,** Union at site of the L osteotomy (Panorex). **L,** Examination in January 1973, reveals stable occlusion relation. (Courtesy General Rose Memorial Hospital, Denver.)

portion is advanced. Special care must be taken to secure it snugly in the glenoid fossa. Transosseous wire is directed so that pull is toward the proximal fragment.

Modified *L* or *C* osteotomy of the ramus and sagittal osteotomy of the mandibular body

Hayes'[41] suggestion for sagittal osteotomy in the body of the mandible as a modification to L or C osteotomy is a significant improvement over the technique that has been described in the immediately preceding pages (Fig. 23-54, *A* and *B*). Byrne and Hinds[17] have endorsed this modification after using it in seven patients. They state that "criteria for technical feasibility including simplicity, surgical repair, operating time, function, preservation of anatomic structures and bone healing have been satisfied in this procedure" and further "that this operation possesses the advantages of the 'parent' procedures without the major disadvantages of either." This is a reference to the extraoral L or C osteotomy and the intraoral sagittal ramus procedure. Fox and Tilson[36] also endorse the Hayes' procedure as offering significant advantages in treatment of mandibular retrognathia and also suggest that the tendency toward relapse can be reduced by installing the coronoid process in the vertical void as a free bone graft. Hayes[41] had suggested sliding a graft of lateral cortical bone posteriorly from the anterior portion of the ramus (Fig. 23-54, *C*).

We are also pleased with the results in the several cases in which we have used this *body sagittal split.* We have, however, encountered one patient in whom the mandible was so thin that the conventional L procedure was utilized as an alternative at the time of surgery. Unfortunately, cephalograms and panoramic x-ray studies do not provide information on the *mediolateral* thickness of the bone. Our adaptation of the sagittal separation has varied somewhat from that reported by Hayes (Fig. 23-55, *A* and *B*).

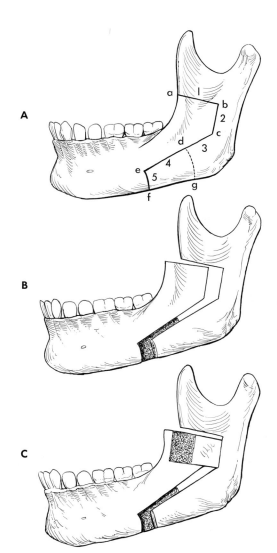

Fig. 23-54. A, Lateral aspects of mandible with lines showing bone sections. From points *a* to *d*, osteotomy is completed through medial and lateral cortices. From points *d* to *e, f,* and *g* and returning to *d* on the medial side (dotted line), saw cuts are through cortex only. Sequence of cutting is shown numerically. **B,** Postoperative corrected relationship of proximal and distal fragments. **C,** Sliding a graft from the lateral cortical plate of the ramus had been suggested by Hayes. (After Hayes.)

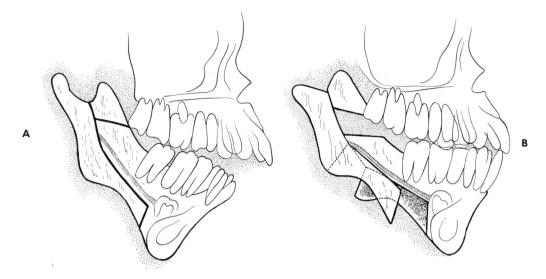

Fig. 23-55. In applying the idea of sagittal separation of the medial and lateral cortices, as suggested by Hayes, Fig. 23-52, we have moved the medial vertical cut, point *d* to *g*, posteriorly to the location of 3 in his drawing and then made that cut in an oblique direction to the angle; thus even more bone is kept in contact as the body of the mandible is advanced anteriorly.

1. The vertical cut on the lateral surface is originated at the mandibular (sigmoid) notch and carried downward to a point just posterior to the mandibular foramen. It is then extended parallel with the posterior border of the ramus to within about 1.5 to 2 cm above the angle of the mandible. The cut from this point is made in the lateral cortex only and is curved anteriorly on the body of the mandible as far anteriorly as planned. This horizontal cut in the lateral cortex may be *over or even superior* to the course of the mandibular canal.

2. The *medial* cut is made *from the angle or even above it* obliquely up and anteriorly to the point where the cut on the lateral surface curves. Thus an extensive approximation of bone is achieved as the bone is split and sagittal sliding osteotomy occurs.

3. All bone cuts are made using burs ranging in size from No. 703 to 701. The cut on the lateral surface is started with a No. 703, which affords better control of penetration of the cortex without risking injury to the nerve. Cuts above the foramen and from the horizontal cut through the lower border are made with a No. 702. The vertical oblique cut on the medial surface is made with a No. 703, while the cut through the cortex along the lower border is done with a No. 701.

4. Final separation may require use of the broad No. 3 Stout chisel or any broad, thin osteotome. The nerve should be intact as separation occurs, even though the lateral cortex is raised, exposing it. Hypothesia is uncommon but may result from stretching as the distal (body) segment is repositioned anteriorly.

Summarizing, we have found sagittal splitting of the body portion of the osteotomy to be a marked improvement in this L technique and have lengthened the mandible as much as 2 cm in one case. We prefer the L shaped cut in the ramus to the C but believe coronoidotomy is essential to ensure against relapse. When grafting is indicated, we usually install fresh autogenous rib since the morbidity from taking it is less than when the ilium is used as a donor (Fig. 23-56). This type of graft is preferable to either the coronoid process or the lateral

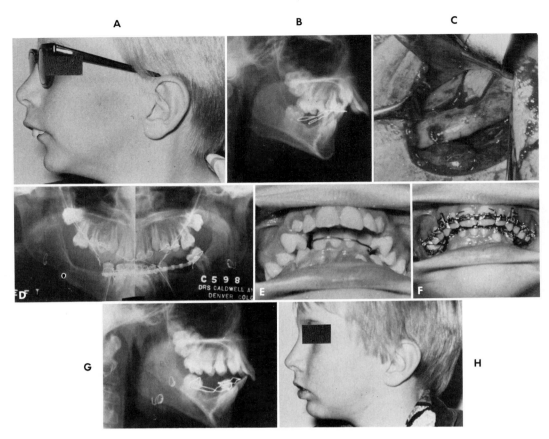

Fig. 23-56. A, Micrognathia in an 8-year-old boy. **B,** He had lost most of his lower posterior teeth earlier in treatment of multiple giant cell tumors, and his mandible was grossly underdeveloped. **C,** Elongation of the jaw was by L osteotomy (with coronoidotomy), sagittal splitting of the body portion, and interposition of a full-thickness graft of fresh autogenous rib in the vertical void. **D,** In the postoperative panogram, the sagittal advancement in the body is visualized better on the left side where position of the vertical cuts is distinct. The rib graft is also evident in the vertical ramus. The occlusion preoperatively, **E,** and postoperatively, **F. G,** The postoperative cephalogram shows normal Class I jaw relation prior to orthodontic correction of the maxillary protrusion. **H,** The patient's profile is improved. His personality also improved, which was reflected in a marked improvement in social adjustment. (Courtesy General Rose Memorial Hospital, Denver.)

cortex since neither of those donor sites yield medullary bone. Medullary (cancellous) bone will hasten repair and regeneration of new bone in the vertical void while free grafts of cortical bone are less apt to survive, and the density of free grafts is unnecessary as a "strut" to maintain the advancement. To date, we have encountered one patient whose mandible was too thin for splitting without risking unplanned fracture.

Z osteotomy

One variant from the usual type of retrognathia is characterized by Class II malocclusion, deep anterior overbite, remarkably decreased anterior vertical dimension (N to Pog), abnormally pronounced labial mental crease, extremely square mandibular angles, and unusual breadth in the lower third of the face. The basic problem is that of a retruded mandible, but the facial and

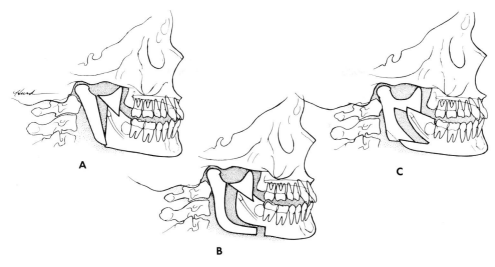

Fig. 23-57. **A,** The vertical osteotomy (Robinson) reduced the gonial angle but left little bone contact and also rotated the condyle forward. **B,** the ∟ osteotomy would suffice but failed to reduce the gonial angle. **C,** The Z design met all objectives—advanced the mandible to Class I relation, increased the N-Pog dimension, and reduced the prominent gonial angle.

skeletal composition places a new requirement for surgical correction. In Figs. 23-59 and 23-60 two case histories and a method of surgery are described and will be summarized herein.

In treating the first patient (Fig. 23-59), there appeared to be three principal objectives: (1) elongate the mandible to correct the Class II relation; (2) increase the N to Pog dimension and eliminate the overbite and at the same time improve the profile; and (3) reduce the prominent gonial angles to overcome the square-faced appearance.

∟ and C osteotomy designs were not applicable; however, further experimentation with "paper cutouts" suggested that a Z-shaped design was adaptable (Fig. 23-57), and all objectives appear to be achieved. From this first design a modification has developed, resulting from technical problems with the horizontal cut above the foramen that extended to the anterior border of the ramus below the coronoid process.

Technique of the Z osteotomy

1. The conventional Risdon approach to the ramus of the mandible is used. When the entire lateral surface of the ramus is exposed, a Thompson retractor is hooked over the mandibular (sigmoid) notch.

2. Coronoidotomy is accomplished in the standard way.

3. The prominence of the mandibular foramen is identified, and the approximate route of the mandibular canal is judged by comparison of the Panorex x-ray film to the lateral surface as it is viewed.

4. With the course of the canal in mind, a curving line is scribed from the mandibular notch vertically downward and back of the foramen and then curving down and forward just below a route judged to be that of the canal.

5. At a point anterior to the antigonial notch and several millimeters above it, the course of the bone cut is reversed at an acute angle and carried horizontally to the posterior border of the ramus, again several millimeters above the angle. The design for this osteotomy as presently used is shown in Fig. 23-58.

6. An interocclusal splint or "wafer" should be available to install between the arches as the mandible is advanced to the

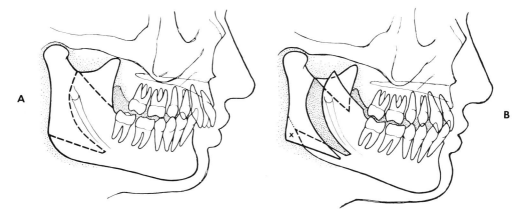

Fig. 23-58. A, Design of the Z osteotomy and coronoidotomy. **B,** As the mandible is advanced, the N-Pog dimension increased. At the same time, the vertical ramus is foreshortened and the prominence of the gonial angle is reduced. It can be reduced even more by excision of bone from the posterior border at point *X.*

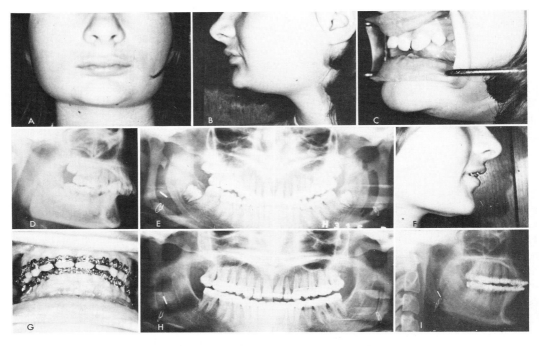

Fig. 23-59. A 16-year-old girl with an unusual facial conformation, including **A,** a short anterior vertical dimension (N-Pog) and a broad, square jaw posteriorly; **B,** a very short N-Pog, pronounced labial-mental creases, and square heavy angles; **C,** extreme crowding of anterior teeth and deep overbite, with lower incisors biting into palate. **D,** Preoperative cephalogram shows retrognathia and Class II occlusion, deep overbite, short anterior vertical dimension, and thick, square rami and gonial angles. **E,** An operation was planned as shown in Fig. 23-57, *C.* However, when it was performed, the distal (body) portion impinged under the coronoid process and could not be advanced, necessitating a cut on each side into the mandibular (sigmoid) notch. The void in the vertical ramus between the fragments filled with new bone. **F,** There is an improved appearance, and the lower third of the face is lengthened vertically. The profile is normal, with retrusion and overbite corrected. **G,** Orthodontics is essential for success in these cases because of the posterior open bite created by surgery. **H,** Postoperative Panorex film shows good bone generation in the rami bilaterally. **I,** Postoperative cephalogram shows a relatively normal profile. (Courtesy General Rose Memorial Hospital, Denver.)

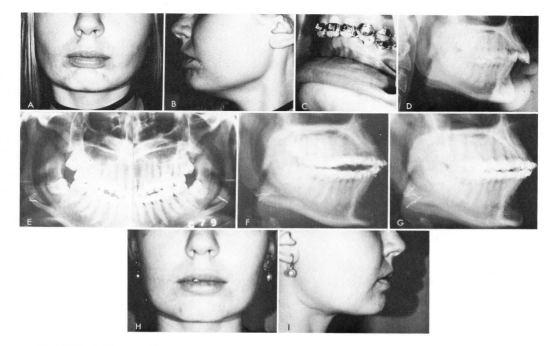

Fig. 23-60. A 21-year-old woman with the same variant of retrognathia as seen in Fig. 23-59 but to a less pronounced degree. **A,** Patient has a less than average N-Pog dimension. Her lower lip rolls out and down over a marked labial mental crease. **B,** Profile shows short anterior vertical dimension and square jaw. **C,** Characteristic Class II malocclusion and deep overbite. **D,** The preoperative cephalogram shows the variant of retrognathia that is being discussed. **E,** The operation was designed as shown in Fig. 23-58 (Z osteotomy with coronoidotomy). A postoperative Panorex x-ray film clearly illustrates the osteotomy. **F,** The surgical treatment is done only in cooperation with orthodontic control and follow-up. In an early postoperative cephalogram the posterior open bite is evident. **G,** In a subsequent postoperative cephalogram the occlusion has been closed in the posterior area by orthodontic treatment. **H,** The most obvious postoperative improvement is in the increased length to the lower third of the face and normal labial-mental fold. **I,** Postoperative profile improved. (Courtesy General Rose Memorial Hospital, Denver.)

desired new position. This is to prevent uncontrolled extrusion of posterior teeth during the period of immobilization and also to ensure placement of the mandible into correct relation with the maxilla.

7. Modest decortication and mortising at some points on both aspects of the Z incision may be necessary to ensure good bone apposition. Small transosseous wire sutures are placed on each side.

8. The jaw should be immobilized for about 6 weeks.

In both cases the results are good at present and seemed to have warranted this tedious procedure. Descriptions of these cases illustrate the problem and the reasoning for the procedure (Figs. 23-59 and 23-60).

MICROGENIA AND GENIOPLASTY

Osteotomy and advancement or lengthening the mandible is not always necessary in receding ''Andy Gump'' facies. Occasionally the occlusion is satisfactory, and all that is needed to improve appearance is addition of substance to the chin or rearrangement of bone already present. At the same time much psychological benefit can result. Occasionally genioplasty is adjunctive to the cosmetic result after one of the previously described osteotomy procedures. Bone, cartilage, tantalum mesh, and alloplastic materials* have been used to build out the mental prominence. Intraoral or extraoral access to the chin is obtained, depending on indications and treatment plan.

The least complicated approach to treatment of this problem is by implantation of a contoured-to-measure piece of silicone rubber inserted intraorally. A short, vertical incision is made at the midline, through which a pocket is formed by blunt dissection. The implant is inserted and properly positioned, and after closure of the wound a semipressure dressing is carefully placed over the chin and lower jaw to maintain the implant in proper position during the immediate postoperative course. Other foreign materials are also "pocketed" supraperiosteally.

The report of Robinson and Shuken[101] in 1969 was discouraging. They reported that 12 of 14 patients with chin augmentation by plastic implants showed some degree of bone resorption on postoperative radiographic follow-up. They recommend a routine procedure for follow-up examinations but do not discourage continued use of this procedure for genioplasty. Silastic implants also tend to be expelled as does cartilage (Fig. 23-62).

Most of the techniques for genioplasty just mentioned have limitations. Alloplastic materials have a tendency to migrate from the position in which they are placed at the time of surgery. Erosion of the chin prominence contiguous with the implant has been reported. Patients have also re-

---

*See references 6, 57, 71, 115, and 123.

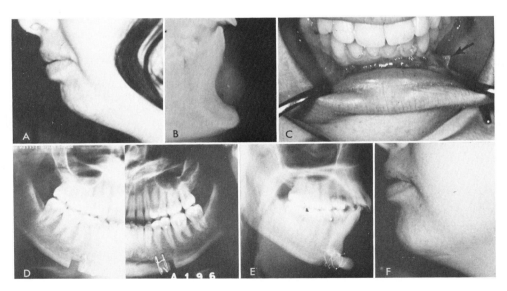

Fig. 23-61. A, A 24-year-old woman had a Silastic implant placed by an intraoral operation 1 year earlier to augment the chin deficiency. **B,** A lateral x-ray film made when she was first admitted showed the preformed silicone rubber implant (Silastic) resting on the supramentale recess. (Note bone resorption that has occurred in 1 year.) **C,** When the patient was first seen, the implant was being expelled (arrow). The surgeon who had placed it tried unsuccessfully to trim the protruding Silastic and close it surgically, using antibiotics to supplement the effort. It was removed, resulting in the appearance exhibited in **A. D,** After a delay of about 6 months, horizontal sliding genioplasty was done through an extraoral submentale approach (Panorex). **E,** Cephalogram shows good protuberance and healing. **F,** Facial profile is improved. (Courtesy General Rose Memorial Hospital, Denver.)

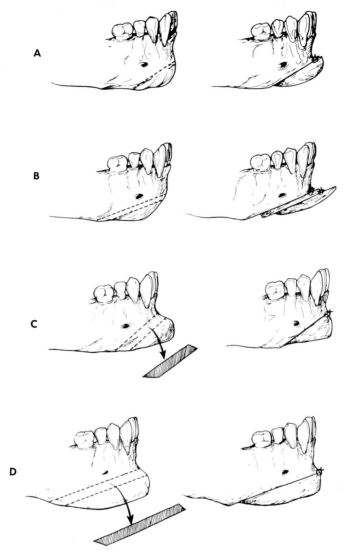

Fig. 23-62. Augmentation and reduction genioplasties. These procedures are all accomplished through the intraoral approach. **A,** Single-section horizontal sliding genioplasty. Transosseous wires are placed to reduce the possibility of relapse. Slight overcorrection is employed. The lateral portions of the osteotomy segment are not contoured at the time of surgery because future resorption would then cause a rounded rather than a gracefully contoured chin prominence to be formed. **B,** Double-section horizontal sliding genioplasty. The additional section allows for greater augmentation of the chin prominence. **C,** The genioplasty for length reduction of the chin prominence. The osteotomy bony incisions are made in a more vertical plane. A section equal to the desired reduction is removed. **D,** Genioplasty for height reduction of the anterior portion of the mandible.

ported unpleasant sensations in the implant region when they were exposed to cold temperatures. We recently removed a Silastic implant device that had migrated into the mental region.

Probably the best way to enlarge the prominence of the chin is to reposition the lower border anteriorly by osteotomy. In 1958 Obwegeser[80] suggested a horizontal sliding osteotomy of the anterior lower border of the mandible that was a modification of Hofer's earlier extraoral procedure (Fig. 23-62).

Augmentation and reduction genioplasty (intraoral)

The intraoral procedure for augmentation and reduction genioplasty is as follows:

1. A paragingival incision is made from the second premolar tooth to the second premolar tooth on the opposite side of the arch.

2. The chin prominence is degloved by elevation of the periosteum anteriorly between the mental foramina.

3. The midline is recorded by scoring the bone with a fine bur in the midsagittal plane across the area of the planned osteotomy.

4. A horizontal osteotomy cut is made in a plane established by three points. The posterior points are set 3 mm below the mental foramina. The anterior midline point is set 2 mm superior to the point of greatest chin prominence.

5. The osteotomy is continued through to the medial cortex with the oscillating Stryker sawblade.

6. The segment is freed of all its attachments.

7. The segment is then placed in the preplanned position and fixed with three transosseous wires, each of which engages the medial cortex for the segment and the anterior cortex of the mandible.

8. The incision is closed, using No. 3-0 polyglycolic suture material (Dexon) in a continuous horizontal mattress format.

9. A pressure bandage is fashioned by placing a folded 10 by 10 cm gauze sponge over the inferior lip, and this is secured with a piece of 2.5 cm tape placed circumferentially around the chin and neck.

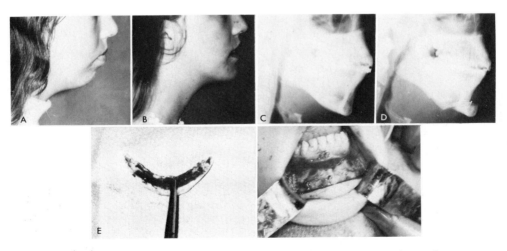

Fig. 23-63. Patient with Class I occlusion (Angle) who had retruded mental protuberance was treated with a horizontal sliding genioplasty (Obwegeser). **A,** Preoperative profile. **B,** Postoperative profile. **C,** Preoperative cephalometric roentgenogram. **D,** Postoperative cephalometric roentgenogram. **E,** Lower border of mandible removed prior to its being replaced as a free graft. **F,** Lower border advanced and fixed with transosseous wires.

This versatile procedure may be modified to correct many deformities of the chin prominence (Fig. 23-63). Abnormally prominent chins may be reduced in size and contour by sliding the segment posteriorly. A narrow, more finely contoured chin may be created by sectioning the segment in the midline and removing a wedge-shaped piece. The length of the lower one third of the face may be reduced by removing a wafer-shaped section superior to the original osteotomy, discarding it, and replacing the segment in the more superior position. Extreme retrusion of the chin may be corrected by using the wafer-shaped section just mentioned as an intermediate between the segment and the mandible. Thus the wafer is wired in a more anterior position, and the segment is wired to it. Corrections between 15 and 20 mm may be secured with this technique.

Augmentation and reduction genioplasty (extraoral)

Essentially, the same changes in bone contour at the lower border of the mandible anteriorly as have been described in the preceding section can be accomplished by

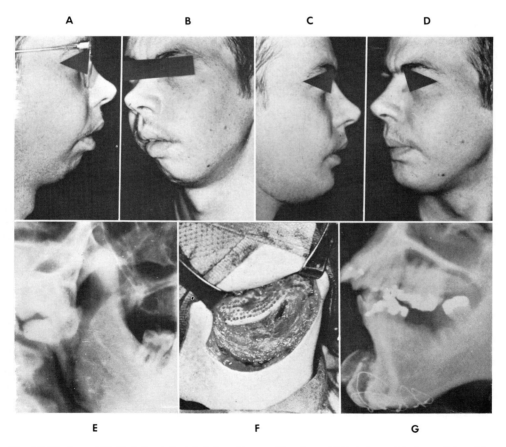

Fig. 23-64. A and **B,** Unilateral facial deformity resulting from birth injury of left condyle with underdeveloped *left* mandible. Class II malocclusion could not be improved on by surgical methods. **C** and **D,** Final cosmetic result. **E,** Deformed *left* condyle. **F,** Bed prepared for correction of deficiency, which will be by addition of a full-thickness bone graft from the ilium to the *right* side of the mandible and symphysis. **G,** Onlay bone graft. (U. S. Army photographs; Letterman Army Hospital.)

an extraoral approach. The extraoral procedure has the advantages of sterile surgical technique avoiding contamination by oral secretions, excellent visualization of the operative site, greater ease of instrumentation, and less postoperative morbidity (edema and ecchymosis), while the only disadvantage is the skin incision and resulting scar (Fig. 23-61).

The incision is made in a curve following the shape of the lower border of the mandible, and dissection is made through each subcutaneous layer so that closure can be achieved with minimal scarring. If there is scarring, it is under the lower border and not visible. The wound is closed in anatomical layers as described for other extraoral operations; however, a pressure dressing is applied to aid in maintaining the segments of bone in position even though transosseous wiring is used.

If large onlays of autogenous bone are needed, an extraoral approach is much preferred and probably safer. The case illustrated in Fig. 23-64, for example, required placement of bone over a large portion of the right lateral surface of the mandible well back of the mental foramen as well as over the symphysis. The incision here was a long one placed well under the shadow of the mandible for two reasons: (1) to place the scar inconspicuously and (2) to have the line of incision well away from the bone graft so that the graft will be well supported. It should be noted in this case that the foreshortened, deformed side was the *left* side, but bone was added to the *right* side and symphysis to develop a symmetrical face. Deformities of this type are ideally corrected in this manner.

Onlay grafts present other problems. If autogenous material is selected, a second surgical site is required from which to take the material. Bank bone or cartilage does not afford the predictability for a good viable graft. Furthermore, the placement of autogenous bone or cartilage grafts requires the use of an extraoral route for placement because of the difficulty of intraoral closure over graft material. A scar results, but placement of the incision well under the symphysis makes it acceptably obscure.

ARRESTED CONDYLAR GROWTH

Arrested condylar growth causing mandibular agenesis (incomplete and imperfect development) to a marked degree, more severe than that seen in the ordinary retrognathic and micrognathic conditions, is rare. Because of this rarity there has been little opportunity to study the problem statistically or in a controlled manner. Variations exist in definition of different entities, and etiology is not entirely clear in all conditions. Similarly, there is not much experience in treating some of these con-

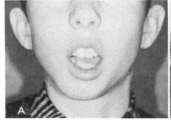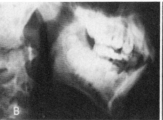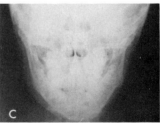

Fig. 23-65. This 11-year-old boy had always had an asymmetrical face, no doubt because of localized condylar growth disturbance, probably resulting from injury at birth. **A,** He has a deviated mandible with proclination of the lower anterior teeth and dentoalveolar structures, a prominent gonial angle, a pronounced antigonial notch, and a shortened vertical ramus and mandibular body. **B** and **C,** These abnormalities are also seen in the Panorex film and lateral skull x-ray film. (Courtesy General Rose Memorial Hospital, Denver.)

ditions, especially those occurring in the first arch syndrome. For treatment planning purposes, Hovell[49] divides mandibular agenesis into two main etiological groups: (1) those conditions caused by a localized disturbance in the condyle growth center and (2) those conditions that are prenatally determined and part of the first arch syndrome.

Mandibular agenesis of the first group may have its onset prenatally or postnatally and may result from several causes, such as intrauterine compression, injury at birth (Fig. 23-65) and subsequent trauma (Fig. 23-66), or infection (Fig. 23-45, *C*). The de-

formity is primarily in the mandible itself in these cases, and for this reason the affected side or sides have a characteristic shape that, according to Hovell,[49] "is absolutely diagnostic of a localized condylar growth disturbance." He attributes the development of this characteristic shape to normal adjacent investing tissues, which in normal molding and growth process exert normal stresses, but to the mandible with arrested growth these normal stresses cause growth dysplasia. This characteristic appearance includes (1) proclination of the lower anterior teeth and dentoalveolar structures, (2) prominent gonial angle, (3) pronounced

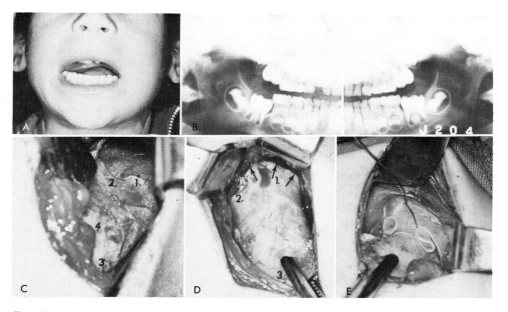

Fig. 23-66. A, This 7-year-old boy could open his mouth 7 mm when first seen for consultation. **B,** Bilateral *ankylosis* is clearly seen in both joint areas of this Panorex x-ray film. The broad, irregular density in the condyles is a typical x-ray finding. **C,** When the patient was operated on, the objective was to free the jaw *without* condylectomy, ostectomy, or other type of conventional arthroplasty. The procedure was by a Risdon approach, which permitted good exposure to the condyle and joint area: *1,* condyle; *2,* mandibular (sigmoid) notch and the coronoid process visible just anteriorly; *3,* gonial angle; *4,* antigonial notch. **D,** A fibrous cleavage line is usually present in all cases of ankylosis in children. It is through this area that movement occurs to allow the slight opening usually seen. It is identifiable surgically. When this is the case in a child or adult, the fibrous cleavage area can be cut through by sharp hand instruments and other leverage. When this is possible, the condylar growth center can be preserved. In this case that cleavage line is pointed to by arrows. It has been dissected free on both sides, and manual opening has been established at almost 40 mm. **E,** A cap of sheet Silastic has been fitted over the condyle head to the medial surface and gathered in around the condylar neck with a small gauge steel wire.

Continued.

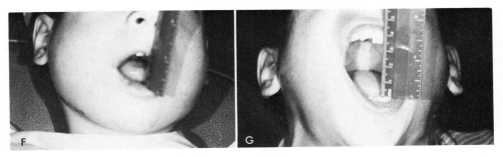

Fig. 23-66, cont'd. F, Much edema and disability follows this surgery, and the main thrust is early function despite pain and rebellion. **G,** Within 6 weeks this patient could open to 35 mm without pain. He has maintained this function for 3 years. Records have been made annually, and normal growth is recorded on the cephalogram. In addition, there appears to be a lengthening of the condyle neck compared to previous Panorex x-ray films. (Courtesy General Rose Memorial Hospital, Denver.)

antigonial notching, (4) shortened antero-posterior dimension of mandibular body, and (5) shortened vertical ramus and variable abnormal growth patterns in the coronoid process, sigmoid notch, and condyle (Fig. 23-65). We have observed this same characteristic appearance in our cases (Figs. 23-65 and 23-66) and note a distinct difference between these and cases of agenesis occasioned by other causes. However, when this retardation or cessation of condylar growth occurs, it results also in extreme maxillary overjet and canting of the occlusal plane in unilateral cases, with a decreased pupillary line to occlusal plane distance on the affected side. Normal excursions of the mandible are not possible because of the lack of function of the lateral pterygoid muscle, which inserts into the anterior surface of the condyle and the articular disk. In young patients, this results in repeated subluxation of the condyle on the normal side when maximum mouth opening is attempted. Lateral excursions toward the normal side are impossible. Only minimal protrusion is possible, and attempts at protrusion result in deviation toward the affected side.

Except in cases of ankylosis, the surgical care of developmental problems associated with localized disturbance in the condyle growth center follows the methods described later.

Ankylosis

Ankylosis of the temporomandibular joint will be discussed now, since the principal etiological factor is interference in some manner with the condyle growth center. Ankylosis untreated during the formative years invariably results in agenesis. Ankylosis may be partial (fibrous) or complete, with bony fusion of the condyle head to the glenoid fossa area of the temporal bone. Fortunately, the majority of patients with ankylosis seek help before complete bony ankylosis occurs. They have a minimal degree of opening, usually in the range of 5 to 7 mm, and x-ray examination will show a broad, flat, irregular vestige of a condyle head. Also an irregular radiolucent line is seen, representing the line of fibrous cleavage, which permits whatever the degree of opening there may be. Above this irregular radiolucent cleavage line and immediately below it at the articular surface of the distorted condyle head, irregular radiopacities are seen in varying degrees.

Historically, treatment of ankylosis has ranged from condylectomy to various arthroplastic procedures, including installation of cartilage, dermal grafts, fascia, alloplastic materials, metal caps, and combinations of foreign substances. In patients afflicted with complete bony ankylosis, there is no choice but to establish a surgical juncture immediately below the mass of dense bone in the former joint area and install a foreign substance such as a Silastic block to prevent reunion. Any technique that will assure mobilization and return to function is satisfactory.

Treatment of partial (fibrous) ankylosis, *especially in children, is entirely different.* Much growth potential is present in the characteristically deformed condyle head, and it must be preserved; however, function is necessary to activate this potential. For years, we have attempted to treat this problem by dissecting through the fibrous cleavage line until complete mobility of the area was established *and then proceeding* with condylectomy and arthroplasty, whether the patient was an adult or a child. We recently reported a case of bilateral ankylosis in a 7-year-old boy who was treated in this manner except that condylectomy was *not* included. Instead, sheet Silastic was capped over the deformed condyle head and in the line of cleavage. Eight years after surgery the patient can open to 35 mm, and his mandible is growing normally.[20] The operative procedure was carried out bilaterally at the same time, which is essential to successful treatment when both sides are involved. It was done through routine Risdon approaches. The preauricular approach is not suitable for these procedures for numerous reasons. Exposure of the entire lateral aspect of the ramus was achieved (Fig. 23-66, *D*) including the coronoid process, sigmoid notch, deformed condyle, accentuated antigonial notch, and prominent gonial angle. The fibrous cleavage line was located and dissection through it carried out using sharp No. 4 Molt curets and heavy manual pressure followed by elevation with a Lane periosteotome, distraction at the angle of the mandible (a good reason for the Risdon access), and leverage by an assistant at the symphysis. Both sides are opened

so that access to both joint areas is available at any point in the operation. Total mobilization, with every vestige of intervening fibrous tissue severed, is essential so that enough completely free space can be created in the cleavage area to slide a sheet of Silastic over it to the medial surface and to secure it in a caplike effect over the whole condylar process (Fig. 23-66, *F*). It is a difficult undertaking but worth the effort in children if by the procedure the growth center can be preserved, function established, and development permitted to occur normally. The case described in Fig. 23-66 has the longest follow-up; however, other children treated since then appear to be developing normally also.

In addition to the actual operative procedure, the following factors must be considered:

1. Anesthesia must include plans for blind nasotracheal intubation, which requires a skilled anesthesiologist, or presurgical tracheostomy as an alternative route to anesthesia.

2. Blood loss may be significant at the time of surgery, especially in children, and there should be plans for replacement if needed.

3. Immediate postoperative tissue reaction should be kept to a minimum by use of steroids such as dexamethasone (Decadron), antibiotic coverage, and ice packs. Antiemetics and analgesics as required and good general supportive care should be prescribed as indicated.

4. Immediate postoperative function is essential to ensure against recurrence of the ankylosis. This is achieved by forced exercise or exercise while the patient is under analgesics. Gum chewing and biting on spring-type clothespins are prescribed in the long course of a regular scheduled program.

The first arch syndrome

As noted previously, the second of Hovell's[49] main etiological groups is mandibular agenesis that is prenatally determined and merely a part of a wider syndrome—*the first arch syndrome* (oral-mandibular auricular syndrome). Because of clinical features, anatomy, and embryology, the following anomalies of the head and neck are considered by McKenzie[69] to arise from abnormal development of the first branchial arch and should be included in this first arch syndrome: (1) Treacher-Collins syndrome (mandibular facial dysostosis), (2) Pierre Robin syndrome (hypoplasia of the mandible with glossoptosis), (3) mandibular dysostosis, (4) cleft lip and palate, and (5) hypertelorism and others. Obviously a multiplicity of developmental skeletal deficiencies are included such as agenesis of the mandibular condyle and hypoplasia of other facial bones, especially the malar, as well as a host of overlying soft tissue malformations, such as macrostomia, auricular deformities (microtia), antimongoloid obliquity of the palpebral fissures, and decreased orotragal and canthotragal dimension. Some of these deformities arise from abnormal development of the second branchial arch as well as the first.

These deformities are challenging problems to anyone interested in reconstructive surgery; however, the oral and maxillofacial surgeon's interest is directed principally to the jaws and dental apparatus. If a deformity in the mandible affects growth in the maxilla, the oral surgeon's interest should extend to that area and so on. Most authorities* agree that surgical intervention should be undertaken early and staged as necessary, the philosophy being that if skeletal growth does not occur in a normal way, then soft tissues will also not grow normally; however, if skeletal enlargement is achieved surgically, then investing soft tissue will grow to accommodate and normal development on the affected side may be maintained. Contrarily, it is well known that scarring is a normal sequela to surgery, and therefore, when serial bone grafting is staged over the years of development, soft

tissue scarring can be expected that in turn may inhibit bone as well as soft tissue growth to some degree.

Surgeons who have endorsed this approach[67,118] perform serial bone grafting with split rib onlay grafts, since the rib cage is a bank of autogenous bone that will replenish naturally. *The iliac crest with its growth center should not be used as a source of bone in children.* Cartilage, banked bone, and dermal grafts have also been used to fill in defects. Stark and Saunders[118] have used bone homografts in patients as young as 18 months. Longacre and associates[67] prefer to start reconstruction before the child is 4 years old to prevent personality and behavior problems. Experience and enthusiasm for early serial allografting in these problems vary. Hovell[49] states ''grafts inserted for cases of first arch dysplasia have entirely resorbed with complete relapse to the preoperative skeletal pattern.'' Well-documented case histories followed up to adulthood are not available except for cases of Hovell, and his were disappointing.

Rowe[102] prompted us to apply the principles set forth in his concept, which did not involve elongation or augmentation by grafting initially but took advantage of bone already present.[27] The hope was that lengthening the affected ramus, stabilized by interocclusal splinting, and orthodontically controlling the postoperative course would stimulate normal maxillary growth on the affected side. Failing this, it was anticipated that maxillary osteotomy with bone grafting could be done to drop the maxilla to proper relation with the mandible.

This concept of surgical treatment of condylar agenesis when it is a part of the first arch syndrome is illustrated in Figs. 23-67 to 23-69. Three cases are reviewed briefly and illustrated. In two of these cases there is no semblance of coronoid and condyloid processes and no sigmoid notch, simply a rounded nub of bone in their place. Our results in this group of patients

---

*See references 49, 67, 69, and 118.

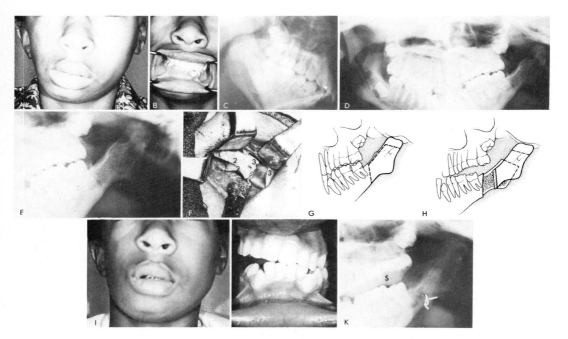

Fig. 23-67. A, A 12-year-old boy with marked facial underdevelopment on the right side, auricular deformity (ear tags), and decreased ostragal and canthotragal dimension. B, He had a slanted occlusal plane. C, Lateral cephalogram shows gross disparity in posterior and lower margins of mandible as well as a markedly retruded pogonion. D, The Panorex film shows the diminutive dimension of the right ramus typically without condyle, sigmoid notch, or coronoid process. E, A closer view of the stubby ramus (one side of Panorex). F, Surgery was in two stages, the first intraorally to start a sagittal split, followed 2 weeks later with extraoral completion of the operation, essentially the same as Dal Pont's. The following are visible: 1, area of gonial angle; 2, area of antigonial notch; 3, area distal to second molar. G, Tracing made from the preoperative Panorex film illustrates the sagittal splitting design (outline). H, Split with lengthening and resulting open occlusion posteriorly. I, Postoperative improved symmetry. J, Occlusion is open on the operated side. This was maintained through the postoperative course with an interocclusal splint, later replaced with a removable retainer, followed by a bite plane only and no interocclusal prosthesis to thus permit maxillary growth. K, Panorex film 3 weeks postoperative with interocclusal splint in place, s. (Courtesy General Rose Memorial Hospital, Denver; drawings by Peter Stone.)

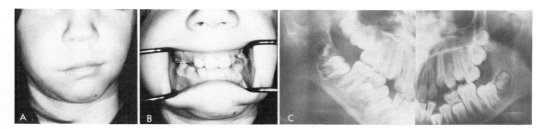

Fig. 23-68. A, A 10-year-old girl with facial underdevelopment on the left side. B, Her occlusion slanted upward on the affected side, and she had microtia with an obliterated ear canal and no hearing on that side. C, The preoperative Panorex film showed an atypical ramus on the left with small condyle, narrow sigmoid notch, broad stumpy coronoid process, and a shortened ramus with a suggestion of antigonial notching. If it were not for other first arch syndrome findings, one might think the cause to be within the condyle growth center only.

Continued.

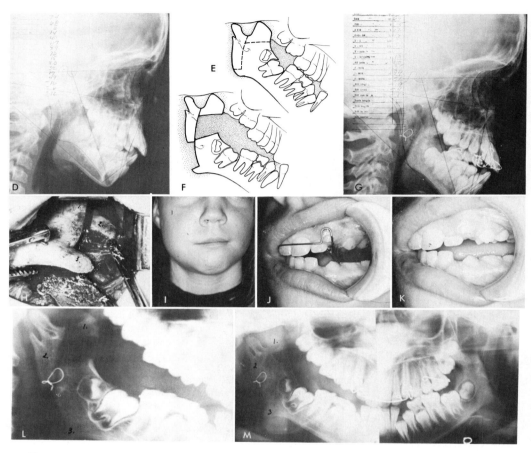

Fig. 23-68, cont'd. D, Preoperative cephalogram that has an overlay clearly traced shows the disparity in mandibular outlines and retrusion. **E,** The operative plan is traced and included a reversed L from the sigmoid notch to a point about 1 cm above the angle and then at a right angle to the posterior border. The objective was to maintain as much bulk for the gonial angle as possible. **F,** Coronoidotomy was planned, but this proved not to be necessary; temporal muscle attachments are so sparse that they can all be stripped off so that the coronoid itself can be distracted downward along with the balance of the distal (body) fragment of the mandible. **G,** Postoperative cephalogram shows tracing of almost perfect alignment of both sides of mandible but with some retrusion. **H,** Surgery was accomplished as designed, the distal (body) fragment *(1 and 3)* is distracted with a Kocher forceps (the gonial angle is labeled *3*) and a sizeable gap is evident between it and the stump of the proximal fragment (at *2*). **I,** Postoperative view of patient with improved symmetry. **J,** Occlusion open on the operated side and maintained at first with a retainer. **K,** Later the patient was fitted with a bite guide but no prosthesis to interfere with maxillary growth. **L,** Close Panorex x-ray view of operative site 5 days after surgery. Note that the coronoid process *(1)* could have been stripped of temporal fibers and distracted downward with the body of the mandible, *3*. **M,** Healing was complete, and remodeling had occurred in the latest Panorex film 4 months postoperatively. (Photographs courtesy General Rose Memorial Hospital, Denver; drawings by Peter Stone.)

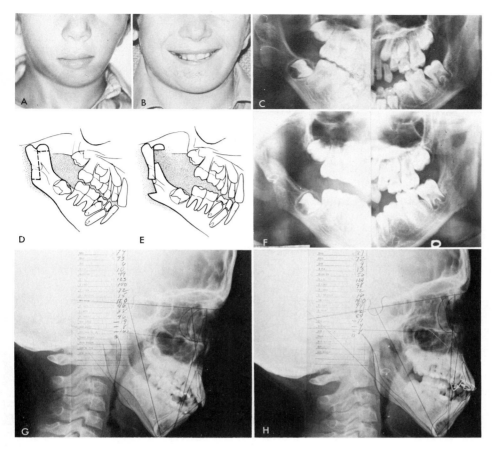

Fig. 23-69. A, A 10-year-old boy with facial asymmetry. Note microtia and micrognathic appearance. **B,** Postoperative appearance. **C,** Preoperative Panorex film shows a typical agenesis as seen in first arch syndrome that was in fact so tiny that reverse L osteotomy without bone grafting was questioned as a suitable approach. **D** and **E,** When traced out, the design appeared to be feasible; here, however, the remnant tip of the coronoid process could have been left, since practically no temporal muscle fibers were attached. **F,** Postoperative Panorex film at 2½ months is significant, showing good healing in the elongated mandible and the desired open occlusion. **G,** Preoperative cephalogram traced shows considerable disparity between the lower borders of the mandible and also a marked retrusion. **H,** Postoperative cephalogram shows some improvement in the dimension on the affected side compared to the normal. (Photographs courtesy General Rose Memorial Hospital, Denver; drawings by Peter Stone.)

treated according to Rowe's concept coincide with Hovell's observations—there has been a tendency toward regression (shrinkage in the mandible and less than normal growth in the maxilla). With 7 years of follow-up, some improvement has been observed but less than hoped for, and at this time we believe all of these patients will need maxillary as well as additional mandibular surgery as they reach maturity.

An article by Ware and Taylor[133] published in 1966 reporting experimental transplantation of cartilaginous growth centers to replace condyles in monkeys was overlooked until after 1970 when the theory was given practical application in children.[131]

We have been encouraged by reports of benefits from transplantation of costochondral junction growth centers to replace defective mandibular condyles in children and have applied this concept in six young patients—one suffering from first arch syndrome and five whose conditions were caused by treatment for ankylosis (Fig. 23-70). This procedure theoretically takes advantage of the growth spurt that occurs in the immediate prepubertal years. Although no conclusions can be drawn from this limited experience, this transplantation process probably offers the best hope for young patients with condylar agenesis, regardless of etiology, that has come to our attention to date. Other reports are inconclusive, but in a recent communication, Ware[132] stated that he has had to reoperate on two patients because of excessive growth from the grafted rib.

There is even more need for positive, definitive methods by which to correct progressive facial asymmetry caused by mandibular growth dysfunction since parental anxiety generated by this problem creates excessive psychological interaction between parent, child, and doctor. During the developmental years when there is minimal or no improvement by orthodontic, sur-

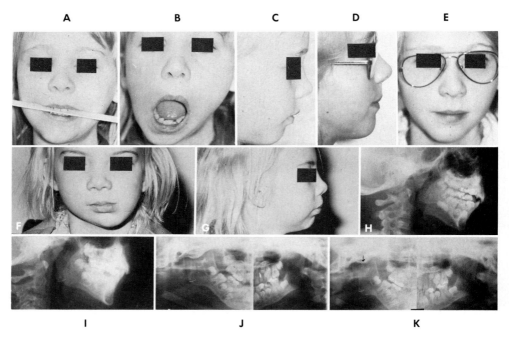

Fig. 23-70. Case I. **A,** A young girl with mandibular growth dysfunction showing the typical canted occlusion and, **B,** facial asymmetry and functional deviation. **C,** She also exhibited moderate mandibular retrognathism. **D,** Two years after costochondral transplantation to the affected mandible, the patient had a relatively normal profile and, **E,** the facial asymmetry was nearly eliminated. Case II. **F,** A 9-year-old girl had arthroplasty including Silastic implant for treatment of temporomandibular joint ankylosis when she was 5, which resulted in loss of growth center and facial asymmetry. **G,** There was associated retrognathia. **H,** Both the retrognathia and growth discrepancy are evident in the preoperative cephalogram. **I,** One year after costochondral transplant, there is improvement in relative size of the mandible. **J,** Immediate postoperative view after removal of Silastic and placement of costochondral junction rib graft. **K,** One year postoperative view showing good calcification in the condylar area, hopefully indicating a resumption of growth (arrow). (Courtesy General Rose Memorial Hospital, Denver.)

gical, or combined orthodontic and surgical treatment, or no treatment at all, the child becomes increasingly more aware of the abnormality until in the pubertal and post-pubertal period, he meets with constant peer assaults. In our opinion, early treatment of an obviously worsening condition aids the parents psychologically and is a confidence stimulator to the child—certainly a better alternative than having the child endure the condition until full growth has been obtained.

Early surgical repositioning of the mandible is necessary in order to take advantage of the enormous growth spurt that occurs in the immediate prepubertal years. The psychological milieu present at that precise time results in many positive advantages. First, there is active growth in the autogenous bone and cartilage used for grafting. Second, the recipient site is in a stage of active bone formation. Third, all growth centers involving the surrounding normal bones are actively increasing in size. The maxillary alveolar processes bilaterally are being driven inferiorly and anteriorly by rapid growth at the maxillary suture lines. As a result, it is only at this precise period in growth that one may consider the use of a procedure that will result in the surgical repositioning of the mandible alone. The canted occlusion is corrected by repositioning the mandible and allowing for the subsequent unrestricted growth inferiorly and anteriorly of the maxillary alveolar process on the affected side.

The technique for costochondral grafting varies somewhat depending on the problem. The lines of osteotomy and placement of the rib as suggested by Ware are illustrated in Fig. 23-71.

1. An incision is made over the surface of the sixth, seventh, or eighth rib from the lateral sternal border to the lateral portion of the chest wall. The rib is exposed from lateral sternal border to the point of greatest curvature on the lateral side, depending on the amount of rib needed. The rib is removed with care taken to *include approxi-mately 1 cm of costal cartilage* and to avoid pleural perforation. The rib is wrapped in a wet gauze sponge and placed on the back table.

2. A standard Risdon approach is made at the angle of the mandible on the affected side. The skin incision must be placed approximately 1 cm more inferiorly than usual in order to preclude closure immediately over the repositioned angle of the mandible.

3. The periosteum lateral to the vertical ramus of the mandible is elevated with a broad periosteal elevator. A Thompson ramus retractor is inserted into the sigmoid notch, but when no notch is present, any broad retractor will suffice.

4. An inverted L osteotomy is accomplished in the standard design with the horizontal cut superior to the mandibular foramen, joining the vertical cut just posterior to it and then extending inferiorly to the lower border of the mandible at the angle. Anomalous anatomy may dictate alteration in design of osteotomy (Fig. 23-67, *C*). The osteotomy can be accomplished with rotary or oscillating cutting instruments (Fig. 23-71, *A* and *B*).

5. A standard oblique osteotomy is usually necessary on the normal side. Both the wounds are packed and draped out of the field while the surgeons enter the mouth to immobilize the mandible in the pre-planned postoperative position employing an interocclusal splint (wafer) and intermaxillary elastics. The splint is constructed in a manner that causes opening of the interocclusal distance on the affected side.

6. After the surgeons change gloves, the wound on the affected side is entered and a bony portion of rib is fitted into position in the newly created space in the inverted L osteotomy (Fig. 23-71, *C*).

7. The remaining portion of the rib containing the cartilage is then cut to a length sufficient to fit from the glenoid fossa area along the posterior border of the mandible and is wired into position. That which is placed in the void created by the osteotomy

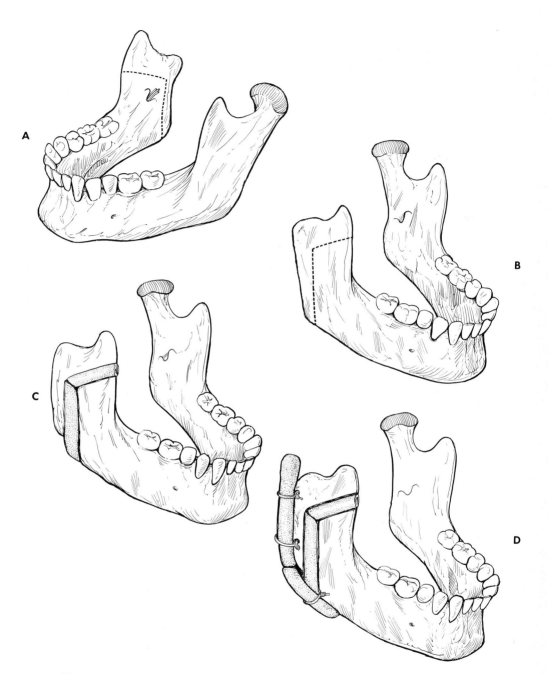

Fig. 23-71. The lines of osteotomy and placement of the rib as suggested by Ware.

is checked for proper position prior to closure (Fig. 23-71, *D*).

8. If indicated, a short portion of rib may be wired into position at the inferior border of the mandible to effectively lengthen the vertical ramus and decrease the mandibular angle.

9. The wounds are closed and a semipressure dressing is applied.

The preceding technique is used where there has been no previous surgical intervention; however, if a prosthesis or other foreign substance has been placed in the condyle area previously, as in Fig. 23-70, Case 2, that substance is removed and replaced with the costochondral graft without osteotomy at all. If the mandible cannot be freely distracted inferiorly to accommodate the interocclusal splint (wafer), coronoidotomy may be helpful.

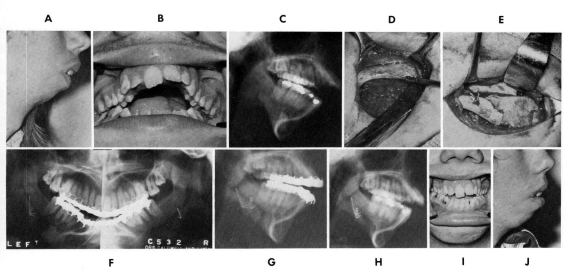

Fig. 23-72. A, The patient was first seen at age 10 years, but because of his many developmental physical disabilities correction of those related to the first arch syndrome were deferred until he was 18. **B,** There was an extreme Class II malocclusion with anterior open bite. **C,** The preoperative cephalogram was typical of this deformity, with prominent gonial angle, marked antigonial notching, shortened vertical ramus, bowed back symphysis, and proclination of the lower anterior teeth. Noted also was a deeply embedded lower canine tooth. **D,** Surgical correction was by an extremely long L osteotomy, the body portion of which extended to the area of the mental foramen. **E,** The embedded canine was removed prior to placement of autogenous iliac bone in the voids created. **F,** The postoperative panogram shows that the ramus portion of the distal (body) fragment was rotated inferiorly and forward as the open bite was closed anteriorly, that cast splints were used to provide a positive means of intermaxillary fixation with minimal damage to teeth, that a circummandibular wire was placed to ensure positive fixation of the splint to the teeth and prevent their extrusion, that transosseous wire was placed in such a direction that it complemented the other steps taken to counter relapse. Note also that the embedded canine tooth has been removed. **G,** The cephalogram also shows the effective direction of transosseous wire, heavy cast splints, circummandibular wire, and intermaxillary wire anteriorly. All combined to hold the mandible in its forward rotated position without harm to the teeth and countering relapse. **H,** In a cephalogram made 9 months after operation, the advanced mandible appears to be stable. **I,** There is an improvement in occlusion and function. **J,** However, the esthetic result is not acceptable. Augmentation genioplasty is indicated, but unless the investing soft tissue is also augmented by grafting, any advancement or addition of bone would doubtless be jeopardized as a result of tissue pressure. The patient declined the cosmetic benefit of additional surgery. (Courtesy General Rose Memorial Hospital, Denver.)

• • •

When patients with condylar agenesis have been treated with unsatisfactory results (Figs. 23-65 to 23-67) or not treated at all during the developmental years, accepted conventional methods are the only recourse. Results of surgery for these patients after growth is completed are not satisfactory as a result of the associated shortage of investing soft tissue, which places a definite limit on the amount of correction physically possible (Fig. 23-72).

APERTOGNATHIA (OPEN BITE DEFORMITY) AND OTHER OCCLUSION AND JAW ABNORMALITIES

Apertognathia, maxillary protrusion and retrusion, and other occlusion and jaw disharmonies and irregularities are correctable

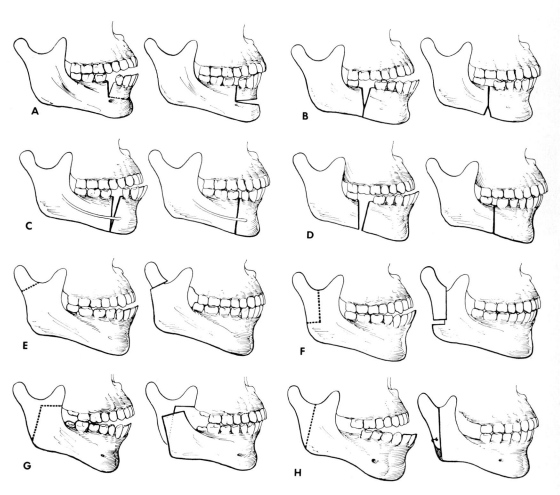

Fig. 23-73. Locations of mandibular osteotomy and ostectomy that have been used to correct anterior open bite deformities. **A,** Hullihen's V-shaped ostectomy. **B,** Thoma Y ostectomy. **C,** Lane and Pickerill V ostectomy. **D,** Thoma's trapezoid ostectomy. **E,** Babcock's osteotomy. **F,** Limberg's osteotomy. **G,** Pichler's and Trauner's osteotomy. **H,** Shira's oblique sliding osteotomy. (After Shira.)

surgically or may be improved sufficiently to greatly facilitate subsequent orthodontic or dental restorative care. Selection of a proper operation for correction of a given problem must be based on a critical examination of the patient's appearance, study of models, and cephalometric analysis. The relationship of the upper lip to the upper incisor teeth in resting, speaking, and smiling positions, correlated with the relationship of segments of sectioned study models, provides the most preoperative information. Murphey and Walker[77] emphasize the benefits of combined orthodontic–oral surgery workup, using photographs, study casts, and cephalometric roentgenograms. Depending on the results of these studies, surgery may be accomplished in the anterior maxilla, posterior maxilla, anterior mandible, mandibular rami, or a combination of more than one site.

A multiplicity of etiological factors exists in this category of deformities and occlusion irregularities. Principal among these causes are interference with the condylar growth center, abnormal tongue habits, and lip and finger sucking. *When the deformity*

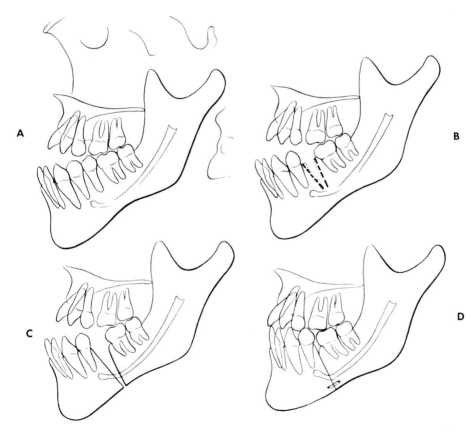

Fig. 23-74. Tracings from cephalograms of a patient with open bite deformity, or apertognathia. **A,** Preoperative relation. **B,** Intraoral V-shaped bone incisions to a level just above the mandibular canal. **C,** V ostectomy completed through an extraoral submandibular approach. **D,** Transosseous wiring at the lower border of the mandible supplemental to dental splinting and intermaxillary fixation.

is caused by habit, corrective surgery should not be undertaken until the habit has been overcome. This is especially the case in apertognathic conditions caused by tongue thrusting and reverse swallowing.

A number of *basic* operations are available for use in correction of these deformities and occlusal disharmonies, and the surgical techniques will be described later in this section. These basic operations, which are now generally accepted and utilized, have evolved over the years since Hulli-

hen's[50] historical first operation was performed in 1849 (Fig. 23-73, *A*). Blair[14] and many others[92,122,124] since then have recommended the procedure or modification of V-shaped ostectomy for correction of open bite (Fig. 23-73, *B* to *D*). Babcock,[5] Limberg,[65] and Pichler and Trauner[91] suggested operations in the ascending rami of the mandible to allow for repositioning of the mandible anteriorly and closure of the open bite relation (Fig. 23-73, *E* to *G*). The principle of vertical sliding osteotomy to lengthen the ramus was suggested in the first edition of this textbook (Figs. 23-75 and 23-76).

When the open bite deformity is associated with prognathism, a different problem presents. Thoma[124] suggested a trapezoid ostectomy in the body of the mandible, with the amount of bone excised determined by geometric measurement of the degree of open bite (Fig. 23-74, *B* to *D*). Shira[111] applied the principles of ramus vertical osteotomy in 8 cases of open bite and reported "gratifying results with little tendency for remission" (Fig. 23-73, *H*). We have also had good success with correction of open bite by vertical (not oblique) sliding osteotomy in the rami but have observed a greater tendency toward relapse than in ordinary prognathic cases. Since the overall vertical length of the ramus is definitely elongated or extended (by vertical sliding), it is our conviction that *decortication, direct transosseous wiring (overcorrected), and coronoidotomy are essential.* At the time of surgery, if anterior open bite cannot be reduced freely and without binding in the operative site, *it may be necessary to detach the sphenomandibular ligament from the lingula below the mandibular foramen.* This can also be done if the operation is being accomplished by intraoral sagittal splitting. *Direct transosseous wiring is virtually impossible if intraoral sagittal splitting or subcondylar (oblique) osteotomy is used in attempting elongation of the ramus.* Furthermore, *subcondylar (oblique) osteotomy is never indicated* as a method

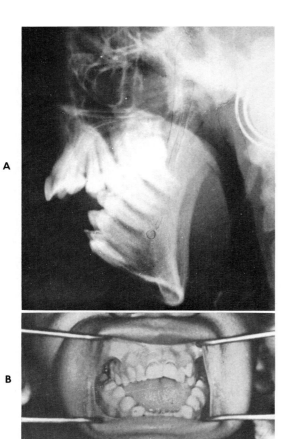

Fig. 23-75. A, Lateral cephalogram of a 10-year-old girl with extreme underdevelopment of the mandible and open bite. She was seen on consultation, but nothing was done at that time (1953) because of her youth. Twenty years later she would be treated surgically in staged procedures as illustrated in Fig. 23-76. **B,** Occlusion of same patient. (U. S. Army photographs; Letterman Army Hospital.)

for correction of anterior open bite. Mohnac[72] suggests "replacing the musculature at a higher point" when closing the soft tissue in these cases. *Also, one should plan for 6 to 8 weeks of immobilization. Most important of all, the abnormal tongue habits must be corrected preoperatively,* and the patient should continue under the care of a speech therapist for several months postoperatively. Many believe that the tongue will adjust further during the period of immobilization after surgery; however, *if there is any noticeable tendency to relapse, there should be no hesitancy to perform*

partial glossectomy at any time. Surgical detachment of the anterior belly of the digastric muscle at its origin on the medial surface of the inferior border of the mandible near the midline may also help overcome a tendency to relapse. Limberg[65] cut the ramus from the mandibular notch obliquely downward to a point near the lower aspect of the posterior border of the ramus above the angle where a short horizontal extension carried the incision to the posterior border. He did not mention any restraining effect that the attachment of the temporal muscle might have but did find it

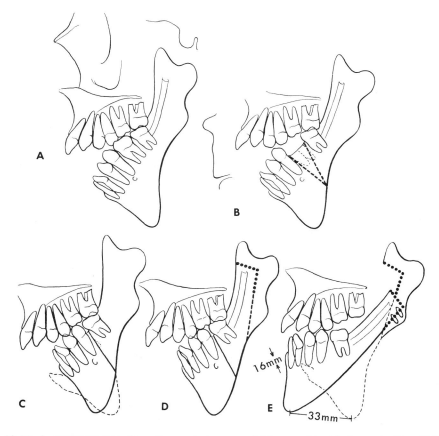

Fig. 23-76. A, Initial tracing from the cephalogram of 10-year-old girl shown in Fig. 23-75. A planned series of operations that can be done at an early age according to present day concepts. **B** and **C,** V ostectomy will close the incisal relationship about 12 mm and move mentum anteriorly about 10 mm. **D** and **E,** L-shaped sliding osteotomy in the ramus (Pichler and Trauner) at a later date will close the incisal relationship about 4 mm more, and by decortication and overlapping of bone ends, mentum will be extended anteriorly an additional 23 mm or a total of approximately 33 mm. Augmentation genioplasty would be a final procedure if indicated.

necessary to detach the stylomandibular ligament to permit downward movement of the body of the mandible. According to Pichler and Trauner,[91] these difficulties were overcome by altering the bone incision. By sectioning the ramus from its anterior border above the foramen (below the coronoid process) horizontally back and then vertically downard, neither the temporalis muscle nor the stylomandibular ligament impeded movement of the sectioned part. Their vertical bone incision was posterior to the foramen, thus avoiding injury to the nerve.

V-shaped ostectomy in the body of the mandible

Technique. The principle and technique for V ostectomy are essentially the same as described of ostectomy in the body of the mandible for correction of prognathism. Unless edentulous spaces are present in appropriate locations, a tooth (usually a premolar) must be extracted bilaterally. Two sets of instruments should be set up, one for the intraoral work and the other for the extraoral. The operation is done as a single procedure, the intraoral being accomplished first.

1. The patient is prepared and draped in the customary manner with curtain drapes to separate the intraoral operation from the extraoral.

2. Generous mucoperiosteal flaps are elevated buccally and lingually, with care exercised to protect the mental nerve.

3. A long-shanked No. 703 carbide fissure bur is used for all bone incisions in this operation.

4. The posterior vertical or transverse incision is made in the bone through the buccal and lingual cortical plates first, to a depth estimated to be just above the nerve.

5. The predetermined amount of bone to be removed is measured with calipers, and the anterior vertical bone incision is made, estimating the degree of angulation necessary to produce the desired V (Figs. 23-74, B to C, and 23-76, B).

6. The intervening bone should be fairly free after the bur cuts are made and can then be removed with end-cutting rongeurs. Thus an effort is made to uncover and identify the inferior alveolar nerve or its mental and incisive branches or both. Although this part of the procedure is tedious and painstaking, it is worthwhile to attempt to save the continuity of the nerves.

7. Both sides should be done before the extraoral stage of the operation is begun.

8. The patient is then repositioned, and the operating team prepares for the submental extraoral procedure.

9. The soft tissue dissection does not differ materially from that already described except (a) the mandibular branch of the facial nerve is more superiorly related in this area and usually will not be encountered, (b) considerable vascularity is present deep to the platysma muscle, but none of these vessels has the caliber of the facial vessels, and (c) progress to the bone is therefore easier and more rapidly accomplished.

10. As soon as the periosteum is reached, it is elevated widely until communication with the intraoral operation is reached and the intraoral bone cuts are in view.

11. The V excision is completed to the lower border, using a No. 703 bur. Once the anterior part of the mandible is mobilized, the segment of bone below the mental foramen can be freed and removed. Trauma to the nerve may result in temporary anesthesia, but even if severed, the nerve usually recovers. Excessive manipulation of the mobilized anterior part of the mandible should be avoided to prevent stretching or tearing of the nerve (Fig. 23-74, C).

12. The bone ends are held firmly with larger Kocher forceps clamped to the lower border as the edges are planed to fit into close approximation. Planing is accomplished with a No. 703 bur principally on the proximal (posterior) fragment. Failure of approximation may occur at the lower border because of the sliding up and

bending back of the distal (anterior) fragment.[122]

13. The mouth is reentered and the occlusion established anteriorly. Intermaxillary fixation is secured. Although not feasible in every instance, satisfactory results have been obtained in using a cast lingual splint on the lower teeth in these cases. This splint is cast to fit a study model that has been sectioned and repositioned. When this stage of the operation is reached, the mandible is moved into position and the teeth in it are wired to the lingual splint or a precast metal labial splint. Orthodontic appliances offer a positive means of fixation also. In any case, firm immobility must be established by some means in the dental arch between the anterior and posterior fragments.

14. The bone ends are then wired together inferiorly and the extraoral wounds closed in anatomical layers as described previously (Fig. 23-74, *D*).

15. Dressings and postoperative care are routine.

16. Healing time is dependent on the accuracy of bone approximation and adequacy of immobilization.

Sliding osteotomy to lengthen the rami (inverted L or vertical)

The osteotomy may be designed in different ways, depending on the problem. The inverted L-shaped osteotomy described by Pichler and Trauner[91] may be indicated, especially in small rami, such as are seen in agenesis (Fig. 23-76, *D* and *E*), or the straight vertical osteotomy (and coronoidotomy) from the mandibular notch may be chosen. However, when the rami are to be lengthened to correct the ordinary anterior open bite problem, the following operation is recommended.

Technique for sliding osteotomy to lengthen the rami

1. The approach to these operations is entirely extraoral and is the same as described previously.

2. If the inverted L or straight vertical osteotomies are selected because of smallness of the ramus, the cuts are outlined on the lateral surface with a No. 702 carbide bur and completed with the smaller gauge No. 701. The entire L or straight cut should be done with these two small burs because of thinness of the bone.

3. From template studies ("paper cutouts") a predetermination is made of the amount of lengthening needed in the ramus to correct the open bite and, if prognathism exists also, the amount of setback that should be anticipated.

4. A *long* vertical cut should be planned to ensure plenty of length to the proximal fragment at a relatively low level on the distal part. This vertical osteotomy may be straight, curved, or angular and is started with a No. 703 carbide fissure bur cut into the lateral cortex from mandibular notch to the angle (Fig. 23-77, *A*).

5. Coronoidotomy is essential and accomplished in the routine way by No. 14 drill perforations and fracture with chisel and mallet (Fig. 23-77, *B*).

6. Decortication is also essential, since success of the operation depends in part on close approximation of the fragments and direct transosseous wiring. The first step in decortication is accomplished by making a second vertical cut in the cortex roughly parallel and anterior to the first. Note the anterior black line in Fig. 23-77, *B,* which was determined by the relation established when the distal (body) part was moved to a desirable occlusion relation in Fig. 23-77, *F.* After both vertical cuts are completed through the lateral cortex, using caution over the approximate course of the mandibular canal, horizontal steps are cut at 6 to 8 mm intervals with a sharp No. 703 carbide fissure bur held at an acute angle to the surface of the bone. Thus steps are placed without risk of penetrating too deeply (Fig. 23-77, *C*). Horizontal steps can be made as far toward the sigmoid notch as necessary. Usually they need be extended only to the level of the foramen. Segments of cortical plate remaining between the horizontal

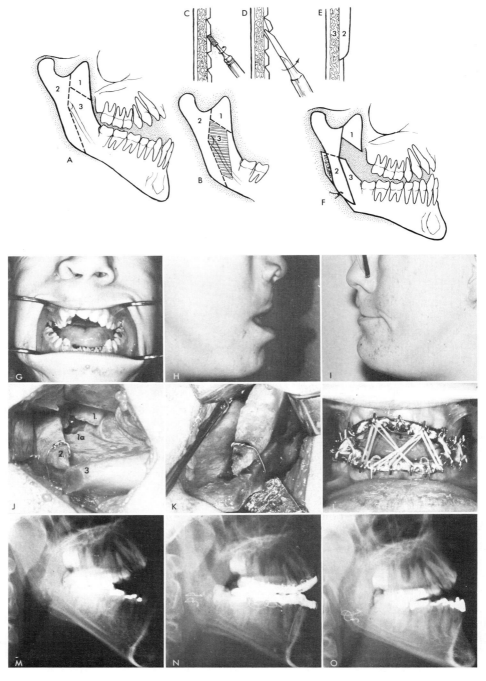

Fig. 23-77. For legend see opposite page.

steps are then excised using a sharp No. 3 Stout chisel *with the bevel down* (Fig. 23-77, *D*). Decortication accomplished in this manner is accurate, fast, and carries little risk of injury to the contents of the mandibular canal.

7. Vertical osteotomy is completed only after decortication and coronoidotomy have been accomplished on both sides. The cut is completed through the medial cortex from the foramen to the lower border first and then on to the mandibular notch.

8. After the vertical osteotomy on both sides has been completed, the oral cavity is entered to be certain that occlusion can be freely established in the incisor relation without restriction or force.

9. If there is any problem in obtaining unrestrained anterior relation, the operative sites are reentered to look for the impediment. One of the following may be necessary: (a) freeing of temporal muscle attachments below the site of the coronoidotomy, (b) detachment of the sphenomandibular ligament from the lingula, or (c) excision of bony interference in the subsigmoid area above the mandibular foramen.

10. Once unimpeded occlusal relation in the anterior area is assured, the mandible is immobilized into the predetermined relation. Cast labial splints or othodontic appliances are preferred to arch bars, since the period of immobilization will be protracted (6 to 10 weeks), and most of the intermaxillary ties will be in the anterior part of the arches, where extrusion of teeth may complicate the postoperative course. Cast splints serve to protect the teeth as

Fig. 23-77. Example of open bite. **A,** Broken lines represent a design of osteotomy required when the ramus is to be elongated to achieve closure of anterior open bite. The vertical cut may be angular, curved, or straight, but it must be extended as low as possible so that the proximal fragment will be long enough to provide ample approximation over the distal fragment. **B,** The shaded area designated by *3* is the area of the ramus on the distal (body) part that should be decorticated to accommodate the proximal fragment *2* overlap. **C,** The procedure for decortication is shown with a No. 703 bur applied at an acute angle to the outer cortex to prevent excessive penetration and chance of damage to contents of the mandibular canal. **D,** After these niches are made at 6- to 8-mm intervals up the "stepladder," a chisel is used to excise intervening segments of the outer cortex. **E,** One way to help reduce the tendency of relapse in open bite involves mortising the proximal part, *2,* on to the decorticated area, *3.* **F,** As the incisor relation is closed anteriorly, a fulcrum is brought into play in the molar region and the ramus portion of the body fragment is rotated downward, thus lengthening the vertical ramus. Obviously coronoidotomy is essential to permit this downward movement. The final relation to expect is shown with the proximal part, *2,* onlaid and mortised into the decorticated area, *3.* **G,** The case of a 17-year-old boy will help illustrate the ramus procedure that is used for correction of anterior open bite in indicated cases. In addition to the open bite that was accentuated by a repaired cleft palate, he had other developmental and organic anomalies and neglected dentition. **H,** He was unable to close his lips except forcibly and on profile view has an exceptionally long vertical dimension in the lower third of his face. **I,** Postoperative view 1½ years later. **J,** After decortication, coronoidotomy, and vertical osteotomy are completed, parts are fixed, that is, the end of the proximal fragment, *2,* is inlaid (mortised) into a notch, *3,* at the lowest extent of the decorticated area and wired into place. Note the gap between the coronoid process, *1,* and the area from which it had been cut, *1a.* **K,** A close view of the mortised joint on the other side. **L,** Cast splints securely fixed to the teeth and heavy anterior intermaxillary elastics for immobilization. **M,** Preoperative cephalogram shows the extreme open bite. **N,** Postoperative cephalogram shows a reduced anterior open bite. The lower splint is also supported anteriorly with two circummandibular wires. **O,** Cephalogram 1½ years postoperative shows some regression, which is not unexpected in this extreme case. Had it been possible to follow up this patient as closely as desired, the regression perhaps could have been controlled. (Photographs courtesy General Rose Memorial Hospital, Denver; drawings by Peter Stone.)

well as provide fixation anchorages. When splints are used, the patient should be instructed to use a Water Pik, since enamel may become hypoplastic if good hygiene is not provided.

11. When occlusion is secure, the operative sites are reentered, and the proximal fragment is adjusted to the decorticated area on the distal (body) part (Fig. 23-77, *E,* area 2 onto area 3). Mortised inlaid result is desirable, with the tip of the proximal fragment neatly fitted into a notch in the cortex (area 2). Some fitting is always needed and readily achieved by using a bur appropriately on the high spots, medial of the proximal fragment and lateral on the decorticated part of the distal fragment (area 2).

12. When fragments are finally well approximated (it is wise to allow for overcorrection), the parts are held in the desired relation, and a small drill hole is placed through both fragments. While the bone is held together, a doubled 0.016-inch stainless steel wire is threaded through. The doubled end is retrieved and cut. One wire is then tied around the posterior border and one carried out through another hole anterior to the first. The proximal fragment is thus securely fixed on both sides (Fig. 23-77, *J* and *K*).

When rami are lengthened as in this case, paresthesia of the lip almost invariably is a sequela because of stretching of the nerve between the foramen ovale at the base of the skull and the mandibular foramen.

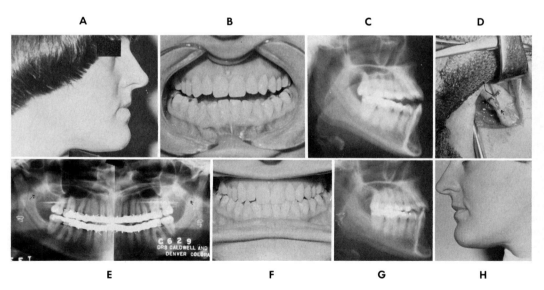

Fig. 23-78. A, This 27-year-old patient had a relatively normal attractive profile with only the slightest suggestion of mandibular prognathism. **B,** Oral examination disclosed total lack of occlusion except on the second molars. **C,** Examination of her cephalogram (and models) revealed a normal plane of occlusion but open from the second molar forward. Models could be placed in normal Class I relation. **D,** Bilateral vertical osteotomies included minimal decortication, notching (arrow), and transosseous wiring to ensure positive position of fragments and early union. **E,** Cast metal splints used for intermaxillary fixation (to prevent injury or extrusion of teeth), the mortised joint at the site of vertical osteotomy, and the wiring and bilateral coronoidotomy (arrow) are seen in the panogram made on the fourth postoperative day. **F,** Two-year follow-up revealed a closed occlusion with all teeth in functional reduction without orthodontics. **G,** Normal cephalogram and, **H,** a good cosmetic benefit with undetectable scarring. (Courtesy General Rose Memorial Hospital, Denver.)

The technique of osteotomy just described must never be modified to place the line of incision through the bone in an oblique direction from the mandibular notch to the posterior border of the ramus above the angle, but the line of incision must always be vertical or even anterior to the angle. Decortication is indicated, especially if prognathism coexists with apertognathia. *Direct wiring with overcorrection is always indicated.* Severing the coronoid process (coronoidotomy) to eliminate the pull of the temporal muscle helps to prevent relapse when a straight vertical cut from the mandibular notch has been made. These extra steps should be routine in correction of anterior apertognathia by this operation in the ramus.

The case illustrated in Fig. 23-77 is not ideal for application of this technique because of the reverse curve in the occlusion. In cases in which there is level occlusion and models can be related without rocking, the results obtained by this method are excellent and dependable (Fig. 23-78).

INTRAORAL SEGMENTAL OSTEOTOMIES
Anterior mandibular segmental osteotomy

Hullihen's[50] procedure for the correction of a mandibular deformity produced by burn scar contractures represents the first anterior mandibular segmental osteotomy. Illustrations of this procedure published in *Dental Cosmos* in 1849 depict an operation not unlike those used today to correct protrusion of the mandibular teeth resulting from dental rather than skeletal malformations. Hullihen completed the case by using a second procedure that excised the scar and placed a skin flap in the defect, thereby improving lip contour.

In 1942 Hofer[47,48] used a similar intraoral approach to accomplish the forward movement of the anterior mandibular segment. In 1910 Babcock[4] described the extraoral operation to accomplish the forward movement of a mandibular segment. Köle[62] re-

ported the use of circummandibular wire in the midline to stabilize the osteotomized segment and a modified intraoral incision, which allowed for unimpeded forward movement of the segment.

Technique for anterior mandibular osteotomy (Hofer)

1. A paragingival incision is made in the free mucosa 2 mm from its junction with the attached gingiva (Fig. 23-79). The incision is initiated at the first molar position and carried forward to the area of planned osteotomy where it passes to the crest of the gingiva. It is then continued from the crest of the gingiva into the paragingival area to the opposite osteotomy site where it again proceeds to the crest of the gingiva. It is completed by an extension paragingivally to the first molar area on the opposite site.

2. A subperiosteal flap is generated, and the chin prominence is degloved from mental foramen to mental foramen.

3. A bony incision is made with a No. 703 bur in the site of the planned osteotomy parallel to the long axis of the cuspid tooth. The incision is carried to a point 3 mm inferior to the apex of the cuspid tooth. A similar incision is made at the opposite osteotomy site. The inferior ends of these incisions are connected across the midline.

4. Teeth in the osteotomy sites are now extracted.

5. A lingual flap from the crest of the gingiva to include a distance of two teeth on each side of the osteotomy site is elevated.

6. A periosteal elevator is inserted to preserve the lingual periosteum while penetrations of the lingual cortical plate are made along the line of the planned osteotomy with a No. 703 bur.

7. The horizontal bony incision is completed from anterior to posterior with an oscillating Stryker saw blade.

8. The vertical osteotomy incisions are now completed with a fine, long-beveled chisel.

9. The freed segment is moved into the preplanned position. All modifications necessary to fit the segment to its new position

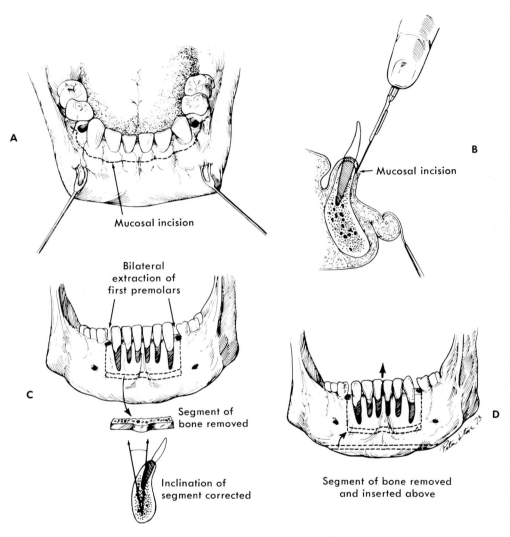

Fig. 23-79. Anterior mandibular segmental osteotomy. **A,** A full paragingival incision is made in the free labial mucosa. **B,** The mucosal incision is made obliquely rather than at right angles to the mucosal surface. **C,** The vertical bony incisions are made in the alveolar bone from which a premolar tooth has been extracted. The horizontal bony incision is placed 2 to 3 mm inferior to the nearest root apices. A segment of bone may be removed to allow for the placement of the segment in a more inferior position. The inclination of the segment may also be adjusted. **D,** Köle modification. A segment of bone removed during the accomplishment of a concomitant horizontal sliding genioplasty is used to graft the space created when the osteotomy segment is placed in a more superior position.

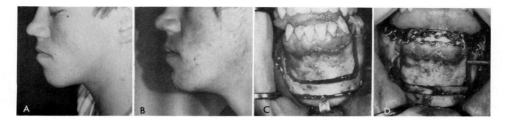

Fig. 23-80. Apertognathia of dental origin was treated by the elevation of a six tooth anterior mandibular segment using the technique recommended by Köle. **A,** Preoperative profile. **B,** Postoperative profile. **C,** Osteotomy bony incisions and incision for the removal of the lower border of the chin prominence. **D,** Segment fixed in cast labial splint and autologous bone graft from lower border in position. (Courtesy General Rose Memorial Hospital, Denver.)

should be made in the mandible, not in the segment. Removal of bone from the segment increases the possibility for damage to the root surfaces or apices of teeth within the segment. All segments being repositioned should go into place without the exertion of pressure.

10. Three 26-gauge transosseous wires are placed along the horizontal osteotomy.

11. A horizontal mattress suture with No. 3-0 Dexon suture material is placed across the gingival crest at each osteotomy site.

12. The surgical splints are wired into place.

13. The soft tissues are closed, using No. 3-0 Dexon suture material in a continuous horizontal mattress format.

14. A pressure bandage of gauze covering the lip and held in place by a 2.4 cm strip of adhesive tape that completely encircles the mandible and neck is placed.

The anterior maxillary and mandibular segmental osteotomies provide the refinement of lip contour and anterior occlusion that orthodontic treatment would provide if it were available or indicated (Fig. 23-80). There are two situations, however, in which surgical movement takes precedence over orthodontic movement. In one situation, an idiopathic resorption of tooth roots occurs after the application of minimal orthodontic forces. Evidence of root resorption appears radiographically after 1 month of attempted

movement. Surgical repositioning will provide the solution to the problems inherent in these cases. Care must be taken to ensure that segments to be moved are completely free before the application of splints to exclude pressures during the stabilization period. In the second situation in which surgical rather than orthodontic treatment is required, there is an anterior open bite of sufficient severity to require the displacement of the teeth with the alveolar process. This type of case, when treated orthodontically, has a proclivity for relapse.

Anterior maxillary osteotomy

Surgery for the maxillary osteotomy may take one of three forms. An initial discussion of the possibilities for surgical intervention was presented by Cohn-Stock[29] in 1921. The single-stage, predominantly labial approach was first reported by Wassmund[134] in 1926. Axhausen[3] added a tunneling procedure on the palate. Schuchardt[106] preferred a two-stage procedure, with the palatal side being treated first and completion of the surgery 4 to 6 weeks later from the labial approach. Wunderer[136] modified Wassmund's original operation in 1962. His single-stage, palatally oriented procedure has many advantages that make it the procedure of choice for most conditions requiring anterior maxillary repositioning. The basic operations are versatile. The segment to be treated may include

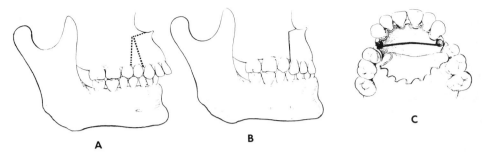

Fig. 23-81. Anterior maxillary osteotomy for correction of maxillary prognathism, retrusion, open bite, and closed bite. **A,** In maxillary protrusion, ostectomy is accomplished in the first premolar area, followed by horizontal osteotomy above the apices of the anterior teeth. **B,** After the palatal osteotomy is completed, **C,** the anterior maxilla is retruded to normal incisal relation. (Modified from Wassmund, M.: Lehrbuch der praktischen Chirurgie des Mundes und der Kiefer, vol. 1, Leipzig, 1935, Johann Ambrosius Barth.)

both premolar teeth bilaterally and all the anterior teeth or any of the various segments within these limits. Furthermore, surgical splitting in the midline permits two segments to be moved independently of each other. The closure of diastemas, recontouring of the anterior maxillary arch, repositioning of segments posteriorly, movement of segments superiorly or inferiorly, rotation of parts, and anterior movement with bone grafting are surgically possible (Fig. 23-81).

Technique for anterior maxillary osteotomy—labial approach (Wassmund)

1. A paragingival incision is made from a point two tooth widths proximal to the area of the planned osteotomy in the buccal sulcus and carried anteriorly to the gingival crest in the area of osteotomy. This incision is continued paragingivally in the labial sulcus to the planned osteotomy site on the opposite side of the dental arch. Here again it is carried to the gingival crest and completed paragingivally two tooth widths proximal to the osteotomy site.

2. A mucoperiosteal flap is generated superiorly to expose the piriform aperture bilaterally and the anterior nasal spine anteriorly.

3. Teeth in the planned osteotomy sites are extracted.

4. Vertical bony cuts are made in the lateral maxillary cortical plate at the midpoint of the planned osteotomy site. These are carried superiorly to a point approximately 3 mm superior to the canine tooth apex. The anterior bony incisions are completed by continuing the cuts medially to a point on the most lateral dimension of the piriform aperture. These bony cuts are preferably made with a narrow, tapered fissure bur, No. 700 (Fig. 23-82).

5. Attention is now directed toward the palatal portion of the procedure, where a subperiosteal tunnel is generated in the areas of the planned palatal osteotomy. This tunneling modification was proposed by Immenkamp.[51]

6. While the palatal tissues are protected with a suitable retractor, the bony incision is carried from the crest of the alveolar bone in one osteotomy site across the palate to the crest of the alveolus on the opposite portion of the arch. Care must be taken to avoid penetration of the nasoendotracheal tube.

7. The remaining bony attachment of the anterior maxillary segment, the nasal septum, is severed with a narrow single-beveled osteotome along the floor of the nasal cavity.

8. The segment is freed manually by cov-

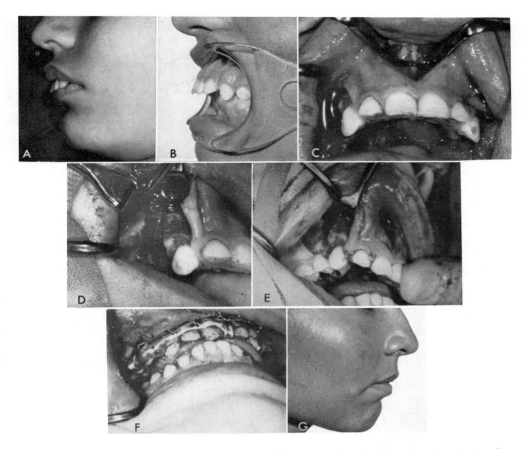

Fig. 23-82. A, Profile of 15-year-old girl with maxillary protrusion. **B,** Class II malocclusion. **C,** Through a vertical midline incision, horizontal osteotomy was accomplished. Although the bone cut *looks* low in this picture, it is placed just below the anterior nasal spine and floor of nasal fossa, well above the apices of the teeth. **D,** The first premolar is extracted, and osteotomy is accomplished in this area from buccal plate right through palate to permit retrusion of the anterior maxilla. **E,** When both horizontal osteotomy and vertical ostectomy are completed, the anterior maxilla is depressed back until space of first premolar is closed or to the previously established correct relation. **F,** Cast labial splint is fitted, soft tissue wounds are closed, and the splint is wired to the the teeth. **G,** Improved incisal relationship and appearance resulted. (Denver General Hospital with Dr. Paul Rowe.)

ering it with a gauze sponge, grasping it, and manipulating it until it is free of all attachments except the palatal pedicle.

9. Any bony portions within the osteotomy sites that resist the placing of the segment into its postoperative position are removed with a No. 703 tapered fissure bur. Relapse is possible if the segment cannot be repositioned with a minimum of effort. A

palatal stent with occlusal and incisal extensions constructed on the postoperative planning models is an excellent aid when employed during the contouring of ostectomy sites.

10. A horizontal mattress suture is placed to reposition labial and palatal tissues over the alveolar crest at each of the osteotomy sites. These sutures are placed

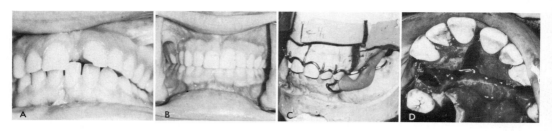

Fig. 23-83. This patient with procumbent anterior maxillary teeth and a 4-mm diastema between the maxillary central incisor teeth was treated by repositioning the two three-tooth anterior segments with an anterior maxillary segmental osteotomy using the technique proposed by Wunderer. **A,** Preoperative occlusion. **B,** Postoperative occlusion. **C,** Model operation with maxillary stabilization splint and mandibular occlusal index appliance. **D,** Palatal sections with segments freed.

at this time because they can be placed more easily and accurately prior to the placement of stabilizing splints.

11. Surgical splints are then fixed into position with circumdental wires.

12. The buccal and labial wounds are closed with a continuous horizontal mattress suture, using No. 3-0 Dexon material.

Anterior maxillary segmental osteotomy (Wunderer)

Wunderer[136] developed his procedure to provide a palatally oriented approach to the sectioning and repositioning of the anterior maxillary segment (Fig. 23-83). Because the segment is pedicled on the labial mucoperiosteum, it is possible to rotate it anteriorly for better visualization of the recipient sites. Hence bony trimming may take place under excellent vision.

Technique for anterior maxillary segmental osteotomy (Wunderer)

1. A 2-cm vertical incision is made one tooth width posterior to the planned osteotomy sites bilaterally. A mucoperiosteal flap is generated to expose the osteotomy sites in the alveolar bone bilaterally. These flaps are extended subperiosteally beyond the extent of the original mucosal incision by tunneling superiorly and medially to the margin of the piriform aperture.

2. Incisions are made in the bony cortex in the area of the planned osteotomies with a fissure bur. These are carried superiorly to a point 3 mm above the adjacent tooth apex and then inclined medially to the piriform aperture.

3. Attention is now directed toward the palate where a paragingival incision is made. This is planned so that it may extend from the first molar teeth anteriorly around the arch with extensions to the gingival crest in the areas of the planned osteotomies.

4. Bony incisions are made in the planned areas across the palate with a fissure bur. If a midline section is contemplated, an osteotomy incision is also extended from the mid palatal point of the first palatal incision to a point 3 mm from the crest of the interradicular bone between the two central incisor teeth.

5. The midline should be fractured with a fine, long-beveled osteotome at this time.

6. The lateral osteotomy incisions are now developed from the labial to the palatal sides with a fine osteotome.

7. The segment is freed completely by covering it with a gauze sponge and, with controlled manual force, fracturing it free of its remaining attachments.

8. The recipient sites are contoured with a bur.

9. The mucoperiosteal flap is replaced across the alveolar crest with a horizontal mattress suture.

10. Stabilization splints are fixed into position.

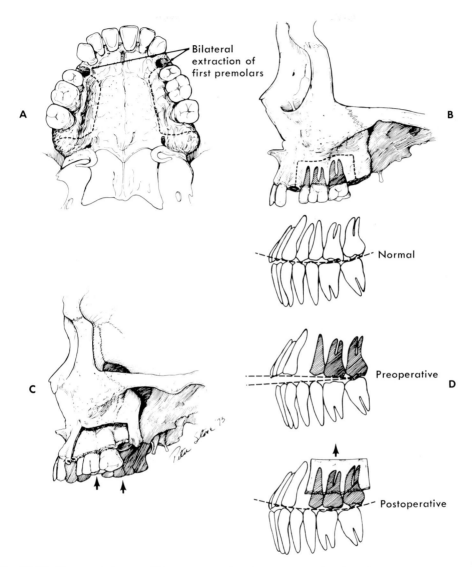

Fig. 23-84. The posterior maxillary segmental osteotomy was developed to correct cases of apertognathia produced by dental interference with closure. Apertognathia resulting from skeletal malformations are best corrected with the mandibular sagittal osteotomy. **A,** This procedure is best done in two stages. The first stage employs a full palatal flap. Either existing space posterior to the cuspid teeth or that created by the extraction of the first premolar teeth bilaterally is used for the anterior vertical alveolar bony incision. A horizontal bony incision superior to the palatal root apices joins the anterior bony incision with a similar incision posterior to the last tooth in the arch or in the pterygomaxillary fissure. **B,** The second stage employs a full gingival lateral flap. Bony incisions are made to correspond with the palatal incisions. **C,** The alveolar segment is displaced superiorly to a height necessary to close the anterior occlusion. **D,** Closure of bite by cephalad repositioning of posterior segments.

11. Soft tissues are closed with a continuous horizontal mattress suture.

12. A stent or gauze pack is placed over palatal tissues to prevent the formation of a hematoma on the palate.

Posterior maxillary osteotomy

Technique. Posterior maxillary osteotomy may be used to expand or narrow the maxillary arch unilaterally or bilaterally and to close vertical dimension posteriorly to correct anterior open bite. It is accomplished in a two-stage operation, the palatal side being completed first (Fig. 23-84).

1. Gingival incisions are made into the interdental papilla from the second molar forward to the central incisor on the palate.

2. Palatal mucoperiosteal tissues are elevated from the gingival margin, exposing the greater palatine foramen and contents. It is unnecessary to strip back the entire palatal covering.

3. Using a No. 703 carbide fissure bur, a cut is made anteriorly from the foramen to the first premolar area, where it is angled downward to the alveolar ridge between the premolar and canine teeth. This cut is kept in a vertical plane parallel with the long axis of the teeth and is carried through the palatine process of the maxilla to the maxillary antrum. The cut is then carefully extended posterolaterally to the pterygomaxillary fissure.

4. The palatal flap is replaced and sutured, and the second stage is delayed 3 to 4 weeks to ensure reestablishment of the blood supply.

5. After the delay a large buccal flap is raised from the gingival margin, exposing the lateral aspect of the maxilla from the canine prominence posteriorly to the tuberosity.

6. A thin, vertical cut is made between the canine and first premolar using a No. 701 or 702 carbide bur. (Occasionally the first premolar must be removed to permit desired placement of the sectioned part.)

7. A horizontal cut is made with a No. 703 bur from the pterygomaxillary fissure anteriorly under the zygomatic process above the apices of the teeth into the maxillary antrum and anteriorly, joining the vertical cut at the canine fossa.

8. If the sectioned part is to be depressed and impacted upward into the sinus, it may be necessary to remove additional bone along the horizontal bone cut.

9. A broad, flat, thin osteotome is usually needed to complete the surgical fracture.

10. A prefabricated labial cast splint is utilized here also to ensure union and resist relapse. Intermaxillary fixation with 0.016 gauge stainless steel wire is applied lightly but only between the anterior teeth.

A case illustrating results of this method for closing open bite deformities is shown in Fig. 23-85.

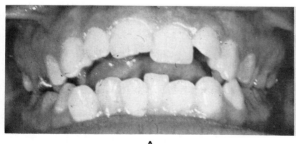 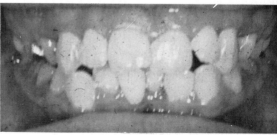

A   B

Fig. 23-85. A, Preoperative malrelation of the anterior teeth with open bite. **B,** Because of high lip line, posterior osteotomy was performed to close the incisal relationship. (Courtesy General Rose Memorial Hospital, Denver.)

Horizontal maxillary osteotomy (Le Forte I procedure)

Early efforts to reposition the entire maxillary alveolar process were directed at correcting traumatically malpositioned maxillary complexes. The dangers of maxillary sinus infections and fistulae as well as the possibility of necrosis of bony segments deterred many surgeons from attempting this correction. Axhausen[3] in 1934 reported the first horizontal maxillary osteotomy. Wassmund[134] followed with a method of advancement that employed a combined surgical-orthodontic movement. The sectioning of the lateral maxillary wall, the lateral nasal wall, and nasal septum was accomplished by a single horizontal incision from the tuberosity across the midline to the opposite tuberosity. Two weeks later elastics were placed on previously attached arch appliances. These were used to draw the partially freed maxillary alveolar process into the desired position. Köle[62] developed a two-stage total maxillary osteotomy. In the first stage he exposed the entire bony palate. An osteotomy in a block U form was made from the posterior border of the palatal bone through the greater palatine foramen, anterior to the second premolar tooth area, then across the palate in the frontal plane to join a similar osteotomy on the opposite side. In the second stage, cuts from the piriform aperture to the pterygomaxillary fissure and along the floor of the nose to detach the nasal septum were made. Recently Paul[87] reported a similar procedure in a single-stage operation. Mohnac[74] used a similar procedure to reposition a malunited maxillary fracture. He modified the palatal osteotomies by continuing them past the second premolar tooth to meet in the midline at the incisive canal. Bell and others* have recently made numerous important contributions to the refinement of maxillary surgical procedures. The "down fracturing" modification of the Le Forte I osteotomy (Fig. 23-86), with its subsequent exposure of the entire superior surface of the distal maxillary fragment, has opened a wide vista of innovations to the surgeon. The distal portion of the maxilla may be surgically segmented into numerous combinations from a superior approach.[68] Good visibility and a substantial palatal pedicle are the two most obvious advantages of this approach.

Technique for horizontal maxillary osteotomy (Le Forte I)

1. An incision is made 2 mm superior to the junction of the free and attached gingiva from the zygomatic process of the maxilla across the midline to the zygomatic process on the opposite side (Fig. 23-87).

2. A mucoperiosteal flap is generated superiorly to the infraorbital foramen, exposing the zygomatic process of the maxilla and the piriform aperture.

3. A bony incision with a No. 703 tapered fissure bur is made from the base of the zygomatic process of the maxilla anteriorly to a point approximately 1 cm above the floor of the nasal cavity. A similar osteotomy cut is made on the opposite side.

4. The periosteum from the base of the zygomatic process to the pterygomaxillary fissure is elevated by a tunneling procedure.

5. The pterygoid plates are fractured

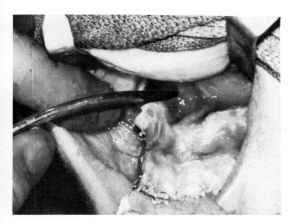

Fig. 23-86. Down-fracturing maxilla. Note excellent exposure of maxillary antrum floor and floor of nasal cavity.

---

*See references 9, 10, 137, and 138.

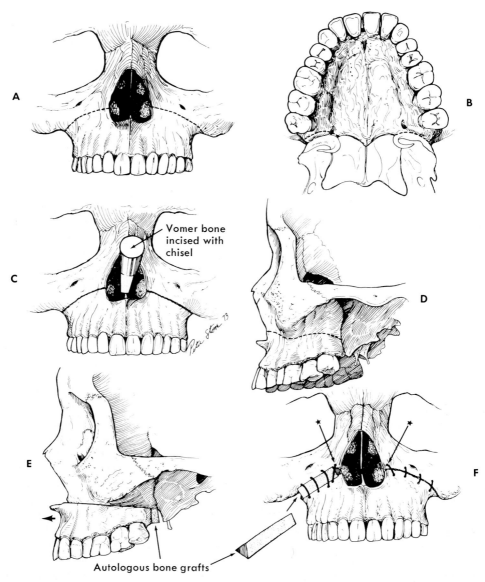

Fig. 23-87. Horizontal maxillary osteotomy. This procedure is employed to correct the position of the entire maxillary alveolar process in three planes. **A,** Lateral horizontal bony incisions are made in the most superior accessible position to place them in thicker maxillary bone. **B,** Bony incisions are made posterior to the maxillary tuberosities bilaterally to separate the maxilla from the pterygoid plates. **C,** The nasal septal cartilage and the vomer bone are separated parallel to the floor of the nasal cavity. **D,** Lateral view of the bony incisions. **E,** Autologous bone from the crest of the ilium is placed bilaterally posterior to the maxillary tuberosity after the placement of the maxillary segment in its postoperative position. The section of bone is cut equal in size to the amount of anterior displacement of the maxillary segment. **F,** A section of autologous bone is placed in the lateral osteotomy bone incisions. Transosseous wires are placed to secure the segment. The most anterior wire on either side must be placed so that it will resist the tendency of the segment to relapse into its preoperative position.

from the posterior portion of the maxilla with a curved Obwegeser osteotome.

6. The nasal septal cartilage and vomer attachments are severed from the maxilla with a fine osteotome. Care should be taken to protect the nasopharyngeal area with a finger because perforation of the nasoendotracheal tube is possible.

7. The lateral wall of the nasal cavity is sectioned at a level below the attachment of the inferior turbinate bone with a fine osteotome.

8. The maxilla may be freed of its remaining attachments by one of four methods. We prefer the use of Rowe forceps. The maxilla may also be fully mobilized by inserting both curved osteotomes or the Tessier instrument posterior to the maxillary tuberosities and rocking it free. In some instances the maxilla may be fully freed by placing a gauze sponge over the teeth and manipulating the segment in all directions with hand pressure. It is of utmost impor-

tance that the freed maxilla go to the new position with minimal force.

9. The teeth are now placed in the postoperative position and intermaxillary elastics used to maintain this occlusion (Fig. 23-88).

10. Rectangular sections of autogenous crest of ilium are cut to a size that is equal to the amount of forward movement of the maxilla on each side, and these sections are inserted between the tuberosity and the pterygoid plates.

11. Transosseous wires are placed across the osteotomy sites in the lateral maxillary walls. These are tagged with hemostats.

12. The lateral osteotomy sites are grafted and the previously placed transosseous wires twisted to fix the maxillary fragments and bone grafts in position. These grafts are triangular in cross section.

13. The incisions are closed with No. 3-0 Dexon suture material in a continuous horizontal mattress format.

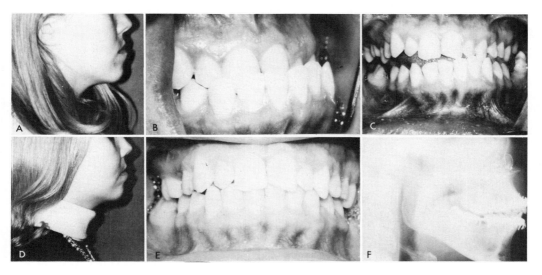

Fig. 23-88. A 23-year-old woman with a normal mandibular skeletal and dental configuration but a retruded maxilla was treated with horizontal maxillary osteotomy (Le Forte I). The total maxillary alveolar segment was moved laterally to the patient's left, rotated to correct the midline discrepancy, lowered 5 mm on the patient's right and 1 mm on the patient's left, and brought anteriorly 4 mm. **A,** Preoperative profile. **B,** Preoperative convenience bite. **C,** Preoperative centric jaw relation. **D,** Postoperative profile. **E,** Postoperative occlusion. **F,** Postoperative cephalometric radiograph.

Indications for horizontal maxillary osteotomy without a deficiency in the infraorbital rims. Retrusion of the maxilla associated with a normal configuration of the mandible is treated best by the repositioning of the entire maxillary alveolar process. In this manner, two of Obwegeser's three basic principles are satisfied. The basilar bone is placed in its proper position, and the dental occlusion is improved. When preoperative or postoperative orthodontic treatment is employed, the third basic principle, which is adjustment of the inclination of the anterior teeth to the basilar bone, is satisfied.

Apertognathia as a result of a malposition or developmental deformity of the maxilla and not associated with a short superior lip may also be corrected by the repositioning of the full maxillary alveolar process. In cases associated with an abnormally short superior lip, the anterior open bite is best treated by repositioning the posterior maxillary segments in a cephalad direction, utilizing the Schuchardt technique.

Residual defects after cleft palate surgery are often also treated by repositioning the remaining maxillary alveolar process. In most cases the residual palatal and alveolar defects are bone grafted as a secondary procedure after the anterior positioning of the alveolar segments. The technique for bone grafting in the palate is technically difficult. Extreme care must be exercised to ensure that a watertight nasal mucosal seal is developed and that both the nasal and palatal flaps are tightly applied to the bone graft material. Thus the possibility of the development of a hematoma between flap and bone is eliminated.

Complications after horizontal maxillary osteotomy. Two complications are frequently associated with the horizontal maxillary osteotomy. Relapse is often reported. Trauner[128] reports that the possibility of relapse is eliminated when sufficient overbite exists in the maxillary anterior teeth to form a locked-in anterior occlusion postoperatively. Another deterrent to relapse is the proper measurement and placement of the bone graft material between the maxillary tuberosity and the pterygoid plates bilaterally. Obwegeser recommends that the most

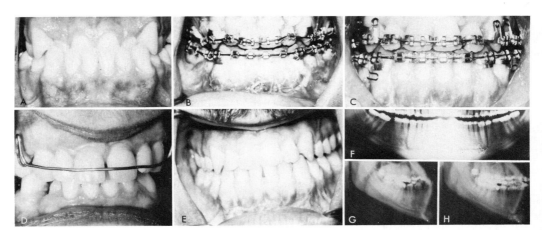

Fig. 23-89. This patient with lingually positioned maxillary incisor teeth and recumbent mandibular anterior teeth was treated with small segment osteotomies of the six maxillary anterior teeth and an anterior mandibular segmental osteotomy. **A,** Preoperative occlusion. **B,** Postoperative band splint stabilization device. **C,** Active postoperative orthodontic movement to refine anterior occlusion. **D,** Retaining device worn for 6 months to maintain position of teeth. **E,** Postoperative occlusion. **F,** Postoperative panographic roentgenogram. **G,** Preoperative cephalometric roentgenogram. **H,** Postoperative cephalometric roentgenogram.

anterior transosseous wires across the horizontal osteotomy sites bilaterally be placed so as to resist the tendency toward relapse of the osteotomized segment.

A frequent and troublesome complication after the maxillary procedure is secondary hemorrhage. The critical period appears to be between 7 and 10 days after the operation. Furthermore, the site of hemorrhage is most often the lateral nasal mucosa. Surgeons reporting fewer hemorrhages in this area section the lateral nasal wall with an osteotome introduced across the maxillary antrum through the osteotomy in the lateral maxillary wall.

Small segment osteotomies

The technique for mobilizing small alveolar segments was developed in an effort to minimize the time required for orthodontic movement (Fig. 23-89). A refinement of the earlier corticotomy technique developed by Bichlmayr[13] and Köle[59] was developed to pedicle the segments on either a labial or palatal flap rather than on the small segment of medullary bone contained within the osteotomy cuts. Bell showed with animal studies that the older corticotomy technique does not provide a sufficient blood supply to the segments. Both one-stage and two-stage approaches have been advocated. Kruger prefers a one-stage technique from a palatal approach. We prefer the two-stage approach.

Technique for small segment osteotomies

1. A full palatal flap is elevated (Fig. 23-90).

2. Bony incisions with a No. 700 bur to

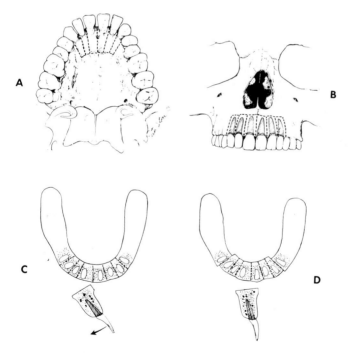

Fig. 23-90. Anterior maxillary single-tooth osteotomy. This procedure is an improved version of the corticotomy. It is best accomplished in two stages. **A,** Stage one is accomplished by a palatal approach. A full palatal flap is raised. Bony incisions are made with a fissure bur. **B,** Second stage completes the procedure. A full labial flap is raised. Bony incisions are made in the interradicular bone. The individual segments are freed with an osteotome. **C** and **D,** Segments are repositioned to close diastemas and correct excess procumbency or recumbency of the teeth.

bleeding bone are made parallel to the long axis of the roots of the teeth to be moved. The incisions are joined across the palate.

3. The flap is repositioned.

4. Four weeks later a full labial flap is elevated.

5. Bony incisions with a No. 700 bur corresponding to those on the palatal surface are made, taking care to limit the bur cut to 2 to 3 mm from the crest of the interradicular bone.

6. The individual segments are fractured free of their bony attachments with an osteotome.

7. The segments are placed into the preplanned position and fixed to an arch-stabilizing appliance.

8. The flap is replaced and sutured.

Techniques for moving small segments of alveolar bone with teeth have enjoyed recent widespread application. As with all new procedures, attempts have been made to broaden the scope of application beyond the inherent limits of the anatomical structures involved. Rapid orthodontics is a myth. The same limitations that apply to larger segments affect small segments. Equally true is the fact that orthodontic forces applied to small segments will cause the same deleterious effects to tooth structure if physiological norms are exceeded. Teeth moved in a small segment require careful follow-up and varying periods of postoperative stabilization with a retainer. We have found the moving of small segments of the mandibular dental arch unfeasible and unrewarding.

COMPLICATIONS (INTRAORAL OPERATIONS)

A discussion of the complications resulting from surgical procedures performed intraorally must be prefaced by an understanding of the true meaning of the terms *complication* and *sequela*. Even medical dictionaries are not entirely lucid on this difference. In our opinion, a complication is an unexpected condition occurring after and associated with an operation. Sequelae

on the other hand are conditions that are commonly expected, occurring after and associated with operations. For instance, infection is a complication, whereas swelling is a sequela of soft tissue surgery. However, sequelae, when they are severe or not controlled with accepted postoperative care and handling methods, may cause complications. Thus the severity of swelling after the accomplishment of the same procedure may vary according to the length of time used to complete the case, the care with which tissues are handled, and the medical and mechanical means used to control postoperative edema.

First and foremost among preoperative measures necessary to eliminate or minimize complications is the history. A complete discussion of the art of history taking is not apropos here because it is presented extremely well in other chapters. The patient must be physically and psychologically able to cope with the surgical insult.

In our opinion, the preoperative administration of appropriate antibiotics and the steroid dexamethasone (Decadron) is de rigueur in all intraoral procedures involving tissues contiguous with the airway. An appropriate antibiotic should be administered preoperatively to all patients on whom major intraoral procedures are to be performed. The steroid and antibiotic may be given intravenously while the patient is on the table prior to the initiation of surgery.

The oral cavity must be cleansed preoperatively. Terry[120] recommends toothbrushing in the operating room as part of the preoperative preparation procedure. All sources of unusual intraoral contamination should be eliminated in the preoperative workup. Cleansing the mouth with aqueous thimerosal (Merthiolate) or povidone-iodine (Betadine) solution should follow the insertion of the throat pack.

Incisions must be positioned so that they afford the surgeon access to and a visualization of the entire operative site. Intraoral incisions are best made in the paragingival position rather than at the gingival crest. Incisions thus placed may be closed easier and with more assurance of a watertight seal. We prefer closing with a polyglycolic acid suture material (Dexon) in a continuous horizontal mattress suture format.

Extreme care must be exercised to restrict the operative field to the periosteal confines. Reports of profuse hemorrhage in most cases occur after the planned or inadvertent perforation of the periosteal covering in regions where there are large vessels contiguous to the operative field. Three areas requiring special care surround the vertical ramus of the mandible. These are the posterior border (retromandibular vein), the premasseteric incisure (facial vessels), and the lingular area (inferior alveolar vessels). Neuropathies also may be associated with perforation of the periosteum. Seventh nerve palsies have been reported. They are most likely caused by perforation of the periosteum at the posterior border of the vertical ramus of the mandible or at the lower border.

We are aware of three cases of profuse hemorrhage associated with large vascular anomalies contiguous to deformed mandibles. All were unilateral deformities. None showed any roentgenographic evidence of bony involvement with the lesion. It would seem prudent then to order vascular studies of the external carotid vessel on the side of contemplated surgery in this type of case.

Preoperative planning and care during surgery must be directed toward the maintenance of a wide vascular pedicle to all segments of bone being treated by osteotomy or ostectomy. Inadvertent stress on the soft tissues or the segment during surgery must be eliminated.

Osteotomy or ostectomy bony incisions must be made in areas as widely separated from tooth roots and apices as surgically possible. It is a wise maxim to make all alterations necessary to reposition maxillary and mandibular segments in the recipient site rather than in the segment itself. Teeth whose apices are inadvertently ex-posed during surgery should be endodontically treated before the operation is completed.

Obwegeser[83] stresses that segments or portions of the maxilla or mandible being moved to new positions should go to position with the least force possible. Thus the entire maxilla freed by the Le Forte I procedure or the entire mandible freed by the sagittal osteotomy may be transported to position with a light tissue forceps. Furthermore, no undue stress should be exerted to place the segments within the confines of the surgical splints. Orthodontic band splints allow for the final, fine adjustment of position of segments without placing damaging stresses on the structures involved. Thus the segments may be placed in positions "besser als Modelen" (better than the models).

Intraoral drainage is recommended after the sagittal osteotomy of the mandible to minimize the large amount of edema associated with this procedure. A No. 10 French catheter is perforated randomly for approximately 8 cm from the end to be introduced into the wound. This is placed with a stab incision anterior to the operative incision so that the tip is at the sigmoid notch. This is attached for 24 hours to low (40 psi), intermittent suction. No pressure dressings are required when this is done. Incisions are closed as stated previously with a biodegradable suture material.

Reports of complications after the sagittal osteotomy of the mandible have been published by Guernsey and DeChamplain[38] and by Behrman.[8] The numbers and severity of complications associated with this procedure indicate that the surgeon must bring more than usual skill and a cursory knowledge of the procedure to the operating room. The technical difficulty dictates that he or she must have observed the execution of the procedure by a surgeon with some successful completions, that is, completions free of severe complications. Furthermore, the precision of the required osteotomy incisions and the limited access because of anatomical confines demand the use of specially constructed instruments. In summary, the sagittal osteotomy of the vertical ramus of the mandible, a worthwhile, useful operation, requires extraordinary preparation.

CONCLUSION

Robinson[99] states that a "standardized outline of surgical technic for prognathism is necessary in teaching residents." We hope this chapter may provide the basis for such an outline in surgical technique. However, training must never become a stereotyped process, otherwise variations from normal may not be coped with adequately when encountered. Students (residents) must be stimulated to think independently and individually and preceptors must teach *all* acceptable methods of corrective jaw surgery, including the more difficult procedures and also those less frequently needed. Imagination and the versatility of many of the operations described herein make possible the correction of almost any conceivable deformity that may be present, but the results will depend largely on how well the operation is planned and on the surgical ability of the surgeon. Blair's classic remark in 1907 that the mandible "is a hoop of bone capable of almost any kind of adjustment" is more realistic in this modern day than ever before. Astute and aggressive as he was, Hullihen would look on the many new innovations in maxillary and mandibular surgery and say, "Well done, but what are your new horizons?"

REFERENCES

1. Akin, R. K., and Walters, P. J.: Experience with the intra-oral vertical subcondylar osteotomy, J. Oral Surg. **33**:342, 1975.
2. Ascher, F.: Zum Problem der chirurgischen Obilisierung des prognathen Oberkiefer-Mittelstückes in kieferorthopaedischer Sicht, Fortschritte der Kiefer und Gesichts-Chirurgie, vol. I, Stuttgart, 1955.
3. Axhausen, G.: über die korrigierende Osteotomie am Oberkiefer, Deutsch. Z. Chir. **248**:515, 1937.
4. Babcock, W. W.: Surgical treatment of certain deformities of jaw associated with malocclusion of teeth, J.A.M.A. **53**:823, 1909.
5. Babcock, W. W.: Field of osteoplastic operations for the correction of deformities of the jaws, Dent. Items Interest **32**:439, 1910.
6. Barsky, A. J.: Principles and practice of plastic surgery, Baltimore, 1950, The Williams & Wilkins Co., p. 312.
7. Batson, O. V.: The temporalis muscle, Oral Surg. **6**:40, 1953.
8. Behrman, S. J.: Complications of sagittal osteotomy of the mandibular ramus, J. Oral Surg. **30**:544, 1972.
9. Bell, W. H.: LeForte I osteotomy for correction of maxillary deformities, J. Oral Surg. **33**:412, 1975.
10. Bell, W. H.: Correction of short-face syndrome vertical maxillary deficiency: a preliminary report, J. Oral Surg. **35**:110, 1977.
11. Bell, W. H., and Kennedy, J. W.: Biological basis for vertical ramus osteotomies—a study of bone healing and revascularization in adult rhesus monkeys, J. Oral Surg. **34**:215, 1976.
12. Bell, W. H., and Schendel, S. A.: Biological basis for modification of the sagittal ramus split operation, J. Oral Surg. **35**:362, 1977.
13. Bichlmayr, A.: Chirurgische Kieferorthopaedie und das Verhalten des Knochens und der Wurzelspitzen nach derselben, Deutsch. Zahnaerztl. Wschr. **34**:835, 1931.
14. Blair, V. P.: Operations on the jaw-bone and face, Surg. Gynecol. Obstet. **4**:67, 1907.
15. Blair, V. P.: Underdeveloped lower jaw, with limited excursion, J.A.M.A. **53**:178, 1909.
16. Bruhn, C.: The surgical-orthopedical removal of the deformations of the jaws, Int. J. Orthod. **13**:65, 1927.
17. Byrne, R. P., and Hinds, E. C.: The ramus "C" osteotomy with body sagittal split, J. Oral Surg. **32**:259, 1974.
18. Caldwell, J. B.: Surgical correction of development deformities of the mandible, U.S. Armed Forces Med. J. **3**:362, 1954.
19. Caldwell, J. B.: Surgical correction of extreme mandibular prognathism, J. Oral Surg. **26**:253, 1968.
20. Caldwell, J. B.: Surgical management of temporo-mandibular joint ankylosis in children. Sixth International Conference on Oral Surgery, Sydney, Australia, May 16-20, 1977, submitted for publication.
21. Caldwell, J. B.: Impaired facial expression secondary to "degloving," a case report, submitted for publication.
22. Caldwell, J. B., and Amaral, W. J.: Mandibular micrognathia, corrected by vertical osteotomy in the rami and iliac bone graft, J. Oral Surg. **18**:3, 1960.

23. Caldwell, J. B., Hayward, J. R., and Lister, R. L.: Correction of mandibular retrognathia by vertical-L osteotomy: a new technic, J. Oral Surg. **26:**259, 1968.

24. Caldwell, J. B., and Hughes, K. W.: Prognathism in edentulous and partially edentulous patients, J. Oral Surg. **16:**377, 1958.

25. Caldwell, J. B., and Letterman, G. S.: Vertical osteotomy in the mandibular rami for correction of prognathism, J. Oral Surg. **12:**185, 1954.

26. Caldwell, J. B., and Lister, R. L.: Retrognathia, a variant surgically corrected by Z osteotomy in the rami, submitted for publication.

27. Caldwell, J. B., Lister, R. L., and Gerhard, R. C.: Surgical lengthening of the mandibular ramus in agenesis (first arch syndrome), submitted for publication.

28. Caldwell, J. B., Lister, R. L., and Gerhard, R. C.: Surgical treatment of mandibular hypertrophy (unilateral macrognathia), submitted for publication.

29. Cohn-Stock, G.: Die chirurgische Immediatregulierung der Kiefer, speziell die chirurgische Behandlung der Prognathie, Vjschr Zahn **37:**320, 1921.

30. Colle, A. J.: Some clinical applications of cephalometric analysis, J. Can. Dent. Assoc. **20:**309, 1954.

31. Dal Pont, G.: Retromolar osteotomy for the correction of prognathism, J. Oral Surg. **19:**42, 1961.

32. Dingman, R. O.: Surgical correction of mandibular prognathism, an improved method, Am. J. Orthod. Oral Surg. (Oral Surg. Sect.) **30:**683, 1944.

33. Dingman, R. O.: Surgical correction of developmental deformities of the mandible, Plast. Reconstr. Surg. **3:**124, 1948.

34. Duformental, L.: Le traitement chirurgical du prognathisme, Presse Med. **24:**235, March 23, 1921.

35. Engel, M. B., and Brodie, A. G.: Condylar growth and mandibular deformities, Surgery **22:**976, 1947.

35a. Epker, B. N., and Wolford, L. M.: Middle third facial osteotomies; their use in correction of acquired and developmental dentofacial and craniofacial deformities, J. Oral Surg. **33:**491, 1975.

35b. Epker, B. N., and Wolford, L. M.: Middle third facial osteotomies; their use in the correction of congenital dentofacial and craniofacial deformities, J. Oral Surg. **34:**324, 1976.

36. Fox, F. L., and Tilson, H. B.: Mandibular retrognathia: a review of the literature and selected cases, J. Oral Surg. **34:**53, 1976.

37. Graber, T. M.: In Salzmann, J. H., editor: Roentgenographic cephalometrics; proceedings of the workshop conducted by the special committee of the American Association of Orthodontists,

Philadelphia, 1961, J. B. Lippincott Co., pp. 21-34.

38. Guernsey, L. H., and DeChamplain, R. W.: Sequelae and complications of the intraoral sagittal osteotomy in the mandibular rami, Oral Surg. **32:**176, 1971.

39. Hall, H. D., Chase, D. C., and Pryor, L. G.: Evaluation and refinement of the intra-oral vertical subcondylar osteotomy, J. Oral Surg. **33:**333, 1975.

40. Harsha, W. M.: Bilateral resection of the jaw for prognathism, Surg. Gynecol. Obstet. **15:**51, 1912.

41. Hayes, P. A.: Correction of retrognathia by modified "C" osteotomy of the ramus and sagittal osteotomy of the mandibular body, J. Oral Surg. **31:**682, 1973.

42. Hebert, J. M., Kent, J. N., and Hinds, E. C.: Correction of prognathism by an intra-oral vertical subcondylar osteotomy, J. Oral Surg. **28:**651, 1970.

43. Hensel, G. C.: The surgical correction of mandibular protraction, retraction and fractures of the ascending rami, Int. J. Orthod. **23:**814, 1937.

44. Hinds, E. C.: Surgical correction of acquired mandibular deformities, Am. J. Orthod. **43:**160, 1957.

45. Hinds, E. C.: Correction of prognathism by subcondylar osteotomy, J. Oral Surg. **16:**209, 1958.

46. Hinds, E. C., and Kent, J. N.: Surgical treatment of developmental jaw deformities, St. Louis, 1972, The C. V. Mosby Co., pp. 64, 176, 185, 190, and 191.

47. Hofer, O.: Die vertikale Osteotomie zur Verlangerung des einseitig verkurzten aufsteigenden Unterkieferastes, Oest. Z. Stomat. **34:**826, 1942.

48. Hofer, O.: Operation der Prognathie und Mikrogenic, Deutsch. Zahn. Mund. Kieferheilk. **9:**121, 1942.

49. Hovell, J. H.: The surgical treatment of some of the less common abnormalities of the facial skeleton, Dent. Pract. **10:**170, 1960.

50. Hullihen, S. P.: Case of elongation of the underjaw and distortion of the face and neck, caused by burn, successfully treated, Am. J. Dent. Sci. **9:**157, 1849.

51. Immenkamp, A.: A. Beiträge zur maxillo fazialen Chirurgie unter besonderer Berücksichtigung der Korrektur von Fehlbildungen des Mittelgesichtes, Fortschritte der Kiefer und Gesichts-Chirurgie, vol. VII, Stuttgart, 1961.

52. Jaboulay, M., and Berard, L.: Traitement chirurgical du prognathisme inferieur, Presse Med., No. 30, p. 173, April 19, 1898.

53. Kaplan, H., and Spring, P. N.: Gustatory hyperhidrosis associated with subcondylar osteotomy, J. Oral Surg. **18:**50, 1960.

54. Kazanjian, V. J.: Surgical correction of defor-

mities of the jaws and its relation to orthodontia, Int. J. Orthod. **22:**259, 1936.

55. Kazanjian, V. H.: The inter-relation of dentistry and surgery in the treatment of deformities of the face and jaws, Am. J. Orthod. Oral Surg. (Oral Surg. Sect.) **27:**10, 1941.

56. Kazanjian, V. H.: The treatment of mandibular prognathism with special reference to edentulous patients, Oral Surg. **4:**680, 1951.

57. Kazanjian, V. H., and Converse, J. M.: Surgical treatment of facial injuries, Baltimore, 1949, The Williams & Wilkins Co., p. 433.

58. Köle, H.: Beitrag zur Beseitigung des tiefer Bisses nach der prognathieoperation, Zahnaerztl. Rundsch. **67:**157, 158.

59. Köle, H.: Corticallisschwachung zur Unterstützung bei der kieferorthopadischen Behandlung, Fortschritte der Kiefer und Gesichts-Chirurgie, vol. IV, Stuttgart, 1958.

60. Köle, H.: Formen des offenen Bisses und ihre chirurgische Behandlung, Deutsch. Stomat. **9:**753, 1959.

61. Köle, H.: Personal communication, International Congress for Maxillo-Facial Surgery, Graz, Austria, May, 1959.

62. Köle, H.: Surgical operations on the alveolar ridge to correct occlusal abnormalities, Oral Surg. **12:**277, 413, 515, 1959.

63. Kostecka, F.: A contribution to the surgical treatment of open bite, Int. J. Orthod. Dent. Child. **20:**1082, 1934.

64. Letterman, G., Caldwell, J. B., Schurter, M., and Shira, R. B.: Vertical osteotomy in the mandibular rami for correction of prognathism—a ten year follow-up study. Excerpta Medical International Congress, Series No. 66, Proceedings of the Third International Congress of Plastic Surgery, Washington, D.C., October, 1963.

65. Limberg, A. A.: Treatment of open bite by means of plastic oblique osteotomy of the ascending rami of the mandible, Dent. Cosmos **67:**1191, 1925.

66. Limberg, A. A.: A new method of plastic lengthening of the mandible in unilateral microgenia and asymmetry of the face, J. Am. Dent. Assoc. **15:**851, 1928.

67. Longacre, J. J., Destefano, G. A., and Holmstrand, K.: The early versus the late reconstruction of congenital hypoplasia of the facial skeleton and skull, Plast. Reconstr. Surg. **27:**489, 1961.

68. Massey, G. B., Chase, D. C., Thomas, P. M., and Kohn, M. W.: Intra-oral oblique osteotomy of the mandibular ramus, J. Oral Surg. **32:**755, 1974.

69. McKenzie, J.: The first arch syndrome, Arch. Dis. Child. **33:**477, 1958.

70. McNeill, R. W., Proffitt, W. R., and White, R. P.: Cephalometric prediction for orthodontic surgery, Angle Orthod. **42:**154, 1972.

71. Millard, D. R.: Adjuncts in augmentation mentoplasty and corrective rhinoplasty, Plast. Reconstr. Surg. **36:**48, 1965.

72. Mohnac, A. M.: Surgical correction of maxillomandibular deformities, J. Oral Surg. **23:**393, 1965.

73. Mohnac, A. M.: Lecture, Rocky Mountain Society of Oral Surgeons, annual meeting, June, 1966.

74. Mohnac, A. M.: Maxillary osteotomy in the management of occlusal deformities, J. Oral Surg. **24:**303, 1966.

75. Moose, S. M.: Correction of abnormal mandibular protrusion by intraoral operation, J. Oral Surg. **3:**304, 1945.

76. Moose, S. M.: Surgical correction of mandibular prognathism by intraoral subcondylar osteotomy, J. Oral Surg. **22:**197, 1964.

77. Murphey, P. J., and Walker, R. V.: Correction of maxillary protrusion by ostectomy and orthodontic therapy, J. Oral Surg. **21:**275, 1963.

78. New, G. B., and Erich, J. B.: The surgical correction of the mandibular prognathism, Am. J. Surg. **53:**2, 1941.

79. Obwegeser, H.: The surgical correction of mandibular prognathism and retrognathia with consideration of genioplasty. I. Surgical procedures to correct mandibular prognathism and reshaping of the chin, Oral Surg. **10:**677, 1957.

80. Obwegeser, H.: Die Kinnvergrosserung, Oste. Z. Stomat. **55:**535, 1958.

81. Obwegeser, H. (Zahnärztliches Institut der Universität, Zürich, Switzerland): Personal communication, November 1959.

82. Obwegeser, H.: Vorteile und Möglichkeiten des intraoraler Vorgehens beider Korrektur von Unterkiefer-Anomalien, Fortschritte der Kiefer und Gesichts-Chirurgie, vol. VII, 1961.

83. Obwegeser, H.: Personal communication, Zurich, Switzerland, 1970.

84. Obwegeser, H., and Gerhard, R. C.: Unpublished data.

85. Parnes, E. I., Torres, I., and Galbreath, J. C.: Surgical correction of maxillary protrusion, J. Oral Surg. **24:**218, 1966.

86. Pascoe, J. J., Hayward, J. R., and Costich, E. R.: Mandibular prognathism, its etiology and a classification, J. Oral Surg. **18:**21, 1960.

87. Paul, J. K.: Correction of maxillary retrognathia, J. Oral Surg. **27:**57, 1969.

88. Perthes, G.: Operative Korrektur der Progenie, Zbl. Chir. **49:**1540, 1922.

89. Pettit, J. A., and Walrath, C. H.: A new surgical procedure for correction of prognathism, J.A.M.A. **99:**1917, 1932.

90. Pichler, H.: Über Progenieoperationen, Arch. Klin. Chir. **1:**11, 1927.

91. Pichler, H., and Trauner, R.: Mund und Kieferchirurgie, part 1, vols. 1 and 2, Wien, 1948, Urban & Schwarzenberg, p. 626.

92. Pickerill, H. P.: Double resection of the mandible, Dent. Cosmos **54:**1114, 1912.

93. Reid, R., Hinds, E. C., and Mohnac, A. M.: Surgical correction of facial asymmetry associated with open bite, J. Oral Surg. **24:**527, 1966.

94. Reiter, E. R.: Surgical correction of mandibular prognathism, Alpha Omegan **45:**104, 1951.

95. Reiter, E. R.: Mandibular prognathism: bilateral osteotomy through the neck of the condyle, lecture course, 36th annual meeting, American Society of Oral Surgeons, Nov. 4, 1954, Hollywood, Fla.

96. Robinson, M.: Prognathism corrected by open vertical condylotomy, J. S. California Dent. Assoc. **24:**22, 1956.

97. Robinson, M.: Micrognathism corrected by vertical osteotomy of ascending ramus and iliac bone graft: a new technique, Oral Surg. **10:**1125, 1957.

98. Robinson, M.: Prognathism corrected by open vertical subcondylotomy, J. Oral Surg. **16:**215, 1958.

99. Robinson, M.: Teaching outline for prognathism surgery at Los Angeles County Hospital, J. Oral Surg. **21:**227, 1963.

100. Robinson, M., and Lytle, J. J.: Micrognathism corrected by vertical osteotomies of the rami without bone grafts, Oral Surg. **15:**641, 1962.

101. Robinson, M., and Shuken, R.: Bone resorption under plastic chin implants, J. Oral Surg. **27:**116, 1969.

102. Rowe, N. H.: Personal communication.

103. Sarnat, B. G., and Engel, M. B.: A serial study of mandibular growth after removal of the condyle in the macaca rhesus monkey, Plast. Reconstr. Surg. **7:**364, 1951.

104. Sarnat, B. G., and Robinson, I. B.: Surgery of the mandible, some clinical and experimental considerations, Plast. Reconstr. Surg. **17:**27, 1956.

105. Schaefer, J. E.: Correction of malocclusion by surgical interference, Am. J. Orthod. Oral Surg. (Oral Surg. Sect.) **27:**172, 1941.

106. Schuchardt, K.: In Bier, Braun, and Kümmel: Chirurgische Operationslehre, vol. II, Leipzig, 1954.

107. Schuchardt, K.: Formen des offenen Bisses und ihre operativen Behandlungsmöglichkeiten, Fortschr. Kiefer Gesichtschir. 1955.

108. Schuchardt, K.: Experiences with the surgical treatment of some deformities of the jaws: prognathia, micrognathia, and open bite, International Society of Plastic Surgeons, Transactions of Second Congress, London, 1959 (Wallace, A. B., editor) Edinburgh, 1961, E. & S. Livingstone, p. 73.

109. Schwartz, A. M.: Lehrgang der Gebissregelung, vol. I, 1958.

110. Shira, R. B.: Personal communication.

111. Shira, R. B.: Surgical correction of open bite deformities by sliding osteotomy, J. Oral Surg. **19:**275, 1961.

112. Sicher, H.: Growth of the mandible, Am. J. Orthod. **33:**30, 1947.

113. Skaloud, F.: A new surgical method for correction of prognathism of the mandible, Oral Surg. **4:**689, 1951.

114. Sloan, A. C.: Intraoral osteotomy of ascending rami for correction of prognathism, Texas Dent. J. **69:**375, 1951.

115. Small, I. A., Brown, S., and Kobernick, S. D.: Teflon and Silastic for mandibular replacement: experimental studies and reports of cases, J. Oral Surg. **22:**377, 1964.

116. Smith, A. E., and Johnson, J. B.: Surgical treatment of mandibular deformations, J. Am. Dent. Assoc. **27:**689, 1940.

117. Smith, A. E., and Robinson, M.: Surgical correction of mandibular prognathism by subsigmoid notch ostectomy with sliding condylotomy; a new technic, J. Am. Dent. Assoc. **49:**46, 1954.

118. Stark, R. B., and Saunders, D. E.: The first branchial syndrome, Plast. Reconstr. Surg. **29:**229, 1962.

119. Taylor, W. H., and Hitchcock, H. P.: The Alabama analysis, Am. J. Orthod. **52:**245, 1966.

120. Terry, B. C.: Personal communication, Washington, D.C., 1973.

121. Tessier, P.: Osteotomies totales de la face, Syndrome de Crouron, Syndrome d'Apert, Oxycéphalies, Scaphocéphalies, Turricéphalies, Ann. Chir. Plast. **12:**103, 1967.

122. Thoma, K. H.: Y shaped osteotomy for correction of open bite in adults, Surg. Gynecol. Obstet. **77:**40, 1943.

123. Thoma, K. H.: Genioplasty with tantalum gauze, Oral Surg. **2:**65, 1949.

124. Thoma, K. H.: Oral surgery; ed. 4, St. Louis, 1963, The C. V. Mosby Co., pp. 1162, 1168, 1169, 1141, 1142, 1147.

125. Thoma, K. H.: Oral surgery, ed. 5, St. Louis, 1969, The C. V. Mosby Co., p. 1144.

126. Trauner, R.: Personal communication, International Congress for Maxillo-Facial Surgery, Graz, Austria, May, 1959.

127. Trauner, R.: Eine neue Operationsmethode bei der Progenie, Dtsch. Zahn. Mund. Kieferheilkd. **49:**77, 1967.

128. Trauner, R.: Personal communication, 1972.

129. Verne, D., Polachek, R., and Shapiro, D. N: Osteotomy of condylar neck for correction of prognathism: study of fifty-two cases, J. Oral Surg. **15:**183, 1957.

130. Walker, D. G.: Personal communication, 1977.

131. Ware, W. H.: Growth centre transplantation in temporo-mandibular joint surgery. In Walker, R. V.: Oral surgery, Transactions of the Third International Conference on Oral Surgery, Edinburgh, 1970, E. & S. Livingstone, p. 148.

132. Ware, W. H.: Personal communication.
133. Ware, W. H., and Taylor, R. C.: Cartilaginous growth centers transplanted to replace mandibular condyles in monkeys, J. Oral Surg. **24:**33, 1966.
134. Wassmund, M.: Lehrbuch der praktischen Chirurgie des Mundes und der Kiefer, vol. 1, Leipzig, 1935, Johann Ambrosius Barth.

135. Winstanley, R. P.: Subcondylar osteotomy of the mandible and the intraoral approach, Br. J. Oral Surg. **6:**134, 1968.
136. Wunderer, S.: Surgical correction of the profile by operation on the maxilla, Proceedings of the Second Annual Meeting Swiss Society of Plastic and Reconstructive Surgeons, Zurich, Switzerland, Nov. 1965.

CHAPTER 24

Surgical aspects of oral tumors

Claude S. La Dow

Tumors, or neoplasms, are new growths of abnormal tissue arising around the oral cavity as in other parts of the body. They may occur in the lips, cheeks, floor of the mouth, palate, tongue, and in the jaw bones. These new growths may be of epithelial tissue, connective tissue, or nerve tissue origin, although neurogenic tumors are rare in the oral cavity.

Tumors may be benign or malignant, depending on their behavior pattern and cellular structure. A benign tumor grows slowly and is usually encapsulated. It enlarges by peripheral expansion, pushes away adjoining structures, and manifests no metastasis. A malignant tumor, on the other hand, endangers the life of its host by its rapid infiltrating extension into surrounding vital structures and the phenomenon of metastasis, which creates secondary growths in distant parts of the body, usually through the lymphatic system and bloodstream.

Treatment of tumors is essentially the extirpation of the mass, although surgical intervention varies with the nature of the neoplasm. Some benign neoplasms of the mouth possess characteristics rarely encountered elsewhere in the body. These characteristics pertain to tumors of dental origin.

Oral tumors may be classified into those of dental origin and those of nondental ori-

gin. Oral tumors of dental origin arise from epithelial inclusions remaining within the jaw bones after tooth formation is completed. This occurs around the teeth and within suture lines of the developing maxillae and mandible. Epithelial tumors may be secreting or nonsecreting, depending on the presence of secretory epithelium, as occurs in cysts.

TUMORS OF THE HARD TISSUES OF THE ORAL CAVITY
Odontogenic tumors

Odontogenic cysts are discussed in detail in Chapter 14. Dental tumors arising in the jaw bones may be broadly classified into odontomas and ameloblastomas.

Odontoma. *Calcified odontomas, simple enamel pearls,* and *cementomas* usually consist of one or more kinds of tooth elements. Enamel pearls consist of enamel. Odontomas consist of dentine. Cementomas are of cementum. Odontomas may be composite by manifesting two or more tooth tissue elements. These simple tooth tumors arise from some aberration of the tooth germ early in life. Surgical intervention is instituted at an early age to prevent derangement of the permanent dentition. In later years multiple cementomas and ossifying fibromas appear frequently near the roots of teeth. The teeth remain vital, with

609

absence of subjective symptoms. Surgical intervention for these tumors is usually unnecessary, since they frequently reach a stage of inactivity and become calcified within the jaw bones without disturbing function and are only apparent in roentgenograms.

Atypical cementomas and cemento-ossifying fibromas can become locally aggressive, causing destruction of anatomical surroundings. These tumors, when occurring in the maxilla, can invade the sinuses. Extensive surgical intervention is necessary for extirpation.

Composite odontomas are excised, since they contain various tooth formations that tend toward destructive cystic change. Some of these masses grow to considerable size in the young, thus interfering with eruption of permanent teeth. They can cause considerable bone destruction. Roentgenographic diagnosis may be the only outstanding evidence of their presence besides a slight aberration of the surrounding structures. Surgical removal of these benign tumors is always conservative. They can be approached by removing the overlying bone (Fig. 24-1). These masses are enucleated from the adjoining bony structures of the jaw with surgical burs or chisels. Controlled sharp dissection is preferred to elevator technique, since the surrounding tissue may be damaged when uncontrolled elevator force is applied. Primary closure of the operative site after obliteration of the cavitation with absorbable packs is the treatment of choice.

Complications after removal of odontomas may include paresthesia of the lower lip and mandible when the tumor mass contacts the inferior dental nerve, hemorrhage from the cavitation when bleeding areas are not controlled, and secondary infection with breakdown of sutures. Recurrence of these benign tumors has not been reported.

Ameloblastoma. The ameloblastoma is a tumor arising from embryonal cells of developing teeth. Although most forms of this tumor simulate other slow-growing, benign tumors, some can develop malignant tendencies. Degeneration of this tumor into carcinoma has occurred. Patients may have few subjective symptoms during tumor growth. Enlargement of the tumor may expand the buccal, lingual, or palatal bone plates. Teeth may loosen, and pressure symptoms may occur, especially in the region of the maxillary sinuses. Roentgenographic examination may demonstrate unilocular or multilocular types. Unilocular ameloblastomas may be confused with benign cysts. The tumor frequently absorbs the alveolus surrounding the roots of teeth and may absorb root ends (Fig. 24-2). They occur in both jaws. Metastasis is rare, but tumor fragments may find their way into the lungs by aspiration. Ameloblastomas grow by extension into adjacent tissues and may perforate the investing bone. A biopsy should precede treatment, since these

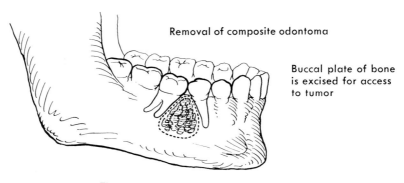

Removal of composite odontoma

Buccal plate of bone is excised for access to tumor

Fig. 24-1. Local excision of benign tumor.

tumors frequently present individual characteristics. Some are slow-growing, expansive tumors, requiring many years to manifest subjective symptoms. Others grow more rapidly and present definite malignant tendencies. Biopsy is satisfactorily performed with the patient under local anesthesia. The overlying cortical bone is exposed through a mucoperiosteal incision, and a portion of bone is carefully removed with surgical burs or chisels. A section of the tumor mass is excised sharply without curettage or trauma. The overlying mucoperiosteum is sutured. The extent of the operative procedure will depend on the histological structure of the tumor and the ex-

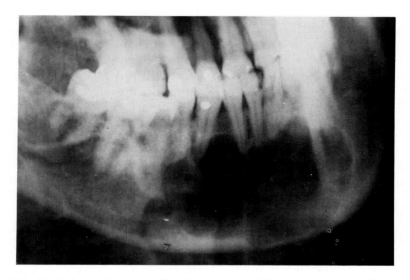

Fig. 24-2. Ameloblastoma of the mandible. Destruction of the alveolar bone and absorption of roots of the incisor teeth.

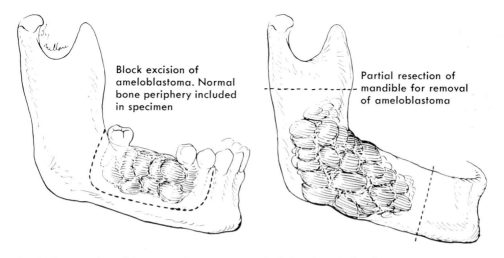

Block excision of ameloblastoma. Normal bone periphery included in specimen

Partial resection of mandible for removal of ameloblastoma

Fig. 24-3. Extension of the tumor through the cortical plate is an indication for partial resection.

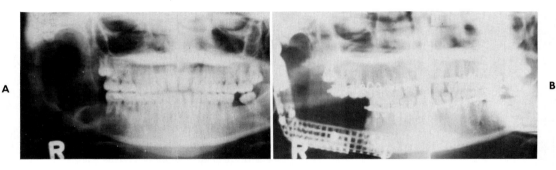

Fig. 24-4. A, Large ameloblastoma of the mandible involving the condyloid and coronoid processes. Lower border of the mandible destroyed by the tumor. **B,** Complete resection of mandible to right premolar region allowing for 12 mm inclusion of apparent normal bone. Replacement of deficient area with titanium mesh packed with cancellous autogenous bone. Adjustable titanium condyle replaced in the glenoid fossa.

tent of involvement of the surrounding tissues.

Methods of treatment include extirpation, radical resection of the jaw, selective block excision, and electrocauterization. Local excision of a small, accessible tumor is indicated in the young, provided they agree to regular follow-up and a radical resection when recurrence occurs. Recurrences are not unusual after curettage. Incomplete surgical treatment may stimulate tumor cell growth.

Ameloblastomas are exposed widely by removing overlying bone, including the buccal plate, as far as the base of the tumor. The buccal plate may be thin because of the expansive enlargement of the underlying tumor. Whenever possible, the inferior border of the mandible is preserved and retained to maintain continuity of the jaw. Block section of the involved bone should extend into and include 10 mm of normal peripheral bone surrounding the tumor mass (Fig. 24-3). Sharp cutting instruments are used to separate this area from normal osseous structures. The entire base and surrounding margins are then electrocauterized to destroy completely the residual tumor cells. Sedative dressing is placed for drainage, to reduce pain, and to allow healing by secondary intention from the bottom of the cavity. The mucoperiosteum is partially approximated, leaving an orifice for

removal and renewal of the dressing. The wound dressing is renewed and gradually reduced in size in small amounts each time the packing is changed during the reparative process.

Ameloblastomas that have extended within the maxilla may perforate palatal mucoperiosteum and nasal mucosa. Radical resection of the tumor and the immediate surrounding osseous structures is the accepted treatment of choice. Since these tumors grow by extension into adjoining tissues, adequate surgical resection is accomplished. Frequently, a stump of normal bone at one periphery of the resection is retained as in the condylar region of the mandible (Fig. 24-3). This bone may be utilized as a base of attachment for reconstruction of the missing section of the mandible by bone grafts. Bone grafts may be inserted at the time of surgical intervention because of the low incidence of metastasis in this type of new growth. Whenever radical procedures (Fig. 24-4) are performed to eradicate the ameloblastoma, conservative efforts are made to maintain function and esthetics.

The ameloblastic fibroma and the ameloblastic adenoma (Fig. 24-5) are also tumors related to dental epithelium. These benign neoplasms grow slowly and expand the cortical plates of the jaws. They may simulate the ameloblastoma in roentgeno-

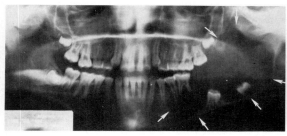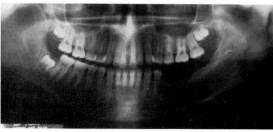

B

Fig. 24-5. A, Extensive ameloblastic fibroma of the left mandible. The second molar and third molar buds have been displaced to the lower border on this 12-year-old child (arrows). Aspiration biopsy and incision biopsy accomplished to establish diagnosis. **B,** One-year follow-up roentgenogram following surgical curettage and chemical cauterization. Displaced teeth removed.

graphic and clinical examinations. These tumors occur most frequently in the second and third decades of life and are painless in the early stages of growth. Surgical treatment is accomplished by complete local excision after a preoperative incision biopsy.

Osteogenic tumors

Neoplasms arising from the jaw bones are classified as osteomas, fibro-osteomas or fibrous dysplasias, myxomas, chondromas, sarcomas, Ewing's tumor, and the central giant cell tumor.

Osteoma. Osteomas of the jaws appear as areas of circumscribed, benign, bony new growths. Osteomas arising from the inner surface of bone cortex are called *enostoses* or *central osteomas*. Tumors of this kind consist of dense cortical bone extending into the spongiosa of the jaw. They can be demonstrated in roentgenograms as circumscribed, dense, bony tumors. Treatment may be unnecessary unless symptoms of pain resulting from pressure on nerve fibers are manifest or superficial ulceration occurs in overlying tissues. All forms of osteoma cast a radiopaque shadow in roentgenograms. Osteomas consisting of spongiosa are much less dense, with outlines more difficult to differentiate from the adjoining bone.

Some forms of osteoma arise from the periosteum proper, from aberrant cartilage cells, and from the cortical plates. These will occasionally assume considerable disfiguring size, in which case surgical removal is indicated to reestablish facial harmony and obviate interference with function. These osteomas are composed of spongy bone with only a thin layer of covering cortex. They cast light shadows on roentgenograms. These tumors may be sharply dissected at their base, where they are contiguous with the bony cortex of the jaws. Osteomas rarely recur after complete excision.

Locally circumscribed bony growths developing outside the cortical plates are called exostoses or peripheral osteomas. These bony outgrowths are benign and slow growing and seem to develop in young adults. They may occur after trauma or irritation. Areas of exostosis may occur at sites of muscle insertion or at the junction of two bones. A frequent site of exostoses is the midline region of the hard palate. This is known as a torus palatinus. A torus mandibularis may occur on the lingual aspect of the mandible in the premolar and molar regions.

Fibro-osteoma. The fibro-osteoma, or ossifying fibroma, a fibrous dysplasia of bone, is a benign, slow-growing tumor of bone that tends to have its greatest growth in the second decade of life. It is a diffuse, poorly differentiated endosteal tumor, replacing the normal spongiosa with fibrous tissue. Increased irregular areas of calcification may occur as new bone formations develop in this tumor. The enlarging neoplasm may displace teeth and expand cortical plates of the jaw bones. A fibro-osteoma tends to occur more frequently in women than in men and is seen more often in the maxilla than in the mandible. This tumor may obliterate the maxillary sinus and may extend into other bone landmarks. It does not invade the nasal structures. This is of diagnostic importance, since in both hyperostoses and Paget's disease the nasal meati are obliterated. This tumor is occasionally confused with the fibrosarcoma because of similar histological patterns.

The fibro-osteoma grows slowly. It usually will begin to develop radiopacity soon after its initial developments, as calcification occurs. Extensive involvement of the mandible will be shown as an enlarged, curved lower border. The tumor mass can be surgically extirpated, providing peripheral normal bone margins are included. Most authors agree that these tumors should be treated conservatively during periods of normal active bone development. Excision of large, active lesions during the second and third decades of life may require resection of the involved segment of the jaw (Fig. 24-6).

Dormant fibro-osteomas that have not demonstrated histological changes or increase in size can be contoured surgically to reestablish normal facial symmetry and maintain masticatory function. They can be approached either through an intraoral or

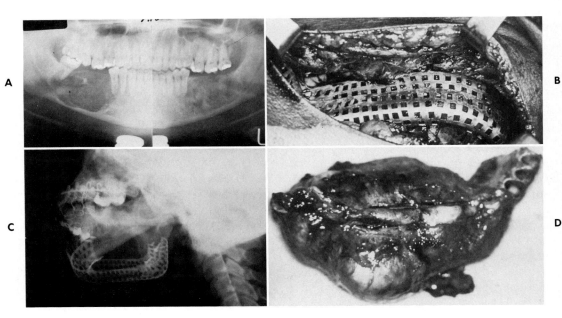

Fig. 24-6. A, Active, aggressive ossifying fibroma growing in right mandible of 34-year-old woman. Dormant lesion on left mandible. No new growth in 15 years. **B,** Titanium mesh support screwed to normal bone at symphysis and ascending ramus. Extraoral approach from 5 cm below inferior border or nearest crease line in neck. Mesh packed tightly with cancellous autogenous bone. Careful intraoral closure and extraoral approach closed in layers allowing room for Hemovac drainage. **C,** Roentgenogram demonstrating titanium mesh and screws. Mandible immobilized with interdental wire fixation on opposite side of the mandible for 4 months. **D,** Photograph of the resected mandibular tumor. Pathological report indicated ossifying fibroma undergoing active growth phase. Anterior teeth removed prior to resection to facilitate resection with Stryker saw.

extraoral approach, depending on which provides proper exposure. Since these tumors tend to bleed freely during contour reduction, pressure packs and electrocoagulation are essential.

The active fibro-osteoma or ossifying fibroma frequently recurs when surgical excision does not include a 10 to 12 mm margin or when treatment has been instituted at an early age. Radical treatment is less likely to lead to a later recurrence. These tumors do not respond favorably to radiation therapy. Osteosarcomas and fibrosarcomas have developed after a long latent period following irradiation treatment to fibro-osteomas.

Myxoma and chondroma. The myxoma and chondroma are closely allied tumors of embryonic tissue origin, developing from immature primitive bone or cartilage cells. The myxoma may simulate a cystic lesion because of its honeycomb appearance in roentgenograms. Expansion of the bone cortex occurs with the appearance of mucoid material replacing bone architecture. The chondroma arises from aberrant fetal cartilage in specific regions of the mandible, such as the symphysis and coronoid and condyloid processes, as well as the alveolomalar and paraseptal cartilages of the maxilla. The chondroma may cast a faint shadow outside of the bone in roentgenograms. A chondroma may calcify and cease to enlarge, in which case it is known as an osteochondroma. Both forms of this precocious tumor occur early in life. Myxomas, chondromas, and the osteochondromas may be detected clinically by pain, swelling,

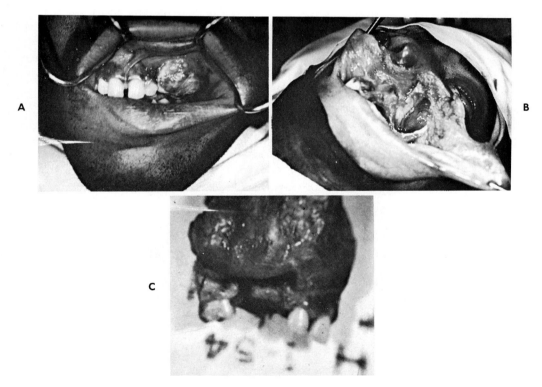

Fig. 24-7. A, Chondrosarcoma of maxilla. Early treatment with x-irradiation and radium application did not demonstrate beneficial results. **B,** Excision of tumor area through external approach. Invasion of the nasal fossa and anterior portion of the antrum had occurred. Exposure was sufficient for extirpation of the tumor. **C,** Specimen consisting of excised tumor and the immediate surrounding structures.

and limitation of motion. These tumors grow slowly. They are extirpated surgically.

Some osteochondromas tend to undergo malignant change, thus becoming chondrosarcomas. Chondrosarcomas consist of cartilagenous masses, areas of ossification, and mucoid degeneration. In young individuals they occur between bone and periosteum in areas of active bone growth. Cortex and spongiosa become secondarily invaded. These tumors are extremely difficult to eradicate; hence conservative surgical intervention is never attempted. The absence of early subjective symptoms leads to undetected progression of the disease. The histopathology of the chondrosarcoma is obscure, thus making early diagnosis difficult. Surgical intervention with its necessary trauma stimulates cellular activity. Radical resection of chondrosarcoma is performed with thoroughness by including in the excision some of the normal bone surrounding the tumor mass (Fig. 24-7). The resulting cavitation is adequately electrocauterized. Although this tumor spreads principally by local extension, it tends to metastasize elsewhere in the body. Radiation therapy does not seem to have any beneficial effects on chondrosarcomas.

Sarcoma. Osteogenic sarcomas originate from bone-producing cells. These highly malignant tumors are rare and generally occur in children during periods of active growth. Three general types are recognized:

1. *Osteolytic* sarcomas, accompanied with considerable bone destruction and immature tumor cells with little new bone formation
2. *Osteoblastic* sarcomas, producing abundant new bone with manifestations of smaller areas of tumor activity interspersed throughout the bone (Fig. 24-8, *A*)
3. *Telangiectatic* sarcomas, highly vascular, developing more rapidly, and invading by extension into the surrounding soft tissue (Fig. 24-8, *B*)

Trauma is considered the main etiological

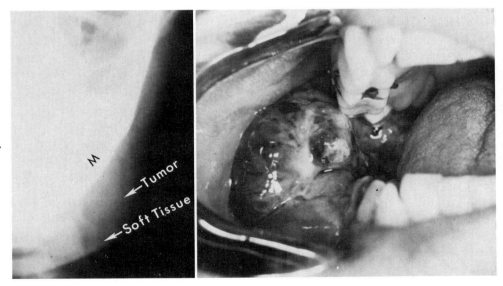

Fig. 24-8. A, Roentgenogram demonstrating osteoblastic activity of the bone sarcoma of the mandible in a 16-year-old boy. **B,** Highly vascularized telangiectatic sarcoma of the right mandible involving bone and soft tissues. This 31-year-old woman was treated with a chemotherapeutic agent only because of metastatic involvement of the lungs. Patient expired after 3 months of treatment.

factor in the history of all osteogenic sarcomas. The subjective symptoms include pain, swelling of the jaw bone, interference with jaw function, and loosening and displacement of the teeth. Anesthesia of the lip and jaw may be present. Roentgenograms reveal a poorly demarcated tumor mass, with areas of bone destruction and areas of new bone formation giving a sort of mottled appearance. The characteristic "sun-rays" appearance in the osteoblastic sarcoma results from the radiating spicules of bone extending outward from the cortex. The more poorly differentiated forms of osteogenic sarcoma develop rapidly and invade surrounding tissues. The sclerosing and osteoblastic forms seem to grow slowly. All types of sarcomas metastasize to the lungs through the bloodstream. Treatment of osteogenic sarcoma is instituted early and consists of radical resection of the bone containing the tumor. The adjoining blood supply leading into the tumor mass is included in any attempts of resection. Roentgenograms of the chest are taken early to detect any metastatic lesions. X-irradiation is given to these metastatic areas. Some clinicians believe preliminary x-irradiation of primary sites is helpful in reducing the incidence of metastatic lesions. Bone grafting of the sectioned portion of the jaw bone is

not indicated at the time of surgical intervention because of the high incidence of metastasis and exposure of the areas to x-irradiation. A prosthetic appliance is positioned immediately after resection to maintain jaw bone continuity until bone grafting is possible (Fig. 24-9). This maintains facial form and aids jaw function. Prognosis is poor, since much depends on the accessibility of the tumor, its state of activity, the presence of metastasis, and the thoroughness of operative intervention.

Ewing's tumor. Ewing's tumor is of obscure etiology. It is believed to arise from the endothelial lining of the blood or lymph vessels or both. Some pathologists regard the tumor as a primary lymphoma of bone. Trauma is the common important factor in its etiology. This neoplasm is seen during the first two decades of life. Subjective symptoms include elevation of body temperature, pain, swelling, and interference with jaw function. The last three subjective symptoms are the usual triad noted with bone sarcomas. Roentgenograms reveal expansion of bone cortex with apparent areas of increased density. The periosteum is thickened and pushed away from the bone. Areas of new bone are formed over areas of bone destruction. Treatment of Ewing's tumor is primarily by x-irradiation, since the

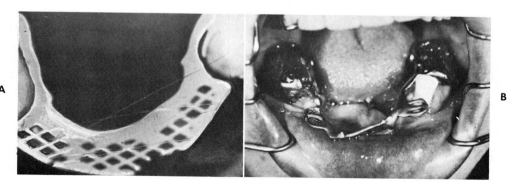

Fig. 24-9. A, Defect after excision of osteogenic sarcoma. Metallic appliance placed to maintain mandibular relation. **B,** Intraoral fixed appliance positioned to maintain mandibular relations and function.

growth is extremely radiosensitive. This may be followed by radical surgical treatment after the acute symptoms caused by x-irradiation subside. Metastasis occurs in almost all cases of Ewing's tumor. Favorite sites for metastatic new growths are the lungs, lymph nodes, spine, and ribs. The prognosis in Ewing's tumor is grave, since less than 20% of patients survive once metastasis has occurred.

Multiple myeloma. Multiple myeloma may occur anywhere in the body, although the first indication of its presence may be apparent in the jaw bone (Fig. 24-10). This tumor is of obscure etiology. It is believed to originate from bone marrow cells. Multiple myelomas are seen in older individuals between 40 and 70 years of age. In 90% of cases the ribs, sternum, clavicles, and vertebrae reveal small, round lesions that appear radiolucent in roentgenograms. The skull and jaw bone are less often affected but should be surveyed roentgenographically in all cases of this disease.

Pain of a wandering type is an outstanding symptom. The presence of Bence Jones bodies in the urine is a diagnostic sign. Alkaline phosphate level is normal in multiple myeloma. Hypercalcemia is frequent. Local biopsy of an accessible lesion confirms the diagnosis. Anemia accompanies this disease. Fractures occur when the long bones, ribs, or mandible become involved. Treatment consists of x-irradiation of involved areas to suppress growth of tumor cells and to alleviate pain. Chemotherapy is used to augment treatment. Hormones and nitrogen mustard are employed as adjuncts in therapy. Hormones aid in alleviating pain. Chemotherapy may retard progress of the disease.

Central giant cell tumor. The central giant cell tumor is a benign neoplasm developing in bone of cartilaginous origin. The symphysis and the angles of the mandible and the canine fossa of the maxilla are typical locations. These tumors occur in the second or third decade of life, with trauma as the suspected factor. Pain and swelling of the mandible with occasional fractures occur whenever the tumor reaches a large size. Expansive enlargement of the jaw reduces the vitality of the tissue, thus precipitating fractures. Roentgenograms show no uniform, clear-cut picture of central giant cell tumor, since the growth appears as multicystic areas with irregularly outlined, fine trabeculations. The teeth are frequently loosened, with evidence of absorption of their roots. Biopsy is essential to establish adequate diagnosis. These tumors destroy spongy bone and tend to thin out the cortical bone to a frail shell, thus leading to ultimate perforation. The tumor tissue is soft and highly vascular and tends to undergo free hemorrhage when traumatized. This tumor may look yellowish red because of blood pigment.

Treatment consists of enucleation of the growth after complete exposure. The walls and bed of the resulting cavitation are thoroughly electrocauterized to destroy possible residual areas leading to regrowth. Since this tumor is benign and slow growing, conservative treatment is carried out for ultimate preservation of the bone continuity of the jaw.

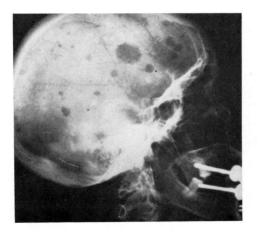

Fig. 24-10. Multiple myeloma with skull involvement in 48-year-old patient. Symptoms of pain and swelling of jaw prior to osteolytic lesions of skull and long bones. Pathological fractures of lower jaw supported by external pin and screw fixation. Local biopsy of jaw established diagnosis.

The central giant cell reparative granuloma is a tumor characterized histologically by many giant cells and seems to occur more frequently in the mandible in the first and second decades of life. Trauma would appear to be an important factor in the etiology of this tumor. Gradual swelling from expansion of the cortical plates encompassing medullary bone neoplasm may be the only objective symptom. Subjective symptoms may be absent, delaying dental consultation. Roentgenographic examinations may demonstrate expansions of the cortical plates and erosion of root surfaces (Fig. 24-13, *C*). Since these examinations are not diagnostic, preliminary biopsy is essential. Surgical treatment consists of enucleation of the thin vascular margins of the tumor after aspiration of the hemorrhagic area. Wide exposure through the expanded buccal cortical plate gives adequate access to the peripheral margins of the tumor. Smaller lesions can be enucleated and permitted to heal by primary intention. Large lesions are packed with medicated gauze and permitted to heal by secondary intention after excision.

TUMORS OF THE SOFT TISSUES OF THE ORAL CAVITY

Papilloma. Papillomas are benign tumors arising from the epithelial tissue of the mucous membranes of the oral cavity. They may be pedunculated or sessile and consist of keratinized epithelium on a connective tissue base. Papillomas are usually small, although they may grow to the size of a grape before the patient seeks treatment. These tumors undergo irritation from the natural dentition or artificial appliances. Malignant changes may occur after trauma. The papilloma is treated by surgical extirpation and electrocauterization of the connective tissue base. Excision is accomplished through a curved incision running around the periphery of the tumor and extending sufficiently into normal tissue to complete removal from the base of attachment (Fig. 24-11). Bleeding may be controlled with electrocautery (Fig. 24-12, *A*). Closure is accomplished with coaptation by means of nonabsorbable sutures. Recurrences are not common if adequate excision has been accomplished.

Fibroma. Fibromas (Fig. 24-12, *B*) are benign tumors arising from the submucous and subcutaneous connective tissues of the mouth and face after trauma. They may arise from the periosteum of the jaws. A fibroma is a sessile or pedunculated tumor. It is usually rounded and firm. Fibromas are more vascular than papillomas. They may assume a considerable size and become traumatized from dentures and mastication.

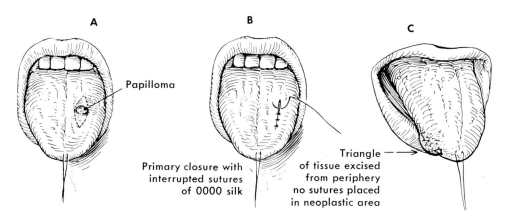

A

B

C

Papilloma

Primary closure with interrupted sutures of 0000 silk

Triangle of tissue excised from periphery no sutures placed in neoplastic area

Fig. 24-11. A and **B**, Excision biopsy. **C**, Incision biopsy.

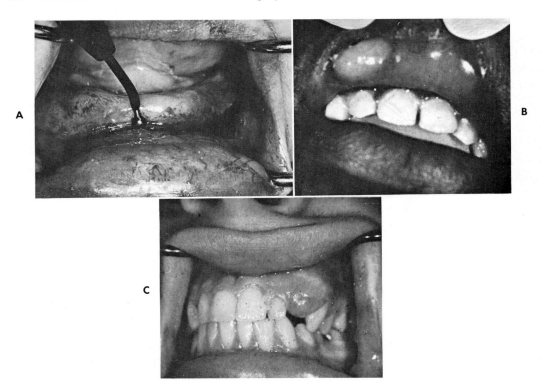

Fig. 24-12. A, Electrocoagulation of bleeding area after excision of small tumefaction of gingiva. Bove ballpoint used with 30 ma. **B,** Fibroma of lip. Irritation caused a connective tissue hyperplasia. **C,** Fibrous epulis. Complete excision may involve the adjoining teeth.

Treatment of the fibroma is surgical excision through a curved incision in the normal tissue surrounding the periphery of the growth. The edges of the resulting wound may require freeing and undermining for some distance to permit coaptation of the edges with nonabsorbable sutures. Fibromas will not recur if complete excision, including the base, is accomplished. A fibroma may arise from the jaw periosteum as well as from the connective tissue of the submucosa. These sessile and pedunculated benign tumors are frequently called fibrous epulides.

Fibrous epulis. Fibrous epulides (Fig. 24-12, *C*) occur around the gingiva frequently and seem to arise from chronic irritation of the bone periosteum or dental periodontium attaching to the teeth. Epulides may reach the size of large grapes and may become

irritated readily from the act of mastication. The treatment of fibrous epulis demands complete excision of the tumor from the surrounding gingival tissues whenever it is of bone periosteum origin. Epulis of dental periodontium origin calls for removal of the tooth involved in the epulis formation to obviate recurrence and ensure proper healing. Although an epulis is benign, it tends to recur if incompletely removed. The exposed bone after excision of the epulis is protected with a covering of surgical cement to permit normal granulation formation and act as a soothing dressing. Surgical packing of this type can be left in position for a period of 7 to 10 days.

Peripheral giant cell tumor. The peripheral giant cell tumor is sometimes called a *giant cell epulis*. It arises from the connective tissues of the dental periodontium that

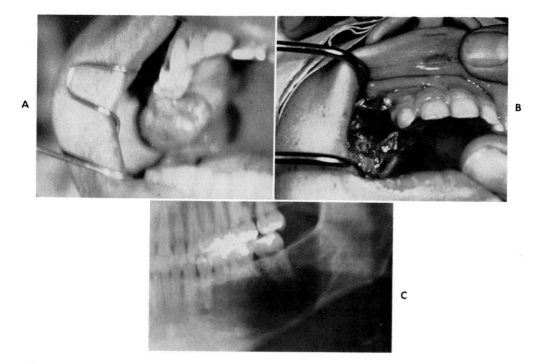

Fig. 24-13. A, Peripheral giant cell tumor. The tumor extends superiorly, eroding alveolar bone. **B,** Cavitation after excision and electrocauterization of base. **C,** Giant cell reparative granuloma of mandible. No subjective symptoms. Treated by intraoral excision.

gives teeth their attachment to the alveolus. This tumor is usually bluish red because of its highly vascular nature. It may be sessile or pedunculated. Peripheral giant cell tumor occurs at any age and seems to be more common among females. It can assume an extensive size when it pushes the teeth from their normal position. It invades the adjoining bone as enlargement proceeds (Fig. 24-13, *A*). Treatment of these tumors is excision. Adjacent teeth should be removed to provide access to the tumor mass. A portion of the sound gingival tissue and bone is included in the excision. The resulting cavitation is electrocauterized to destroy any residual remnants and to control bleeding. The cavitation is finally filled with a sedative pack to permit normal granulation and alleviate pain. Peripheral giant cell tumor does not recur after complete excision.

Pregnancy tumor. Pregnancy tumors arise on the gingival tissues of the jaw bones as pedunculated growths during pregnancy as a result of an obscure hormonal reaction. They appear about the second or third month of pregnancy and persist until parturition, when they begin to disappear. A pregnancy epulis consists of highly vascular connective tissue. It is bluish red, fading slightly on compression, occurring in either dental arch and bleeding readily on the least trauma. Pregnancy tumors attain considerable size, are unsightly, and may interfere with mastication. Treatment of a pregnancy tumor is local excision followed by electrocoagulation when the tumor is large enough to disturb the patient's state of mind. Surgical intervention offers better results after parturition whenever these tumors persist, since the stimulating hormonal factor is then absent. Pregnancy tumors may be multiple.

Hemangioma and lymphangioma. Hemangiomas and lymphangiomas arise in connection with the blood vessels and lymphatics. They are benign tumors, seem to exhibit a congenital trend, and appear in the young. Their etiology is obscure, being attributed to aberrant remains of developing blood and lymph tissue elements within areas in which they are not usually found.

Hemangiomas may be classified into capillary and cavernous types. Capillary hemangioma is known as "port-wine stain." It may occur on the face or within the mouth. This tumor fades on compression and has a dark, bluish red hue. The cavernous hemangioma has large blood sinuses and tends to invade the soft tissue or erode the adjoining bony structures by pressure. A pulsation may be detected in the cavernous types. Preliminary biopsies of these bluish, pulsating lesions should never be attempted in the office because of extensive hemorrhage.

Capillary hemangioma has been treated by local excision when the tumor was small. Injection of boiling water into the afferent vessels has been employed to sclerose the vessels. Radium applications and x-irradiation have been used to accomplish the same results. Conservative measures are followed in children. Excision and skin grafting is the treatment of choice whenever surgical intervention is justified. Radium applications and x-irradiation are deferred in infants whenever possible, to obviate injury to developing teeth and jaws.

Cavernous hemangiomas involving soft tissues of the oral cavity may be excised with a scalpel or endothermy knife. The excision should extend around the tumor in normal tissue. Feeding vessels are isolated and ligated prior to extirpation of the tumor. Sclerosing solutions have been successfully employed to reduce the size of larger hemangiomas prior to surgical treatment by fibrosing the blood supply. A 5% solution of sodium morrhuate is injected into the immediate surrounding areas in multiple, small applications. The resulting reduction in size of the tumor lessens injury to adjacent vital structures and enhances esthetic results.

Interosseous hemangiomas do not present a clear radiographic appearance and may simulate other osseous lesions such as giant cell tumors, traumatic bone cysts, fibrous dysplasias, and ameloblastomas. Changes in normal bony architecture are poorly defined, with lytic areas in the medullary portion. A history of swelling, pigmentation of a bluish red color, spontaneous bleeding without severe trauma, and mobility of teeth should be an admonition that uncontrollable hemorrhage will occur after the most insignificant surgical procedure in the suspected area.

Preoperative examination of undiagnosed central bony lesions of questionable vascular etiology should include objective symptoms of a bruit heard by stethoscope, compression of overlying tissues that are decompressed by the vascular system, and tooth movement in harmony with peripheral pulses (Fig. 24-14). Selective arteriography must be accomplished to determine anomalous arteriovenous circulations and extensions of tumor beds (Fig. 24-15).

Management of these vascular neoplasms may be accomplished by several divergent methods. Control and reduction of the tumor bed and its blood supply may be attempted by application of x-irradiation or radium proximal and to the vascular area in adult patients. The resulting fibrosis may eliminate the neoplasm or allow resection without excessive blood loss. Wide resection with necessary blood replacement while the patient is under hypotensive anesthesia and ligations of major blood vessels are usually employed. Cryotherapy, which freezes the tumor bed and causes subsequent necrosis, is a new technique. Selective embolization with macerated, striated muscle to occlude proximal circulation and the tumor bed with resulting fibro-osteolytic consolidation is used. Embolization using

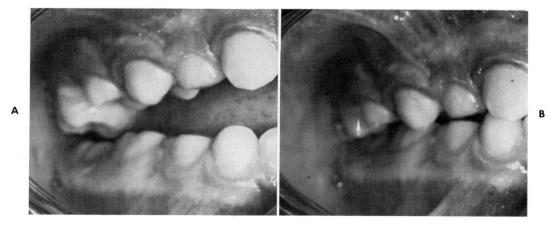

Fig. 24-14. A, Tooth extrusion of the first molar while the jaws are open and relieved of occlusal pressures. Vascular tumor superior to the tooth has destroyed alveolar bone and depresses the tooth. **B,** Normal position of the first molar tooth following occlusal contact of the jaws. Small spurts of blood may accompany this closed position because of pressure on hemangiomatous tumor superiorly positioned. (Arrow at first molar gingiva.)

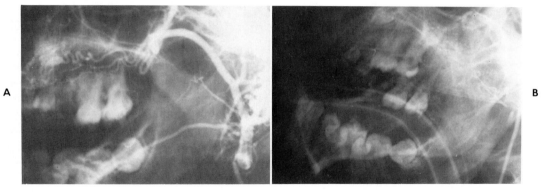

Fig. 24-15. A, Enlarged and tortuous vessels supplying maxillary tumor bed visualized through angiographic studies by means of maxillary artery catheterization with opaque dye. **B,** Blockage of dilated and anomalous vessels with silicone pellets by means of catheterization and selective embolization of tumor bed and arterial blood supply.

selected, main arterial feeders with 0.5 to 1 mm barium impregnated silicone pellets to accomplish a similar occlusion has been successful (Fig. 24-15, *B*).

The *lymphangioma* is a benign tumor frequently occurring on the lips and cheek, but it may occur in the nasopharynx and tongue. It presents a soft, doughy texture of the tissues. The overlying skin tends to present a wrinkled appearance. Distortion oc-

curs as a result of periods of active growth followed by formation of fibrous tissue. Treatment of the lymphangioma is surgical excision when the tumor has not assumed a large size. Large tumors may be reduced surgically by partial excision in succeeding operations. Sclerosing solutions have been employed with some success for further reduction of drainage channels to these tumors. The lymphangioma is radioresistant. No recurrence follows complete excision, but this is rarely accomplished.

Lipoma. Lipoma is a benign tumor consisting of adipose tissue, developing anywhere in the oral cavity where fat tissue is present. The lips and cheeks are favorite sites for this tumor. The overlying mucosa may be stretched by the pressure enlargement of the lipoma. A lipoma is a firm and freely movable mass, yellowish in color. It is demonstrable roentgenographically as a hazy mass within soft tissues. Lipoma may be single or multiple and may present extensions into adjoining soft tissues. This tumor grows slowly.

Treatment of the lipoma is surgical extirpation. The tumor is dissected easily from surrounding soft tissues. Primary closure is accomplished with nonabsorbable sutures in the mucosal tissue and absorbable sutures in the deep layers of tissues, such as muscle.

Myoma. Myomas are benign, well-defined, muscle tissue tumors commonly occurring in the tongue, lips, and soft palate. They appear as firm, sessile masses that may not be encapsulated. A myoma has few subjective symptoms. The patient may be aware of a painless "lump" in the tongue, cheek, or lips. The tumor is readily traumatized by mastication. Surgical excision is the treatment of choice. The growth is bluntly freed from surrounding structures through an incision in the overlying mucosa or skin. The wound is closed with coaptation sutures. Myomas rarely recur after complete excision.

Pigmented nevus. Pigmented nevi are benign, epithelial tumors seen occasionally in the oral cavity on the buccal mucosa, gingiva, and tongue. They contain melanin pigment. Nevi in the mouth may vary in color from a light blue to black. They may be flat, sessile, or papillary in form. A nevus may simulate pigmented papilloma, hemangioma, or the normal pigmented areas present in people from tropical climates. This tumor can exhibit malignant changes in later life as a result of continued chronic irritation. Symptoms of malignant change are rapid increase in growth rate, darkening in color, superficial ulceration, and bleeding on the least trauma. The nevus usually precedes the malignant melanoma. Incisional biopsy should never be attempted. The malignant melanoma can metastasize early through the lymphatic channels to the lungs and liver. Treatment consists of wide excision and complete dissection of the regional and related lymph nodes early in the course of the disease. This tumor is radioresistant. Prognosis is poor despite extensive radical excision.

Mixed tumor. Mixed tumors are new growths arising from salivary gland tissue. They may occur in the lips, cheeks, floor of the mouth, or soft and hard palates within the area of distribution of the major or minor salivary glands. Almost 90% of all mixed tumors occur in the parotid gland. Most clinicians agree that these tumors are of epithelial origin. Lymphoid and mucin-producing cells may be present in these epithelial patterns. The mixed tumor is encapsulated and can be defined from normal structures on palpation. It may be lobulated, firm, and slightly movable. The tumor may be attached by stalks to the normal gland tissue or present extensive protrusions of the capsule into surrounding structures. Large mixed tumors of the oral cavity and major salivary glands tend to recur after removal, a result of further growth from remnants of these extensions. The growth rate is slow, but incomplete surgical intervention tends to activate recurrences. Although mixed tumors of the oral cavity are essentially benign, some may become malignant, since the occurrence of regrowth is common.

The diagnosis of mixed tumor is accomplished by clinical examination and biopsy. The presence of an encapsulated, firm, lobulated tumor with well-defined borders and a history of slow growth usually indicates mixed tumor. Confirmation of the diagnosis is established by biopsy.

Treatment of mixed tumor is complete

surgical removal after adequate exposure of the tumor mass; most of these tumors are radioresistant. Mixed tumors known as papillary cystadenomas (Fig. 24-16) can be easily extirpated, including their capsular extensions. Cylindromas (Fig. 24-17), on the other hand, are difficult to extirpate completely, since they tend to recur because of their highly malignant nature. Electrocauterization may be necessary in

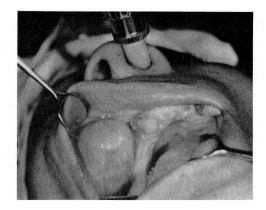

Fig. 24-16. Mixed tumor, papillary cystadenoma type. Local excision with careful dissection of the capsule is the treatment of choice.

some cases to destroy all residual tumor cells. Prognosis depends on the pathological characteristics of the mixed tumor and its wide excision.

Adenocarcinoma. Adenocarcinoma is a highly malignant tumor usually arising from salivary gland tissue. This tumor can occur in aberrant gland tissues of the lips, cheeks, palate, and oropharynx as well as in the major salivary glands. Primary adenocarcinoma may be differentiated from the benign mixed tumor by the rapidity of growth, early pain from sensory nerve pressure, anesthesia of tissue peripheral to neoplasm, and immobility of the tumor mass from extensions into adjacent tissues. Adenocarcinomas metastasize to regional lymph nodes, lungs, and the skeletal system. Diagnosis is established from biopsy. Roentgenograms of the chest are advisable to determine the presence of metastatic lesions. Treatment of adenocarcinoma includes radical excision of the tumor and its accessible extensions. Irradiation therapy may be employed to treat distant metastatic lesions when present. Prognosis is much less favorable when metastasis has occurred.

Adenocarcinoma metastasizing to the jaws from the prostate gland in men and the

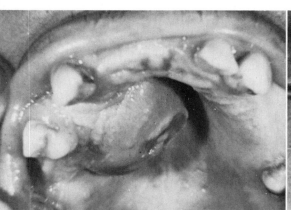
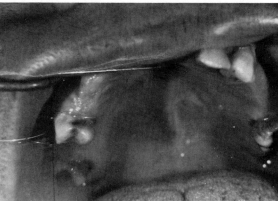

| A | B |

Fig. 24-17. A, Mixed tumor (cylindroma). This malignant tumor spreads locally with many extensions in all directions. Involvement of the palate may simulate a lytic lesion over roots of teeth. Mucoperiosteal extension of this tumor may be palpated as a rubbery, firm mass. **B,** One-year follow-up photograph after wide excision and electrocoagulation. Teeth were utilized for stent to aid in healing and support a surgical gauze dressing.

breast tissues in women is not an unusual sequela. It may be present without early roentgenographic evidence. Anesthesia of the lip on the involved side of a patient with a history of prostate or breast surgery may be an important indication of metastasis. Careful scrutiny of the past medical history and selective bone biopsies should be instituted.

Sarcoma. Sarcomas of the soft tissues are generally classified according to their cell of origin. They arise from poorly differentiated mesenchymal tissue of fat, muscle, vascular epithelium, and connective and fibrous nature. The most frequently encountered soft tissue sarcomas in the head and neck regions are the rhabdomyosarcomas and neurogenic fibromas. Surgical excision and postoperative irradiation reduces recurrence of these malignant tumors.

Fibrosarcomas are rarely encountered in the soft tissues of the oral cavity. The most common sites are in the cheeks and pharyngeal regions. Wide local excision is the recommended treatment. Additional investigative efforts with the newer chemotherapeutic agents such as bleomycin and actinomycin could enhance present methods of treatment for the sarcomas.

NEURILEMOMA (SCHWANNOMA) AND GANGLIONEUROMA. Neurilemoma and ganglioneuroma are rare nerve tumors. These tumors occur principally around nerve tissue in the maxilla and mandible. Usual roentgenographic studies are negative. Tomograms and myographic studies may help localize the tumor area (Fig. 24-18). Subjective symptoms are vague. Myalgia and anesthesia in areas of involvement of the peripheral nerves may be an indication of tumor activity. Since these tumors are potentially malignant, they should be biopsied promptly. Malignant variations of these nerve neoplasms are difficult to eradicate. They creep into every foramina in the skull, following nerve roots, and may cause many bizarre subjective symptoms. Surgical treatment necessitates wide exposure and vigorous and extensive excision.

CARCINOMA OF THE ORAL CAVITY

Carcinoma arises in connection with the cutaneous surface of the face and mucous membrane of the mouth. The *basal cell* form of carcinoma develops on the skin of the lips and face. *Squamous cell* carcinoma occurs on the vermilion borders and mucosa of the mouth. Carcinoma of the mouth accounts for approximately 5% of all carcinomas occurring in man. Carcinoma of the oral cavity develops as a result of invasion of malignant epithelial cells through the normally intact basal cell layer into subcutaneous and submucosal tissues. The etiology is obscure, although certain contributing factors may be present. *Chronic irritation* from overexposure of the lips to sunlight and traumatism by jagged teeth and ill-fitting dentures are among the predisposing factors in some individuals. The use of *tobacco* is considered an etiological factor. Areas of leukoplakia are frequently present

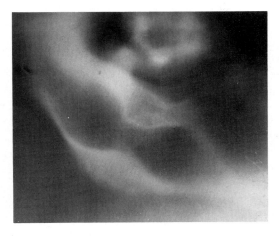

Fig. 24-18. Neurilemoma of the mandible. Tomogram demonstrating tumor extending to mental region. Skull x-ray films demonstrated enlargement of the foramen ovale. This benign tumor was removed through intracranial and submandibular approach. The latter approach was facilitated by decortication of the buccal plate of the mandible. (Courtesy James A. Tatoian, Jr., Philadelphia.)

as premonitory lesions in the history of squamous cell carcinoma. Leukoplakia is a lesion of the mucous membranes, appearing as a painless, hard, bluish-white, shiny patch. It occurs in older patients after continued, chronic irritation. Patches of leukoplakia may undergo malignant change by malignant cells in the mucosa invading the underlying tissue (Fig. 24-19, *A*).

Clinical staging and grouping of carcinoma of the oral cavity may be accomplished by careful examination of the local and regional area prior to biopsy. Objective findings with the magnifying lens, gentle palpation of the tumor and peripheral tissues, and bilateral palpations of the regional lymph nodes will elicit important information. Subjective symptoms of local or re-

ferred pain, trismus of the jaw, fixation of local musculature, and paresthesia are aids in clinical staging of the neoplastic disease.

The TNM system advocated by the American Joint Commission for Cancer Staging was modified in 1977. Current definitions are shown on the form on p. 628.

Carcinoma may have an ulcerative or verrucous lesion (Fig. 24-19, *B*). Squamous and basal cell carcinomas invade submucosa and subcutaneous tissues, including bone. They may arise insidiously, with little pain in their early growth. The patient may be aware of a "blister" on the lip or an ulcer or "lump" in the mouth that persists. Clinical examination may demonstrate an ulcerated area presenting raised or rolled borders, with infiltration and induration about

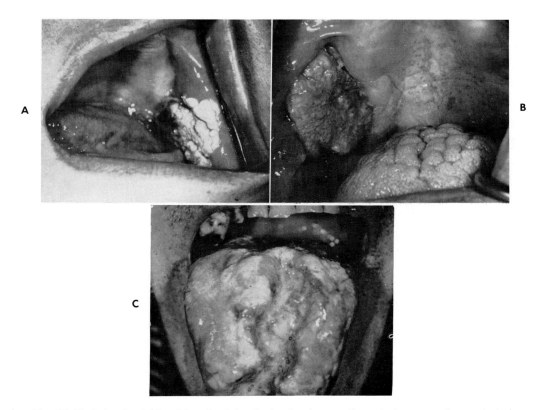

Fig. 24-19. A, Leukoplakia of the cheek beginning to show malignant change as demonstrated by the indurated, leathery appearance and fissuring of the surface. **B,** Squamous cell carcinoma, verrucous type, of buccal mucosa. X-irradiation and interstitial radium implantations constitute the treatment. **C,** Carcinoma of dorsum of tongue and overlying syphilitic lesion.

TNM CLASSIFICATION

Primary Tumor (T)

TX   Tumor that cannot be assessed **by rules**
T0   No evidence of primary tumor
TIS   Carcinoma in situ
T1   Tumor 2 cm or less in greatest diameter
T2   Tumor greater than 2 cm but not greater than 4 cm in greatest diameter
T3   Tumor greater than 4 cm in greatest diameter
T4   Massive tumor greater than 4 cm in diameter with deep invasion to involve **antrum,** pterygoid muscles, root of tongue, or skin of **neck**

Nodal Involvement (N)

NX   Nodes cannot be assessed
N0   No clinically positive node
N1   Single clinically positive homolateral node less than 3 cm in diameter
N2   Single clinically positive homolateral node 3 to 6 cm in diameter or multiple clinically positive homolateral nodes, none over 6 cm in diameter
    N2a: Single clinically positive homolateral node, 3 to 6 cm in diameter
    N2b: Multiple clinically positive homolateral nodes, none over 6 cm in **diameter**
N3   Massive homolateral node(s), bilateral nodes, or contralateral node(s)
    N3a   Clinically positive homolateral node(s), none over 6 cm in diameter
    N3b   Bilateral clinically positive nodes (in this situation, each side of the neck should be staged separately; that is, N3b: right, N2a; left, **N1)**
    N3c   Contralateral clinically positive node(s) **only**

Distant Metastasis (M)

MX   Not assessed
M0   No (known) distant metastasis
M1   Distant metastasis present
    Specify _____
    Specify sites according to the following notations:

Pulmonary - PUL	Bone Marrow - MAR
Osseous - OSS	Pleura - PLE
Hepatic - HEP	Skin - SKI
Brain - BRA	Eye - EYE
Lymph Nodes - LYM	Other - OTH

HISTOPATHOLOGY

Predominant cancer is squamous cell carcinoma

GRADE

Well-differentiated, moderately well-differentiated, poorly to very poorly differentiated, or numbers 1, 2, 3-4

STAGE GROUPING

Stage I   T1 N0 M0
Stage II   T2 N0 M0
Stage III   T3 N0 M0
    T1 or T2 or T3, N1, M0
Stage IV   T4, N0 or N1, M0
    Any T, N2 or N3, M0
    Any T, Any N, M1

Residual Tumor (R)

R0   No residual tumor
R1   Microscopic residual tumor
R2   Macroscopic residual tumor
    Specify _____

the margins. Induration of the surrounding tissue may not be present in early stages. Superficial ulceration or areas of leukoplakia may precede the neoplasm. Inflammatory lesions may complicate carcinoma of the tongue (Fig. 24-19, *C*). Carcinoma of the mouth metastasizes to regional lymph nodes during its extension. Metastasis to the cervical nodes may be detected by bimanual palpation of the local sites of lymphatic drainage. Metastatic nodes may be discrete and difficult to palpate, but lymphatic dissemination of the neoplasm has progressed. Large, extensive, fixed metastatic nodes indicate an advanced primary tumor.

Diagnosis is established from a biopsy, which is taken as early as possible with little trauma. Local anesthesia is indicated for biopsy, provided the injection is not delivered into the tumor area. Excision biopsy is done if the lesion is small. When the lesion is large, an incision biopsy is performed prior to surgical intervention. This is accomplished by removing a wedge-shaped segment of the tumor, using the scalpel or the electrocautery (Fig. 24-11, *C*).

The electrocautery is advantageous for controlling hemorrhage, since it seals off the bleeding vessels and prevents passage of tumor cells into the circulation. Sutures are avoided to prevent extension of the neoplasm. Multiple sampling may be necessary from the perimeter of the tumor for accurate diagnosis. The biopsy material should extend into submucosal tissues as demonstrated in Fig. 24-20. Aspiration biopsy is useful in cases of deep, inaccessible sites of metastasis. Aspiration biopsy is performed by employing a specially constructed, large-caliber needle and glass syringe. Some tumor cells are drawn or aspirated into the syringe after the tip of the needle is introduced into the tumor bed. This technique is difficult, even in the hands of an experienced clinician.

Biopsy material may be obtained by rubbing the tumor site gently with a tongue blade, thus transferring some of the tumor cells to the sponge for histological examination. This is an adequate method when screening large numbers of patients with suspicious oral lesions. It has been employed with satisfactory results in gynecol-

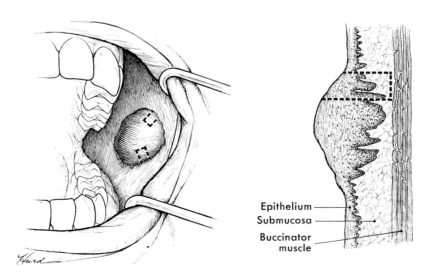

Fig. 24-20. Biopsy technique: Incision from area of active growth. The incision should extend through the mucosa down to the muscle layer to determine the extension of the tumor in the submucosal layers. Multiple sampling may be necessary to demonstrate histologically the characteristics in different areas of the tumor.

Epithelium
Submucosa
Buccinator muscle

ogy and is known as the Papanicolaou test. A negative pathological report could be misleading because the tumor surface may contain only inflammatory exudate or necrotic tissue. A positive report would still require an incision or excision biopsy for confirmation of the diagnosis.

Treatment

Treatment planning for malignant tumors will depend on the histology of biopsy, location of the neoplasm, its radiosensitivity, the degree of metastasis, and the age and physical condition of the patient.

The location of the tumor in the oral cavity may complicate treatment (see Table 24-1). Neoplasms in the posterior part of the mouth are less accessible and frequently encroach on vital structures. Adjunctive irradiation therapy may be indicated in certain cases. Eighty percent of cancers of the lip may be successfully treated by prompt therapy, but carcinoma of the floor of the mouth, tongue, and gingiva presents a poorer prognosis. Carcinoma arising in the posterior part of the mouth is not always diagnosed and treated early in the course of the disease. These carcinomas infiltrate rapidly into adjacent structures and metastasize early to cervical lymph nodes. Less

than 25% of these neoplasms may be successfully treated after extensive metastasis.

The age and physical condition of the patient are important in the treatment plan. Aged, debilitated patients can withstand extensive surgical procedures only after careful preoperative preparation. This may delay treatment and permit progression of the disease.

Irradiation therapy. Sensitivity of the tumor to irradiation therapy influences treatment. Radiosensitive tumors may be advantageously treated with x-ray or radium emanations alone or in combination with surgery.

Treatment of carcinoma is the responsibility of a team consisting of the pathologist, radiologist, internist, oncologist, and oral surgeon. Irradiation therapy for treatment of malignant neoplasms is based on the fact that tumor cells in stages of active growth are more susceptible to radiation than adult tissue. The more undifferentiated these cells appear histologically, the more radiosensitive the tumor is likely to be. The more the cells appear like normal adult cells, the less their reaction to irradiation. Mode of action on the active, growing neoplasm by irradiation is the immediate or delayed death of the tumor cells and a suppression

Table 24-1. Distribution of 14,253 cases of oral carcinoma by anatomical site, age, sex, and race of patients*

Anatomical site	Number in group	Percentage of total in group	Age range (years)	Cases in males (% of total)	Cases in females (% of total)	Cases in blacks (% of total)
Lower lip	5,399	38	14-99	97.5	2.5	0.6
Tongue	3,117	22	14-99	92.5	7.5	7.8
Floor of mouth	2,479	17	15-99	90.4	9.6	7.0
Gingiva	923	6	20-99	93.6	6.4	8.4
Palate	786	5.5	14-99	85.9	14.1	6.1
Tonsil	673	5	20-89	93.4	6.6	8.0
Upper lip	553	4	20-99	92.3	7.7	0
Buccal mucosa	245	2	20-99	78.7	11.3	1.7
Uvula	78	0.5	40-79	96.9	3.1	5.5
Total	14,253	100.0				

*From Krolls, S. O.: Squamous cell carcinoma of the oral soft tissues: a statistical analysis of 14,253 cases by age, sex and race of patients, J. Am. Dent. Assoc. **92**(3):572, 1976. Copyright by the American Dental Association. Reprinted by permission.

of reproduction. Agents employed for irradiation are the short-wavelength roentgen rays or the gamma rays of radium. Although these agents have a selective effect on active neoplastic tissues, normal tissue must be protected.

Three methods are generally used for application of irradiation. The emanations are delivered to the tumor area from a distance, the radioactive agents are implanted into the tumor bed, or a combination of both methods may be used with or without surgery.

X-irradiation is frequently used to sterilize the tumor from a distance outside the oral cavity. Filters of aluminum and copper may be employed to protect tissues. Intraoral cones have been devised to increase tumor dosage and reduce exposure of normal tissues. Newer methods of treatment include other radioactive metals. Radioactive cobalt is used extensively to irradiate tumor sites. Increased kilovoltage of roentgen equipment is now employed so that undesirable side effects of irradiation are reduced.

Radioactive agents such as radium, radon gas, or activated iridium can be implanted directly into the neoplasm (Fig. 24-21, *A*). Radium and radon gas are enclosed in gold or platinum to reduce immediate tissue necrosis and permit even distribution of the emanations. Careful irradiation treatment planning is essential so that proper distribution of the radioactive agents is accomplished to sterilize the tumor. Consideration of the surrounding normal tissue is given, since it receives some of the emanations.

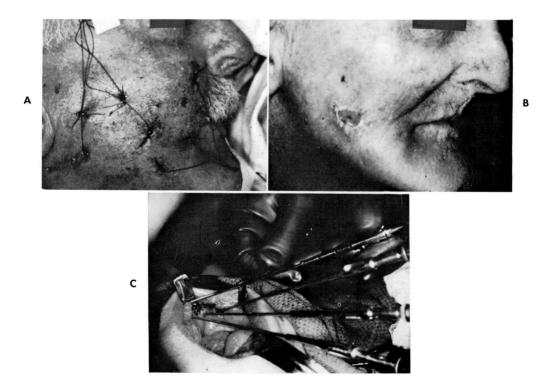

Fig. 24-21. A, Interstitial implantation of radium needles for squamous cell carcinoma of the buccal mucosa. **B,** Erythema of the skin 4 weeks after use of interstitial radium implant. **C,** Radon seed implantation by means of applicators to neoplasm on mucosa of cheek. Insertion is made to a predetermined depth and at calculated distances from the center of the neoplasm.

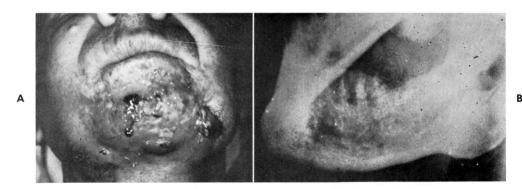

Fig. 24-22. A, Radio-osteomyelitis of the mandible with draining sinuses in the overlying soft tissues. **B,** Early osteoradionecrosis 5 years after x-irradiation of the tonsillar region. No protection was given to the osseous structures during therapy.

Areas of irradiation develop erythema (Fig. 24-21, *B*), and normal tissue function is impaired. Skin tolerance to irradiation must be determined to avoid severe injury. Necrosis of bone also occurs after intensive treatment. Osteoradionecrosis may follow irradiation therapy because of the interference with normal bone nutrition by the radioactive agents in the presence of infection (Fig. 24-22). Progressive necrosis can involve the entire jaw, necessitating sequestration or resection. Teeth in the irradiated area should be removed prior to therapy so that this retrograde process is avoided.

Surgical treatment. Surgical treatment of malignant tumors of the oral cavity requires wide excision. Squamous cell carcinoma of the oral mucosa invades adjacent tissues and metastasizes more readily than cutaneous carcinoma. Prompt, adequate treatment is essential to eradicate the growth. Wide excision is important, since growth of the tumor extends into surrounding normal tissues with considerable invasion, which may not be visible clinically. Scalpel and electrocautery are employed to excise the tumor. Primary healing does not always occur after excision with the electrocautery, since scar tissue formation is extensive in this case. Scar tissue is removed after successful treatment of malignant disease because extensive scar formation interferes with function.

Extension of the neoplasm into the periosteum and bone requires complete or partial resection of the jaw. Resection can be extensive when the bony cortex is invaded. Partial resection may be indicated whenever the periosteum alone is involved. Malignant tumors can involve the medulla of bone, thus revealing osteolytic areas in roentgenograms. Infiltrating carcinoma of the jaw may cause paresthesia by invading branches of the trigeminal nerve. Extensive resections of the jaws for squamous cell carcinoma should include an adequate resection of blood vessels of the affected side. The adjoining soft tissue should be supported whenever possible by prosthetic appliances attached to the bone stumps (Fig. 24-23, *B*). Immediate bone grafting is not advisable after radical resection for carcinoma. A period of observation is necessary to ensure no recurrence.

Squamous cell carcinoma may metastasize to the cervical lymph nodes early in the progress of the disease. Regional lymph nodes become enlarged and can be detected by palpation. These lymph nodes are excised widely before further extension occurs. Skin flaps are reflected widely to expose underlying involved tissues (Fig. 24-24). Although some lymph nodes within the operative field may appear normal, their removal in continuity with fascial attachments is imperative. Some normal struc-

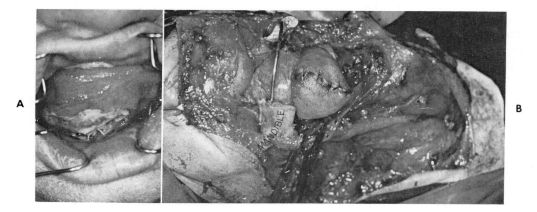

Fig. 24-23. A, Ulcerative carcinoma with infiltration of intrinsic and extrinsic tongue muscles. Metastasis to the cervical lymph nodes occurred on both sides. **B,** Resection of anterior third of tongue and floor of mouth and partial resection of mandible in continuity with bilateral neck dissection. Zimmer pin placed for stability of mandible.

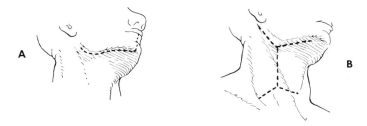

Fig. 24-24. A, Incision line for hemisection of mandible. Extension through lip is optional when an anterior segment of bone is resected at the symphysis. **B,** Incision lines for skin flaps for radical dissection of the cervical lymph nodes. The superior incision exposes the entire lower border of the mandible and its associated structures.

tures are sacrificed in this procedure. Ligations and excisions of some blood vessels are necessary to control hemorrhage and completely extirpate contiguous lymph tissues. Closure is accomplished with nonabsorbable coaptation sutures after drains have been positioned to reduce hematoma formation. Pressure bandages are useful to aid healing.

Chemotherapy. New advances in therapy, better patient management, and advanced anesthetic technique have improved the prognosis of oral carcinoma. Infusion of chemotherapeutic agents into major blood vessels supplying tumor areas around the

oral cavity has been successful in some cases. These agents seem to have a predilection for anaplastic cells and destroy the tumor. A promising group of synthetic chemical agents used for treatment of oral cancer are the antimetabolites. These chemicals interfere with the metabolism of the rapidly growing and dividing cancer cells. Agents such as methotrexate and 5-fluorouracil are infused under controlled pressure into the arterial stream nourishing the tumor site. The quantity of the chemical compound necessary for consistent cancericidal effect may have to be reduced in concentration because of depressant effects on the hemopoietic system of the patient. Oral administration of these agents may also need to be increased or reduced according to the results of frequent complete blood counts and clinical and histological examinations of the tumor site following initial arterial infusion.

Nausea, vomiting, and general malaise are anticipated subjective symptoms. Remission of tumor activity occurs, and the local site usually sloughs. Follow-up treatment may be threefold and consist of additional chemotherapeutic agents, x-irradiation, and surgical extirpation of a smaller and less aggressive tumor.

Cryosurgery. Recent improvements in freezing of selected tissues have given new impetus to the treatment of benign and malignant neoplasms, and cryosurgery has recently been successfully attempted in treatment of tumors. The technique of freezing selected areas in the oral cavity is accomplished by a probe tip contacting neoplastic tissue after liquid nitrogen has entered the tip in controlled amounts. The temperature of the contacted tissues is lowered to around $-180°$ C. Cell injury and death occur as a result of this brief contact. Usual sequelae of swelling, necrosis, and slough of affected tissues follow this treatment.

The advantages of using chemotherapeutic infusion agents and selective cryosurgery are inclusion of the poor-risk patient with advanced neoplastic disease in treatment, conservation of bony support to contiguous soft tissues involved with tumor tissue, minimal blood loss because of more conservative treatment, and less postoperative pain and cosmetic deformity.

COMMENT

The dentist has the opportunity to regularly examine patients for all aspects of oral diseases. He should maintain a high index of suspicion regarding any changes in the character of the oral mucosa. Recognition of early malignant changes in oral tissues should be a challenge and stimulate continued study to improve diagnostic ability. Prompt referral of patients for definitive treatment is most important for satisfactory results.

REFERENCES

1. Ackerman, L. V., Del Regato, J. A., and Spjut, H. J.: Cancer: diagnosis, treatment and prognosis, ed. 5, St. Louis, 1977, The C. V. Mosby Co., chap. 10.
2. Anderson, W. A. D.: Pathology, ed. 4, St. Louis, 1961, The C. V. Mosby Co., p. 1319.
3. Bennett, J., and Zook, E. G.: Treatment of arteriovenous fistulas in hemangiomas of face by muscle embolization, Plast. Reconstr. Surg. **50:**84, 1972.
4. Bhaskar, S. N.: Oral tumors of infancy and childhood: a survey of 293 cases, J. Pediatr. **63:**195-210, 1963.
5. Bhaskar, S. N., Cutright, D. E., Beasley, J. D., III, and Perez, B.: Giant cell reparative granuloma (peripheral): report of 50 cases, J. Oral Surg. **29:**110, 1971.
6. Bitter, K.: Pharmacokinetic behavior of bleomycin-cobalt-57 with special regard to intraarterial perfusion of the maxillofacial region, J. Maxillofac. Surg. **4:**226-231, 1976.
7. Blair, V. P., and Ivy, R. H.: Essentials of oral surgery, ed. 4, St. Louis, 1951, The C. V. Mosby Co., pp. 342, 507, and 533.
8. Bojrab, D. G., and Topazian, R. G.: Large myxoma of the mandible, J. Oral Surg. **29:**371, 1971.
9. Cade, S.: Malignant disease and its treatment by radium, vol. 1, Baltimore, 1948, The Williams & Wilkins Co., p. 167.
10. Cahn, W. G.: Cryosurgery of malignant and benign tumors, Fed. Proc. **24:**S 241, 1965.
11. Catlin, D., Das Gupta, T., McNeer, G., and others: Noncutaneous melanoma, CA **16:**75, 1966.
12. Conley, J.: Treatment of malignant tumors of the salivary glands, Bull. N.Y. Acad. Med. **46:**511, 1970.
13. Conley, J.: Radical neck dissection, Laryngoscope pp. 1344-1352, 1974.
14. Conley, J., and Dingman, D. L.: Adenoid cystic carcinoma in the head and neck (cylindroma), Arch. Otolaryngol. **100:**81-90, 1974.
15. Conley, J., and Janecka, I. P.: Neurilemmoma of the head and neck, presentation by Commission on Surgery, Seventy-Ninth Annual Meeting of the American Academy of Ophthalmology and Otolaryngology, Dallas, October 6-10, 1974.
16. Crowe, W. W., and Harper, J. C.: Ewing's sarcoma with primary lesion in mandible, report of a case, J. Oral Surg. **23:**156, 1964.
17. Cundy, R. L., and Matukas, V. J.: Solitary intraosseous neurofibroma of the mandible, Arch. Otolaryngol. **96:**81, 1972.

18. Curphey, J. E.: Chondrosarcoma of the maxilla: report of a case, J. Oral Surg. **29**:285, 1971.

19. De Lathouwer, C., and Brocheriou, C.: Sarcoma arising in irradiated jawbones, possible relationship with previous non-malignant bone lesions: report of six cases and review of the literature, J. Maxillofac. Surg. **4**:8-20, 1976.

20. Doner, J. M., Granite, E. L., Laboda, G., and Finkelman, A.: Primary oral carcinoma with pulmonary metastasis, report of a case, J. Oral Surg. **25**:173, 1967.

21. Eller, D. J., Blackemore, J. R., Stein, M., and Byers, S. S.: Transoral resection of a condylar osteochondroma: report of a case, J. Oral Surg. **35**:409-413, 1977.

22. Emmings, F. G., Koepf, S. W., and Gage, A. A.: Cryotherapy for benign lesions of the oral cavity, J. Oral Surg. **25**:321, 326, 1967.

23. Emmings, F. G., Neiders, M. E., Greene, G. W., Koepf, S. W., and Gage, A. A.: Freezing the mandible without excision, J. Oral Surg. **24**:145, 1966.

24. Esser, E., Schumann, J., Wannenmacher, M.: Irradiation treatment of inoperable squamous cell carcinoma of the oral cavity and oropharynx after partial synchronisation, J. Maxillofac. Surg. **4**:26-33, 1976.

25. Gingrass, P. J., and Gingrass, R. P.: Lymphangioma of the oral cavity: report of three cases with long-term follow-up, J. Oral Surg. **29**:428, 1971.

26. Hattowska, H., and Borowicz, K.: Histologic evaluation of treatment of epidermoid carcinoma in the oral cavity with methotrexate and 5-fluorouracil, J. Oral Surg. **32**:508-512, 1974.

27. Henefer, E. P., Borghesani, E. P., and Sacks, F. R.: Liposarcoma of the cheek, J. Oral Surg. **34**:1039-1043, 1976.

28. Kelly, D. E., Terry, B. C., and Small, E. W.: Arteriovenous malformation of the mandible: report of a case, J. Oral Surg. **35**:387-393, 1977.

29. Kennett, S., and Cohen, H.: Central Giant cell tumor of the mandible: report of a case, J. Oral Surg. **29**:492, 1971.

30. Kennett, S., Jr., and Curran, J. B.: Giant cemento-ossifying fibroma: report of a case, J. Oral Surg. **30**:513, 1972.

31. Krausen, A. S., Gulman, S., and Zografakis, G.: Cementomas: aggressive cemento-ossifying fibroma of the ethmoid region, Arch. Otolaryngol. **103**:371-373, 1977.

32. Krausen, A. S., Pullom, P. A., Gulman, S., Schenck, N. L., and Ogura, J. H.: Cementomas: aggressive or innocuous neoplasms? Arch. Otolaryngol. **103**:349-354, 1977.

33. La Dow, C. S., Henefer, E. P., and McFall, T.: Central hemangioma of the maxilla with Von Hipple's disease, a case report, J. Oral Surg. **22**:252, 1964.

34. Leban, S. G., Lepow, H., Stratigos, G. T., and Chu, F.: The giant cell lesion of jaws: neoplastic or reparative? J. Oral Surg. **29**:398, 1971.

35. Lewin, R. W., and Cataldo, E.: Multiple myeloma discovered from oral manifestations, report of a case, J. Oral Surg. **25**:72, 1967.

36. Lichtenstein, L., and Jaffe, H. L.: Fibrous dysplasia of bone, Arch. Pathol. **33**:783, 1942.

37. Longacre, J. J., Benton, C., and Unterthiner, P. A.: Treatment of facial hemangioma by intravascular embolization with silicone spheres, a case report, Plast. Reconstr. Surg. **50**:618, 1972.

38. Luessenhop, A. J., Kachmann, R., Jr., Shevlin, W., and Ferrero, A. A.: Clinical evaluation of artificial embolization in management of large cerebral arteriovenous malformations, J. Neurosurg. **23**:400, 1965.

39. Malcolm, P., Thompson, L. W., and Duncan, M., Jr.: An ossifying fibroma of the coronoid process: a case report, J. Plast. Reconstr. Surg. **60**:118-120, 1977.

40. Marchetta, F. C., Sako, K., and Camp, F.: Multiple malignancies in patients with head and neck cancer, Am. J. Surg. **110**:538, 1965.

41. Martin, H.: Surgery of head and neck tumors, New York, 1957, Hoeber-Harper, pp. 246, 248.

42. Martis, C. and Karakasis, D.: Central fibroma of the mandible, J. Oral Surg. **10**:758, 1972.

43. Matsumura, T., Hasegawa, K., Isono, K., and Kawakatsu, K.: Congenital fibromyxoma: report of a case, J. Oral Surg. **35**:313-315, 1977.

44. Matsumura, T., and Kawakatsu, K.: Verrucous carcinoma of oral mucosa: histochemical patterns and clinical behaviors, J. Oral Surg. **30**:349, 1972.

45. Matsumura, T., Sugahara, T., Wada, T., and Kawakatsu, K.: Recurrent giant cell reparative granuloma: report of case and histopatterns, J. Oral Surg. **29**:212, 1971.

46. Meyer, I., and Giunta, J. L.: Adenomatoid odontogenic tumor (adenoameloblastoma): report of a case, J. Oral Surg. **32**:448-451, 1974.

47. Morgan, J. F., and Schow, C. E., Jr.: Use of sodium morrhuate in the management of hemangiomas, J. Oral Surg. **25**:363-366, 1974.

48. Piercell, M. P., Waite, D. E., and Nelson, R. L.: Central hemangioma of the mandible, intraoral resection and reconstruction, J. Oral Surg. **33**:225-232, 1975.

49. Robinson, H. B. G.: Ameloblastomas—survey of 379 cases from the literature, Arch. Pathol. **23**:831, 1937.

50. Roser, S. M., Nicholas, T. R., and Horose, F. M.: Metastatic chondrosarcoma to the maxilla: review of literature and report of case, J. Oral Surg. **34**:1012-1015, 1976.

51. Rush, B. F., Jr., and Klein, N. W.: Intra-arterial infusion of the head and neck, anatomic and distributional problems, Am. J. Surg. **110**:513, 1965.

52. Schmaman, A., Smith, I., and Ackerman, L. V.: Benign fibro-osseous lesions of the mandible and

maxilla: a review of 35 cases, Cancer **26**:303-312, 1970.

53. Schroll, K.: Results of tumor operations in the Department of Oral Surgery of Graz, Oest. Z. Stomat. **66**:191, 1969.
54. Seldin, H. M., Seldin, D. S., Rakower, W., and Jarrett, W. J.: Lipomas of the oral cavity, report of 26 cases, J. Oral Surg. **25**:271, 1967.
55. Seymour, R. L., Bray, T. E., and Irby, W. B.: Replacement of condylar process, J. Oral Surg. **35**:405-408, 1977.
56. Sherman, R. S., and Sternbergh, W. C.: The roentgen appearance of ossifying fibroma of bone, Radiology **50**:595, 1948.
57. Smith, D. B., and Weaver, A. W.: Cryosurgery for oral cancer—a six year retrospective study, J. Oral Surg. **34**:245-248, 1976.
58. Smith, I.: Recurrent ameloblastoma of the mandible, J. Maxillofac. Surg. **4**:1-7, 1976.
59. Sullivan, R. D.: Continuous intra-arterial infusion chemotherapy for head and neck cancer, Trans. Am. Acad. Ophthalmol. Otolaryngol. **66**:111, 1962.
60. Sullivan, R. D., and McPeak, G. J.: A favorable response in tongue cancer to arterial infusion chemotherapy, J.A.M.A. **179**:294, 1962.
61. Taylor, G.: Ameloblastomas of the mandible: a clinical study of 25 patients, Am. Surg. **34**:57, 1968.
62. Thoma, K.: Oral surgery, ed. 5, St. Louis, 1969, The C. V. Mosby Co., pp. 1042, 1044, 1119.
63. Treggiden, R.: Mandibular metastasis from carcinoma of the bladder, J. Oral Surg. **35**:1016-1018, 1976.
64. Ward, G. E., and Hendrick, J. W.: Diagnosis and treatment of tumors of the head and neck, Baltimore, 1950, The Williams & Wilkins Co., pp. 315, 324-326, 351, 738, 747.
65. Ward, T. G., and Cohen, B.: Squamous carcinoma in a mandibular cyst, Br. J. Oral Surg. **1**:12, 1963.
66. Wilde, N. J., Tur, J. J., and Call, D. E.: Hemangioma of the mandible: report of a case, J. Oral Surg. **24**:549, 1966.

CHAPTER 25

Salivary glands and ducts

Donald E. Cooksey

STRUCTURE OF THE SALIVARY GLANDS

Salivary glands may be divided for purposes of description into major and minor glands. The major salivary glands are the parotid, submandibular, and sublingual glands. The minor salivary glands are those smaller glands and groups of glands in the palate, buccal mucosa, and floor of the mouth that secrete primarily mucus. Since the salivary glands have frequently been described in detail in various texts on anatomy, histology, and surgery, this discussion is limited to such descriptions as are pertinent to oral surgical problems.

Gross anatomy

Parotid gland. The parotid gland (Fig. 25-1, *A*) is a paired, bilobular serous gland overlying the masseter muscle. It extends upward to the level of the auditory canal and downward to, and frequently below, the lower border of the mandible. Posteriorly it wraps itself around the posterior border of the mandible, and anteriorly it extends into the buccal fat pad, where it gives off its excretory duct. In the fat substance a small lobule of gland usually attaches itself to the duct. The superficial lobe and the deep lobe are connected by an isthmus at the posterior border of the gland.

The motor portion of the seventh cranial, or facial, nerve emerges from the stylomastoid foramen and passes laterally and anteriorly to the isthmus, where it divides into two main branches. These branches pass above and below the isthmus between the lobes, branching and rejoining along their course. Thus the seventh cranial nerve is deep to the superficial lobe of the parotid gland and passes between the lobes rather than within the parotid substance. As a result, it is possible to remove the superficial lobe without sectioning the nerve.

The parotid duct passes anteriorly and medially from the gland along the lateral border of the masseter muscle and turns at a right angle around the anterior border of the masseter muscle. It then penetrates the buccinator muscle and the oral mucosa and opens, at the level of the neck of the maxillary second molar, into a small caruncle. Thus from 1.5 to 3 cm of the duct is accessible from the mouth. Dissection through the mouth past the right angle turn at the anterior border of the masseter muscle is most difficult; and an element of risk is present, since portions of the seventh cranial nerve may be encountered at this level.

Submandibular gland. The submandibu-

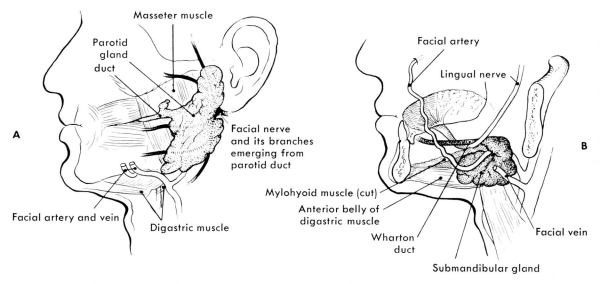

Fig. 25-1. **A,** Anatomical relations of parotid gland and duct. **B,** Anatomical relations of submandibular gland and duct.

lar gland (Fig. 25-1, *B*) is a paired muco-serous gland lying in the submandibular space. It extends inferiorly to the digastric muscle, superiorly to the mylohyoid muscle, anteriorly to the midbody of the mandible, and posteriorly to the angle of the mandible. It is bordered laterally by the medial border of the mandible and medially by the hyoglossus muscle. Inferolaterally it is covered by the skin and platysma muscle.

At the posterior border of the mylohyoid muscle the submandibular gland turns up and forward, entering the sublingual space and giving off its excretory duct. The duct passes anterosuperiorly in the sublingual space and opens into the mouth beneath the anterior portion of the tongue at a caruncle lateral to the lingual frenum. In its course the duct travels from lateral to medial and from below upward, crossing beneath the lingual nerve at the level of the third molar and then above the lingual nerve at about the level of the second molar. Thus, in a transoral procedure for removal of a stone, the lingual nerve would be encountered above the duct posteriorly but beneath the

duct or not at all from the second molar forward.

The facial artery passes from behind and medial to the gland up and over the gland to emerge from the submandibular space laterally and proceeds into the face at the level of the anterior border of the masseter muscle. Thus the facial artery would not be encountered in the incision for removal of the gland but would have to be located by dissection. Its location is usually indicated by the presence of two lymph nodes, the pre-vascular and retrovascular nodes, which overlie it at the level of the inferior border of the mandible. Superior and deep to these nodes is the marginal mandibular branch of the seventh cranial nerve, and posterior to the nodes is the facial vein. Since the facial vein is lateral to the gland, this vein may be cut in the incision and cannot be depended on as a landmark once it has been disturbed.

Just medial to the course of the facial artery, at the superior pole of the gland and at the posterior border of the mylohyoid muscle, are several ganglionic connections from the lingual nerve. The submandibular gan-

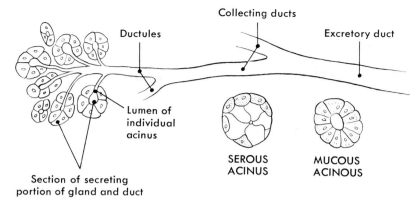

Fig. 25-2. Microscopic anatomy of salivary glands.

glion is included in this plexus but is seldom identified at surgery. The lingual nerve may be identified above these connections and follows an anterior and medial course into the sublingual space in proximity to the submandibular duct.

The hypoglossal nerve and sublingual vein cross the lateral surface of the hyoglossus muscle in the medial wall of the submandibular niche. They are separated from the gland capsule by a thin layer of fascia, through which they may be identified, and therefore need not be disturbed. The hypoglossal nerve and sublingual vein, together with the posterior border of the mylohyoid muscle and the pulley of the digastric muscle, form a triangle having the hyoglossus muscle as its floor. By spreading the fibers of the hyoglossus muscle at this point, the lingual artery may be exposed.

Sublingual gland. The sublingual gland is a paired mucous gland lying in the sublingual space, above the mylohyoid muscle, in a line parallel to the course of Wharton's duct. Its landmark is a ridge called the *plica sublingualis*, which runs anteroposteriorly in the floor of the mouth. It secretes principally mucus from a series of small short ducts, which vary in number from person to person, and seldom becomes involved in the problems of its fellows, the submandibular and parotid glands. Occasionally glands normally occupying the anatomical

position of the sublingual gland attach to the submandibular duct and open into it rather than into the mouth.

Minor salivary glands. The minor salivary glands are scattered throughout the oral mucous membrane and are simply clusters of mucous acini attached to short ducts that open into the mouth. They are sometimes clustered in groups, as are those beneath the tongue, and their ducts emerge in large numbers in relatively small areas. These glands are superficial, lying just beneath the mucosa.

Microscopic anatomy

Microscopically these glands are all similar in construction, being composed of mucous or serous acini or combinations of both. The primary differentiating characteristic in any given fragment of tissue is the relative number of mucous or serous forms, the parotid gland being almost entirely serous.

Since the minor glands and the sublingual glands are simple systems, their epithelium-lined excretory ducts are small and short. The parotid and submandibular duct systems are composed of a series of small ducts that drain a single acinus and join to make larger ducts. These larger ducts drain lobes and in turn join the principal excretory duct to the mouth. Thus, if the ductal pattern were seen in its entirety, it would resemble a leafless tree with the termination of each twig an individual acinus, the branches the lobular ducts, and the trunk the main excretory duct (Fig. 25-2).

The principal tissue elements seen microscopically are glandular epithelium representative of the secretory portion of the gland, cuboidal epithelium lining the ducts, connective tissue compartments dividing the individual lobes, and a capsule of connective tissue.

Anatomical weaknesses

Study of the salivary glands reveals several distinct anatomical weaknesses. The minor glands and the sublingual glands, having short, straight, simple duct systems, are seldom affected by inflammatory conditions but may react to anything causing partial closure or rupture of the duct. A mucocele is the usual result. Complete closure produces atrophy of the gland.

The other systems have more serious weaknesses. First, the entire submandibular gland and duct system lies in a dependent position, which predisposes it to retrograde invasion by oral flora. Second, both the submandibular duct and the parotid duct are slightly larger along their course than at their caruncle. This permits storage of secretions so that a ready flow may be available on stimulation without waiting for the secretory process. This relatively static reservoir, however, permits settling out of epithelial cells and inspissation of salivary fluids, which tend to form obstructions and are a ready nidus for bacterial activity. Third, both the submandibular and the parotid ducts make a radical turn along their course. The submandibular duct turns sharply at the posterior border of the mylohyoid muscle, just anterior to the hilus of the gland. The parotid duct turns sharply at the anterior border of the masseter muscle, fairly close to the caruncle. These two areas are favorite points for lodgment of obstructions, just as the mechanical aspects of the arrangement would suggest. Finally, since both glands are dependent on one

mode of disposal of secreted fluids, anything tending to reduce the flow tends also to alter the composition and function of the glands.

DISEASES OF THE SALIVARY GLANDS
Inflammatory diseases
Acute sialadenitis

Any acute inflammation of the salivary glands may be termed acute sialadenitis. What is discussed in this instance, however, is the nonspecific acute adenopathies not related to any other condition.

Symptoms. These swellings are usually sudden in onset, although they may be the acute phase of some chronic condition. The gland becomes sore and tense, usually on one side only, and pus may be seen at the orifice of the duct or may be milked from the duct system. The patient's temperature may rise, and the blood picture will reflect the relative toxicity of the infection. If uncontrolled, these infections will sometimes localize beneath the skin and require incision and drainage.

Etiology. Smears and cultures to determine the predominant organism reveal a wide range of bacteria, most of which are normally found in the oral cavity. These include *Streptococcus salivarius,* viridans streptococci, *Diplococcus pneumoniae,* and *Staphylococcus aureus.* Occasionally yeast forms are found. Thus evidence does not indicate any specific cause or predominant pathogen. Acute stomatitis seldom plays an appreciable role in the onset of such conditions.

Treatment. Treatment of these infections is by medicinal means. Antibiotics or sulfonamides to control the acute infection are indicated. If a sample of pus is obtainable, tests for specific antibiotic sensitivity are of great help. Care should be taken when making the culture to obtain the secretions of the duct rather than samples of the oral flora.

After the acute phases of the infection subside, or the patient is under adequate antibiotic control, the duct may be dilated with a blunt probe to assist drainage. Sialograms aid in assessing the cause or amount of damage and frequently are of great assistance in treatment because of the antimicrobial effect of the iodized solution used to make them. Adequate hydration of the patient is important, and the use of sialogogues to increase the salivary flow and produce a washing action may be beneficial.

Prognosis. Once established, this condition tends to recur. Frequently, the recurrent disease takes the form of a chronic or subacute type, and later in the course of the disease, obstructions may appear in the duct or cavitations may appear in the gland structure.

Differential diagnosis. Occasionally one sees conditions that may be confused with acute sialadenitis and vice versa. Unilateral epidemic parotitis, for example, is always a consideration in differential diagnosis. Often one sees cases of what has been termed idiopathic parotitis or submandibular adenitis for want of a better understanding of the condition. In these instances the gland has become hard and tender. No increase in temperature and no pus formation occurs. Sialograms reveal no evidence of disease, and the gland and duct substances appear normal. This condition is recurrent and subsides variously after administration of antibiotics, antihistaminics, or lemon drops, after massage, or on neglect. Two possible explanations have been advanced for this phenomenon: (1) that it is caused by the presence of small mucous plugs, which eventually pass out of the salivary caruncle when placed under enough pressure, and (2) that it is caused by the transmission of noxious stimuli to the sympathetic nerves supplying the mucous acini, which produces hypersecretion of mucus and relative stasis as a result of increased viscosity.

Not infrequently the lymph nodes within the submandibular gland substance become enlarged. This enlargement may be accompanied by adenopathy of the adjacent pre-vascular and retrovascular nodes and is usually the result of infection higher in the head or jaws; still, it simulates inflammation of the submandibular gland. On palpation the vascular nodes can be separated from the gland and trapped against the mandible; however, the intraglandular node stays with the gland and is difficult to differentiate from glandular adenopathy except by the size and texture of the remainder of the gland. A similar situation obtains with the parotid gland, a frequent cause being minor infections of the eye.

Chronic sialadenitis

Any of the acute salivary gland infections just described may become chronic. The chronic disease, however, is most frequently found behind an obstruction that has produced long periods of stasis. In this condition the duct system dilates and exerts pressure against the adjacent gland. Obstruction and stasis increase the pressure, and atrophy and fibrosis of the gland occur. The gland becomes firm and hard and may or may not be tender, depending on the phase of the inflammatory change and the degree of chronicity. Abscesses and cysts that require drainage may occur in the gland substance, or they may smolder for years in a series of remissions and recurrences. Conservative treatment in the form of removal of the obstruction, dilation of the duct, and diagnostic and therapeutic sialography may abate the condition. Unfortunately, recurrence is not unusual, and surgical removal of the gland may be necessary.

Chronic sialadenitis may also occur after long periods of general anesthesia, general debilitation, pneumonia, or other diseases involving high febrile courses, or any factor possibly tending to produce long periods of dehydration; all these permit bacteria to retrograde and incubate in the duct system. The resultant sialodochitis produces strictures of the duct, stasis, dilation, and chronic infection that resists permanent cure.

Diseases due to obstruction
Sialolithiasis

The series of events leading to both gross and microscopic chronic inflammatory changes in salivary glands is somewhat obscure. It is well known, however, that one of the most prominent signs is the production of a salivary stone, or sialolith. The most popular theory of sialolith formation is that an accretion of mineral salts forms in and around a soft plug of mucus, bacteria, or desquamated epithelial cells. This theory seems to be well founded in that some sialoliths are radiopaque and well calcified, whereas others are soft and rubbery and are not demonstrable radiographically. Sialoliths occur in a wide variety of sizes and shapes, a fact indicating that their development is progressive once they become lodged in the duct. The development of a sialolith inevitably leads to stasis and infection of the duct system and produces the changes described under chronic sialadenitis.

Symptoms. Symptomatically the gland involved may swell, especially at mealtimes, and may become tense and sore. This swelling and tenderness may subside, only to recur later. Pus may be seen at the orifice of the caruncle, which may be inflamed, and pus or cloudy saliva may be obtained by milking the gland. The stone may be palpable by bimanual manipulation and may be movable up and down the duct. The stone may be visualized in radiographs, and dilation at the site of the stone and of the ducts of the gland will be evident in a sialogram.

Management. Management of these stones is surgical. Generally the stone can be removed transorally; however, extreme damage to the gland or recurrence of the disease after transoral removal of the stone may indicate removal of the gland (Fig. 25-3).

Sialoangiectasis

This term is employed to describe a gland and duct system vastly dilated by stasis of salivary secretion resulting from obstruction. The most frequent cause is a sialolith, although a simple stricture may be the cause. It is not unusual to observe glands

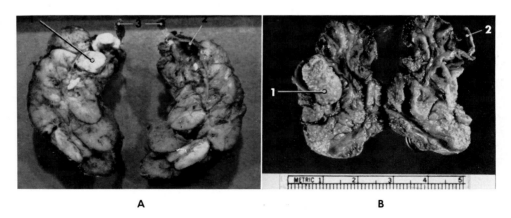

A **B**

Fig. 25-3. A, Surgical specimen of a submandibular salivary gland containing several large stones. *1,* Clump of four stones in the pelvis of the gland; *2,* gland pelvis showing dilation of the pelvis from the stones; *3,* submandibular duct demonstrating the relative size of the stones compared to the duct. **B,** Surgical specimen of submandibular salivary gland containing one large stone. *1,* Solitary stone in the pelvis of the gland; *2,* duct of the gland demonstrating difference in size of duct and stone. Stones such as are shown in **A** and **B** are difficult to remove transorally and not infrequently do sufficient damage to the gland during their tenure to require the ultimate removal of the gland.

with a long history of chronic infection from no obvious cause that demonstrate this extensive dilation.

The prognosis for such glands is poor, since their natural history is one of repeated acute attacks, ultimately resulting in removal of the gland.

Retention cysts

Retention cysts result from rupture of a duct into the gland parenchyma. This rupture fills with salivary secretion and is eventually encapsulated with fibrous connective tissue. A complete or partial epithelial lining may or may not be present.

Since these cysts seal themselves off from the duct system, they do not fill with radiopaque contrast medium in sialography; instead, they demonstrate themselves radiographically as nonfilling, space-occupying defects in the gland substance. They may have an obscure opening into a duct that permits them to drain and refill periodically but that does not admit the radiopaque oil. For this reason, they are prone to enlarge and subside (a characteristic that readily differentiates them from mixed tumors, which do not subside). On palpation they are usually soft and may be doughy or fluctuant and they are sometimes tender. (Mixed tumors are hard and seldom tender.)

Treatment. Surgical removal is the treatment of choice. This is necessary not only to eliminate the lesion but to establish the diagnosis as well. Incision and drainage usually result in eventual recurrence. Exteriorization should not be considered.

Atrophy

Degree plays an important part in the effect of obstruction on glandular tissue. Partial obstruction results in sialoangiectasis; obstruction with rupture of the duct produces retention cysts; partial obstructions are usually accompanied by infection; and complete obstruction produces atrophy. Complete obstruction productive of atrophy is rare and is usually the result of surgical accident in which the main excre-

tory duct is tied and all avenues for the escape of fluid are obliterated. Another prominent cause of salivary gland atrophy is heavy doses of irradiation, usually in the treatment of malignant tumors.

The loss of one salivary gland because of atrophy or excision is of little importance. The loss of several of the major glands, however, produces xerostomia and atypical caries.

Lack of salivary secretion, collapse of the duct, and inability to receive iodized oil for sialography are typical of this condition. No treatment is available once the atrophy has occurred.

Tumors of the salivary glands

Like tumors in most locations, primary tumors in the major and minor salivary glands can be roughly classified as benign and malignant. Even this classification will be disputed, since at least two tumors, the mixed tumor and the mucoepidermoid tumor, although benign in biological behavior at the outset, are well known to undergo malignant changes. In addition, at least one developmental defect, the branchial cleft cyst, so simulates a tumor clinically as to defy differential diagnosis short of formal biopsy. For this reason these tumors will be discussed according to their biological behavior when observed clinically. For a better understanding of these lesions, further study of the extensive literature on this subject should be carried out.

Benign tumors

Salivary adenoma. This tumor is a benign neoplastic proliferation of secretory cells in a salivary gland. It is usually confined to the substance of the parotid gland. It is firm, painless, usually well encapsulated, and slow growing, and it is readily moved from its growth site on pressure and returns to its original position on release. This is an important sign, since most malignant growths are indurated and cannot be so displaced. Few, if any, visible changes appear in the sialogram, and differential diagnosis is not positive without biopsy. This tumor is regarded as biologically benign. Management is surgical.

Papillary cystadenoma lymphomatosum (Warthin's tumor). This benign and slow-growing tumor may occur anywhere in or near the parotid gland, usually in the region of the angle or ramus of the mandible or beneath the ear lobe. It is firm and nontender and may be sufficiently circumscribed to be readily movable. Changes in the sialogram are minimal until the tumor has attained sufficient size to display nonfilling, space-occupying, tissue-displacing tumor substance. Even then, differential diagnosis is questionable without biopsy. Warthin's tumor occurs most frequently in males in their fifth decade, but it may occur in either sex and somewhat earlier or later. Management is surgical.

Branchial cleft cyst. A branchial cleft cyst is a nonneoplastic and nonmalignant developmental anomaly, originating from epithelium that is enclaved between branchial arches at the time they fuse. It usually manifests itself as a swelling on the lateral aspect of the neck or in the floor of the mouth; but it is known to develop in sites adjacent to or within the major salivary glands, in such fashion as to defy differentiation from tumors of the gland by clinical means. A branchial cleft cyst is firm but softer, as a general rule, than any of the true neoplasms. It may undergo periodic recessions, a sign that is never present in a true neoplasm. Movement may be possible, but this is not always a characteristic, since the cyst may be attached to structures that move with difficulty, or it may have had a previous inflammatory episode that has produced circumferential fibrosis. During its tenure it may become tender to palpation, at which time it is usually tense and firm.

A branchial cleft cyst appears in the sialogram as a space-occupying, nonfilling defect, similar in many respects to other solid or cystic lesions of the salivary glands. Usually, however, it does not exhibit the typical "ball-in-hand" deformity common to mixed tumors.

Mixed tumors. Wide disagreement is present among pathologists as to the essential nature of mixed tumors and among surgeons as to the proper method of treating them. For clinical purposes, the most arguable question is: Are they malignant or benign? Perhaps the best way to answer this question for the clinician is to point out that since mixed tumors do not generally metastasize or, when untouched, do not invade until late in their development, they may be regarded as benign. Unfortunately, they have a strong propensity to recur. The recurrences are probably the result of either incomplete excision at operation or multicentric origin of the lesion; they are frequently more serious than the primary lesion because pathways of invasion are opened. Some say that a mixed tumor may undergo metaplasia after surgical intervention and recurs as a true malignant neoplasm. This theory leads to differences among surgeons, who variously recommend enucleation, wide excision, or radical resection of the gland, seventh cranial nerve, integuments, and lymph node–bearing tissues that furnish drainage to the area. The best solution probably lies in the middle course, in which the lesion, together with a portion of the gland supporting it, is widely excised. It is seldom necessary to sacrifice the seventh cranial nerve in this procedure, and cure is the rule rather than the exception. When reoperation becomes necessary because of recurrence, seventh cranial nerve damage is more common and the incidence of cure is reduced. This fact emphasizes the need for adequate management at the original operation.

Clinically mixed tumors are hard, probably, in part, because they are composed variously of epithelial and connective tissue elements. They are usually loosely encapsulated in fibrous tissue and are readily movable, although as they advance in size, involving more tissue, they may become firmly fixed and even give the impression of induration. Recurrences, on the other hand, almost without exception are firmly fixed. Mixed tumors are generally nodular to palpation and give the impression of being composed of one or more globular masses.

Mixed tumors occur most frequently in the parotid gland, usually at the angle of the mandible or beneath the ear lobe. They occur less frequently in the submandibular gland but occur often in the minor salivary glands of the palate and lips. (I have not encountered this tumor in the sublingual glands, although no reason is known why these should not be affected.)

Mixed tumors are painless and slow growing and are usually brought to the patient's attention by touch while shaving or applying make-up. Frequently, they are thought to be wens by the patient because of their proximity to a common epidermoidal cyst–bearing area. For this reason some mixed tumors are large when first seen, whereas others are relatively small.

It is difficult to differentiate mixed tumors from the several other benign tumors of the area or from hyperplastic lymph nodes. Tissue examination is the most reliable method, and diagnosis can usually be rendered by means of frozen section,

with sufficient accuracy to guide the surgeon in completing the procedure. In dealing with suspected mixed tumors of minor salivary glands, biopsy by total excision is the method of choice (Figs. 25-4 and 25-5), since these lesions are usually of manageable size when first discovered. Sialography in problems of the minor glands is not useful.

Sialograms of major glands may show displacement of the glandular structure, particularly of the superficial lobe of the parotid gland. As a result of this displacement the collecting ducts curve around the lesion, giving the appearance of a hand carrying a ball. Unfortunately this characteristic is not limited to mixed tumors, and its presence requires that the tumor be of sufficient size to produce the deformity. For this reason, as with most tumors extrinsic to the duct system, sialograms are of limited benefit in the diagnosis of mixed tumors.

Treatment is always surgical. Since these lesions do not metastasize unless they have undergone metaplasia and are behaving like a true malignant tumor, dissection of the lymph node–bearing area appears to be excessively radical. On the other hand, in view of the well-known tendency toward

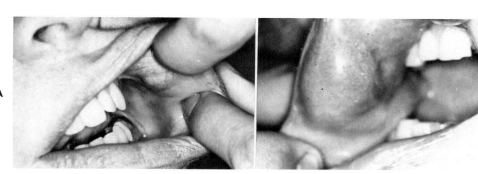

Fig. 25-4. A, A benign mixed tumor (pleomorphic adenoma) of minor salivary gland origin in a 24-year-old woman. The tumor was hard, slow growing with a history of 3-years' duration, and readily movable. It was totally excised with adequate normal tissue margins clinically and microscopically. These procedures are easily done in the office, employing local or outpatient general anesthesia. Closure is done primarily. **B,** Benign mixed tumor of the lip in a 48-year-old man. The primary clinical feature in differentiation between mucocele and mixed tumor is the hard nodular consistency of the neoplasm.

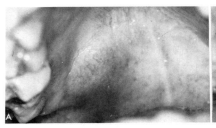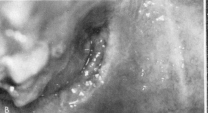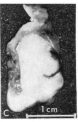

Fig. 25-5. A, Mixed tumor of the palate in a 28-year-old man. These tumors should be widely excised rather than enucleated, since they tend to recur. The presence of a capsule is illusionary, and tumor can frequently be demonstrated outside what seems to be a capsular membrane. **B,** The defect may be difficult to close primarily and must heal by secondary intention, as this has in a week's time. A prosthetic guard may add to patient comfort. **C,** Surgical specimen of the lesion seen in **B** after sectioning through its center. These tumors are frequently larger than superficial appearances suggest. Lobulations are frequent. Periosteum must frequently be taken in the excision. The known duration of this tumor was 4 months.

recurrence, an original attempt at enucleation seems dangerously conservative. Thus wide, adequate excision of the area, with efforts toward preservation of vital structures, seems the technique of choice. Mixed tumors do not respond to irradiation.

Neurilemoma (schwannoma). Neurilemoma is included in this discussion, not because it occurs in salivary gland tissue, but because it occasionally affects branches of the seventh cranial nerve and because it bears such a similarity to mixed tumors clinically that differentiation is almost impossible.

This tumor is benign, slow growing, and asymptomatic. It is encapsulated and readily movable.

No sialographic findings appear until the tumor reaches a large size; then the sialogram shows displacement of gland substance, similar in all respects to that of the mixed tumor.

The primary problem inherent in a tumor of this type is its removal. A neurilemoma is firmly attached to the sheath of the nerve that it involves, and although the tumor has no special effect on the function of the nerve, its removal usually results in damage or section of the nerve at the point of attachment. Since this lesion does not ordinarily undergo malignant transformation, it would be better left alone if the diagnosis

of neurilemoma were established. All too often, however, the damage to the nerve occurs at the time of investigation, and the diagnosis arrives too late. A neurilemoma does not respond to irradiation.

Malignant tumors

Mucoepidermoid tumors. Mucoepidermoid tumors have been variously subdivided in the past into two groups, malignant and benign. Even now, reasons seem adequate to believe that some are of a higher degree of biological activity than others and therefore more malignant than others. The class in general, however, is malignant and should be regarded and treated as such.

Mucoepidermoid tumors may grow either rapidly or slowly. They seldom exhibit pain unless infection or invasion of vital structures occurs. They occur most frequently in the parotid gland but may occur anywhere salivary gland tissue exists. On palpation they feel firm, indurated, and bound down to the surrounding structures; they do not move readily.

Since mucoepidermoid tumors involve the ductal and acinar structures of the gland, changes may be observed in the sialogram. Evidence of cavitations may appear where necrosis has occurred or of hyperplastic glandular activity with new duct formation or of a stricture caused by the filling of a duct with neoplastic tissue. Because any of these findings may also be typical of inflammatory disease, care should be taken to coordinate the clinical and sialographic findings accurately before risking a diagnosis. In the final analysis, tissue examination is the only method by which an accurate diagnosis may be reached.

Treatment of these tumors is surgical. Resection may of necessity be more radical than in the mixed tumors, depending on the extent of the tumor. Conservative management of the seventh cranial nerve must not be considered important; instead, the surgeon should be governed by the extent to which the lesion has invaded adjacent tissue. This is not to imply that the nerve must always be sacrificed. If conservation of the nerve jeopardizes a surgical cure, however, sacrificing the nerve is indicated. Radical neck dissections are not generally indicated unless evidence exists of regional node metastasis, although some schools of thought regard prophylactic neck dissection at the original operation as the mode of choice.

Irradiation may be of benefit in controlling metastasis or in palliative therapy, but it is not thought by most to afford a cure or to be indicated as a postsurgical prophylaxis.

Squamous cell carcinoma. Like the mucoepidermoid tumors, squamous cell carcinomas originate from the epithelium lining the salivary glands and ducts. Unlike the mucoepidermoid tumors, however, no doubt exists about the malignancy of carcinomas, only about the relative degree of their malignancy. Although it is thought that these tumors probably originate within the ducts, invasion of the surrounding glandular tissue occurs promptly. Metastasis to the regional lymph nodes may occur early or late, depending on the individual behavior of the tumor.

The symptoms, signs, and sialographic evidence of these tumors are similar to those of mucoepidermoid tumors, and no clear-cut clinical differentiation may be made.

Treatment is also similar in all respects, with radical neck dissection figuring more prominently in the treatment by most surgeons.

Irradiation has a noticeable effect in the control of these lesions and their metastasis, particularly in the control of the more anaplastic types. However, control and palliation, rather than cure, are the usual goals of irradiation.

Adenocarcinoma. A large number of lesions, bearing an even larger number of names and subclassifications, may be grouped under the general heading of adenocarcinoma. Included in these are the pseudoadenomatous basal cell carcinoma (adenocystic basaloid mixed tumor or cylindroma), papillary adenocarcinoma, serous cell adenocarcinoma, mucous cell adenocarcinoma, malignant oncocytoma, and malignant mixed tumor. These and many other terms serve largely to confuse the clinician. For the sake of clarity in thinking of these lesions, it should be understood that all are malignant, all are potential killers, and all require some form of radical surgery or cancericidal irradiation if they are to be cured.

The symptoms of these lesions, with the notable exception of cylindroma, are generally those seen in mucoepidermoid tumor and squamous cell carcinoma. A cylindroma is usually a slow-growing lesion, and its mild-appearing histological characteristics and growth history may lead the surgeon to believe that it is not an aggressive lesion. Actually, it has a powerful propensity for recurrence and extensive invasion with local destruction, frequently leading to successive, disfiguring operations and ultimately metastasizing to distant sites late in the disease.

Other adenocarcinomas may grow with great rapidity and may be so anaplastic in their microscopic characteristics as to defy subclassification.

Sialographic identification of an adenocarcinoma is questionable, since the appearance of its internal structure may be similar to that of any other lesion that produces spaces resulting from central necrosis. In some of the more slowly growing tumors, however, attempts by the tumors to form tissue morphologically similar to the parent tissue produce abnormal acinar structures that are capable of receiving the iodized oil and simulate hypertrophic glandular substance.

The treatment of choice is usually radical surgery. Radical neck dissection may be performed when indicated.

Irradiation is effective in individual cases but by no means effective in all cases. Cylindroma in particular is radioresistant. If the tumor is accessible to effective irradiation, it is usually accessible to surgery. For this reason, irradiation is usually reserved for control, palliation, and, in some cases, prophylaxis rather than for primary treatment—the condition and life expectancy of the patient and the size, grade, and location of the lesion all being factors for consideration.

DIFFERENTIAL DIAGNOSIS OF SALIVARY GLAND LESIONS

A principal problem associated with the treatment of salivary gland lesions is the decision of the clinician regarding the type of lesion being treated and its anatomical location in relation to the various associated structures. Cytological examination is becoming increasingly important in diagnosis because of improvements in technique and understanding of the specimens obtained. The validity of this examination and of needle biopsy depends largely on the accuracy of the technique by which the tissues were obtained and on the training and ability of the pathologist responsible for analyzing the tissues. Formal biopsies are dependable, but they involve openings on the face and are contraindicated in inflammatory diseases. It rests with the clinician to decide with the nonsurgical means at hand what, if any, further steps are required to secure an accurate diagnosis. The means available are principally the history, the physical examination, and the radiographic examination. From these a rational course of treatment or further diagnostic needs can be determined. Occasionally clinical laboratory examinations may aid in making the decision.

History

A history of the lesion concerned frequently aids in the determination of its nature.

Duration. The duration of a lesion is an important factor. If a lesion is old and has a history of remission and exacerbation, it is probably of an inflammatory nature. If it is old and has a history of slow, steady growth, it is usually a benign or low-grade malignant tumor. If it is a new lesion with acute symptoms, inflammation is suggested. A new lesion with a painless swelling, however, is suggestive of early malignancy.

Nature of onset. The nature of the onset may offer some clue. If the onset is gradual and painless but continuous, tumor is suggested. If it is sudden and painful, the diagnosis of inflammation is more proper, although rapidly growing tumor with overlying infection cannot be discounted.

Rapidity of growth. The rapidity of growth is an important diagnostic point and indicative of the degree of malignancy. A slow but continuously growing lesion is seldom inflammatory or of a high grade of malignancy. A rapidly growing lesion may be either; but pain, exudate, inflammation, fever, or alterations in the differential blood count toward immaturity usually accompany inflammations. (It is to be remembered that tumors as such are not painful until they either invade surrounding sensitive structures or become infected.) Rapidly growing lesions with a history of resolution and remission are odds-on favorites to be inflammations. Slowly growing lesions with a history of remissions are usually cysts or other retention phenomena.

It is not typical of any true neoplasm to remit or regress, although some will have periods of biological inactivity.

Coincidental conditions. A history of other conditions coincidental to the present complaint frequently offers a clue or an explanation of the problem. A history of juvenile tuberculosis or tuberculosis in the family may explain the presence of a calcified body in the region of a salivary gland when no connection with the gland is demonstrable. A history of pneumococcal pneumonia or other acute febrile disease may mark the beginning of chronic sialadenitis, particularly of the parotid gland. Long general anesthesias, usually with the employment of antisialogogues, are pertinent to the observation, as would be the coincidental presence of any cachectic or dehydrating condition.

Physical examination

A proper physical examination is the most important single factor in the differential diagnosis of any given condition. In addition to a general physical survey to detect systemic factors that might be contributory, a careful appraisal of the adnexa of the glands should be carried out. It is important to remember that both the submandibular and parotid glands have adjacent lymph nodes and nodes within the glandular structure itself. Adjacent infections or tumors in the drainage areas of these nodes frequently cause swellings that only appear to be primary in the glands. Typical of such infections are those of the eye that produce enlargement of the parotid nodes or those of the teeth that cause enlargement of the submandibular nodes. Tumors of the facial skin such as melanoma, of the oral cavity, and of the facial structures may all produce enlargements of the lymph nodes of the head and neck. Metastasis from more distant parts is relatively rare, although involvement of these nodes by malignant lymphomas is common.

Bimanual appraisal of these lesions is a necessity, and much information can be transmitted to the examining finger. Manual examination is correctly done by placing one finger into the mouth and the opposite hand over the lesion. Careful manipulation with both hands is calculated to estimate the following circumstances.

Location of the lesion. Ductal lesions are best palpated from within the mouth when the lesion is in the submandibular duct or in the anterior third of the parotid duct. Lesions in the hilus of the submandibular gland just superior to where it passes beneath the mylohyoid muscle are also best palpated from within the mouth. Most salivary stones fall into this category.

Lesions lateral to the musculature of the mouth can be displaced laterally by the intraoral finger and can be more readily felt by the extraoral hand. Portions of the gland itself can be displaced and its texture more readily felt. Nodes and swellings can be fixed and identified. Lesions not palpable or movable from within the mouth are then better related as to the relative position they bear.

Milking the gland and duct bimanually offers an estimate of the nature of the secretion and hence of the location of the lesion. Extraductal lesions seldom produce pus within the duct system unless they are so far advanced as to occlude the ducts by pressure.

Consistency of the lesion. Circumscribed lesions such as mixed tumors, enlarged inflammatory nodes, and schwannomas are readily movable. The inference from this phenomenon is that the lesion has not invaded surrounding tissues and is not surrounded by diffuse inflammatory exudate. Acutely inflamed areas, abscesses, invasive malignant tumors, or their lymphatic spread are not readily movable, a result of the infiltration of the surrounding tissues by the disease. An exception is the lymph node involved in early metastasis that has not yet lost its capsular integrity.

Indurated lesions bear a graver prognosis. Although the primary differential sign between a malignant lesion and an indurated inflammatory lesion is the presence or absence of pain, this sign is not always dependable, since overlying infection may be involved in any advanced malignant growth. In general, however, induration and boardlike hardness of the area in question is a grave sign, particularly if the cardinal signs of infection are absent or not in proportion to the extent and history of the change. Induration is typical of invasive malignant lesions, and this sign must be considered diagnostic until proved otherwise.

Consistency of the remainder of the gland is essential. Malignant lesions rarely involve the entire gland unless they are infected or far advanced. Thus a portion of the gland should feel normal to the examining hand. Infections, conversely, usually produce tenseness throughout the entire gland, as does ductal obstruction.

Separation of the gland from lesions not actually involving the gland is also an important sign. In many cases, swellings may seem to involve the gland, but palpation and fixation by finger pressure of either the gland or the lesion demonstrate that the lesion bears only an anatomical rather than a histological relation to the gland. This characteristic is particularly true of branchial cleft cysts, dermoid cysts, nodes, and inflammatory swelling primary in the teeth. In these cases the consistency of the uninvolved gland will be normal.

Many conditions have a typical consistency. Abscesses are usually fluctuant; dermoids and other thick-walled cysts are usually doughy; stones are dense and may be stellate; and infected or obstructed glands are usually firm and tense. It becomes obvious that the consistency of the lesion is an important differential sign.

Subjective response. The subjective response of the patient to the bimanual examination frequently varies in accordance with the nature of the disease. Inflammatory conditions are usually accompanied by pain. This pain is increased with manipulation and is reliable. At the risk of repetition, it should be remembered that tumors that have become infected or have invaded sensory nerve–bearing structures may also be painful, but that pain is usually a late rather than an early sign of malignancy.

Benign tumors, low-grade malignant tumors, and early malignant tumors are seldom painful. Manipulation may be carried out without complaint from the patient until it has continued long enough to become nettlesome.

The tissues overlying a salivary stone, on the other hand, are almost always tender because of the incompressibility of the stone, the sharp processes sometimes present, and the inflammation occurring in the ducts surrounding it.

Radiographic evaluation

Ordinary radiographs are of little value except in the presence of a calcified stone or advanced invasion of nearby bony structures. For this reason routine radiography may be omitted unless the examiner has reason to suspect one of these conditions. When a salivary stone is suspected, the mandibular occlusal and the lateral oblique jaw views are of the most value in locating submandibular stones (Fig. 25-6). The posteroanterior and lateral views of the face, coupled with an occlusal film placed in the buccal parietes and shot with a very short (½ to ¾ second) exposure, may be of value in locating parotid stones. A submentovertex view outlining the zygomatic arch may also be useful.

The sialogram offers more diagnostic information. This special study is carried out by instilling radiopaque oil into the duct system of the gland and taking such views as are indicated. Many techniques and forms of equipment to accomplish this study have been described. One that I have found successful is illustrated (Fig. 25-7).

Materials. The following materials are required:

1. Several sizes of polyethylene tubing about 18 inches in length, one end of

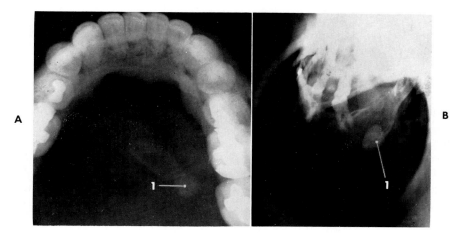

Fig. 25-6. A, Submandibular stone (sialolith, *1*) in the posterior portion of the duct demonstrated in the occlusal view. **B,** Submandibular sialolith *(1)* in the gland pelvis demonstrated by a lateral oblique jaw radiograph.

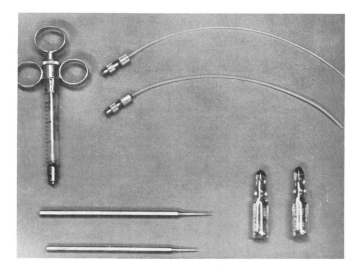

Fig. 25-7. Setup for sialography.

which has been sharply and smoothly beveled
2. A Luer-Lok connector of the type employed in continuous spinal anesthesia
3. A ring-handle 3 ml Luer-Lok syringe
4. A broken explorer, the end of which has been rounded and polished, to be used as a dilator
5. Any radiopaque oil contrast medium

Method. A length of polyethylene tubing of suitable caliber is selected and fitted into the connector. The syringe is filled with contrast medium and attached to the connector. All air is removed from the system. Extra oil will serve as a lubricant.

The syringe is detached, and the duct in question is cannulated. If pain is encountered, a few drops of local anesthetic around the caruncle may be used. If cannulation proves difficult, the explorer may be introduced to dilate the duct opening. Factors leading to difficulties in cannulation are as follows:

1. Too large caliber tubing
2. Rough bevel on tubing
3. Short or blunt bevel on tubing
4. Lack of lubrication on tubing

The tubing is inserted well into the duct. In the parotid duct an anatomical block is usually encountered where the duct turns posteriorly around the anterior border of the masseter muscle. In the submandibular duct a distance of 3 to 4 cm is usually sufficient.

The patient is then asked to close his mouth, and the tubing may be held in place through any convenient embrasure without being crushed. The syringe is reconnected, and the patient is instructed to hold it against his chest. In this way, the patient may be moved and positioned at the convenience of the radiologist. When the radiologist has positioned the patient satisfactorily, injection of the contrast medium is started. The patient is instructed to raise his hand when pressure is felt and again when definite pain is felt. Amounts of solution used are subject to individual variation, and symptomatic filling is usually more reliable than predetermined amounts.

Pressure is maintained for 10 seconds after pain is elicited, and then the sialogram is taken. Light pressure is maintained during repositioning for additional views. Postero-anterior and lateral skull views may be taken at the discretion of the operator.

After all views are taken, the tubing may be removed, and the patient is instructed to assist in emptying the gland by massage. Residual oil in the gland and duct system is not harmful and may be beneficial in some low-grade inflammatory conditions.

A great deal may be learned from the sialogram, especially if the information is accurately integrated with the clinical findings. Not all lesions have typical sialographic findings, however, and in many cases the final diagnosis depends on formal biopsy techniques. Fortunately, most inflammatory conditions display fairly typical findings when these are coupled with the clinical course, whereas tumors are frequently characterized by the singular ab-

Text continued on p. 657.

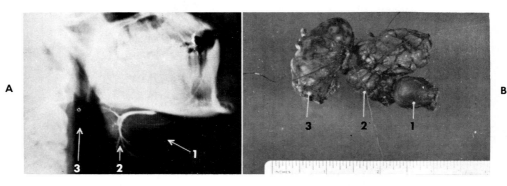

Fig. 25-8. This patient had a marked swelling of the submandibular region. There were no laboratory findings or other physical findings of note. **A,** Preoperative sialogram demonstrated marked displacement of the gland architecture *(1)* by some tumefaction. The gland was otherwise normal. Major swelling *(2)* posterior to this area is not noted in the sialogram. The lesion *(3)* proved to be marked lymphoid hyperplasia when investigated surgically. **B,** Surgical specimen of the submandibular gland and two associated lymph nodes. The preglandular node *(1)* is the same as *1* in **A.** The salivary gland *(2)* is slightly deformed anteriorly by the hypertrophy of the preglandular node. The retroglandular node *(3)*, since it was not tightly confined, did not distort the gland.

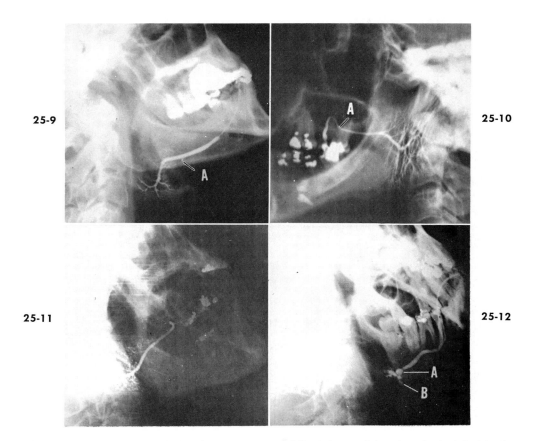

Fig. 25-9. Normal submandibular gland. In the normal film it is noted that the principal duct is of greater caliber than any of the smaller collecting ducts. The presence of ancillary connections *(A)* with small glands in the sublingual area is not unusual. The collecting ducts are noted to be of comparatively small size, and the terminal acini fill without dilation. A follow-up film in 20 minutes reveals little, if any, residual oil in the gland if proper secretory function is present.

Fig. 25-10. Normal parotid gland. The course of the excretory duct around the anterior edge of the masseter muscle is well demonstrated *(A)*. The parotid duct is usually somewhat smaller in caliber than the submandibular duct, and its volume may not appear to be equal to the total volume of the collecting ducts. The acinar structure looks much like a leafless tree, and the collecting ducts are fine. (Accessory gland tissue frequently present in the buccal fat pad is not demonstrated in this figure but can be readily demonstrated in Fig. 25-19.)

Fig. 25-11. Sialadenitis. This sialogram demonstrates the typical "leafy tree" appearance in which the terminal acini of the parotid gland are dilated. This is the early manifestation of inflammation as seen in the sialogram and is usually reversible under proper therapy.

Fig. 25-12. Sialolith. This sialogram demonstrates a small submandibular salivary stone *(A)* at the hilus of the gland effectively blocking the glandular secretions and producing a "link sausage" dilation *(B)* of the collecting ducts behind the stone.

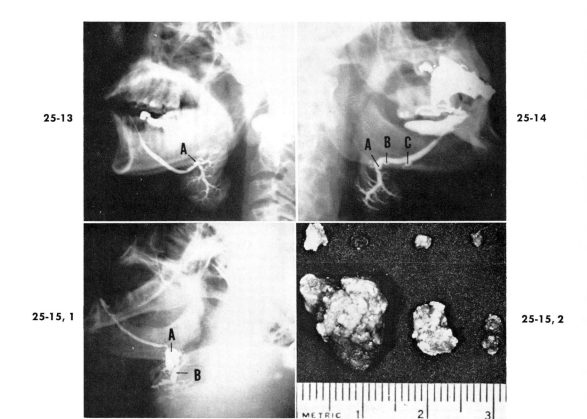

25-13

25-14

25-15, 1

25-15, 2

Fig. 25-13. Sialolithiasis of submandibular gland. The dilated space *(A)* at the hilus of the gland represents a small, poorly calcified stone that impairs but does not prevent excretion. There is slight dilation of the duct system behind the obstruction. Transoral sialolithotomy is the treatment of choice in such cases. Access to stones this far distal is frequently technically difficult.
Fig. 25-14. Sialolithiasis, multiple, of submandibular gland and duct. This patient had several stones in the duct and gland and had undergone repeated probings and surgical procedures for their removal. Dilation *A* at the hilus of the gland represents the principal salivary stone. Dilations *B* and *C* of the ancillary sublingual ducts are typical of obstruction further forward and represent residual defects resulting from previous stones. Considerable sialoangiectasis is noted in the collecting ducts. This gland continued to be suppurative and symptomatic following the removal of the principal stone and eventually had to be extirpated.
Fig. 25-15. 1, Sialolithiasis; an example of an extremely large submandibular salivary stone *(A)* occupying the hilus of the gland; marked dilation of the ducts *(B)* noted behind the obstruction. This patient was successfully treated by transoral sialolithotomy. **2,** Some of the larger stones removed from the gland shown in **1.** Note the marked stellate formation of these calcified foreign bodies. Such a rough configuration prohibits the movement of stones within the duct.

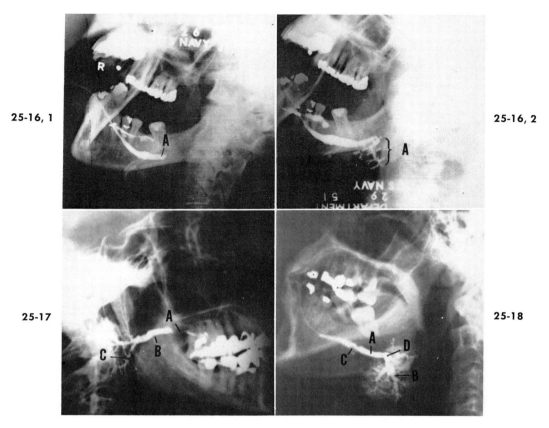

25-16, 1

25-16, 2

25-17

25-18

Fig. 25-16. 1, Sialolith. This patient had symptoms of submandibular gland obstruction. The sialogram failed to disclose the gland because of the inability to force the contrast medium past the obstruction *(A).* Seven salivary stones were removed transorally. **2,** Postoperative sialogram of case illustrated in **1.** Note the vastly dilated duct, as well as the clubbing and dilation of the collecting ducts *(A).* In spite of the extreme damage to this gland, it was not necessary to remove it.

Fig. 25-17. Obstructive parotitis with sialolith and sialoangiectasis. The interruption *(A)* in the main excretory duct, just behind the second molar, represents a poorly calcified sialolith that totally occupies the lumen of the duct. Extreme dilation of the duct *(B)* is noted behind the defect. The interruptions *(C)* in the collecting ducts represent inspissated salivary fluid, which, it is believed, may well form the nidus for additional stones. This obstruction was accessible to the surgical procedure described later.

Fig. 25-18. Sialoangiectasis resulting from sialolith and stricture. Large dilation of the excretory duct *(A)* is noted, with concomitant dilation of the collecting ducts *(B).* The nonfilling defect *(C)* in the midportion of the excretory duct represents a stricture, whereas the large dilation *(D)* in the hilus of the gland represents a smooth sialolith. This stone could be moved by bimanual manipulation from its posterior position forward to the stricture. It was removed transorally from the anterior position after first being fixed by means of a suture passed posterior to it. The patient has remained asymptomatic, in spite of the fact that there appears to be greater structural change in this gland than in the gland shown in Fig. 25-14. Such differences in individual response are difficult to explain, and a decision to remove a gland must be based on the presence of symptoms.

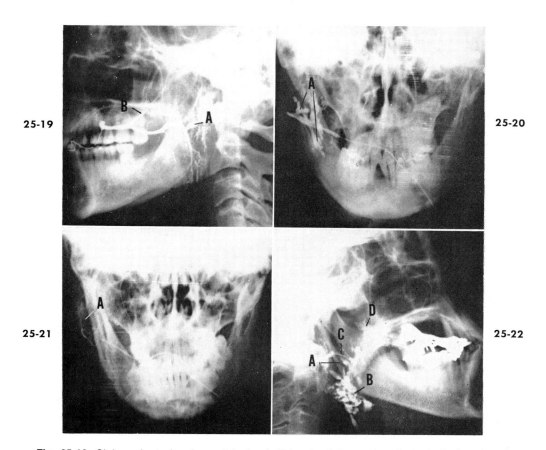

Fig. 25-19. Sialoangiectasis of parotid gland. This glandular pattern is typical of a chronic sialadenitis with areas of sialoangiectasis in the duct system. The rather large filling defect *(A)* represents destruction of the gland parenchyma by abscess formation. These areas of destruction may be much larger or smaller, depending on the severity of the disease. Dilation and clubbing of the terminal acini gives the collecting ducts the overall appearance of coarseness typical of salivary stasis. An incidental finding in this sialogram is the presence of the accessory gland structure *(B)* in the buccal fat pad. This is a fairly common anatomical variation and is in no way abnormal.

Fig. 25-20. Sialoangiectasis with chronic sialadenitis. Marked destruction caused by abscess formation *(A)* is noted in this parotid gland. This was a chronic, recurrent condition that eventually required removal of the gland. The condition was bilateral and followed a severe bout of pneumonia with dehydration and a high febrile course.

Fig. 25-21. Retention cyst of parotid gland. The small nonfilling defect *(A)* in the parenchyma of the parotid gland has displaced the normal architecture. At operation this defect proved to be a retention cyst filled with salivary fluid.

Fig. 25-22. Developmental cyst of parotid gland. This patient had a soft mass in the parotid gland that varied in size and was tender when it became enlarged. A large nonfilling defect *(A)* has pushed aside a part of the gland parenchyma. The remainder of the gland, particularly the inferior pole *(B)*, is greatly dilated, suggesting that the mass obstructs the drainage ducts and prevents excretion. The superior pole is more nearly normal in appearance, and the duct course can be seen passing around the superior pole of the cyst *(C)*. Accessory glands *(D)* are noted along the entire course of the duct. On removal this lesion was noted to have all the histopathological characteristics of a branchial cleft cyst. The sialoangiectasis was incident to the blocking action caused by the enlargement of this cyst. Retrograde infection followed the blocking.

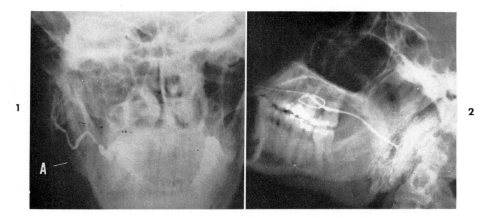

Fig. 25-23. 1, Mixed tumor, parotid gland. The parotid gland in this case is normal insofar as the sialogram is concerned. The stricture seen in the anterior third of the duct is technical rather than anatomical. The only noticeable feature is that the gland appears to be separated from the angle of the mandible *(A)* by some nonfilling mass that has displaced the superficial lobe of the gland. The inference from such a picture is that of extraductal involvement, which may result from a swollen lymph node, a developmental cyst, a mixed tumor, or any other tumefaction that tends to displace parotid structures. **2,** This lateral view of the patient shown in **1** offers no clue to the presence or identity of the lesion, which in this case was a mixed tumor of the parotid gland, but could have been any one of several extrinsic tumefactions. Sialography in such cases does not offer diagnostic evidence, as it may in conditions that invade the gland or duct system, but there is always some clinical manifestation that can be seen or palpated. Sialograms may or may not tend to support clinical impressions, yet the absence of sialographic findings is of value in determining that the disease is extraductal or extraglandular in nature.

sence of sialographic evidence. An example of misinterpretation of equivocal findings is seen in Fig. 25-8.

Sialographic interpretation is best studied by integrating sialographic findings with clinical and historical findings and a knowledge of the basic anatomy and pathoses of the region. For this purpose a group of typical cases is presented in which the sialographic findings and the clinical and historical findings were sufficiently clear to reach an accurate diagnosis (Figs. 25-9 to 25-25).

Laboratory procedures

Several laboratory procedures are useful in the differential diagnosis of salivary gland lesions. Mumps, infectious mononucleosis, and acute sialadenitis, which tend to resemble one another in the early stages, may be differentiated by an examination of the blood and blood serum. Infectious mononucleosis usually displays a high percentage of atypical lymphocytes as well as an increased overall lymphocyte count in the blood examination. Sialadenitis, if acute, may show an increase in the number of immature polymorphonuclear leukocytes in the blood examination. A heterophil agglutination test of the blood serum is of benefit in distinguishing infectious mononucleosis.

Most laboratories regard cytological smears as undependable in the differentiation of extraductal salivary gland lesions. Aspiration or needle biopsies are difficult to read because of the small amounts of tissue they offer. Frozen sections and formal biopsies, however, are highly dependable and complete the generally used clinical laboratory examinations.

A complete blood count and a differential blood count may offer some clue as to the

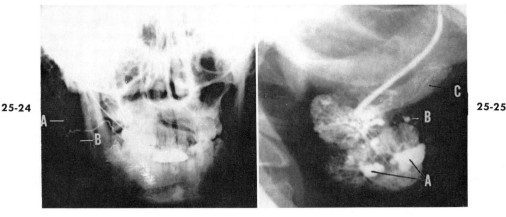

Fig. 25-24. Mixed tumor of parotid gland. This sialogram shows the typical ball-in-hand deformity *(A)*. There is considerable displacement of the superficial lobe of the parotid gland, causing it to stand away *(B)* from the body of the mandible and curve around the tumor mass.
Fig. 25-25. Squamous cell carcinoma, primary in the submandibular gland, which is obviously involved with neoplastic disease, has invaded the gland parenchyma. The duct is normal, but the gland substance displays an unusual network pattern suggesting complete arborization of the gland parenchyma. The numerous spaces filled with radiopaque fluid *(A)* are typical of necrotic areas destroyed by tumor. In one area the gland capsule has ruptured sufficiently to permit radiopaque fluid *(B)* to enter the surrounding space. Of interest is the large sublingual extension of glandular tissue *(C)* (which represents hypertrophic extension) that was also invaded by the tumor, as were the mandible and the contiguous lymph nodes of the neck. It is impossible to predict the cell type in such tumors, but this sialographic picture, coupled with the clinical findings of a firm, indurated, nonpainful submandibular mass of several years' duration, makes the diagnosis of malignant lesion of the submandibular gland reasonably obvious. Before biopsy it was thought that this might well be either an adenocarcinoma or a mucoepidermoid carcinoma, either of which might well display this clinical and sialographic picture. Accurate diagnosis can be established only by formal biopsy.

relative toxicity of the disease, but they are in no way specific, since they demonstrate only the blood's response to an infectious process.

Cytological examination may be carried out if malignant involvement of the duct system is suspected. It is to be remembered, however, that simple saliva from the mouth is not a useful sample, and material for this examination should be obtained from the duct of the suspected gland by cannulation. The applications of this examination are limited, and, if results are negative, they are by no means conclusive.

Smears, cultures, and antibiotic sensitivity tests are valuable when the type of organism and the specific antibiotic to be employed are at issue. Again, the sample must

be taken from the cannulated duct to avoid oral contamination.

SURGICAL PROCEDURES

With the possible exception of the surgical management of retention cysts such as mucoceles and ranulas, the transoral sialolithotomy is the most frequent operation performed on the salivary system (Fig. 25-26). It is a simple operation, frequently overlooked by medical practitioners untrained in oral surgery in favor of enucleation of the gland. If the stone is favorably located, its removal through the mouth preserves the gland and hence the function of the gland. Although sialoliths are known to recur and glands may be so badly damaged by infection as to require subsequent or

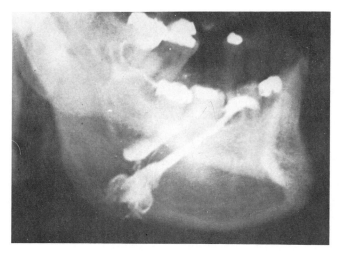

Fig. 25-26. Retained sialolith after incomplete surgery. This patient's submandibular gland was removed by a general surgeon before any effort was made to remove the stone transorally. Symptoms persisted and pus was constantly discharged from the salivary caruncle. The sialogram shows why. The patient still has the salivary stone and part of the gland that lies above the mylohyoid muscle. It is apparent that the underlying condition that produced the glandular dysfunction has not been dealt with. It is usually prudent to attempt the removal of stones transorally before condemning the gland. If it becomes necessary to remove the gland, the operator must assure himself or herself of adequate operative procedure to section the duct above the area occupied by the stone.

eventual enucleation, the more conservative course is usually indicated at the original operation because of its widespread success in the hands of most operators.

The submandibular gland can be enucleated without sequelae if the operation is properly accomplished. Before removing this gland, however, thought should be given to the results of the loss of its function, although in most patients with normal salivary secretion in the remaining glands, its removal is of no consequence.

Removal of the parotid gland is of greater consequence. Danger to the seventh cranial nerve is always present, although careful surgery permits the removal of this gland with only transient weakness in most instances.

The removal of either gland results in slight facial deformity. In the case of the submandibular gland a scar plus a depression or, more accurately, a lack of fullness in the submandibular region results. When the parotid gland is involved, a retromandibular scar plus a loss of some facial contour is experienced. These factors are not significant if the operation is necessary but contraindicate such procedures when conservative methods would suffice.

Transoral sialolithotomy of submandibular duct

Transoral sialolithotomy is best done with the patient under local anesthesia and in a sitting position.

The stone is first located accurately by radiography and palpation. If possible, and especially if the stone is small and smooth, a suture is passed through the floor of the mouth, below the duct and behind the stone, and tied to prevent the stone from sliding backward. A towel clamp is placed through the tip and, if necessary, the side of the tongue to obtain retraction and control of this member. This step is especially important in obese persons or in those who are unable to control their tongue voluntarily. In slim or especially cooperative persons the tongue can be held in a gauze sponge. How the tongue will be retracted and controlled should be determined at the time of examination, but towel clips should be included in the armamentarium in any case.

The gland is then palpated extraorally and pushed upward toward the floor of the mouth to fix the intraoral tissues under tension and make the stone easier to palpate.

When the incision is made, consideration is given to two structures, the lingual nerve and the sublingual gland. Posteriorly the lingual nerve is superior and lateral to the duct, crossing beneath it at the posterior end of the mylohyoid ridge and passing medially and deep. Thus, if the stone is posterior, the incision is shallow and blunt dissection is employed immediately to prevent injury to the lingual nerve. If the stone is more anterior, the incision must be made medial to the plica sublingualis (Fig. 25-27), or the operator will find the sublingual gland

between his instrument and the stone, and a portion of the gland will be transected. Thus the incision for an anterior stone is designed to be over the stone and medial to the plica.

As soon as the operator progresses through the mucosa, blunt dissection is used. Both the incision and the opening obtained by spreading the tissues should be large enough to permit the entrance of the examining finger, since reorientation is frequently necessary. Dissection is continued bluntly through the loose tissues of the space until the duct is encountered. If the lingual nerve is encountered in the incision, it must be retracted gently but never cut. Bleeding is seldom a problem, but, if it occurs, it should be controlled by ligation before proceeding.

The duct is best identified at the point where the stone is lodged. If difficulty arises at this stage, a probe may be passed into the duct to aid in its location. When the duct is located, a longitudinal slit is made directly over the stone. The duct should not be cut

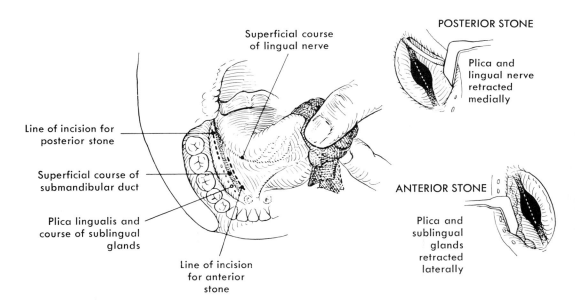

Fig. 25-27. Intraoral landmarks and lines of incision for transoral sialolithotomy of the submandibular duct.

transversely because retraction may complete the division and a fistula may result. The opening should reveal the stone and should be of sufficient length to permit its removal. The stone can usually be carefully removed with small forceps, but large stellate stones may have to be broken by crushing them with a forceps. After the stone is removed, a small aspirating cannula may be passed toward the gland to remove any pus, mucous plugs, or satellite stones that remain. A probe is then passed from the caruncle to the surgical opening to ensure patency of the anterior end of the duct.

No effort is made to close the duct proper. The wound edges are sutured at the level of the mucosa only, and recanalization occurs without further intervention.

Transoral sialolithotomy of parotid duct

The approach to calcifications in the parotid duct may be more difficult than to similar lesions in the submandibular duct. The reason for this is the anatomical peculiarity of the parotid duct. After following a short, superficial course from its caruncle, the parotid duct turns laterally and rounds the anterior border of the masseter muscle, proceeding posteriorly to join the gland. A direct cut-down on stones in this duct therefore is possible only when the stone is anterior to the anterior border of the masseter muscle. Since most parotid duct stones lodge at or posterior to this point, a direct cut-down is seldom effective. Splitting the duct to follow the channel posteriorly frequently so damages the duct and caruncle that strictures are produced, which lead to new stasis and stone formation.

The suggested procedure therefore involves making a semilunar incision running from above downward in front of the caruncle (Fig. 25-28, *A* and *B*). The caruncle, mucosal flap, and duct are then retracted medially, the cheek is retracted laterally, and free access is gained to the more posterior segments of the duct by simply following the duct with blunt dissection. This

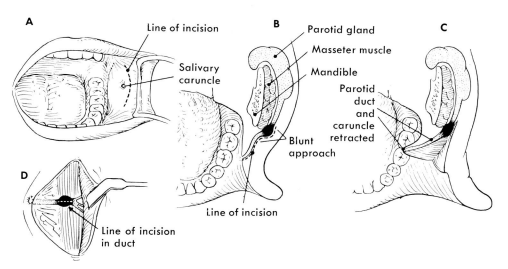

Fig. 25-28. A, Intraoral view of line of incision for transoral sialolithotomy of the parotid duct. **B,** Sectional view of line of incision and blunt approach for transoral sialolithotomy of the parotid duct. **C,** Retraction for removal of parotid duct stone, sectional view. **D,** Retraction and duct incision for removal of parotid duct stone, intraoral view.

procedure also permits the duct to be retracted anteriorly so that the stone can be delivered into the wound. When the stone becomes accessible, a longitudinal incision is made in the lateral side of the duct, and the stone is delivered (Fig. 25-28, *C* and *D*). The duct need not be sutured, since simply closing the mucosal flap with deep mattress sutures will serve to produce recanalization of the duct.

Removal of submandibular gland

Occasionally, because of previous damage from stasis and chronic infection, removal of the submandibular gland is necessary. Usually this is not done until conservative means have been exhausted.

The extraoral incision parallels the course of the digastric muscle. To deter-

mine this course, the surgeon palpates the mastoid eminence, the lateral surface of the hyoid bone, and the genial tubercle. A curving line connecting these three landmarks represents the course of the anterior and posterior bellies of the digastric muscle. A 5-cm incision is made along this curving line (Fig. 25-29) directly over the inferior pole of the gland, and the platysma muscle is sectioned.

The first structure encountered is the facial vein, which is ligated and cut. At the level of the deep fascia the cervical ramus of the seventh cranial nerve is encountered where it communicates with superficial cervical nerves from the cervical plexus. This ramus can usually be retracted posteriorly by passing a hernia tape around it, although cutting it represents no serious

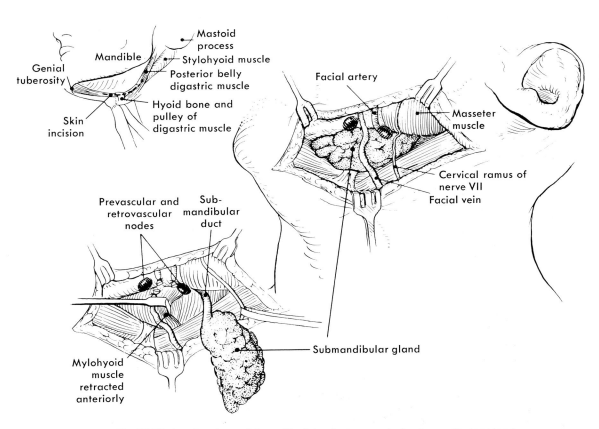

Fig. 25-29. Landmarks and line of incision for removal of submandibular gland.

loss, since it provides only partial innervation to the platysma muscle on one side only.

Beneath the fascia lies the submandibular niche. Blunt dissection between the pulley of the digastric muscle and the gland will free the anterior and inferior portions of the gland. The dissection is continued around the posteroinferior pole, leaving the superior and medial portions of the gland attached.

Vital structures to be considered at this point are the facial artery, the lingual nerve, and the submandibular duct. The facial artery curves up and over the superior aspect of the gland and emerges on the lateral side of the mandible at the anterior border of the masseter muscle. This artery can usually be located by the presence of the prevascular and retrovascular lymph nodes that lie on either side of the vessel. In most instances it is wise to identify and double ligate the facial artery below the gland and to separate it before proceeding with the dissection because its connections with the gland are usually short and difficult to tie and the vessel is frequently buried within the gland.

The gland may then be retracted posteriorly and detached from its ganglionic connections with the submandibular ganglion. The lingual nerve can be identified at this point, but the ganglion is seldom seen at surgery.

As the dissection proceeds bluntly, the submandibular duct may be noted passing superiorly and anteriorly over the roof of the submandibular niche, which is formed by the mylohyoid muscle. This muscle should be retracted anteriorly, the duct retracted posteriorly, and a ligature placed anterior to the ductal pathosis if such exists. A second ligature is placed posterior to the first but still anterior to the ductal pathosis, and the duct is sectioned between the ligatures. This procedure prevents seepage of infected material into the wound from either the residual duct or the gland. The gland may then be removed and consideration given to the closing of the wound.

Dead space resulting from removal of the gland must be closed or drained. Closure can usually be accomplished by approximating the fasciae of the digastric, stylohyoid, hyoglossus, and mylohyoid muscles with absorbable catgut sutures. If this cannot be done and a dead space remains, or if it is believed that the crypt has become contaminated or is infected, a Penrose drain should be inserted into this area. A second layer of absorbable sutures should be used to close the deep fascia and platysma muscle. A third layer of subcutaneous or subcuticular absorbable sutures is used to close the skin, and the skin edges are then carefully approximated with interrupted silk sutures, size No. 4-0 or smaller.

The wound should always be covered with a pressure dressing. The drain, if one is placed, should emerge from the wound at the most dependent point, which is usually at the posterior aspect of the wound. This drain may be removed after 24 to 48 hours if no suppuration is present. After 4 days the pressure dressing may be discontinued and half of the sutures may be removed. The incision should be bridged with adhesive butterflies or with a firm collodion dressing. The remaining sutures may be removed on the fifth to seventh day, but the wound should continue to have bridging support for at least 2 weeks.

Removal of parotid gland

In general, removal of the parotid gland is not considered to be within the purview of the oral surgeon. By virtue of special training or because of local circumstances, however, the oral surgeon may include this operation in his or her repertoire. In any case the surgeon should have some knowledge of the problems involved in order to make decisions regarding treatment.

Because of certain inherent risks of permanent damage to the seventh cranial nerve, this operation is not usually done without strong indications. The presence of a tumor or suspected tumor or of chronic inflammatory disease resistant to conservative treatment is the primary reason for such an undertaking. Most surgeons make every attempt to conserve the seventh cranial nerve by careful dissection or partial removal of the gland. A malignant lesion, however, suffers no compromise, and when attacked surgically, it must be extirpated without regard for the possible resultant deformity.

The incision runs from the superior attachment of the pinna downward, turns anteriorly at the angle of the mandible, and stops at the hyoid bone. A second incision, which may be made posterior to the pinna, joins the first at the inferior margin of the pinna (Fig. 25-30). The ear is retracted from the operative field, and the skin flap is developed on the cheek side of the incision.

The facial nerve may be located in either of two ways: (1) by finding the peripheral portion where it emerges from the anterior edge of the gland and then dissecting backward or (2) by dissecting directly down the posterior aspect of the gland and identifying the main trunk between its entrance into the gland substance and the stylomastoid foramen (Fig. 25-1, *A*). An electric stimulator is of great assistance in this maneuver. After the nerve has been identified, the course of the trunks is followed and the superficial

lobe is freed from its attachments. The duct is ligated and cut. Some of the smaller connections between the main trunks may be destroyed in this process, with resultant postoperative facial weakness. Preservation of the main branches of the nerve, however, ensures eventual return to full function.

After the superficial lobe of the gland has been freed and the main branches of the facial nerve have been identified, the deep lobe may be approached. This lobe wraps around the posterior border of the mandible, and dissection in this confined space is facilitated by posterosuperior retraction of the ear. Care should be taken to protect the external carotid artery and the retromandibular vein during this operation. Ligation of these vessels may be prudent because either or both of them may be embedded in the gland substance in a part of their course and because hemorrhage from the rather large maxillary branch of the external carotid artery may be difficult to control as a result of its relative inaccessibility.

The parotid capsule is tough along its posterior attachment, particularly where the gland encounters the sternocleidomastoid muscle and the acoustic meatus. Care must be exercised, while the pinna is retracted, not to incise the acoustic meatus during separation of the gland.

Most dead space may be closed by careful suturing after removal of the gland. A drain may be indicated in the wound, especially if a portion of the gland is removed and salivary accumulation is expected.

CONCLUSION

An essential part of the mission of oral surgery is the diagnosis and treatment of certain diseases of the salivary glands. Careful diagnosis is the key to success and usually indicates the method of treatment. The ability to distinguish those diseases and conditions the treatment of which is a part of oral surgical training and those the treatment of which is within the province of one of the medical specialties is of paramount

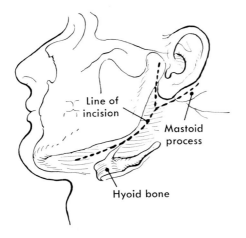

Fig. 25-30. Landmarks and line of incision for removal of parotid gland.

importance. A knowledge of the anatomy of the salivary glands, an adequate examination, a thorough history, and diagnostic radiographs are a necessity. Clinical laboratory procedures may be of some assistance. Formal biopsy is the only sure method of establishing a firm diagnosis when a malignant condition cannot otherwise be ruled out.

REFERENCES

1. Abaza, N. A., El-Khashab, M. M., and Fahim, M. S.: Adenoid cystic carcinoma (cylindroma) of the palate, Oral Surg. **22:**429, 1966.
2. Alaniz, F., and Fletcher, G. H.: Place and technics of radiation therapy in the management of malignant tumors of the major salivary glands, Radiology **84:**412, 1965.
3. Blatt, I. M.: Systemic diseases and their relation to the major salivary glands, Trans. Am. Acad. Ophthalmol. Otolaryngol. **69:**1115, 1965.
4. De la Pava, S., Karjoo, R., Mukhtar, F., and Pickren, J. W.: Multifocal carcinoma of accessory salivary gland; a case report, Cancer **19:**1308, 1966.
5. Eisenbud, L., and Cranin, N.: The role of sialography in the diagnosis and therapy of chronic obstructive sialadenitis, Oral Surg. **16:**1181, 1963.
6. Frank, R. M., Herdly, J., and Philippe, E.: Acquired dental defects and salivary gland lesions after irradiation for carcinoma, J. Am. Dent. Assoc. **70:**868, 1965.
7. Frazell, E. L., Strong, E. W., and Newcombe, B.: Tumors of the parotid, Am. J. Nurs. **66:**2702, 1966.
8. Garusi, G. F.: The salivary glands in radiological diagnosis, Bibl. Radiol. **4:**1, 1964.
9. Huebsch, R. F.: Acute lesions of the oral cavity, Dent. Clin. North Am., p. 577, Nov., 1965.
10. Kashima, H. K., Kirkham, W. R., and Andrews, J. R.: Postirradiation sialadenitis; a study of the clinical features, histopathologic changes and serum enzyme variations following irradiation of human salivary glands, Am. J. Roentgenol. Radium Ther. Nucl. Med. **94:**271, 1965.
11. Morel, A. S., and Firestein, A.: Repair of traumatic fistulas of the parotid duct, Arch. Surg. **87:**623, 1963.
12. Moskow, R., Moskow, B. S., and Robinson, H. L.: Minor salivary gland sialolithiasis, report of a case, Oral Surg. **17:**225, 1964.
13. Prowler, J. R., Bjork, H., and Armstrong, G. F.: Major gland sialectasis, J. Oral Surg. **23:**421, 1965.
14. Rosenfeld, L., Sessions, D. E., McSwain, B., and Graves, H., Jr.: Malignant tumors of salivary gland origin; 37 year review of 184 cases, Ann. Surg. **163:**726, 1966.
15. Ross, D. E., and Castro, E. C.: Recurrent inflammatory swellings of the salivary glands: emphasis of sialangiectasis, Am. Surg. **30:**434, 1964.
16. Simons, J. N., Beahrs, O. H., and Wollner, L. B.: Tumors of the submaxillary gland, Am. J. Surg. **108:**485, 1964.
17. Wallenborn, W. M., Sydnor, T. A., Hsu, Y. T., and Fitz-Hugh, G. S.: Experimental production of parotid gland atrophy by ligation of Stensen's duct and by irradiation, Laryngoscope **74:**644, 1964.
18. Waterhouse, J.: Inflammation of the salivary glands, Br. J. Oral Surg. **3:**161, 1966.
19. White, N. S.: Sjögren's syndrome, J. Oral Surg. **22:**163, 1966.

CHAPTER 26

Neurological disorders of the maxillofacial region*

John M. Gregg

The neurological apparatus of the maxillofacial region is unique in many respects. It has special anatomical characteristics such as the highest sensory innervation density in the body[71] and a peripheral intermingling of major cranial nerve branches whose central connections do not follow the orderly segmentation typical of spinal cord innervation. Developmentally, oral tissues are the first to respond reflexly to in utero tactile stimulation.[58] These tissues simultaneously perform the vital processes of feeding, sensory perception, respiratory activity, and external communication by means of facial expression and speech. In spite of their importance to the organism, maxillofacial nerves course tortuously through bony crevices and canals and run dangerously close to cutaneous and mucosal surfaces where they are vulnerable to various injuries. The terminal branches must coexist with local tissues that have an extremely high pathological incidence: the paranasal sinuses, the teeth, and the peri-odontium. Therefore, it is not surprising that the maxillofacial neurological apparatus is a prime target for characteristic pathology that is frequently different from neuropathology in other body regions.

There are maxillofacial neurological disorders of somatic sensation and visceral and motor activity. Many are responses to acute lesions in adjacent tissues, such as partial seventh nerve paralysis that results from advancing parotid gland carcinoma. Others are part of systemic disease states such as diabetic trigeminal neuropathy. The pathological condition may be primary to the nerve tissues, as in trigeminal neuralgia caused by multiple sclerosis. Finally, when there is chronic facial pain, the symptoms themselves may take on the dimensions of a disease process, since neurological disorders in the facial region carry an especially high emotional impact for many individuals.

The diagnosis of maxillofacial neurological problems depends on an orderly process of (1) interpreting the symptoms and signs of altered neurophysiology, (2) determining the anatomical localization of the disease process, (3) understanding the basic pathological processes that exist, and (4)

*This investigation was supported by NIH Research Grant No. DE 02668 from the National Institute of Dental Research and by NIH Grant No. RR 05333 from the Division of Research Facilities and Resources.

when possible, identifying the etiological or precipitating factors. Treatment of these problems is a challenge to practitioners from many disciplines, and effective action may depend on a team approach. However, the dentally educated clinician is in a position to make a strong contribution in this field because of his extensive knowledge of maxillofacial symptomatology, anatomy, physiology, and pathology.

PSYCHOPHYSIOLOGY

Terminology. The clinical effects of altered nerve physiology are identified by certain useful terms. *Paralysis* means loss of or impairment of motor function in a body part, and *paresis* is incomplete paralysis. Although these terms are usually reserved to describe neuromuscular deficits, they may also be applied to malfunction in autonomic nerves. *Anesthesia* refers to the loss of any and all sensation and should be distinguished from the loss of specific sensations, such as *ageusia,* the loss of taste, and *analgesia,* the loss of sensitivity to painful stimuli. *Hyperesthesia* means excessive sensitivity, and *hypoesthesia,* also called *hypesthesia,* refers to diminished sensitivity, usually to touch. *Hyperalgesia* is an excessive sensitivity to painful stimuli, and *hypoalgesia* implies lowered pain sensitivity.

In cases of altered sensitivity, the concept of thresholds is introduced, and two clinically useful pain thresholds have been described: pain detection and pain tolerance thresholds. The *pain detection threshold,* which is the lowest level at which a given stimulus is considered painful, is known to be remarkably similar for most humans and is influenced little by minor environmental factors. The detection threshold is altered in rarely occurring cases of congenital insensitivity to pain and in neuropathological conditions such as hyperalgesia resulting from incomplete nerve regeneration. The *pain tolerance threshold* is the level of maximally tolerated stimulus and is highly variable between individuals

as well as for a given person tested at different times. Tolerance is greatly influenced by cultural, psychological, and environmental factors, and it is this pain threshold that is often changed therapeutically by pharmacological and hypnotic techniques.

Sensory dissociation refers to a loss of certain senses with the simultaneous maintenance of other senses. For example, sensory dissociation is seen in incomplete local anesthetic block, in which fine tactile and pinprick sensitivity is lost, although proprioception and deep pain awareness persist. The terms paresthesia and dysesthesia are both used to describe abnormalities of sensory quality and both occur spontaneously. A *paresthesia* represents any altered sensation and may be described as itching, tingling, numbness, crawling, or feelings of tissue fullness or swelling. A *dysesthesia* is a painful paresthesia and may be reported as burning, boring, or stabbing and occasionally may be a sensation of "phantom" pain such as the awareness of a previously extracted tooth or a burning tongue after glossectomy.

Components and mechanisms of pain. Pain may be defined as an unpleasant experience that involves three main components: (1) perception, (2) affect or emotion, and (3) reaction (Fig. 26-1). The first proposed component, somatic sensory perception, raises the question of whether pain is really a specific sensation like vision, touch, and taste, which have specific forms of energies in the environment, specialized receptors that may be excited by chemical mediators, and transmission along precise pathways to isolated brain centers. Clinical support for this specificity theory of pain comes from the observation that pathology and surgery at many levels of the nervous system may induce a sensory dissociation in which pain is eliminated and other primary sensations retained. Indeed, a class of nerve fibers of relatively small diameter, 1 to 5 μ, have been identified as *nociceptors,* or fibers that respond specifically to noxious stimuli, meaning stimuli that have

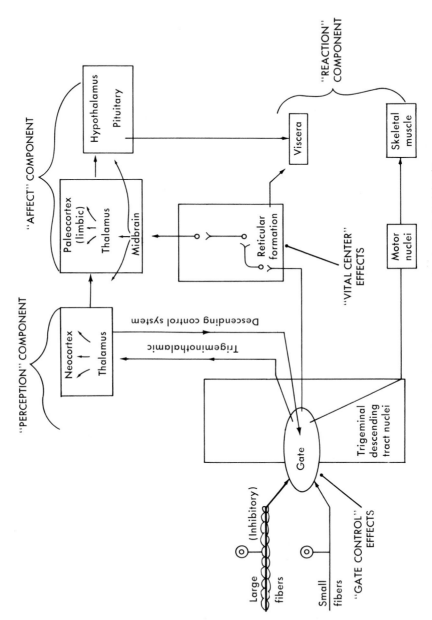

Fig. 26-1. Mechanisms and components of maxillofacial pain.

the potential to produce tissue damage.[60] It is generally agreed that the nociceptors are unmyelinated or thinly myelinated fibers of the *A delta* and *C* type that are activated by specific biogenic amines such as serotonin and prostaglandin AG.[131] Current theories stress that transmission of "pain impulses" to higher integration centers is greatly influenced by the balances and interactions between the A delta and C fiber nociceptors and the larger A alpha and beta fibers.[50,87] The net effect of large fiber activity on the transmission of nociceptive information beyond the primary brain stem trigeminal synaptic region is an inhibitory one.[27] Conversely, the smaller incoming fiber components, if unchecked by the inhibitory larger fibers, would tend to encourage the transmission of pain impulses to higher centers. This physiological phenomenon is known as "afferent inhibition" and is a basic tenet of the gate control theory of pain as described by Melzack and Wall.[87]

A key point of afferent inhibition for the maxillofacial region and the "gate" through which pain information must pass is thought to be located in the caudal portions of the brain stem trigeminal synaptic regions, specifically in the subnucleus caudalis of the descending trigeminal tract.[27,91] From this theory it follows that any process that disturbs the inhibitory balances of incoming small and large fiber populations that arrive at the subnucleus caudalis would have the effect of changing the amount and nature of pain information transmitted to higher centers. Later it will be shown that many conditions of maxillofacial neuropathology may upset the balances of incoming fiber populations. More recent extensions of the gate control pain theory have stressed that afferent inhibition at the brain stem gate also may be influenced by the activity of fibers that converge on this area from other brain regions such as the reticular formation and the cortex (see *Descending control system,* Fig. 26-1).[21,35] The descending control neurons converge on the trigeminal "gating" neurons of subnucleus caudalis from a number of higher centers in the brain stem, particularly from the reticular gray substance surrounding the aqueduct of the midbrain.[95] The midbrain periaqueductal gray (PAG) region is important because it is a well-studied part of the *opiate receptor* system, the sites of action of the opiate analgesics.[102,116] The PAG region is also of interest because it is activated not only by exogenous opiates but also by a recently discovered class of endogenous polypeptides, the endorphins, or endogenous morphinelike substances.[57] The endorphins appear to originate as products of the hypothalamus, are secreted by the anterior pituitary in response to stress and excitement, and are distributed throughout the body as well as to the opiate receptors.[46,53] One of the functions of the endorphin system, therefore, appears to be an intrinsic changing of pain threshold levels at the gating level brought about by an activating of the opiate receptor–descending neurons.

There is another very important link to the opiate receptor–descending control system. A bidirectional pathway links the midbrain PAG region with the limbic paleocortex, the seat of human emotion, arousal, and memory functions.[11,50,93] These connections provide a partial anatomical explanation for the well-known influence that emotion, personality, learned behavior, psychopathology, and culture have on pain threshold responses.[85,118]

When pain impulses pass through the "threshold" gate in the trigeminal system, they travel rapidly and directly along discrete ventral secondary ascending tracts in the brain stem to synapse in the lateral thalamus and finally distribute diffusely to many areas of the neocortex (see *Perception component,* Fig. 26-1). Neurosurgical sectioning of the trigeminothalamic tracts eliminates the perceptive and informative phase of the pain experience.[135] But, as is unfortunately demonstrated in many of these cases, the perceptive phase of pain does not constitute all the pain experience.

The second major component of pain, affect or emotion, is also inseparable from the pain experience. Perception of a noxious stimulus without feeling emotion is not recognized as pain by the individual. It is suspected that the affective phase of pain is carried in entirely different anatomical pathways and reaches brain integration regions that are far different from the perception component. Specifically, fiber projections from the nucleus of the descending tract of the trigeminal nerve enter the reticular formation at many levels of the caudal brain stem core where they activate diffuse and multisynaptic fiber groups.[119] The reticular formation in these regions also contains the vital centers for maintenance of consciousness and for control of basic cardiac and pulmonary function. These anatomical associations may explain why painful stimuli evoke profound reflex changes, both in conscious attention levels and in heart and lung function (see *Vital center effects,* Fig. 26-1). Anterior to these vital centers in the midbrain gray matter and in the medial thalamus are reticular formation nuclei that probably receive pain-related fiber projections and whose stimulation brings about an extreme aversion response.[16] These reticular centers project forward to many regions of the paleocortex in the ventral core of the brain, known collectively as the limbic lobes. The limbic cortex has long been considered an important integration center for human emotion. It is also known to exert a powerful influence over the hypothalamus to initiate endorphin release as previously described (see *Affect component,* Fig. 26-1). Therefore, by way of complex projections of the brain stem reticular formation to the limbic cortex, the hypothalamus, and the pituitary, pain information gains access to the seat of human emotion and to the central nervous system sources of both the autonomic nervous system and major endocrine glands. In this way, an emotional response becomes a direct part of the pain experience and a "visceral" reaction also spreads throughout the body. It may be these associations

that link chronic pain with widespread systemic and visceral diseases of a "psychosomatic" nature, such as gastric hyperacidity and vascular headache.

The third component of pain, reaction, therefore includes an automatic visceral phase that can often be detected clinically by observing such signs as pulse and blood pressure elevations, pupillary dilation, sweating, and changes in saliva consistency. There is also a skeletal muscle reaction phase of the pain response that is more obvious (see *Reaction component,* Fig. 26-1). Painful stimuli evoke reflex facial grimaces, turning of the head, and protective clenching of masticatory muscles. Skeletal muscle reactivity to chronic pain may also set up secondary pain foci, such as in the temporomandibular joint myofascial pain dysfunction syndrome.

• • •

In summary, the experience of pain is the most common problem in maxillofacial neuropathology and should be viewed as more than a predictable specific sensation or a warning sign of disease. Rather, pain may become a disease syndrome in itself. Pathological factors that disturb peripheral and central inhibitory-excitatory balance must be detected, and the relative strengths of perception, emotion, and reaction components must be considered for each individual. Having accomplished this, one can best tailor control of the pain problem to offset each of the affected pain components.

ANATOMICAL FEATURES

Gross sensory supply. Somatic sensation from the maxillofacial region is mainly carried by branches of the maxillary and mandibular divisions of the trigeminal nerve, which extensively branch before entering the skull. Because of this peripheral separation of branches, acute lesions (such as infection, compression, and neoplasia) frequently cause highly specific symptoms that aid in localizing the disease. However, neurological symptoms felt in peripheral tissues may also result from lesions as far central as the trigeminal ganglion and its sensory root because the peripheral fields of innervation are known to project precisely onto specific regions of the central trigeminal system. This concept is called *somatotopic organization* and may explain the mimic effect of peripheral disease and the highly localized "trigger points" that are part of many trigeminal neuralgia states. For example, certain forms of acute and highly localized trigeminal neuralgia may be caused by the irritation and destruction of specific fiber groups in the trigeminal ganglion overlying a carotid artery aneurysm.[68] In spite of the occasional specificity of neurological symptoms, it is more typical for subacute or chronic maxillofacial lesions to produce poorly localized symptoms. They are often changeable or inappropriate for the stimulus and may even be *referred,* a situation in which symptoms are felt in distant tissues and are unrelated to the true pathological site. These characteristics may be partially explained on the basis of anatomical features in the brain stem trigeminal complex. All sensory input from the maxillofacial region has its primary synaptic termination in a laterally placed columnar region, the descending tract nuclei of the trigeminal system, which extends from the rostral pons to the third or fourth cervical spinal cord levels. It is typified by many fibers that synapse on one another and bring about considerable overlap and convergence of fibers on common secondary neurons.[69] These complex interplays and convergences may help explain the diffuseness and also the referred nature of maxillofacial symptoms. For example, an irritative pathological condition from an alveolar osteitis in a third molar socket may cause pain anterior to the ear because the same irritated inferior alveolar brain stem synaptic regions are also shared by converging fibers of the auriculotemporal nerve. Similarly, pain accompanying angina pectoris may be referred to the supraclavicular and mandibular angle regions because incoming fibers of the cervical plexus are known to converge in the caudal portions of the descending trigeminal nucleus.[69]

Microscopic sensory supply. The maxillofacial somatosensory tissues also have unique microanatomical features that help explain pathology in the region. On the basis of fiber size, trigeminal nerve branches contain the largest proportion of myelinated axons and the smallest proportion of unmyelinated axons in the entire somatic sensory system.[72] This leads to the prediction that primary diseases affecting the myelin sheaths will show some predisposition for the trigeminal system. This does appear to be the case in multiple sclerosis, a demyelinating disease in which trigeminal neuralgia occurs in up to 5% of cases.[109] A preponderance of myelinated fibers in peripheral nerves is also significant in those systemic disease states in which vascular pathology is a significant feature because the Schwann cells that are responsible for laying down and maintaining the myelin sheaths are known to be especially vulnerable to ischemia.[128] This is the case in diabetes mellitus, in which trigeminal nerves may display *polyneuropathy,* defined as a symptomatic degeneration of many nerves.

The trigeminal ganglion cells themselves are known to be significantly larger on the average than the spinal ganglion cells. This may explain the high incidence of viral disorders in the trigeminal ganglion, such as trigeminal herpes zoster in which the inclusion bodies preferentially inhabit the larger cell bodies of the ganglion.[94] A selective effect on a specific trigeminal cell population may be significant in certain congenital disorders such as the Riley-Day syndrome and in congenital insensitivity to pain.[1] It has been suggested that these conditions result from an interference with the maturation of a particular segment of the sensory ganglion. In the case of the trigeminal ganglion, it seems that ganglion cells may develop from at least two separate sources, the neural crest and the epidermal placode.[65] A teratological influence may act preferentially on one of these cell sources.

Autonomic supply. The *sympathetic* nerve supply to the maxillofacial region originates in the cervical spinal cord and, following synapse in the superior cervical chain ganglion, distributes to glands and smooth muscles by coursing in network fashion along the arteries of the head and neck. Lesions of the sympathetic fibers at any point distal to the cervical ganglion may produce signs and symptoms in the maxillofacial region. For example, an interruption of sympathetic functions in the orbit may result in Horner's syndrome, which is characterized by lid ptosis, pupillary constriction, and local anhidrosis. Horner's syndrome may result from lesions as diverse as a carotid sinus tumor, cellulitis in the infratemporal fossa, and retro-orbital edema after facial trauma.

The perivascular location of sympathetic nerve nets also makes them vulnerable to reflex stimulation by inadvertent stimulation during local anesthetic administration. Mechanical contact of the nerves with the anesthetic needle or intra-arteriolar deposit of solution with vasoconstrictor may trigger a severe spasm distal to the point of contact with the perivascular nerve fibers. This produces rapid pain and tissue blanching followed occasionally by an edema response. This phenomenon is perhaps most common with infraorbital nerve blocks in which stimulation of autonomic and also sensory fibers at the infraorbital foramen triggers a firing of autonomic branches by axon reflex.

Parasympathetic neurons to the maxillofacial region arise in brain stem cell columns designated as portions of the third, seventh, and ninth cranial nerves. Nerve processes course outward to synapse in the ciliary, sphenopalatine, otic, submandibular, and other smaller ganglia before distributing to smooth muscle, salivary glands, and lacrimal glands. These fibers are small in diameter and reach their final destinations by coursing with the larger nonautonomic branches of cranial nerves, primarily the trigeminal. For this reason, lesions of somatic nerves also affect parasympathetic function as in submandibular and sublingual gland dysfunction, which may result from the severance of the lingual nerve in the retromolar region. Because of the complexity of autonomic fiber distribution, there are occasional errors in nerve regeneration patterns, which may result in bizarre reflex syndromes. For example, the *gustatory sweating syndrome* may follow interruption of the auriculotemporal nerve and its associated autonomic fibers caused by trauma in the mandibular fossa, parotid gland injury, or condylar fracture.[26] In this syndrome a sweating and uncomfortable flushing of the face occurs over the distribution of the auriculotemporal nerve in response to a taste stimulus. This is probably a result of an inappropriate regrowth of the ninth nerve parasympathetic fibers along vacant sympathetic pathways that terminate in sweat glands rather than salivary acini.

Motor supply. Conscious control of skeletal muscle in the maxillofacial region, which includes extraocular, masticatory, facial, lingual, and palatopharyngeal groups, originates in the cerebral cortex as "upper motor neurons." These nerves descend in both crossed and uncrossed tracts to many levels of the brain stem, where they terminate on secondary motor nuclear groups of "lower motor neurons" (Fig. 26-2). It is these latter neurons that send out peripheral extracranial processes to skeletal muscle and constitute the cranial nerves. The cranial nerves diverge from the brain at points widely separated from one another and range from the midbrain to the cervical spinal cord. It is for this reason that patients presenting with signs of multiple cranial motor nerve deficit probably are not suffering a lesion of the lower motor neurons. Rather, the diagnostician should suspect a lesion of upper motor neurons in the more rostral brain stem or cerebral tissues where the upper motor neuron tracts are more grouped. In addition, since all the lower motor cranial

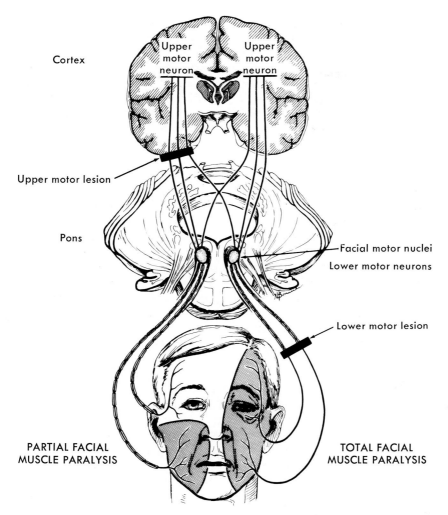

Fig. 26-2. Motor nerve lesions.

nerves except the fourth nerve are completely uncrossed in their courses to skeletal muscles, any lesion of the lower motor nerves produces a deficit in all the muscles supplied by that nerve. For example, lesions of the seventh nerve on one side will cause deficits in all ipsilateral facial muscles equally, whereas a lesion of the upper motor neurons that course to the motor nuclei of the seventh nerve causes a deficit primarily in the lower facial muscles, sparing upper facial muscle activity. This results

from the patterns of crossing and uncrossing by the upper motor nerves that result in double innervation to some portions of the facial motor nucleus (Fig. 26-2).

Most cranial motor nerves are anatomically well shielded from damage. For example, the trigeminal nerves to the masticatory muscles branch from the deeply located mandibular nerves and are rarely affected by peripheral pathological conditions. Therefore, if there are signs of masticatory neuromuscular deficit, the diagnostician should suspect a centrally located pathological condition, probably within the cranial cavity. Unfortunately the seventh nerve is not well protected and is especially vulnerable to lateral facial trauma. For example, seventh nerve paresis may result from compression over the mastoid process and at the mandibular angle during general anesthesia using the face mask.[117] The seventh nerve is also known to be especially prone to the effects of ischemia, perhaps because of its long course within the non-expanding facial bony canal. This may explain the occasional transitory facial palsy resulting from mandibular block anesthesia, in which intravascular injection has produced an ischemia in the posterior auricular and stylomastoid artery distributions.[117] The facial nerve is also responsive to hypocalcemia as demonstrated by the use of the Chvostek test for systemic hypocalcemia, in which tapping over the nerve trunks elicits a tetany of facial muscles.

HISTOPATHOLOGY

Although symptomatic maxillofacial neurological disease may be caused by a wide variety of lesions acting at many levels of the nervous system, certain basic histopathological processes help explain both the disease course and the associated clinical picture.

Reversible lesions. In the peripheral nerves, many common irritative lesions caused by mild trauma, chemical irritation, and necrotic infection may induce transient paresthesias as well as mild muscle paresis. A typical incident is the compression of inferior alveolar nerve branches during tooth extraction or the excessive blunt retraction of seventh nerve branches. The essential histopathological process in these cases involves tearing, hemorrhage, microinfarcts, and cellular infiltrates of the epineural and perineural sheaths without damage to endoneural tissue. Because these lesions involve no significant damage to the nerve axons or myelin sheaths themselves, they are reversible if the irritating factors are promptly removed.

Degeneration. There are two forms of degeneration seen in peripheral nerves that produce specific clinical symptomatology and that may result in irreversible neurological changes: segmental demyelination and wallerian degeneration. *Segmental demyelination* is a selective dissolution of the myelin sheath segments and is characterized by a slowing of conduction velocity as nerve impulses travel slowly along denuded axons. The clinical picture is frequently one of *polyneuropathy,* which is characterized by simultaneous involvement of many nerve branches, and the distribution of symptoms tends to be ''patchy'' and to cross natural neuroanatomical boundaries. The symptoms are typically those of paresthesia or dysesthesia in which certain of the sensibilities, such as deep pain, are retained, but others, such as fine tactile and pinprick sensitivity, are absent or delayed. Segmental demyelination is most often associated with vascular and connective tissue disorders that produce small infarcts in the ischemia-susceptible, myelinated nerve segments.

Wallerian degeneration is a disease process demonstrating disintegration of both the peripheral nerve fibers and myelin sheaths that spread distally from the point of first degeneration. Breakdown products are rapidly phagocytized, leaving prominent Schwann cell columns that once contained the nerve elements. Although these responses are best known as an invariable response to traumatic nerve section, they may be caused by any destructive lesion that attacks the peripheral nerve, including ischemia, inflammation, or tumor. In addition, wallerian degeneration of peripheral nerve processes may occur whenever the neuron cell bodies are diseased and unable to maintain their peripheral nerve cytoplasms. For example, necrosis of trigeminal ganglion cells resulting from invasion by herpes zoster virus is also accompanied by a wallerian degeneration of peripheral trigeminal nerves. A cerebrovascular accident in the pons adjacent to the motor nucleus of the seventh nerve may also result in degeneration of the peripheral nerve branches in the face. In some cases a peculiar form of wallerian degeneration may occur in which degeneration begins in the most peripheral nerve tissues and progresses centrally from that point. This condition, known as "dying back" neuropathy, has been associated in the trigeminal system especially with metabolic intoxications caused by heavy metal poisoning, with isoniazid and penicillin therapy, and with conditions of malnutrition.[1,114] In these cases anesthesia and paresthesia appear peripherally, and, as the disease progresses, more centrally located nerve branches become symptomatic.

These degenerative changes all take place within the first 48 hours after the primary lesion, and clinically the tissues distal to the point of degeneration become rapidly unreactive. In denervated zones the monosynaptic reflexes, such as the jaw-jerk reflex, disappear, sweating ceases, salivation decreases, and a zone of anesthesia develops immediately. Initially, the acute zone of anesthesia consists of a central *autonomous* zone that is absolutely free of sensation and a narrow surrounding *intermediate* zone of hypoesthesia, which results from the overlap of fibers of adjacent intact nerves. Within the first few days after denervation, the diameter of the autonomous zone becomes smaller because of the "sprouting" of new sensory terminations from adjacent normal nerves into the autonomous zone.[56] A similar phenomenon may occur in denervated flaccid muscular regions as neuromuscular end plates sprout from adjacent intact nerves. This has the effect of partially reducing the size of the completely flaccid zone.

Neurotrophic effects. If tissues remain denervated for longer periods of time, certain clinical changes take place, called *neurotrophic effects.* In skeletal muscles the early spontaneous muscle spasms are followed by a flaccid paralysis with progressive atrophy and lack of muscle definition and tone. Denervated skin and mucosa may typically become cold, dry, and inelastic, with a greater susceptibility to injury and

poor healing capacity. Keratinization is irregular, and skin surfaces may become caked and scaly, with a shiny cyanotic appearance. Joint structures may deteriorate, especially if subjected to intermittent stress. Although many of the neurotrophic tissue effects may be results of the interruption of efferent sympathetic fibers concerned with vasoconstriction, a missing neurohumoral nutritional factor has also been postulated to account for neurotrophic effects.[34] Because of the potential for destructive neurotrophic effects, all efforts should be made to protect the denervated tissues from damage and to stimulate artificially the remaining intact structures until proper reinnervation can take place. Classic physical and occupational therapy techniques should be applied in these cases, such as lubrication and protection of surface tissues from trauma, manual stimulation of glandular tissues, warming and temperature control for assuring effective circulation, and electrical stimulation of intact motor units.

Normal regeneration. Peripheral nerve regeneration may begin within 24 hours if the cause of the original degeneration has been eliminated. The central nerve stump of the interrupted nerve sends out a swollen tangle of newly sprouted fibers, called a *growth cone,* that advances through the scar area of original degeneration seeking contact with the residual and now vacant Schwann cell tubes of the degenerate peripheral nerve. If the growth cone fibers reach the distal passages, they enter in random fashion, grow distally at a rate of approximately 1.5 mm daily, and finally make contact with terminal receptors and neuromuscular end plates. The thin fibers will then gradually thicken to approach their original diameters, and the investing Schwann cell will elaborate new myelin sheaths. Clinically the advance of the regenerating growth cone can be detected by observing *Tinel's sign,* in which a tapping on the growth cone or proximal stump will elicit paresthesias. As functional contacts are made, the autonomous zone of anesthesia gradually shrinks in size, first with the return of proprioception and a response to deep pressure pain stimulus that may be poorly localized and is itching, burning, or "bursting" in character; however, responses to fine tactile and pinprick stimulation are lacking. Although these neurological imbalances usually disappear as the regenerated nerves continue to mature, a persistence of this sensory pattern may occur and is called *hyperpathia*.

Abnormal regeneration. Unfortunately many other factors may detract from the return of proper function in regenerated peripheral nerves. For example, the successful bridging of the gap between the in-tact central stump and the distal Schwann cell passageways may be hampered by scar and foreign body barriers. When this happens the growth cone may continue to proliferate at the scarred junction in an aimless tumor of small fibers that constitute a *traumatic neuroma* (Fig. 26-3). In other cases poorly myelinated tubular regions in the regenerated nerve, called *neuromas in continuity*, may result and resemble in many respects the discrete lesions of segmental demyelination. Because the nerve tissues of peripheral neuromas rarely mature and myelinate properly, their stimulation may result in painful bursts of intermittent pain and bizarre paresthesias. This phenomenon

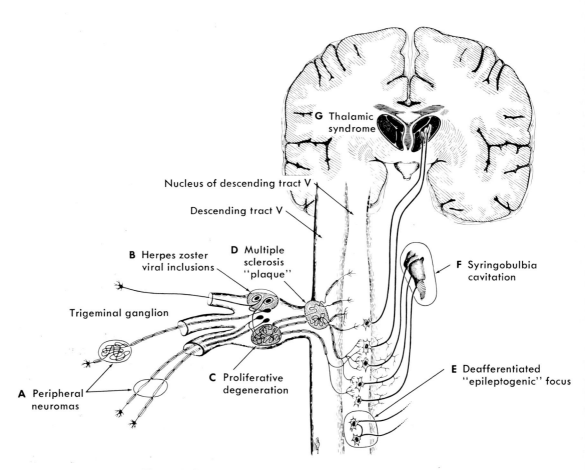

Fig. 26-3. Sites and pathogenesis of maxillofacial neuralgias.

may be explained on the basis of the setting up of *artificial synapses,* in which impulses in one demyelinated fiber may excite neighboring demyelinated fibers, resulting in an abnormal chain reaction to the original stimulus.[49] The concept of the artificial synapse occurring in pathological peripheral nerve zones, as suggested by White and Sweet,[135] may be a common explanation for many trigeminal neuralgias, such as those accompanying multiple sclerosis lesions and the paroxysmal shocking pain of tic douloureux (Fig. 26-3). A similar explanation has been used to explain the deep burning pain of posttraumatic *causalgia,* which may be caused by the excitation of demyelinated sensory nerve segments by adjacent unmyelinated sympathetic fibers.[33] In addition to neuroma formation, there are other potential accidents of regeneration. It is known that the relocation of growth cone fibers in the distal Schwann cell passages is largely a nonspecific selection process, and the identical matching of new regenerating fibers with their former tissue receptors may not occur. Fibers may come to innervate the wrong tissues. When this occurs in reinnervated skeletal muscle and glands, motor control is inappropriate. Little is known about similar accidents in sensory tissues. It is also known that regenerated fibers rarely attain their original diameters, and the distances between nodes of Ranvier are shorter in regenerated nerves.[96] These two factors may lead to reduced nerve conduction velocities as well as disproportionately high numbers of smaller fibers. According to the gate control theories of pain and sensory modulation outlined previously, such imbalance in the afferent fiber diameters could lead to sensory abnormality such as hyperpathia.

In addition to imbalances that may be induced by histopathological conditions in the peripheral nerve fibers, significant imbalances may also be caused by selective effects on the nerve cell bodies themselves. For example, there is considerable evidence that trigeminal ganglion cell bodies may be selectively lost as a result of many life and disease processes.[94] Neuron necrosis occurs more readily in immature cells, and possibly in larger cells, from such diverse causes as trauma, metabolic disease, and viral infection. In those circumstances in which the neuron cell bodies are unable to survive, there is not only a wallerian degeneration of peripheral nerve but also a disintegration of the central nerve processes. This has the effect of severing functional synaptic connection with the secondary transmission, reflex, and integration centers in the central nervous system. In sensory systems the loss of peripheral fibers and synaptic contacts that normally arrive at the primary synaptic regions is called *deafferentation,* and it is now known that trigeminal deafferentation may induce both morphological and physiological changes in the nuclei of the descending trigeminal tract.[134] Deafferentated brain stem regions take on bizarre and stereotyped electrical characteristics that have been called *epileptogenic foci* because they resemble the EEG patterns that typically initiate seizure activity (Fig. 26-3). It has also been postulated that these epileptogenic firing patterns may represent the physiological change responsible for paroxysmal and atypical neuralgia states.[2] Deafferentation effects may eventually explain the cause of such poorly understood conditions as trigeminal neuralgia, postherpetic neuralgia, and phantom limb pain.

NEURALGIAS

Neuralgia may be defined as paroxysmal, intense intermittent pain that is usually confined to specific nerve branches of the head and neck. It is the modern view that paroxysmal, bursting maxillofacial pains may have a common histopathology, which is a breakdown in the insulating mechanisms between axons without destroying them.[135] This primary condition may occur in peripheral nerve branches, in the sensory ganglion tissues, or in the posterior roots. There is good evidence that these peripheral lesions may cause pain by creating afferent imbalances and setting up abnormal pools of secondary central neurons in the trigeminal descending tract nuclei, possibly the epileptogenic foci type (Fig. 26-3).[2]

Idiopathic trigeminal neuralgia. The most dramatic and well-known neuralgia is *tic douloureux,* which displays the classic and diagnostic features of paroxysmal pain that is (1) extreme, "stabbing," or "shocking," lasting seconds to minutes, (2) rapidly provokable by gentle stimulation over surface "trigger zones," (3) confined to the distributions of trigeminal nerve branches, (4) unilateral and does not cross the midline for any given paroxysm, and (5) without objective sensory or motor loss in the affected region. (See Table 26-1.) In some cases atypical neuralgia features may be superimposed on this clinical picture, including an unprovoked burning or aching that persists between the paroxysms, pain that may radiate into the neck and posterior scalp, and the occurrence of mild hypesthesias. Idiopathic trigeminal neuralgia occurs most frequently in the sixth decade of life and more frequently in women (over 58%), has a predilection for the right side (over 60%), and may be cyclic or seasonal with more than 50% of patients experiencing early remissions of greater than 6 months before return of active pain.[135] Pain occurs most often in the maxillary peroral tissues, which are grossly and microscopically normal, and the pain may be triggered by gentle touching or by facial movements during talking or mastication. Although the pain of the trigger zones and pain fiber distributions often mimic pain of odontogenic or sinus origin and cause patients to seek indiscriminate dental extractions, there have been no proved correlations between dental or antral sepsis and the occurrence of tic douloureux.

The histopathological lesion of idiopathic trigeminal neuralgia has now been established as a hypermyelination, segmental demyelination, and microneuroma formation that is localized in ventral portions of the trigeminal ganglion and its adjacent posterior root fibers.[5] It has been theorized that such a lesion would act pathophysiologically as an artificial synapse by setting up abnormal volleys throughout the tangle of demyelinated fibers.[135] Also, according to the gate control theory of the pain mechanism, the selective degeneration of the largest myelinated fibers in these lesions could have the effect of lowering pain inhibition of smaller fibers in the brain stem trigeminal nuclei.

The cause of this disease process is unknown. Vascular factors such as transient ischemia and autoimmune hypersensitivity responses have been proposed as causes of the demyelination. Mechanical factors have also been postulated, such as the action of aneurysms of the intrapetrous portion of the internal carotid artery that may erode through the floor of the intracranial fossa to exert a pulsatile irritation on the ventral side of the trigeminal ganglion.[68]

More recently, an anomaly of the superior cerebellar artery has been described that has been shown to lie in contact with the sensory root of the trigeminal nerve.[62] This anomaly has been implicated as a cause of demyelinating pathology. Surgical elevation of the vessels away from the sensory root has been highly successful in relieving paroxysmal pain in cases of idiopathic trigeminal neuralgia.

The diagnosis of this syndrome is based primarily on recognizing the clinical features. Diagnostic local anesthetic blocks applied at the point of triggering should eliminate all paroxysms of pain and help differentiate atypical neuralgia and other forms of trigeminal neuralgia or neuritis conditions. Treatment of this condition is both medical and surgical. However, analgesics, sedatives, and the formerly advocated vitamin B_{12} injections have no significant therapeutic effect on tic douloureux pains. The best medical results have been gained with antiepileptic agents such as phenytoin (Dilantin), which decreases the pain symptoms approximately 50% of the time, and more recently carbamazepine

Table 26-1. Diagnostic features of major maxillofacial neurological disorders

	Myofascial pain dysfunction	Idiopathic trigeminal neuralgia (tic douloureux)	Periodic migrainous headache (cluster headaches)	Migraine headache	Post-traumatic neuropathy	Systemic disease neuropathy
Age at onset	Young adult	Middle to old age	Young adult	Puberty	—	Middle to old age
Sex factor	Female (strong)	Female (slight)	No	Female (strong)	No	No
Hereditary	—	No	No	Yes (moderate)	No	Variable
Emotion factor	Yes (strong)	No	Yes (slightly)	Yes (strong)	No	Variable
Symptom duration	Variable	Seconds to minutes	5 to 20 minutes	Hours to days	Variable	Variable
Symptom stimulus	Mastication	Surface tactile	Vasodilation	Vasodilatation	Deep pressure	Spontaneous
Common location	Preauricular, gonial	Right V_3 division	Midfacial	Upper lateral face	Injury site	Appendages, extraocular muscles, alveoli
Sensations	Aching, tightness	Sharp, electric pain	Burning, aching	Throbbing, aching	Phantoms, burning, numb	Variable by region
Sensory signs	No	No	No	No	Dysesthesias	Dysesthesias
Autonomic signs	Rare	No	Local discharge (strong)	Systemic discharge (strong)	Variable	Variable (moderate)
Systemic effects	Other psychosomatic effects	No	Rare, variable	Gastrointestinal	No	Metabolic (strong)
Special features	Malocclusion	Paroxysms	Seasonal	Prodromal sensory visceral effects	Neurotrophic effects	Neurotrophic effects
Diagnostic block effect	Muscle mass—partial relief	Trigger zone—total relief	Pterygopalatine fossa—total relief	Relief with pressure on carotid artery	Nerve block—partial relief	Nerve block—little relief
Systemic medication effect	Analgesics, supportive tranquilizer—partial relief	Analgesics—ineffective; antiepileptics—effective	Analgesics—little relief; systemic vasoconstrictors—effective	Analgesics—little relief; systemic vasoconstrictors—effective	Analgesics—partial relief	Analgesics—effective

(Tegretol), which affords significant or total pain relief in a high percentage of cases, as much as 100% in some of the series reported.[107] The effectiveness of antiepileptic agents in the control of paroxysmal pain lends support to the concept of the epileptogenic focus as a factor in the pathophysiology of paroxysmal pain. Reports on the use of carbamazepine have reversed early concerns about its toxicity, although its effectiveness for long-term pain control is not yet known.

Surgical approaches for maxillofacial neuralgias are varied and will be discussed in greater detail in a later section (Fig. 26-4). They consist of (1) temporizing procedures such as alcohol injection and peripheral neurectomy for eliminating the peripheral trigger effects, (2) decompression and complete resection of ganglion posterior root fibers, and afferent trigeminal tracts, and (3) interruption of central trigeminal ascending pathways. In addition, neurophysiological stimulation techniques based on the gate control theory of the pain mechanism appear to hold promise for the future control of tic douloureux.

Vagoglossopharyngeal neuralgia. Formerly called glossopharyngeal neuralgia, the syndrome of *vagoglossopharyngeal neuralgia* occurs less than one-eightieth as often as idiopathic trigeminal neuralgia and is an affliction of sensory, autonomic, and motor fibers of the ninth and tenth cranial nerves.[108] The onset is usually in the fourth decade, with there being no apparent predilection for either sex. The left side is involved more frequently than the right, and both bilateral pain or combinations with idiopathic trigeminal neuralgia are rare. The pains are felt in the base of the tongue, the adjacent tonsillar pillars, and occasionally the soft palate and external auditory canal. The paroxysms may be of lower intensity than trigeminal tic pain, with intermittent refractory periods. Pain triggering is most often caused by swallowing or surface stimulation in the tongue or pharynx, and occasionally pain will follow taste stimulation

by spicy or bitter foods. As part of the paroxysmal attack there is also excessive salivation, lacrimation, mild vertigo, and involuntary movements of the pharynx and larynx, which may result in severe coughing and vomiting. Syncope may occur as well as a progressive hypotension and bradycardia; in extreme cases ECG recordings have demonstrated asystoles of over 1 minute, and there are records of associated cardiac arrest.[108]

The histopathological finding is similar to that described for idiopathic trigeminal neuralgia, and the complex clinical features can most easily be explained on the basis of an indiscriminant artificial synapse lesion of mixed ninth and tenth cranial nerve components. The pain fiber distribution to the tongue and pharynx and the taste fibers from the posterior third of the tongue are known to be components of the ninth nerve. Irritation of the greater petrosal nerve branches explains the increased function of the parotid gland, and the pharyngeal-laryngeal motor reflexes suggest involvement of the ninth and tenth nerve pharyngeal plexuses.[135] Most significantly, the extreme cardiovascular effects of this syndrome reflect an affliction of the nerve of Hering, which is responsible for initiating carotid sinus reflex activity.

Possible causes include posterior root demyelination from the pressure of intracranial aneurysm, and correlations have also been made with preceding paratonsillar infection. Neuralgia association has also been demonstrated with an elongated ossified stylohyoid ligament, causing *Eagle's syndrome*, in which chronic and functional pressures may be exerted on the vagoglossopharyngeal nerve complex in the region of the foramen spinosum.[36] The firm and enlarged stylohyoid ligament in these cases can be seen radiographically, may be palpable in the lateral soft palate or anterior tonsillar pillar, and will often precipitate the paroxysmal pain if the head is turned toward the affected side. In one retrospective study an ossified stylohyoid ligament

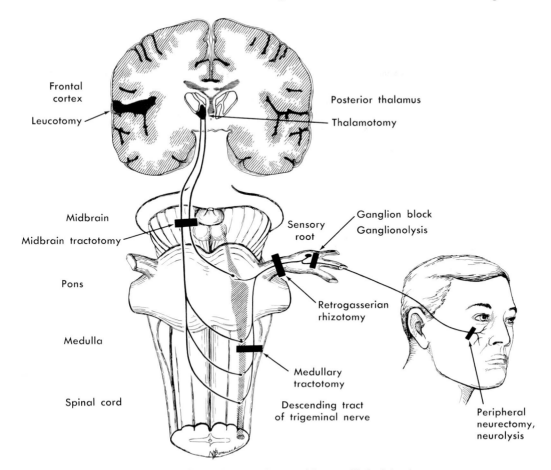

Frontal
cortex

Leucotomy

Posterior thalamus

Thalamotomy

Midbrain

Midbrain tractotomy

Sensory
root

Ganglion block
Ganglionolysis

Pons

Retrogasserian
rhizotomy

Medulla

Medullary
tractotomy

Spinal cord

Descending tract
of trigeminal nerve

Peripheral
neurectomy,
neurolysis

Fig. 26-4. Sites of surgical control for maxillofacial pain.

was found in 70% of cases of vagoglosso-pharyngeal neuralgia, and intraoral osteotomy of the styloid process has brought about a cure in 11 of 12 patients reported in the literature.[135]

Drug therapy similar to that used to manage trigeminal neuralgia has also been effective in this condition. Surgical peripheral neurectomy procedures have not been effective for relief in these cases, and most attention has focused on intracranial rhizotomies of the ninth and tenth nerves' posterior roots as well as the tractotomy procedures identical to those used in the control of trigeminal neuralgia (Fig. 26-4).

Intermedius (geniculate) neuralgia. A rare

paroxysmal pain, described as a "red-hot poker" felt deep within the external auditory canal, the auricle, and occasionally the soft palate, is attributed to involvement of the sensory or intermedius portions of the seventh cranial nerve. This unilateral condition, also known as the *Ramsey-Hunt syndrome,* has a strong predilection for women, no preference for right or left side, and has its usual onset in young to middle adulthood.[59] The pains are typically longer in duration than the paroxysms of idiopathic trigeminal neuralgia, and they are often nonprovokable, although trigger zones have been identified in the pinna of the ear. Other unusual clinical features may include excessive salivation and nasal secretions, tinnitus, mild vertigo, and a bitter taste. Diagnosis may be confirmed by stimulating the tympanic plexus and chorda tympani nerves in the middle ear of the awake patient. After the specific involved nerve branches have been identified by stimulation, the pain may be relieved by neurectomy of these branches.

Periodic migrainous neuralgia. Periodic migrainous neuralgia, known also as "cluster headache" and "histamine cephalgia," also encompasses the syndromes of ciliary neuralgia, vidian neuralgia, and sphenopalatine (Sluder's) neuralgia.[135] Its clinical features are intermediate between trigeminal neuralgia and migraine headache in that it combines painful paroxysms with prominent facial autonomic disorder (see Table 26-1). The pain is burning or aching and usually begins deep within the midface behind or beneath the eye and then "migrates" unilaterally to the forehead, temple, and then to the lower face. The attacks increase in severity for 5 to 20 minutes before subsiding and occur in groups or "clusters" over a 2- to 3-month interval, followed by pain-free remission intervals of weeks to years. The overall incidence is lower than for classic migraine and has no known hereditary basis. Although the role of psychogenic factors is disputed, there is a common association with both emotional stress and compulsive personalities.[137] There is no known trigger point or point of provocation, although alcoholic intake and subcutaneous injections of histamine will precipitate attacks. Along with pain attacks, there is a rapid injection of the conjunctival and nasal mucosal vessels, heavy lacrimation and salivation, and often the development of a transient Horner's sign of ptosis and miosis. The temporal vessels become dilated and tender, the eyelids and oral mucosa may swell, and the face may flush a brilliant red.

It is generally agreed that this disorder is a result of an arterial dilation as in classic migraine headache, but in periodic migrainous neuralgia the point of neuropathology is somewhere along the course of the greater superficial petrosal nerve, either intracranially, in its tympanic and petrous course, in the vidian canal, or in the sphenopalatine ganglion itself. The pain and autonomic signs typical of this syndrome appear to be explained on the basis of abnormal excessive discharges in this mixed parasympathetic nerve.

Diagnosis and pain relief can be aided by local anesthetic block of the sphenopalatine ganglion through the greater palatine foramen. Although petrosal neurectomy may be indicated in certain refractory cases, good relief of neuralgia attacks is usually gained by using either ergotamine tartrate or methysergide (Sansert, Deseril), which appears to act through vasoconstriction and serotonin antagonism.[38] Carbamazepine appears to be of no benefit.

Multiple sclerosis neuralgia. A paroxysmal maxillofacial neuralgia, in which the pain is indistinguishable from the pain of idiopathic trigeminal neuralgia, may occur as a feature of multiple sclerosis.[109] The pains are precisely confined, have a shocking or stabbing character, and may be triggered by tactile stimulation. However, in contrast to idiopathic trigeminal neuralgia, multiple sclerosis neuralgia more often involves multiple trigeminal divisions and more often becomes bilateral. Although paroxysms may be the initial symptom of the disease process, they usually are associated with the other progressive and various disorders that characterize this disease. In some cases the paroxysmal pains have followed an initial transient facial numbness and loss of taste on one side; late in the disease process the facial pain may become constant as secondary central pain tracts become diseased.

Multiple sclerosis is a degenerative disease prevalent in northern climates, and its cause is unknown. It runs a varied episodic course over a 10- to 30-year period and involves progressive widespread sensory and motor disability. The acute onset is usually in the third decade and appears typically as a weakness of the lower limbs, disturbed vision, and objective sensory loss in about half the cases. These early signs are typically followed by long remissions. The histopathological lesion in multiple sclerosis is the sclerotic "plaque," a discrete focus of myelin loss with maintenance of axon segments and glial proliferation. The plaques may be seen in widely divergent brain tissues, but the trigeminal neuralgia paroxysms seem to be associated specifically with plaques that span the junction of the posterior trigeminal root entry to the pons (Fig. 26-3).[135]

The differential diagnosis of this disorder depends on identifying the features of a multiple nervous system disorder. There is no known cure for the basic disease process, but the facial pain can be effectively controlled by the same surgical techniques used for idiopathic trigeminal neuralgia. Carbamazepine relieves the pain of multiple sclerosis trigeminal neuralgia in approximately 80% of cases.[107]

POSTTRAUMATIC SENSORY DISORDERS

Trauma to the peripheral nerves of the maxillofacial region is a common consequence of daily life, whether the damage is caused by accident or iatrogenic sources. Because of unique features of nerve tissue degeneration and regeneration, a wide range of posttraumatic pathological conditions may result.[56] The clinical problems may range from barely perceptible paresthesias caused by small neuromas-in-continuity to a profound neuralgia with phantom characteristics that reflects central nervous system pathophysiology.

Posttraumatic trigeminal neuropathy. Maxillofacial trauma is now recognized as a common factor in facial pain syndromes that in the past may have fallen in the catchall "atypical facial pain" class. (See Table 26-1.) The type of trauma that precedes this syndrome usually involves direct tearing or intense compression of peripheral sensory nerves; repetitious trauma is of particular importance even with moderate force. Specific examples that have been cited are fractures of the maxillofacial bones such as basilar skull, supraorbital, and zygomatic fractures involving the infraorbital nerves and displaced mandibular fractures in which the traumatized nerves are associated with disrupted bony canals.[135] In many cases of fractures that precede neuropathy, the displaced bony segments are not firmly fixed, permitting continued mobility and repeated injury to the regenerating sensory nerves. The development of neuropathy may be associated with indirect or iatrogenic trauma such as maxillary and frontal sinus-lining ablation, chronic denture flange irritation, cured infections of the masticator spaces, alveolar osteitis, and, most common of all, damage to the inferior alveolar nerve during third molar extraction.[47] Although an acute onset of the pain syndrome at the time of injury has been reported, there is more often an initial period of anesthesia over the traumatized nerve zone, followed by a gradual onset of symptoms 2 months to 15 years after injury. Any of the cranial or sensory nerve distributions may be involved, although the third division of the trigeminal nerve is most commonly affected. The accompanying pain is aching, burning, boring, or pulling in character, is poorly localized along anatomical lines, and spreads out from the zone of original nerve injury. It is usually not provokable or triggered but is sustained and builds gradually, although in some cases bursts of paroxysmal pain may be superimposed. The neurological examination of the pain areas is significant in that there are often reduced fine tactile and pinprick sensitivities as well as paresis and neurotrophic effects, such as masticator muscle atrophy.

The spreading, nonprovokable nature of the pain and its delayed onset suggests a central nervous system focus of hyperexcitability, similar perhaps to the epileptogenic focus previously described (Fig. 26-3). However, it has been emphasized that more peripheral sites of pathology such as the traumatic neuroma may also result in abnormal sensation. Therefore all efforts should be made to identify any sources of peripheral nerve irritation such as bone fragments displaced into neurovascular canals, occluded nerve foramina, or foreign bodies such as transosseous wires impinging on nerve bundles.

Although peripheral neurectomy procedures may benefit some cases, the sustained burning quality in this syndrome is often refractive even to retrogasserian rhizotomy. Medical treatment with carbamazepine has been effective in the more paroxysmal forms of posttraumatic pain but less successful in relieving the overall neuropathy syndrome.[107]

Causalgia. As a syndrome, causalgia means literally "burning pain" and occurs in the appendages as a result of penetrating missile wounds of mixed peripheral nerves.[33] Pain begins after a postinjury delay of at least 2 weeks with a deep aching or burning that spreads out from the injured zone and beyond natural nerve boundaries. It is neither paroxysmal nor triggered, although attacks are brought on by mild pain or touch stimulation of the region, by drying of tissues, or by environmental stimuli such as loud noises. The affected tissues sweat excessively, may be either very warm or cold, and show color and degenerative trophic changes. All the symptoms are intensified by emotional stress. There is no apparent sexual or racial predilection, and the syndrome is most often seen in vigorous middle-aged people.

Major causalgia has been described only rarely for the maxillofacial region, yet minor causalgia-like states may account for some of the rather common complaints of persistent, focal posttraumatic burning of the gingiva, palate, tongue, and lips.[39] Perhaps most common are complaints of persistent burning in postextraction sites, which occurs along with subtle vasomotor and trophic changes that are made more intense by emotional stress. The specific

mechanism of causalgia pain may be the artificial synapsing of efferent sympathetic fibers with somatic sensory fibers within neuromas that have formed at the site of original nerve injury. The initiation of sympathetic impulses for this bizarre nerve firing pattern probably takes place in the limbic-hypothalamic axis that normally regulates general sympathetic activity. This interaction may explain the influence of emotional factors in heightening the pain. Maxillofacial causalgia pathological lesions are likely to be located at sites of sympathetic and somatic sensory nerve intermingling in nonexpansile bony canals such as the supraorbital, trochlear, and infraorbital and mandibular canals, where mixed nerve bundles are found.

The differential diagnosis of causalgia-like lesions in the maxillofacial region includes psychalgia or hysteria reactions, persistent local pathological conditions, and the more diffuse tissue changes such as surface hypersensitivities. Selective blocking of tissues with vasoconstrictor alone may aid in the diagnosis because true causalgia attacks are relieved by sympathetic blockade. Major causalgia has been treated effectively with sympathectomy, and although minor causalgias have been occasionally cured by identifying and excising neuromas, the best treatment for minor maxillofacial causalgia-like conditions has not been determined.

Phantom facial pain. Patients who have undergone excision of a body part often experience a sense of awareness of the missing part called the *phantom phenomenon*. In cases of limb amputation, in which the phantom phenomenon is best known, the phantoms are painful in approximately 30% of cases and persist in 5% to 10%. Paroxysms are of approximately 10 minutes' duration and are described as stabbing, with extreme itching or deep burning and pressure of the missing part. They may be triggered by tactile stimulation and usually are relieved by local anesthetic block of the peripheral nerve stumps. Although little is known of the incidence and pathogenesis of phantom pain in the maxillofacial region, it should be given consideration in the differential diagnosis of facial pain and not dismissed as evidence of psychological disorder. Complaints can be anticipated from patients who have undergone radical excisions as in orbital-antral exenterations, glossectomy, and mandibulectomy operations for cancer control. Complaints of toothache and of "phantom teeth" in dental extraction sites are not unusual, especially when the teeth have been chronically symptomatic before removal.

Although neuromas occurring at the regenerated nerve stump surface may contribute to this syndrome, it appears that the primary site of pain mechanism is in the brain stem. After limb amputation about half the associated neurons die, and the regenerated fibers of the stump are usually small, poorly myelinated, and slow conducting.[135] Stimulation of these stump tissues therefore may have the effect of activating an imbalanced gate control mechanism in the brain stem and cause inappropriate sensory phenomena such as phantom pain. Palpation and diagnostic block may reveal the presence of a contributing neuroma, and reamputation of nerves at more proximal levels may be successful in these cases. In more severe cases the pain can be eliminated by anterolateral cordotomy, although the awareness of phantom tissues is seldom eliminated. Carbamazepine therapy results in varying degrees of success, and supportive care and reassurance is often adequate in less severe cases because phantom pain seems to diminish with time.

Anesthesia dolorosa. When the afferent fibers of the cranial nerve sensory roots are divided central to the ganglion in rhizotomy procedures, there is a profound and permanent numbness of the denervated tissues. However, the majority of these patients experience some type of paresthesia within the anesthetic zone, and, for an unfortunate few (3% to 15%), these sensations

become intolerably painful.[100] The pain, called *anesthesia dolorosa,* has a gradual onset in the weeks to months after rhizotomy, is constant, burning, pressuring, "crawling or grinding" in sensation, occurs most often in the ophthalmic regions, and is not provokable. The likelihood of anesthesia dolorosa occurring for a patient can be accurately predicted by observing effects of long-term trial denervations with peripheral neurectomy or alcohol blockade of nerves. The site of the disorder is probably in the central nervous system, possibly in the cortex, and medical management is of questionable value. The most effective treatment to date seems to be bilateral frontal lobe leukotomy and lesions of the trigeminothalamic tracts.

INFECTIOUS DISORDERS

Few primary infections involve the nerves of the maxillofacial region. Leprosy is the only known direct infection of peripheral fibers, but herpes infections of the cranial nerve ganglia are proved viral infections, and rare fungus infections of the trigeminal ganglion are also known. However, numerous infections involve the central nervous tissues secondarily because they cause peripheral symptoms and signs and thus are of concern, since these infections may arise in the maxillofacial tissues and spread intracranially.

Herpes zoster (postherpetic trigeminal neuralgia). *Herpes zoster,* commonly known as shingles, may occur in the sensory nerve distributions of the trigeminal, seventh, ninth, and tenth cranial nerves. Herpes zoster is associated with sensory abnormality in its acute disease phase but, more significantly, may result in a severe postherpetic facial neuralgia that is difficult to treat. The acute disease involves the trigeminal nerve in 18% of cases, which is second to the thorax in disease frequency.[124] Outbreaks are most commonly seen in the ophthalmic division. The acute eruptions are discrete painful vesicles with erythematous bases that correspond in distribution to the particular nerve branches, which may involve skin, mucosa, and corneal surfaces. It appears mainly in older people, although a life-threatening neonatal variety is known. It is probably contagious and appears to have peak seasons. The disease may arise after a systemic toxicity or metabolic disorder but most often follows trauma to peripheral sensory nerve branches. In the maxillofacial region, for example, herpes zoster may follow inferior alveolar nerve damage from dental extraction. Herpes zoster is the only definite viral infection of the peripheral nervous system and may be caused by a reactivation of varicella viruses that are latent in the tissues with a specific infection of the larger neuron cell bodies of sensory ganglia (Fig. 26-3). This selective effect in some cases has resulted in a relative loss of the larger trigeminal nerve fibers and a shifting of the postherpetic fiber spectrum toward the small elements.[94] Based on gate control concepts of pain mechanism, this phenomenon may explain the occasional complication of postherpetic neuralgia. Clinically this condition is a constant burning or aching often associated with a deep aggravating anesthesia within the region of the original herpetic outbreak. In addition, severe paroxysmal stabbing pains may be elicited by light touch stimulations. Unfortunately postherpetic neuralgia has been extremely refractive to surgical treatment, and most efforts toward pain management with carbamazepine have been unsuccessful.

Infectious meningitis. It is well established that foci of infection in the maxillofacial tissues may spread into the intracranial cavity. When the process is acute, it may lead to death within 10 days, and some experts feel that chronic forms of central nervous system infection from maxillofacial foci may be responsible for bizarre forms of epilepsy and also contribute to multiple sclerosis.[120] Exacerbations of the infection, causing inflammation and scarring of the cranial nerve rootlets that pass through the meninges, may cause focal neurological disease such as extraocular muscle paresis and may result in transient trigeminal and facial nerve (Bell's) palsy. Clinical signs of acute meningitis are progressive headache with nuchal rigidity and neck flexion and a decreasing level of consciousness with memory deficits. Later in the course, focal signs appear such as hemiparesis, loss of extraocular muscle tone, vertigo, papilledema, and facial pain. Lumbar puncture will usually reveal a leukocytosis in the cerebrospinal fluid, and angiograms and brain scan may reveal an expansile abscess mass. A direct culture of identical organisms from both the brain abscess and the maxillofacial infection will confirm the diagnosis.

The main pathways of infection are venous routes and direct extension, although perineural spread and lymphatic and arterial bacteremias may also infect the brain.[55] The most common route of venous spread is from anterior maxillary foci along the facial angular veins to anastomoses with the inferior and superior ophthalmic veins. Because the facial veins lack valves, these infectious emboli may reach the cavernous sinus along this route. A similar spread may occur from infratemporal space infections that involve the pterygoid venous plexus and that readily communicate with the intracranial venous sinuses adjacent to the temporal lobes. Temporal lobe abscesses may also result from a direct erosion of the temporal bone by cellulitis in the infratemporal and temporal fossae.[125] Direct pulsations of organisms into the subarachnoid space occur almost routinely in basilar skull fractures. Likely sites of seeding in these cases are the frontal lobes superior to the cribriform plates and the temporal lobes adjacent to the middle ear cavity. The most common maxillofacial foci for venous spread and direct invasion are the maxillary teeth, pericoronitis in the mandibular third molars, the palatine tonsils, and contaminated needles introduced into the pterygomandibular space. Prevention of intracranial spread depends on establishing early dependent drainage, wound culture, and attaining high blood levels of antibiotics, preferably penicillin. However, craniotomy and direct abscess drainage may become necessary to avoid brain necrosis and high intracranial pressures.

Leprous neuropathy. Leprosy is the most common neuropathy in the world and is caused by a communicable infection by the acid-fast bacillus, *Mycobacterium leprae,* which enters at skin or mucous membrane surfaces and invades peripheral nerve branches with the capacity to ascend as high as the sensory ganglia.[29] It has a special affinity for the cooler body parts, especially the maxillofacial region where disfiguring lesions appear, including subcutaneous nerve nodules on the eyebrows, nares, and cheeks and cauliflower ears and depigmentation of the skin. A patchy paresis of the seventh cranial nerve branches often leads to drooping of the eyelid and oral commissures, and spotty anesthetized areas over the trigeminal nerve division make the patient vulnerable to trauma.

The essential histopathological lesion is the leprous nodule, a granuloma of bacterial colonies, epithelioid and fibroblastic cells, and plasma cells. The nodule surrounds an area of demyelination and eventually causes wallerian degeneration of the nerves. Leprous nodules can be differentiated from similarly appearing tuberculosis and actinomycosis by analysis of nasal scrapings or nerve biopsy. Modern chemotherapy with sulfones prevents further nerve destruction by these organisms.

Diphtheritic neuropathy. Diphtheria is an acute neuropathy caused by the exotoxin of *Corynebacterium diphtheriae,* which spreads along the peripheral perineural channels to produce a segmental demyelination.[40] Most of the cranial nerves may be affected, producing facial palsies, extraocular muscle paresis, nerve deafness, and hypoglossal paresis. In over 75% of cases of diphtheritic neuropathy there is an unexplained predilection for the motor fibers of the vagus that supply the skeletal muscles of the palate, pharynx, and larynx. Suscep-

tible children are infected by droplets in the palatine tonsil and nasopharyngeal tissues, producing a gray pseudomembrane in these areas. Early symptoms include hypernasality, nasal regurgitation associated with a deviated uvula, and absence of palatal elevation in the gag reflexes. The disease may progress to include a myocarditis and may be complicated by pneumonia. Active immunization is routinely induced in the first year of life, but if the acute disease is encountered, diphtheria antitoxin should be administered. After recovery there may be a postdiphtheritic cranial nerve palsy in the palate that requires speech aid.

Neurosyphilis and tabes dorsalis. Neurosyphilis occurs in 10% of persons infected by *Treponema pallidum,* and the organism may reach the nervous system in the primary stage before the development of any cutaneous lesions.[6] In the secondary stage of the disease process, headaches are common as are ocular palsies. Occasionally a polyneuritis occurs that may involve cranial nerves. It is the tertiary form of neurosyphilis, however, that may lead to the most serious maxillofacial neurological dysfunction. The essential pathological lesion is a vascular inflammation, which results in a necrotic and granulomatous response of the meninges called *gumma.* Gummatous lesions of the meninges may secondarily affect the cranial roots and typically cause palsy of the third, fourth, and sixth nerves as well as partial or total paralysis of the seventh nerve. The trigeminal nerve may also be involved, causing spontaneous paroxysmal pain that is poorly localized and spreading. The diagnosis of tertiary syphilis depends on recognizing the widespread neurological symptoms, and obtaining accurate history and a positive VDRL test.

A particular form of chronic tertiary neurosyphilis, called *tabes dorsalis,* involves a selective degeneration and demyelination of the largest fibers of the dorsal roots and cranial nerve afferent tracts that project through the dorsal columns of the spinal cord and brain stem. The pain of tabes dorsalis is described as "lightning" with a burning or "tearing of the flesh" character that persists for seconds and then shifts to another location. Although tabetic pain occurs most commonly in the extremities, the trigeminal and glossopharyngeal nerves may be involved. Examination may reveal loss of deep pain and proprioceptive sensitivity, with occasional loss of taste and smell. The treatment of tabetic pain is symptomatic.

MAXILLOFACIAL NEUROPATHIES OF SYSTEMIC ORIGIN

A broad range of common systemic disease states including metabolic and nutritional disorders, intoxication, and connective tissue diseases may affect neurological function in the maxillofacial region. These manifestations are typically less predictable in location, intensity, and course than primary neuropathological conditions, and they often simultaneously involve motor, sensory, and autonomic functions. Neuropathies may result from segmental demyelination, wallerian degeneration, or dying-back processes, and clinical features may be confusing because nerve degeneration and regeneration often exist side by side.

Connective tissue disease neuropathies. Trigeminal neuropathies have increasingly been linked with the major collagen disorders, including lupus erythematosus, Sjögren's syndrome,[67] rheumatoid arthritis,[48] scleroderma,[7] polyarteritis nodosa,[4] and diabetes mellitus.[106] The grouping of these diseases is not coincidental; their association with trigeminal neuropathy is based on a rather common mode of pathogenesis. A randomized vasculitis occurs in the nutrient vessels of the peripheral nerves, causing microinfarcts and ischemia to the nerve segments. A segmental demyelination develops rapidly, with initial preservation of the nerve fibers. The haphazard positioning of pathological areas in more peripheral tissues and the selectivity for myelinated portions of the nerves help explain some clinical features. Patchy regions of pares-

thesia occur, often described as "creeping" or "tightening" numbness with infrequent shooting pains. The disturbances are often multifocal and involve motor, sensory, and autonomic nerves regionally and may change position gradually as nerve regeneration occurs in some areas. The trigeminal neuropathies are often preceded by weeks or years by the appearance of Raynaud's phenomenon, a condition in which the fingers and toes respond to cold and emotional stress with pallor, cyanosis, and trophic skin changes caused by vasospasms. The combination of Raynaud's phenomenon and trigeminal neuropathy is significant because of the strong correlation with the development of refractory postextraction dry socket.[15]

Neurological examination of the collagen trigeminal neuropathies reveals reduced vibratory, pinprick, temperature, and light touch sensibilities and an unpleasant hyperpathia that is brought on by deep pressure stimulation. Clinical tests and nerve conduction studies may reveal that deep tendon reflexes such as the blink reflex to glabellar tapping and the jaw-jerk reflex are depressed. Vasomotor deficits may be observed in some cases.

The disease state most commonly associated with neuropathies of all types is diabetes mellitus.[106] Trigeminal diabetic neuropathies tend to be scattered sensory and motor dysesthesias, and, as in the pure collagen disorders, the neurological disorders may be only slightly improved by controlling the underlying disease processes. Systemic steroid therapy may check the progression of trigeminal neuropathies, but circumstantial evidence exists that steroids themselves may act as neurotoxic agents.

Toxic and nutritional neuropathies. In conditions of severe nutritional deprivation and in reactions to foreign substances, the nerve cell metabolism may be so disturbed that it can no longer maintain its peripheral processes, and a dying-back wallerian degeneration results.[104,128] These metabolic neuropathies are characterized by numbness and paresthesias that begin in the more distal portions of nerves and branches of nerves most acutely affecting vibratory and position senses.

The nutritional neuropathies usually occur in the appendages but may involve the maxillofacial region. They are usually related to mixed deficiencies of the vitamin B complex.[98] Deficiencies of vitamin B_1 (thiamin) cause beriberi and may result in nerve deafness, laryngeal paralysis, and a patchy trigeminal paresthesia or anesthesia. This syndrome may also be seen as part of Wernicke's encephalopathy, which is caused by thiamin deficiency in chronic alcoholism.[132] Pellagra, a result of niacin (vitamin B_2) deficiency, is characterized by stomatitis, glossitis, erythematous dermatitis, diarrhea, and a randomized trigeminal sensory neuropathy. Pernicious anemia neuropathy is caused by incomplete absorption of vitamin B_{12} by the small intestine and may cause burning paresthesias in the orofacial region.

Heavy metal intoxications are known to specifically induce necrosis in sensory ganglia, including the trigeminal and the geniculate.[43] The metals that have been most frequently associated with maxillofacial neuropathies have been mercury, lead, cadmium, bismuth, and arsenic.[18]

Among the nonmetals that are known to intoxicate the nervous system, a few have specific preference for the trigeminal system. Trichloroethylene, formerly used extensively in obstetrical analgesia, produces a trigeminal neuropathy by a selective necrosis of ganglion cells. Triorthocresyphosphate ("Jamaica Ginger"), an occasional contaminant of bootleg liquor, produces polyneuropathy in many body regions including the face.[23] A transient trigeminal neuropathy with peroral paresthesias has also been linked to acute ethyl alcohol intoxication.[111]

Finally, trigeminal sensory neuropathies have been linked with a number of well-known therapeutic drugs, including penicillin, cortisone, Stilbamidine, isoniazid, and nitrofurantoin.[48,128]

HEADACHES

More than 90% of the population have experienced maxillofacial headache, and most headaches result from combinations of both organic and psychic factors that act cyclically and potentiate one another.[137] The most frequent kinds of major headaches are vascular in origin, resulting from excessive vasodilation of extracranial or intracranial vessels as in the migraine headaches, or direct vessel wall pathology such as temporal arteritis. Most common mild headaches are "tension headaches," caused by abnormal skeletal muscle contractions. A most common tension headache is the temporomandibular joint–related syndrome of myofascial pain dysfunction.

Coronary artery disease may cause referred pain headaches in the lower face and neck, and hypertensive disease may induce chronic, diffuse headaches. Severe cranial trauma may produce both acute and chronic posttraumatic headaches, and distinctive head pains are known to follow both lumbar puncture and spinal anesthesia. Nonlocalizing headaches may signal progressive intracranial disease such as infection or tumor. Finally, radiating maxillofacial headaches are a frequent by-product of acute neuritis in nasal, paranasal, otological, ocular, and dental tissues.

Migraine. True migraine headaches are "sickening," often debilitating pains that throb and ache unilaterally in the temporal region.[137] Women are affected twice as often as men, and the onset is usually before 16 years of age. There is a 57% familial tendency, and the stereotyped migraine personality is anxious, rigid, perfectionistic, and may be resentful and appear fatigued. The attacks last minutes or as long as a few days, and headaches may be separated by weeks or months and precipitated by menstruation or intake of certain foods or by alcohol. The attacks are preceded by a prodroma or "aura" of vertigo, facial flushing or pallor, and a spotty blindness or flashing of lights in the visual fields. As the headache progresses, there is increasing psychic irritability, nausea, vomiting, and constipation or diarrhea.

Migraine is caused by excess vasodilation of the extracranial vessels, such as the maxillary artery, and the dural portions of the middle meningeal, both of which are innervated by the trigeminal nerve. The prodromal symptoms are probably produced by a preparatory vasoconstriction of these same vessels. The diagnosis can be substantiated by noting rapid pain relief after digital pressure over the common carotid or external carotid arteries and also by obtaining relief with ergotamine tartrate. This condition must be differentiated from trigeminal neuralgia, periodic migrainous neuralgia, and myofascial pain dysfunction. (See Table 26-1.) Its treatment is almost entirely medical; aspirin may help in milder cases by acting on the peripheral vasodilation mechanisms. However, the more severe forms usually respond to systemic ergotamine tartrate, a vasoconstrictor that may be combined with caffeine (Cafergot).[38] The syndrome may be prevented in some cases by using the serotonin antagonist methysergide (Sansert). Psychological counseling is also of benefit in many cases.

Temporal arteritis. Temporal arteritis is a primary arterial disorder that appears most commonly in women between 55 and 80 years of age.[28] It causes intense, unilateral boring headaches over the lateral maxilla, zygoma, preauricular region, temporal region, and occipital region. A referred diffuse pain is felt over the scalp. The pain is initiated by mastication in over 50% of cases, it may be aggravated by lying down or stooping, and digital pressure applied over the external carotid will produce temporary relief of the pain. There is a tenderness over the courses of the superficial temporal, transverse facial, and supraorbital arteries, and palpation may reveal pulseless, tortuous nodules over these ves-

sels. Because the ophthalmic and retinal arteries may also be diseased, there is a gradual onset of blindness in more than one third of the cases.

The pathological characteristic is an arteritis with giant cell and chronic inflammatory infiltrates, intimal thickening, and frequent thromboses. Treatment with cortisone and adrenocorticotrophic hormone (ACTH) results in successful control of the headaches and, if instituted early in the disease course, will prevent blindness. In extreme cases the pain can also be relieved by selective resection of small portions of the diseased vessels.

Coronary disease headache. The referral of a deep pressing pain to regions of the head and neck is a confusing manifestation of heart disease. It is not difficult to recognize the association between face pain and heart disease when pain begins during exertion or emotional stress and spreads from the chest up the neck to the angle of the mandible, its most common facial location. However, facial pain may also occur without any of the classic anginal signs of chest and left arm pain, and symptoms may be localized to the maxilla, cheek, mandibular body, orbit, or occiput and may persist for longer periods of time than the typical anginal attack.[97]

As in classic angina pectoris the pain is thought to originate from stimulation of cardiac afferent fibers by myocardial ischemia. These fibers then converge onto a common synaptic region with somatic sensory fibers that arrive from a different body region. In this case the convergence of cardiac fibers is with cervical plexus and trigeminal fibers in the upper cervical spinal cord segments. As in other forms of anginal pain, these referred headaches can be controlled by the use of nitroglycerine tablets.

Myofascial pain dysfunction. Most neuralgia-like headaches of the lower face are caused by muscle spasm in the masticatory apparatus.[23] In their acute form, these spasms produce trismus, deviation of the mandible to the affected side, inability to occlude the teeth, and a sharp pain brought on by clenching. The pain is most often felt directly over the temporomandibular joint or above the gonial angle and less frequently over the zygoma, temporal, submandibular, or occipital regions. There may be tender palpable "knots" in the masseter and temporal muscles that can be relieved by injecting local anesthetic directly into the muscles. The acute syndrome often follows trauma such as subluxation or dislocation of the mandible and radical changes in the chewing patterns, but the most important precipitating factor appears to be emotional stress. Chronic forms of this syndrome also correlate well with underlying emotional tensions that may promote injurious jaw habits and amplify the effects of occlusal disharmonies. The chronic symptoms are most gradual in onset, appear four times as often in women, and occur most often in early adulthood, during puberty, and at the menopausal ages. Joint clicking and jerky mandibular movements are common, and sharp pains are superimposed on a dull, aching, and "drawing" pain in the lower face.

The myofascial pain syndrome must be differentiated from true osteoarthritis, migrainous neuralgias, and temporal arteritis and from acute neuritides such as maxillary sinusitis and referred odontogenic pain. Primary temporomandibular osteoarthritis may produce acute clinical features identical to acute myofascial pain. Differentiation is made by radiographically observing the hypocalcification and lipping of the condylar head, resorption of the articular tubercle, and dystrophic joint calcification.

Treatment of the acute phase of myofascial pain is aimed at interrupting the muscle spasm cycle by (1) *supportive* therapy with analgesics, tranquilizers, and muscle relaxants such as diazepam and physiotherapy such as local moist heat and (2) *disengagement* of the masticatory apparatus by consciously avoiding stressful clenching, by injecting the tender muscles with local anesthetics, and by using temporary occlu-

sal splints. The need for rest and the beginning of psychological counseling should be stressed at this time. Treatment of the chronic problems will rely even more heavily on psychological counseling to identify and compensate for abnormal muscle habits. Correction of occlusal discrepancies should proceed only after the acute myospasms have been controlled. Surgical treatments, such as cortisone joint injections, arthroplasty, and condylectomy, are indicated only after the presence of osteoarthropathy or ankylosis has been confirmed.

MAXILLOFACIAL NEURITIS

The often misused term *neuritis* means literally "inflammation of nerve" and will be used here to identify acute, reversible irritations of maxillofacial nerves. Neuritis may occur in sensory, motor, or autonomic nerves and results from peripheral pathology that infects, compresses, entraps, or erodes the adjacent nerves. Neuritis is significant because it is a signal of an acute pathological condition and because neuritis that is allowed to persist may eventually progress to degenerative and irreversible neuropathy. Sensory neuritis is almost always manifested as pain, but its character depends on the location and nature of the primary lesion. It is also characterized by a lowering of the pain thresholds, probably as a result of alterations in the central gate control mechanisms. For example, with chronic neuritis from a periapical abscess, irritation of the smaller pain-sensitive fibers seems to have the effect of sensitizing the brain stem synaptic regions to respond more readily to any kind of incoming stimulation. This slight opening of the gate may explain why tactile or light pressure stimulation of tissues around periapical abscesses will result in pain responses, even in the locally anesthetized state.

Bell's palsy. Bell's palsy is an isolated facial paralysis of sudden onset caused by a neuritis of the seventh nerve within the facial canal.[130] It occurs often in the young adult man with a history of recent exposure to local cold, such as sleeping next to an open window, or in some cases it occurs after infections of the nasopharynx or masticator spaces. The clinical appearance is a unilateral flaccidity of all facial muscles with loss of eyebrow and forehead wrinkles, drooping of the eybrows, flattening of the nasolabial furrow, sagging of the corner of the mouth, and collection of food in the buccal vestibule. Patients are unable to frown or raise their eyebrows, and they cannot close their eyes or purse their lips. If the neuritis has extended as far centrally as the point at which the chorda tympani nerve joins the facial nerve trunk, then taste will be impaired over the anterior two thirds of the tongue on that side. Patients may also complain of loud noise intensification because of damage to the nerve of the stapedius muscle. The histopathological sign of Bell's palsy is edema in the nonexpansile facial canal. It is not known whether the precise source of inflammation is in the nerve fibers themselves, in related connective tissues, or in the periosteum of the canal walls. After its sudden onset the paralysis begins to subside within 2 to 3 weeks, and gradual complete recovery occurs in over 85% of patients. It is necessary to differentiate between the isolated lower motor neuron lesions of Bell's palsy and the more complex upper motor lesions that may result from vascular lesions or neoplastic lesions in the pons. In these central "upper motor" lesions, upper facial muscle function is spared. (See Fig. 26-2).

In the early stages of Bell's palsy, inflammation may be suppressed by using systemic cortisone or ACTH. Surgical decompression of the facial canal may also aid in edema control if it is performed during the first few days.[24] Galvanic stimulation of facial muscles may counteract the neurotrophic effects. The cornea must be protected from abrasion by applying lubricants or in some cases by suturing the eyelids. If paralysis is permanent, the facial tissues may be given artificial support by means of prosthetic devices or by subcutaneously grafted masseter or fascia lata slings. In some cases a surgical redirection of the accessory nerve into the degenerate seventh nerve tissues has been effective in restoring some facial muscle function.[83]

Other cranial motor neuritides. A rare trigeminal neuritis has been described that is similar to and in some cases accompanies Bell's palsy.[37] This neuritis is unilateral and results in total anesthesia or pain, usually over the mandibular division. It is also associated with a unilateral total loss of function in the masticatory muscles supplied by the trigeminal nerve. The cause is unknown, and gradual complete recovery has been reported for most cases.

Cranial nerves three, four, and six are often affected by traumatic lesions, either directly by damage or indirectly by orbital edema. Third nerve neuritis is confirmed by observing the features of Horner's syndrome, which include ptosis, pupillary constriction, and anhidrosis. Upward gaze is also deficient with this lesion. Trochlear neuritis appears as an inability to rotate the eyeball down and outward. Paralysis of the sixth cranial nerve results in impaired lateral gaze. In each of these cases the primary neuritis can be differentiated from local muscle entrapment by a forced duction of the individual muscles.

Paranasal sinus neuritis. Less than 5% of all headaches are related to paranasal sinusitis, and these painful neuritides are usually accompanied by symptoms of nasal discharge, epistaxis, otalgia, and fullness in the ears.[13] The maxillary sinus is most frequently involved, and tapping over the infraorbital and zygomatic regions elicits a dull aching response. However, the pain may also be referred to the maxillary teeth. The diagnosis of sinusitis is usually confirmed by observing pus in the middle meatus and detecting radiographic air-fluid cloudiness in the sinuses.

Salivary gland and mucosal neuritis. The most common causes of salivary gland neuritis are infection of the glands and obstruction of the ducts by bacterial plugs or sialoliths. In both cases dull pain and pressure sensations are correlated with eating or "milking" the gland.

Mucosal neuritis has many local causes. For example, an intense mucositis with stinging pain may be caused by acute drug idiosyncrasy. An itching neuritis is typical of neuritis from overuse of systemic antibiotics. Galvanism, a result of the presence of adjacent, dissimilar restorative metals, may also result in a burning ulceration.

Odontogenic neuritis. Pulpal disease is the most common cause of dental pain, and in the initial hyperemia phase, pain is often severe and exaggerated in response to stimulation by heat or cold. As pulpal disease progresses, pulpitis pain becomes more spontaneous, sharp, and throbbing because of the inflammation of poorly myelinated nerves in the rigid-walled pulp chambers. As the pulps become necrotic, however, the pain is less intense and is most likely to be elicited by tapping or pressing on the affected tooth because the nerve irritation is now primarily caused by fluid pressures in apical and periapical tissues.

The pain of periodontal disease is usually less intense, dull, and gnawing in character and is without the pulsations that occur with pulpal neuritis. Extension of pericoronitis along adjacent muscle and fascial planes may cause symptoms of neuritis, although the clinical picture in these cases may be dominated by signs of trismus and myofascial spasm. Acute periosteal and alveolar disease may set up referred neuritis such as the preauricular pain that occurs during dry socket in the mandibular third molar region.

CENTRAL DISORDERS

Most central nervous system pathology is vascular in origin, and strokes at many levels of the brain may cause neurological disorder in the maxillofacial region. For example, the frequent occlusion of basilar artery branches interrupts the blood supply to the emerging rootlets of the third to seventh cranial nerves as well as the long sensory and motor tracts that course in the ventral pons. This produces simultaneous neurological deficits in many cranial nerves along with hemiparesis and hemianesthesia, a pattern that helps to differentiate this lesion from more isolated peripheral diseases. The symptoms of intracranial neoplasia vary greatly and also may mimic peripheral disease. Differentiating features, however, include constant progressive headaches, mental deterioration, and spreading seizures. Among the more localized intracranial tumors, the lesions of neurofibromatosis (von Recklinghausen's disease) may involve sensory cranial nerves.[25] The acoustic neuromas often produce secondary pareses of trigeminal and facial nerves by compression. Primary trigeminal tumors are extremely rare.[63] There are other forms of intracranial disease that may present problems in the differentiation of maxillofacial neurological disorder. They include multiple sclerosis, tertiary neurosyphilis, syringobulbia, thalamic syndrome, meningitis, and psychalgia.

Syringobulbia. Syringobulbia is a slowly progressive and degenerative disease of the medulla oblongata that causes a great range of maxillofacial neurological change.[2] The most striking clinical feature is a dissociated sensory loss in which there is a loss of pain and thermal sensibilities with retention of touch. Other classic signs include lingual atrophy, vertigo, palatal paralysis, nystagmus, facial weakness, Horner's syndrome, and especially hoarseness. Although pain and paresthesias are uncommon, there may be spontaneous trigeminal burning and aching that resembles the pain of tabes dorsalis. Men are more often affected, usually before age 30, and after an insidious onset the disease develops rapidly in the first few weeks.

The histopathology of both syringobulbia and the related syringomyelia is a cavitation and gliosis that begins near the central canal of the brain stem or spinal cord and then enlarges ventrally to gradually interrupt the large sensory and motor fiber tracts that cross over in these ventral regions (Fig. 26-3). The cavitations (syringes) most often begin in the cervicothoracic regions (syringomyelia) and cause sensory loss and wasting of small muscles of the head. The cavitation often then spreads rostrally into the medulla (syringobulbia) to involve first the twelfth and tenth cranial nerve nuclei and eventually the other cranial nerve nuclei. The cause is unknown but there are indications that the lesions arise congenitally. The main differential diagnosis in syringobulvia is with multiple sclerosis, poliomyelitis, and tabes dorsalis. There is no satisfactory treatment, and, because of the condition's slow course, preventive physiotherapy and dental care should be actively pursued.

Thalamic syndrome. The thalamic syndrome is a rare pain condition caused by damage to the lateral thalamic nuclei on the side opposite the symptoms.[135] The pains are aching, burning, and gnawing; they spread unilaterally and are felt deeply in wide facial and trunk regions. The threshold for pinprick is raised in this condition, but many types of stimuli, especially deep pressures, will evoke the delayed and inappropriate pain. In this respect the thalamic syndrome resembles the hyperpathia seen in postraumatic neuropathies of the peripheral nerves. The pathogenesis is unknown, but traumatic and vascular lesions that involve diencephalic and cortical tissues have been implicated. This condition must be differentiated from causalgia, peripheral neuromas, and intracranial tumors. Treatment with narcotics is only partially effective, and prefrontal leukotomy may be effective in some cases (Fig. 26-3).

Psychalgia. The incidence of maxillofacial psychalgia, which is pain of mental and truly nonorganic origin, is unknown, but to the patient, it may be severe and real. These pains tend to be vague and nonspecific, shifting over poorly defined nerve distributions, and usually cannot be elicited by specific stimulations. Although pain is the common complaint, hysterical conversions may result in anesthesia, paresthesia, blindness, deafness, and such objective signs as flaccid facial paralysis, tics, dermatological outbreaks, vomiting, and even angioneurotic edema.[74] Symptoms are strongly correlated with emotional stress, and other signs of character disorder or psychosis may be prominent. Almost any form of medical or surgical treatment, even placebo, will yield temporary symptom relief, and these patients will often prescribe their own treatment and even seek multiple deforming surgeries. Because of the high incidence of character disorders related to psychalgia, psychological screening tests such as the Minnesota Multiphasic Personality Index (MMPI) may be helpful. The only effective treatment is psychotherapeutic.[103]

The diagnosis of psychalgia should not be made lightly or as a last resort. It should be recognized that maxillofacial neurological problems, especially pain, are almost always complicated by an emotional component. (See Fig. 26-1.) The identification of even a strong psychological component should not be the signal to abandon the search for and treatment of organic problems. Nor should those patients whose symptoms seem bizarre or even humorous ("crawling, puffing, inside-out") be quickly relegated to the psychalgia category. Facial sensation is a personal matter, and the honest patient may not "feel" his abnormality in textbook terms.

DIAGNOSIS

In the process of making a final diagnosis of maxillofacial neurological problems, the history and examination should lead to a description of four basic disease elements: (1) *symptoms,* (2) *pathology,* (3) *location,* and (4) *etiology* (see following outline).

 I. History
   A. Symptom classification
    1. System
      a. Sensory (pain, numbness, paresthesia)
      b. Motor (weakness, spasm)

c. Autonomic (nasal, ocular, cutaneous, gastric)

d. Special sense (visual, auditory, olfactory, taste)

2. Quality
   a. Strength (mild, moderate, severe)
   b. Onset (spontaneous, induced, triggered)
   c. Duration (momentary, minutes, days, constant, paroxysmal)
   d. Nature (dull, aching, burning, pulsing, sharp, itching)

3. Localization
   a. Precise (V_1, V_2, V_3, VII, IX, other)
   b. Unilateral or bilateral
   c. Migrating, spreading, radiating
   d. Diffuse

4. Influences
   a. Movement or function (face, jaw, body)
   b. Position (head, jaw, body)
   c. Activities (exertion, eating, talking)
   d. Time of day, month, or season

5. Symptom course
   a. Unchanged
   b. Response to therapy (drug, surgery, other)
   c. Changes in character

B. Systemic and environmental factors
   1. Metabolic disorders (anemia, diabetes mellitus, uremia)
   2. Connective tissue disorders (arthritis, scleroderma, lupus erythematosus, Sjögren's syndrome)
   3. Toxicities (heavy metal, organic chemical, food, drug, alcohol)
   4. Nutritional disorders
   5. Infectious disorders (herpes zoster, meningitis, syphilis, leprosy, diphtheria)
   6. Vascular disorders (coronary artery disease, temporal arteritis, Raynaud's syndrome, hypertension)

C. Primary neurological and psychiatric disorders
   1. Neuralgia (trigeminal, vagoglossopharyngeal, intermedius, periodic migrainous)
   2. Migraine
   3. Central disorders (syringobulbia, thalamic syndrome, seizure disorders)
   4. Neuroses (psychalgia)

5. Psychoses
6. Multiple sclerosis

D. Neuritis factors
   1. Maxillofacial trauma (facial fracture, prosthetic irritation, iatrogenic)
   2. Infection (odontogenic, periodontal, facial)
   3. Paranasal sinusitis
   4. Otalgia
   5. Salivary gland disorders (sialolith, adenitis)
   6. Mucosal disorders (mucositis, herpetic ulcers)
   7. Motor neuritides (Bell's palsy, ocular palsies, Horner's syndrome, myesthesia)
   8. Myofascial dysfunction

II. Examination
A. General cerebral function
   1. Consciousness level
   2. Gross movements

B. Cranial nerve function
   1. Motor functions
      a. III, IV, VI (extraocular muscle function)
      b. V (masticator muscle function)
      c. VII (facial muscle function)
      d. IX, X (palatal, pharyngeal, laryngeal function)
      e. XI (sternocleidomastoid, trapezius function)
      f. XII (tongue function)
   2. Somatosensory functions (V, VII, IX nerves)
      a. Pinprick sensitivity
      b. Pressure pain sensitivity
      c. Pulp tester sensitivity
      d. Fine and two-point tactile
      e. Vibratory sensitivity
      f. Hot, cold sensitivity
   3. Special functions
      a. I (smell)
      b. II (vision)
      c. VII, IX (taste)
      d. VIII (hearing)
   4. Autonomic functions
      a. Sympathetic (pupillary dilation, eyelid tone, sweating, vasoconstriction, salivation)
      b. Parasympathetic (pupillary constriction, serous salivation)

C. Special reflexes or tests
   1. Corneal reflex

2. Jaw-jerk
3. Electromyography
4. Nerve conduction studies
5. Minnesota Multiphasic Personality Index
D. Acute maxillofacial neuritis lesions
  1. Odontogenic (caries, periodontal disease)
  2. Osteal-periosteal (cysts, osteomyelitis)
  3. Myofascial
  4. Salivary glandular (ductal obstruction, adenitis)
  5. Mucosal (mucositis)
  6. Paranasal sinus
  7. Vascular
E. Diagnostic blocks
  1. Placebo effects
  2. Vasoconstrictor effects
  3. Anesthetic effects

History

Chief complaint and present illness. Disease symptoms should first be expressed in the patient's own terms and then evaluated by the clinician to determine whether the problem seems to be motor, sensory, autonomic, or a combination and to establish the basic nature, intensity, location, onset, and course of the complaint. At this time a tentative *symptom diagnosis* may be made (such as neuralgia, headache, paralysis, dysesthesia).

Past history. The neurological history should begin with a questioning about systemic disease and environmental conditions that have known neurological effects in the maxillofacial region. Next, patients should be questioned about the past history of major neurological and psychiatric disorders. Once the systemic, environmental, primary neurological, and psychiatric disease factors have been considered, questioning should turn to the incidence and nature of direct lesions in the maxillofacial tissues themselves. On the basis of information gained in the neurological history alone, it may be possible to make a tentative *pathology diagnosis* (such as infectious, degenerative, arteritic, or demyelinating) or an *etiology diagnosis* (such as posttraumatic, odontogenic, psychogenic, or diabetic).

Examination

Major goals of the examination for maxillofacial neurological disorders should be detection of acute lesion sources of neuritis within the tissues and location of the disease process and site of pathology. The disease is located by examining first the general and then the more specific functions. The examination should begin with an observation of cerebral functions such as level of consciousness and gross movements and continue with a study of specific cranial nerve reflex functions. In addition to the classic techniques of inspection, tissue palpation, and reflex stimulation, the diagnostician may benefit from the use of special tests such as electromyography, nerve conduction studies, EEG, and lumbar puncture. Personality screening such as the MMPI can also be done at this time. Finally, a detailed search for specific and local sources of acute neuritis should be done, using all routine dental diagnostic skills and aids such as inspection, palpation, radiography, and electrodiagnosis.

Diagnostic nerve blocks

A simple and most revealing technique for locating and characterizing neurological lesions is the diagnostic block. The level of a particular lesion may be determined by depositing small amounts of local anesthetic solution, first at the most superficial nerve levels and then at progressively more central levels. After each injection the patient should be carefully questioned regarding change of symptoms, especially in response to direct stimulation of trigger points or sensitive tissues. These blocks may lead directly to a localization diagnosis. For example, blocks of the sphenopalatine ganglion by injecting deeply within the descending palatine canal may be diagnostic for periodic migrainous neuralgia. Diagnostic blocks are also helpful in differentiating between the precise superficial trigger zones of classic neuralgias and the deeper, more diffuse loci of neuritides and neuropathies. Diagnostic nerve blocks may also define for the clinician the specific type of nerve fiber that is initiating the pain response.[136] A rigid protocol is recommended in which placebo (saline) nerve block is injected in the region of pain complaint. Relief of pain with placebo for more than a few minutes suggests a possible psychogenic basis for the pain. If pain persists, however, a second injection should be made with 0.25% procaine or lidocaine. Relief of pain after this injection indicates that pain is initiated by small, nociceptor fibers or autonomic fibers and therapy should be pointed toward correcting this neuropathy. If pain is still persistent after the second, small-fiber nerve block, then a final block of both small and large fibers should be given, using 1% to 2% procaine or lidocaine. Pain relief after this block indicates larger fiber mediation of pain reflexes, commonly seen in myofascial pain syndromes. If pain is unrelieved, even after total nerve block, a central nervous system lesion or a psychogenic basis for pain or both should be suspected.

• • •

In summary, when the neurological history and examination of a patient with a maxillofacial neurological disorder has been completed, a differential diagnosis can be developed (Table 26-1). In each case, the four key elements of the diagnosis should have been investigated. A sample, all-inclusive diagnosis would be posttraumatic neuralgia associated with infraorbital neuroma (etiology, symptom, location, and pathology).

TREATMENT

Because nervous tissues often do not withstand or recover completely from repeated insults by infection, inflammation, metabolic toxicity, and especially trauma, preventive treatment should begin by removing sources of acute neuritis and bar-

riers to nerve regeneration. It is also clear that neurological problems of the maxillofacial region are varied, since they encompass motor, autonomic, and sensory systems along with the diverse components of pain (Fig. 26-1). Effective treatment therefore must have a similar broad base of medicine, surgery, physiotherapy, and psychotherapy.

Medical treatments

Analgesics. The type of analgesic selected for pain control is determined by the severity and the nature of symptoms as well as the location of the neurological lesion. Mild, chronic neuritis caused by inflammation in the skin, mucosa, and joints or when vasculitis and edema are present are best managed by mild analgesics, such as salicylates, propoxyphene, or para-aminophenols, for which the suspected site of action is in the peripheral tissue and paravascular receptors.[103] Potent analgesics such as narcotics, narcotic antagonists, and synthetic agents such as pentazocine are indicated for more severe pain when the suffering and the affect component of pain are predominant. Because these agents seem to act in subcortical, reticular, and limbic cortex regions, they are more effective against more diffuse and central pains such as visceral and periosteal pains, nerve invasions by carcinoma, neuropathies, syringobulbia, and the thalamic syndrome. However, not even the most potent narcotics are effective in the relief of true paroxysmal pain such as trigeminal, intermedius, or vagoglossopharyngeal neuralgias. They are of marginal value in postherpetic pain, migraine, posttraumatic neuralgias, tabes dorsalis, and periodic migrainous neuralgia. Because of the potential for addiction, chronic pain syndromes should not be managed solely by narcotic analgesics.

A number of studies have now shown that the timing and approach to an analgesic drug may be more important than the particular type of analgesia used.[9,41,118] When analgesics are used for acute or postoperative pain they are most effective when used frequently, in small doses, and early in the pain cycle on an "as needed" basis. In chronic pain syndromes, however, the "as needed" approach should be replaced by a strict "time contingency" schedule of drug use. In this manner a reasonable blood level of analgesic is maintained, and patients take medication "by the clock" rather than "as they feel." In this manner cyclical pain phenomena are more likely to be controlled and problems of drug habituation or addiction are minimized.[9,42]

Anticonvulsants. Based on the concept that many paroxysmal pains are produced by the epileptiform mechanism (Fig. 26-3), anticonvulsant agents have proved effective in the treatment of severe neuralgia. Phenytoin (Dilantin), administered in doses of 100 mg four times daily, has controlled the pain of idiopathic trigeminal neuralgia in approximately 50% of cases.[10] Although phenytoin has been a safe agent for chronic use, it has not been as effective in the later stages of the neuralgia. It is known to act on peripheral nerve transmission and by a depression of brain stem trigeminal nuclei function. However, within the last 5 years the anticonvulsant drug of choice for severe neuralgia states has become carbamazepine. This agent acts similarly to phenytoin as a depressant of peripheral nerve transmission but has a more potent effect on polysynaptic systems in the trigeminal descending tract in the medulla and ultimately in the thalamic nuclei related to head and neck pain transmission.

In a large number of clinical series, carbamazepine administered in doses of 200 to 800 mg daily has been effective in controlling tic douloureux in 85% to 100% of cases.[107] This drug has also been useful in the control of intermedius, vagoglossopharyngeal, multiple sclerosis, and posttraumatic neuralgias. However, it has been less than 50% effective in postherpetic neuralgia, phantom pain, and periodic migrainous neuralgia.

Side effects including slight sedation, dizziness, nausea, and occasional rash are seen with carbamazepine. Although the incidence of complications is low, agranulocytosis, thrombocytopenia, and trigeminal paresthesias have been reported in approximately 7% of cases; these toxic effects seem to be most prominent in older, debilitated patients. In spite of promising results reported with carbamazepine, trigeminal neuralgia pain returns in approximately 10% of patients.

Systemic vasoconstrictors and antihistamines. Classic migraine and other vascular headaches have been managed by ergotamine tartrate, which is known to counteract directly the painful dilation of craniofacial arteries. Methysergide preparations, which may act as a serotonin and histamine antagonist, have also been effective in as many as two thirds of cases of periodic migrainous neuralgia.[38] Recent clinical studies have also shown that the beta-adrenergic blocking agent Propanolol (Inderal) is effective in relieving vascular facial pain disorders.[30] The usual trial dosage is 40 mg given three times daily.

Corticosteroids. Agents such as ACTH and adrenal corticosteroids are indicated when the neurological disorder is a result either directly or indirectly of inflammation. They may be helpful in the early stages of seventh nerve neuritis (Bell's palsy) to prevent degeneration of the nerve trunk within the facial canal.[130] Steroids may also be indirectly effective in preventing further degeneration when vasculitis is a factor, such as in connective tissue diseases, diabetic neuropathy, and temporal arteritis.

Tranquilizers. Minor tranquilizers such as the benzodiazapines (Valium, Librium) have no direct analgesic effects but may be helpful as an adjunct in the overall management of chronic pain in which the affect is a strong pain component. They may also be useful in relieving the acute stages of tension headaches and myofascial pain dysfunction because of the indirect skeletal muscle relaxation effects of these agents.

Antidepressant and psychotropic drugs. Because of the nearly universal association of chronic pain and emotional disorder, antidepressant and major tranquilizer drugs are necessary and effective treatment for many patients. Many studies have documented the therapeutic value of tricyclic antidepressants given for depression-related chronic pain, especially myofascial pain disorders.[9,44] This class of drugs is contraindicated in patients with significant cardiovascular disease and in patients with latent schizophrenia. Primary agents that have proved effective are amitriptyline, imipramine, and doxepin given in dose ranges of 75 to 150 mg daily for 4 to 6 months.[8]

In more severe forms of psychopathology, in which facial pain may represent a conversion hysteria or a ''mask'' for psychosis, major tranquilizers such as chlorpromazine (Thorazine) or fluphenazine (Prolixin) have been effective.[126,127]

Surgical control of maxillofacial pain

In the surgical control of maxillofacial pain, manipulations are made at four main levels of the sensory nervous pathway: (1) the peripheral nerves, (2) the sensory ganglia and their roots, (3) the brain stem, and (4) the thalamus-cortex (Fig. 26-4). Surgery can be performed by using decompression, simple nerve section, selective thermal lesions, cautery, cryosurgery, and mechanical and chemical necrosis.

Formerly, the objective of most of these techniques was denervation of the pain regions. Although rapidly effective in relieving pain in many cases, denervation, rhizotomy, and tractotomy surgeries also have the potential to result in secondary neuroma formations, causalgia, anesthesia dolorosa, and phantom pains. Recent years, therefore, have seen the emergence of less destructive and more selective thermal lesions and decompression procedures for the control of pain.

Treatment of nerve injuries. Although injuries to nerves often cannot be prevented, it is possible to decrease the incidence and severity of clinical problems by taking steps to avoid aberrant regeneration (see section on histopathology). For example, a major hindrance to proper regeneration is secondary irritation to injured nerves. Therefore, attempts should be made to avoid nerve compressions from sources such as displaced root tips, fragments of alveolar bone, or prosthetic devices that impinge on nerve branches. After facial fracture the nerves should be protected from entrapment by malplaced bone segments, irritation from transosseous wires, and shearing effects caused by mobile fractures. Other steps in the treatment of nerve injuries are encouragement of the regeneration of nerve fibers into their appropriate distal tissues and prevention of the formation of barriers to regeneration such as scar tissue.

Severed nerves that can be directly exposed should be sutured immediately by first cutting back in both the proximal and distal nerve stumps until a symmetrical cross section of nerve is obtained that bleeds freely. Then the perineural sheaths of both prepared nerve cylinders are engaged by fine linen (No. 10-0 Tevdek) or wire suture, with the two ends oriented properly to one another, while the remaining nerve circumference is sutured.[54] To protect the repair site further from the ingrowth of foreign scar tissue, it is recommended that the nerve be wrapped in Millipore filter.[88] The repaired nerve should then be stabilized by suturing it loosely into adjacent soft tissues. Although the optimum time for nerve suture is usually at the time of acute injury, if the wound has been grossly contaminated with significant tissue loss, it may be advisable to label the cut nerve ends with sutures and delay the nerve repair at least 10 days. When there has been no evidence of returning nerve function within 4 to 6 weeks after injury, it is advisable to explore the injury site. The objectives of this exploration are to decompress the nerve by evacuating hematoma, removing impinging bone fragments or foreign bodies, and resecting the neuroma segments and, finally, to rejoin the nerve segments using the suture techniques just described.

The prognosis of good function returning after nerve injury is less when motor nerves have been injured and when long segments of nerve have been lost. Although nerve grafting has been used successfully in the maxillofacial region to repair large nerve deficits, little is known at this time about the ideal conditions and the prognosis of this procedure.[83] In all cases of nerve damage, it is important to protect and maintain the nonneurological tissues that have been denervated to assure their maximum function when regeneration does occur.

Therapeutic anesthetic blocks. Blocks of peripheral nerve, myofascial, or neurovascular trigger zones by anesthetic agents are of considerable value in managing pain syndromes.[14] They have value as diagnostic aids as outlined previously. They are also useful as a palliative procedure to achieve instant relief for a suffering patient and to "buy time" for the clinician to establish more definitive therapy or to make a more thorough diagnosis. Palliative blocks with long-acting anesthetics such as 0.5% bupivacaine with epinephrine, for example, may be given daily or at longer intervals to control acute triggered paroxysms of trigeminal neuralgia while effective levels of anticonvulsant drugs are being attained.

Nerve blocks have prognostic value. They may indicate whether permanent denervation or neurolysis would be effective and whether a given patient can tolerate paresthesias during everyday functions. Blocks may also be used in therapy, particularly for pain disorders of a cyclical nature in which remissions are common such as the major neuralgias, posttraumatic pain, and certain myofascial pain syndromes. Using anesthetic blocks for therapy is highly controversial because it is seen as strictly symptomatic (and not curative) treatment and because no scientific basis has been established for its effectiveness. Neverthe-

less, anesthetic blocks given for a wide variety of pain syndromes in many body parts have repeatedly brought pain relief for longer than the known pharmacologic action of the drug itself.[14,17] Blocks are given at 48-hour to weekly intervals into nerve distributions and particularly into zones of previous trauma and neural or muscular trigger foci.

Peripheral denervation. The objectives of peripheral denervation are to give prompt and sustained relief from severe pain, either as a temporary palliative measure or to avoid the hazards of radical craniotomy procedures. It is indicated in old and debilitated patients, in cases in which the first and second divisions of the trigeminal system are involved, in neuralgias with a greater likelihood of bilateral pain such as multiple sclerosis and carcinoma, and in retarded patients who cannot cooperate to the extent needed to perform more conservative neurolysis. It is especially indicated for the patient with short life expectancy resulting from painful invasive cancers. Interruption of the peripheral nerves may be brought about by injecting a 95% solution of ethanol into the affected nerve branch or by surgical exposure and sectioning of the branch. Although both techniques effectively bring about wallerian degeneration of the peripheral branches, the direct severance techniques may be preferred to alcohol injections because they are more precise and because repetitive neurectomies are more easily done.[105] The specific objectives of peripheral neurectomy are to eliminate as much as possible of the affected nerve branch and also to attempt to block its regeneration. Therefore, after the nerve has been exposed and before it is cut, dissection should be carried distally into the terminal tissues as far as possible. Proximally the maximum amount of nerve tissue should be avulsed by rolling the nerve around a hemostat. Finally, the nerve foramen should be obliterated with sterile wooden pegs, amalgam, or bone plugs to block further nerve regeneration.

In the third trigeminal division, inferior alveolar and lingual nerves are commonly resected (Fig. 26-5). The lingual nerve can most easily be exposed at the inner surface of the mandible in the third molar region by making a vertical incision along the internal oblique ridge. This same incision can be used to approach and cut the inferior alveolar nerve at the mandibular foramen (Fig. 26-5, *A*). However, an extraoral approach to inferior alveolar resection is simpler and has the advantages of avoiding damage to the lingual nerve and permitting direct obliteration of the mandibular canal (Fig. 26-5, *B*). In this procedure, a 1-cm incision is made at the inferior border of the mandible in the antegonial notch region. Dissection is carried directly to bone, and, by use of a nasal speculum to retract the masseter, the outline of the mandibular canal can be seen with the aid of intraoral transillumination. The lateral bony plate of

the canal is removed, the nerve is avulsed, and the canal is finally obliterated. When this procedure has been combined with mental nerve resection (Fig. 26-5, *C*), the entire intramandibular length of the inferior alveolar nerve can often be removed intact.

Most clinicians prefer the intraoral approach for infraorbital neurectomy (Fig. 26-5, *D*). Both the superior labial and lateral nasal branches of the nerve should be dissected free, and then the infraorbital foramen can be clearly visualized. After avulsion, canal obliteration, and suture, a firm pressure should be maintained over the infraorbital region for at least an hour to prevent the profuse bleeding that may follow this procedure.

Branches of the first trigeminal division, including the supraorbital, frontal, and supratrochlear nerves, may be exposed through an incision in the midportion of the unshaven eyebrow (Fig. 26-5, *E*). Care

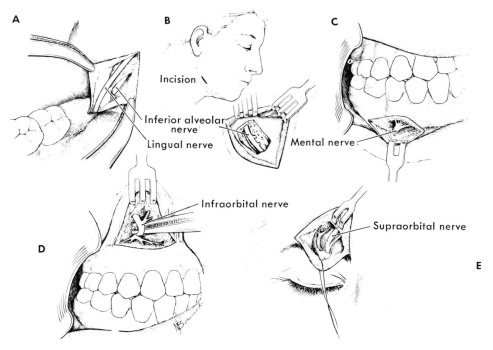

Fig. 26-5. Techniques of maxillofacial neurectomy.

should be taken to avoid damaging the lacrimal gland in the lateral roof of the orbit.

Peripheral neurectomies are minor operations that may be performed comfortably with local anesthesia and sedation since there is little risk even in elderly or debilitated patients. This operation may be completely effective in some cases, especially if repetitive neurectomies are done, and over 60% of patients can expect to be pain free for 4 years after neurectomies have been started. However, pain usually does recur slowly as axonal regeneration takes place, and because neurectomies may serve to delay an inevitable radical treatment, it is important that cases be selected carefully.

Selective thermal lesions. In the past 5 years the surgical treatment of choice for paroxysmal trigeminal neuralgias has become radiofrequency (RF) thermal lesions performed most often at the level of the trigeminal ganglion and sensory root.[79] Pre-

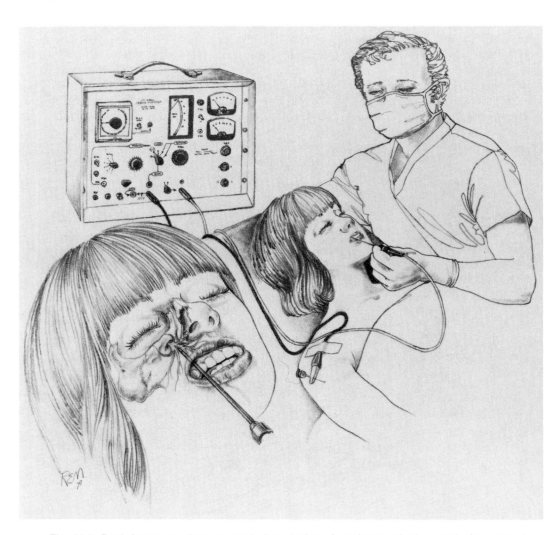

Fig. 26-6. Radiofrequency thermoneurolysis technique for microsurgical control of neurological-based trigeminal pain. (From Gregg, J. M., Banerjee, T., Ghia, J. N., and Campbell, R.: Radiofrequency thermoneurolysis of peripheral nerves for control of trigeminal neuralgia, Pain **5**:231-243, 1978.)

liminary research had shown that RF thermal lesions of 60° to 70° C, when applied to peripheral nerves, have the effect of selectively destroying small nerve fibers but at the same time retaining the larger nerve fibers.[75] In clinical application, this has had the effect of eliminating abnormal pain and triggering functions yet preserving normal tactile sensation for the patient. It therefore represents a major improvement over previous neurectomy or alcohol or rhizotomy lesions, which produced a disturbing total loss of sensory function.

In the most common RF *thermoganglionolysis* technique a 22-gauge needle, insulated except at its tip, is inserted through the skin of the cheek, passed medial to the mandibular ramus and through the foramen ovale to come to rest at the ventral aspect of the trigeminal ganglion in Meckel's cavity.[122] After fluoroscopic checking of location, the patient, still awake, is given a mild electrical stimulus through the needle tip to elicit paresthesias and determine whether the needle is in the proper position for nerve lesion. When this is assured, a general anesthetic or deep sedative is given to the patient and one or two thermal lesions of 60° to 70° C are made for 30 seconds each. Results of these lesions have been very good, with a high control rate of pain, minimal complication, and a pain recurrence rate of approximately 20% per year.[79]

Recently, RF lesions of more peripheral nerves, including occipital, inferior alveolar, infraorbital, and supraorbital branches, have produced very good results (Fig. 26-6).[12,52] In these techniques the same basic approach is used as described previously except that the lesions can be made in the outpatient setting, general anesthesia is not required, there are no risks of damaging vital intracranial structures, and lesions can be repeated more easily if necessary. The selective thermal lesions may, in the near future, open a new era in less destructive surgeries for controlling neuropathic pain, replacing in part the pharmacological approaches.

Craniotomy procedures. The most precise lesions of the sensory ganglia and root tissues are made by means of direct craniotomies. With these techniques, a simple incision of the dural sleeve that surrounds the ganglia and sensory roots is made, followed by a gentle freeing and manipulation of the ganglion and its roots. For unknown reasons, this manipulation alone has the surprising effect of pain elimination with retention of tactile and proprioceptive senses.[123]

More recently, a major modification has been made in decompression procedures at the level of the trigeminal sensory root.[62] In this operation, using a posterior fossa approach, the superior cerebellar arteries are elevated away from the sensory root and a Teflon sponge barrier is placed between the root and the vessels. This operation has proven highly effective in a large series of cases of neuralgia. However, the long-term recurrence rate of these central decompressions is not known.

The most definitive technique for eliminating severe pain, such as tic douloureux, continues to be the retrogasserian rhizotomy[66] (Fig. 26-4). With this technique, the sensory root fibers are selectively lesioned at some point between the ganglion and its point of root entrance into the pons. Rhizotomy is most often accomplished by a temporal approach to the middle cranial fossa, although a more hazardous posterior fossal approach is also effective. Root fibers are selectively lesioned by cutting, electrocoagulation, or cryosurgery, which results in a complete and permanent degeneration of nerve cell bodies and their centrally projecting fibers. In spite of the apparent permanence of this procedure, there is a neuralgia recurrence rate of 13% to 15% that may be a result of either incomplete nerve lesion or the action of aberrant sensory fibers in the motor trigeminal root.[135] This operation may be complicated by painful herpes zoster lesions, corneal ulcerations, a variety of trophic lesions, and the painful anesthesia dolorosa paresthesias. In addition to neuralgia associated with the trigeminal nerve, rhizotomy is also indicated for controlling intermedius and vagoglossopharyngeal neuralgia, periodic migrainous neuralgia, and uncontrolled neoplasms of the head and neck. Rhizotomy procedures, although useful in selected cases, have largely been replaced by the more conservative radiofrequency and decompression techniques described previously.

Tractotomy procedures. The primary descending tracts of trigeminal, as well as eighth, ninth, and tenth nerve sensory fibers, may be interrupted by lesions placed 4 mm below the obex in the medulla[135] (Fig. 26-4). A desirable sensory dissociation often results from this operation, in which tactile senses are retained but pain sensitivity is lost. It is especially indicated when pain is bilateral or when many cranial nerves are involved simultaneously. However, medullary tractotomy has a significantly higher mortality than rhizotomy, and it has been found that pain may recur in as many as 50% of patients within 1 year of the operation.[135]

Tractotomy may also be performed at the level of the pons or midbrain to control maxillofacial pains such as postherpetic neuralgia (Fig. 26-4). However, none of the tractotomy procedures described here have been effective in eliminating the suffering or affect component of pain (Fig. 26-1). Therefore these once highly regarded procedures have gradually come into limited use in the past decade and have given way to either rhizotomy or to surgical lesions made in the thalamus or cortex.

Thalamotomy and cortical leukotomy procedures. Selective lesions in the thalamus and cortex are the only known surgical treatments for most varieties of central pain such as phantom pain, thalamic syndrome, tabes dorsalis, and postherpetic facial neuralgia[133] (Fig. 26-4). Lesions of the posterior medial thalamus are made by RF electrodes that are left implanted for a period of time to allow repetitive enlargement of the original lesion, thus adapting the lesion size to

compensate for spreading of the pain disease.[20]

Cortical leukotomy consists of white matter lesions of the frontal lobes and has the interesting result of decreasing the suffering or emotional component of pain without causing any significant change in the perception thresholds. Patients do not complain of pain spontaneously but will describe the painful stimulus in great detail if questioned about it. It is for this reason that this technique is indicated when fear and suffering are prominent features of the disease, which is often the case in patients with malignant tumors of the oral and pharyngeal regions; their pain is accompanied by fear of suffocation and exsanguination. An important danger with leukotomy procedures is the potential to induce significant personality defects and loss of "social senses." For this reason these procedures are usually reserved for cases of central suffering pain that cannot be managed by peripheral neurectomy, sensory rhizotomy, or medical psychiatric therapy.

New approaches to treatment

Even though current medical and surgical techniques are effective for many neurological problems, many of these approaches afford only partial or temporary control, and often the available techniques, such as central nervous system surgery, are too drastic to be applied to the numerous milder syndromes found in the maxillofacial region. The side effects of traditional therapies may be more troublesome than the original disease problems. For these reasons there is a continuing search for new treatments of neurological disorders, especially for chronic, idiopathic pain conditions.

Physiological inhibition of pain. The use of physiological counterstimulation to inhibit chronic pathological pain grew out of the gate control concept of pain threshold. The earliest applications included the technique of dorsal column stimulation in which subcutaneous electrical transmitters have brought about pain relief in over half the cases of chronic back pain as well as in difficult cases of phantom limb pain and pain from invasive carcinoma.[92] Daily stimulation by similar transmitter-electrode systems that have been placed adjacent to the trigeminal rootlets has also proved effective in relieving paroxysmal pains.[113] Even peripheral nerve stimulations have shown promise by use of this technique. For example, low-voltage RF waves have been passed through the surface and needle electrodes that were implanted into the infraorbital, lingual, and auriculotemporal nerves of patients with idiopathic trigeminal neuralgia.[121]

Transcutaneous neural stimulation. The most widely used and effective stimulation approach, however, is transcutaneous neural stimulation (TNS). With TNS, cutaneous bipolar surface electrodes are placed in the painful body regions and low-voltage electrical currents are administered by the patient.[80] Best results have been obtained when intense stimulation is maintained for at least an hour daily for more than 3 weeks. TNS portable units are in widespread use in pain clinics throughout the world, and TNS has proved most effective against neuropathic pain such as phantom limb pain and nerve injury pain. It has been effective in a smaller percentage of patients with facial pain but, when successful, is an excellent noninvasive treatment.[51]

Acupuncture. Serious consideration must now be given to acupuncture as a physiological parapsychological approach to pain control and neurological treatment. Acupuncture theory is based on an invisible system of communication between various organs of the body that is distinct from the circulatory, nervous, and endocrine systems known to Western medicine. The few objective reports and available statistics are impressive. In one series, surgical anesthesia by acupuncture was "successful" in 90% of 1,500 patients undergoing a wide variety of operations, including thoracotomy, orthopedic procedures, and craniotomy for

brain tumor.[30] Thyroidectomy has been performed on 504 consecutive cases with an anesthesia success rate of 98%. As a surgical anesthetic technique acupuncture has the advantage of convenience, great safety, stability of vital functions, no interruptions of patient hydration, no nausea or vomiting, and no postoperative respiratory complications. Pathological pains have also been controlled in cases of appendicitis, peptic ulcer, hepatic abscess, and renal biliary colic, and toothaches have been completely relieved by needling at the dorsum of the wrist (the "hoku" point).[82]

In the technique of acupuncture, slender needles of any metal type are twirled and moved vertically over selected points of more than 800 acupuncture sites. Recently the need for hand needling has been eliminated by attaching phasic electrical currents of 6 to 9 V at 105 cpm to the needles. In some cases, drugs such as morphine have been injected at the needle sites, and most patients receive small amounts of intravenous meperidine.

Patients apparently sense a "numbness, distension, heaviness and hotness" at specific sites in addition to a generalized raising of the thresholds of pain.[82] Other remarkable physical effects include increased circulation time and transient leukocytosis. In experimental animals, profound shock has been reversed and sleep EEG patterns have been induced by needling.[30]

The reason why each of the stimulation techniques is effective in reducing pain is still not clear, although two mechanisms are most likely.[45] First, stimulation may selectively amplify the large inhibitory nerve fibers and suppress the effects of small fibers. Second, stimulation may act indirectly through the opiate receptor–descending control system (Fig. 26-1). Objective evidence of this latter mechanism has come from recent experiments when analgesia induced in experimental animals with either TNS or acupuncture was reversed when the animals were given the narcotic antagonist, naloxone.[84]

Psychological approaches

Significant control over pain and other sensory complaints may be gained through psychophysiological techniques such as relaxation therapy, biofeedback, hypnosis, and psychotherapy.[85,118]

Many of the chronic, episodic pain syndromes such as myofascial pain dysfunction, vascular headaches, and atypical burning mucosa are known to be markedly influenced by the patient's response to stress. The techniques of *progressive relaxation* originally developed by Jacobson and the related techniques of *autogenic biofeedback* are now gaining wide acceptance as pain therapies.[42,86] Biofeedback techniques have been especially useful for the pain of migraine and other vascular headaches in which the patient is trained to control cranial vascular dilation through a technique of hand temperature control.[89] The widest use of biofeedback has been in the control of painful muscle spasms, however, using electromyogram (EMG) feedback.[19,32] In these techniques, microvoltage signals from muscles such as the frontal or the masseter are used to train the patient in reducing tension and relieving muscle tenseness, clenching, bruxism, and other pain-producing habits. Hypnosis is another paraphysiological technique with primary action on pain tolerance thresholds that holds promise for the control of chronic facial pains.[112] Carefully selected patients may, with training in autosuggestion, come to effectively deny or accept their pain.

Much of the psychological management of patients with neurological problems, especially pain, must be directed toward prevention. Curable pain should be relieved promptly and not allowed to become chronic because pain that persists longer than 6 months in a neurotic individual often becomes too valuable in interpersonal relations to give up easily. Because there is known to be a higher incidence of maxillofacial pain in paranoic and psychopathic deviates, the clinician should remain alert for signs of personality disorders. In consultation with a clinical psychologist or psychiatrist, patients with susceptible personalities can be identified, often with the help of screening techniques such as the MMPI. Patients must not be allowed to become overly dependent on a given therapist. Demands for repetitive or irrelevant treatments should be tactfully opposed. It is often helpful to discuss openly with patients the nearly universal role of psychological components in neurological problems, especially in pain disorders, so that counseling and psychotherapy can be included in the overall treatment.

SUMMARY

It is obvious that maxillofacial neurological problems require a wide range of professional expertise. Future treatment may rely heavily on referral centers, computer-assisted diagnostic services, and multidisciplinary pain clinics to meet the challenges in this field. The dental clinician has an important role in developing and using these new approaches to manage maxillofacial pain.

REFERENCES

1. Aguayo, A. J., Nair, P. V., and Bray, G. M.: Peripheral nerve abnormalities in the Riley-Day syndrome, Arch. Neurol. **24:**106, 1971.
2. Anderson, L. S., Black, R. G., Abraham, J., and Ward, A. A.: Neuronal hyperactivity in experimental trigeminal deafferentation, J. Neurosurg. **35:**444, 1971.
3. Appleby, A., Foster, J. B., Hankinson, J., and Hudgson, P.: The diagnosis and management of the Chiari anomalies in adult life, Brain **91:**131, 1968.
4. Ashworth, B., and Tait, G. B. W.: Trigeminal neuropathy in connective tissue disease, Neurology **21:**609, 1971.
5. Beaver, D. L.: Electron microscopy of the gasserian ganglion in trigeminal neuralgia, J. Neurosurg. **26**(Suppl.):138, 1967.
6. Beerman, H., Nicholas, L., Schamberg, I. L., and Greenberg, M. S.: Syphilis: review of the recent literature, Arch. Intern. Med. **109:**323, 1962.
7. Beighton, P., Gumpel, J. M., and Cornes, N. G.: Prodromal trigeminal sensory neuropathy in progressive systemic sclerosis, Ann. Rheum. Dis. **27:**367, 1968.

8. Berger, F. M.: Depression and antidepressant drugs, Clin. Pharmacol. Ther. **18:**241, 1975.

9. Black, R. G.: The chronic pain syndrome, Surg. Clin. North Am. **55:**999, 1975.

10. Blom, S.: Tic douloureux treated with a new anticonvulsant, Arch. Neurol. **9:**285, 1963.

11. Bloom, F., Segal, D., Ling. N., and Guillemin, R.: Endorphins: profound behavioral effects in rats suggest new etiological factors in mental illness, Science **194:**630, 1976.

12. Blume, H. G.: Radiofrequency denaturation in occipital pain: a new approach in 114 cases, Adv. Pain Res. Ther. **1:**691, 1976.

13. Boles, R.: Paranasal sinuses and facial pain. In Alling, C. C., editor: Facial pain, Philadelphia, 1968, Lea & Febiger.

14. Bonica, J. J.: Clinical applications of diagnostic and therapeutic nerve blocks, Springfield, Ill., 1959, Charles C Thomas, Publisher.

15. Bonnette, G. H., and Arentz, R. E.: Raynaud's disease and extraction wound healing, J. Oral Surg. **26:**185, 1968.

16. Bowsher, D., Mallert, A., Petit, D., and others: A bulbar relay to the centre median, J. Neurophysiol. **31:**288, 1968.

17. Brena, S.: Current status of regional analgesia for diagnosis and therapy, Clin. Anesth. **2:**167, 1969.

18. Browne, R. C.: Metallic poisons and the nervous system, Lancet **1:**775, 1955.

19. Budzynski, T. H., and Stoyva, J. M.: An electromyographic feedback technique for teaching voluntary relaxation of the masseter muscle, J. Dent. Res. **52:**116, 1973.

20. Carr, E. M.: Chronically implantable radiofrequency electrode for lesion production, J. Neurosurg. **35:**495, 1971.

21. Casey, K. L.: Pain: a current view of neural mechanisms, Am. Sci. **61:**194, 1973.

22. Casey, K. L., and Melzack, R.: Neural mechanisms of pain: a conceptual model. In Way, E. D., editor: New concepts in pain and its clinical management, Oxford, 1967, Blackwell Scientific Publications, Ltd.

23. Cavanagh, J. B.: The toxic effects of tri-ortho-cresyl-phosphate on the nervous system, J. Neurol. Neurosurg. Psychiatry **17:**163, 1954.

24. Crabtree, J. A.: Facial nerve decompression, Arch. Otolaryngol. **95:**395, 1972.

25. Crowe, F. W., Schull, W. J., and Neel, J. V.: Multiple neurofibromatosis, Springfield, Ill., 1956, Charles C Thomas, Publisher.

26. Daly, R. F.: New observations regarding the auriculotemporal syndrome, Neurology **17:**1159, 1967.

27. Darian-Smith, I.: Presynaptic component in the afferent inhibition observed within trigeminal brain-stem nuclei of the cat, J. Neurophysiol. **28:**695, 1965.

28. Das, A. K., and Laskin, D. M.: Temporal arteritis of the facial artery, J. Oral Surg. **24:**226, 1966.

29. Dastur, D. K.: The peripheral neuropathology of leprosy. In Antia, N. H., and Dastur, D. K., editors: Symposium on leprosy, Bombay, 1967.

30. Diamond, S., and Medina, J. L.: Double blind study of propanolol for migraine prophylaxis, Headache **16:**24, 1976.

31. Dimond, E. G.: Acupuncture anesthesia; Western medicine and Chinese traditional medicine, J.A.M.A. **218:**1558, 1971.

32. Dohrmann, R. J., and Laskin, D. M.: An evaluation of electromyographic biofeedback in the treatment of myofascial pain-dysfunction syndrome, J. Am. Dent. Assoc. **96:**656, 1978.

33. Doupe, J., Cullen, C. H., and Chance, G. O.: Post-traumatic pain and the causalgic syndrome, J. Neurol. Neurosurg. Psychiatry **7:**33, 1944.

34. Drachman, D. B.: Is acetylcholine the trophic neuromuscular transmitter? Arch. Neurol. **17:**206, 1967.

35. Dubner, R., and Sessle, B. J.: Presynaptic modification of corticofugal fibers participating in feedback loop between trigeminal brain-stem nucleic and sensorimotor cortex. In Dubner, R., and Kawamura, Y., editors: Oral-facial sensory and motor mechanisms, New York, 1971, Appleton-Century-Crofts.

36. Eagle, W. W.: Elongated styloid process; symptoms and treatment, Arch. Otolaryngol. **67:**172, 1958.

37. Eggleston, D. J., and Haskell, R.: Idiopathic trigeminal sensory neuropathy, Practitioner **208:**649, 1972.

38. Ekbom, K., and Olivarius, B. F.: Chronic migrainous neuralgia-diagnostic and therapeutic aspects, Headache **11:**97, 1971.

39. Elfenbaum, A.: Causalgia in dentistry: an abandoned pain syndrome, Oral Surg. **7:**594, 1954.

40. Fisher, C. M., and Adams, R. D.: Diphtheritic polyneuritis: a pathological study, J. Neuropathol. Exp. Neurol. **15:**243, 1956.

41. Fordyce, W. E.: An operant conditioning method for managing chronic pain, Postgrad. Med. **53:**123, 1973.

42. Fowler, R. S.: Operant therapy for headaches, Headache **15:**63, 1975.

43. Gabbiani, G.: Action of cadmium chloride on sensory ganglia, Experientia **22:**261, 1966.

44. Gessel, A. H.: Electromyographic biofeedback and tricyclic antidepressants in myofascial pain-dysfunction syndrome: psychological predictors of outcome, J. Am. Dent. Assoc. **91:**1048, 1975.

45. Ghia, J. N., Mao, W., Toomey, T. C., and Gregg, J. M.: Acupuncture and chronic pain mechanisms, Pain **2:**285, 1976.

46. Goldstein, A.: Opioid peptides (endorphins) in pituitary and brain, Science **193:**1081, 1976.

47. Goldstein, N. P., Gibilisco, J. A., and Rushton, J.

G.: Trigeminal neuropathy and neuritis, J.A.MA. **184:**458, 1963.

48. Good, A. E., Christopher, R. P., and Koepke, G. H.: Peripheral neuropathy associated with rheumatoid arthritis, Ann. Intern. Med. **63:**87, 1965.

49. Granit, R., Leskell, L., and Skoglund, C. R.: Fibre interaction in injured or compressed region of nerve, Brain **67:**125, 1944.

50. Gregg, J. M.: Functional anatomy of facial pain. In Alling, C. C., and Mahan, P., editors: Facial pain, Philadelphia, 1977, J. B. Lippincott Co.

51. Gregg, J. M.: Post-traumatic trigeminal neuralgia: response to physiologic, surgical and pharmacologic therapies, Int. Dent. J. **23:**43, 1978.

52. Gregg, J. M., Banerjee, T., Ghia, J. N., and Campbell, R.: Radiofrequency thermoneurolysis of peripheral nerves for control of trigeminal neuralgia, Pain, in press, 1978.

53. Guillemin, R., and others: Beta-endorphin and adrenocorticotropin are secreted concomitantly by the pituitary gland, Science **197:**1367, 1977.

54. Hausamen, J. E., Samii, M., and Schmidseder, R.: Restoring sensations to the cut inferior alveolar nerve by direct anastomosis or by free autologous nerve grafting, Plast. Reconstr. Surg. **54:**83, 1973.

55. Hollin, S. A., Hayashi, H., and Gross, S. W.: Intracranial abscesses of odontogenic origin, Oral Surg. **23:**277, 1967.

56. Hubbard, J. H.: The quality of nerve regeneration: factors independent of the most skillful repair, Surg. Clin. North Am. **52:**1099, 1972.

57. Hughes, J., and Kosterlitz, H. W.: Opiate peptides, Br. Med. Bull. **33:**157, 1977.

58. Humphrey, T.: Reflex activity in the oral facial area of the human fetus. In Bosma, J. F., editor: Second symposium on oral sensation and perception, Springfield, Ill., 1970, Charles C Thomas, Publisher.

59. Hunt, R.: The sensory field of the facial nerve: a further contribution to the symptomatology of the geniculate ganglion, Brain **38:**418, 1915.

60. Iggo, A.: Cutaneous receptors. In Hubbard, J. I., editor: The peripheral nervous system, New York, 1974, Plenum Publishing Corp., pp. 347-404.

61. Jaeger, R.: The results of injecting hot water into the Gasserian ganglion for the relief of tic douloureux, J. Neurosurg. **16:**656, 1959.

62. Jannetta, P. J.: Microsurgical approach to the trigeminal nerve for tic douloureux, Prog. Neurol. Surg. **7:**180, 1976.

63. Jefferson, G.: The trigeminal neurinomas with remarks on malignant invasion of the Gasserian ganglion, Clin. Neurosurg. **1:**11, 1955.

64. Jefferson, G.: Trigeminal root and ganglion injections using phenol in glycerine for the relief of trigeminal neuralgia, J. Neurol. Neurosurg. Psychiatry **26:**345, 1963.

65. Johnston, M. C., and Hazelton, R. D.: Embryonic origins of facial structure related to oral sensation and motor functions. In Bosma, J. F., editor: Third symposium on oral sensation and perception, Springfield, Ill., 1972, Charles C Thomas, Publisher.

66. Kahn, E. A.: Trigeminal rhizotomy: the temporal approach, J. Neurosurg. **25:**242, 1966.

67. Kaltreider, H. B., and Talal, N.: The neuropathy of Sjögren's syndrome: trigeminal nerve involvement, Ann. Intern. Med. **70:**751, 1969.

68. Kerr, F. W. L.: The etiology of trigeminal neuralgia, Arch. Neurol. **8:**31, 1963.

69. Kerr, F. W. L., and Olafson, R. A.: Trigeminal and cervical volleys; convergence on single units in the spinal gray at C-1 and C-2, Arch. Neurol. **5:**171, 1961.

70. Khodadad, G.: Microsurgical techniques in repair of peripheral nerves, Surg. Clin. North Am. **52:**1157, 1972.

71. King, R. B.: Interaction of peripheral input within the trigeminal complex. In Bosma, J. F., editor: Second symposium on oral sensation and perception, Springfield, Ill., 1970, Charles C Thomas, Publisher.

72. Kruger, L.: A critical review of theories concerning the organization of the sensory trigeminal nuclear complex of the brain stem. In Dubner, R., and Kawamura, Y., editors: Oral-facial sensory and motor mechanisms, New York, 1971, Appleton-Century-Crofts.

73. Laskin, D. M.: Etiology of the pain-dysfunction syndrome, J. Am. Dent. Assoc. **79:**147, 1969.

74. Lesse, S.: Atypical facial pain syndromes; a study of 200 cases, Arch. Neurol. **3:**100, 1960.

75. Letcher, F. S., and Goldring, S.: The effect of radiofrequency current and heat on peripheral nerve action potential in the cat, J. Neurosurg. **49:**42, 1968.

76. Lewis, D. C.: Systemic lupus and polyneuropathy, Arch. Intern. Med. **116:**518, 1965.

77. Lim, R. K. S.: Revised concepts of the pain mechanism. In Knighton, R. S., and Dumke, P. R., editors: Pain, Boston, 1964, Little, Brown & Co.

78. Lim, R. K. S.: A revised concept of the mechanism of analgesia and pain. In Knighton, R. S., and Dumke, P. R., editors: Henry Ford Hospital International Symposium on Pain, Boston, 1966, Little, Brown & Co.

79. Loeser, J. D.: The management of tic douloureux, Pain **3:**155, 1977.

80. Long, D. M.: Electrical stimulation for the control of pain, Arch. Surg. **112:**884, 1977.

81. Man, P. L., and Chen, C. H.: Acupuncture 'anesthesia'—a new theory and clinical study, Curr. Ther. Res. **14:**390, 1972.

82. Mann, F.: Acupuncture: the ancient Chinese art of healing, New York, 1962, Random House, Inc.

83. Marmor, L.: Nerve grafting in peripheral nerve repair, Surg. Clin. North Am. **52:**1177, 1972.

84. Mayer, D. J., Price, D. D., and Rafii, A.: Antagonism of acupuncture analgesia in man by the narcotic antagonist naloxone, Brain Res. **121:** 368, 1977.

85. Melzack, R.: The puzzle of pain, New York, 1973, Basic Books, Inc., Publishers.

86. Melzack, R., and Perry, C.: Self regulation of pain: the use of alpha-feedback and hypnotic training for the control of chronic pain, Exp. Neurol. **46:**452, 1975.

87. Melzack, R., and Wall, P. D.: Pain mechanisms: a new theory, Science **150:**971, 1965.

88. Merril, R.: Oral-neurosurgical procedures for nerve injuries. In Walker, R. V.: Oral surgery. Transactions of the Third International Conference on Oral Surgery, Edinburgh, 1970, E. & S. Livingstone.

89. Mitch, P. S., McGrady, A., and Iannone, H.: Autogenic feedback training in migraine: a treatment report, Headache **15:**267, 1976.

90. Morosko, T. E., and Simmons, F. F.: The effect of audio-analgesia on pain threshold and pain tolerance, J. Dent. Res. **45:**1608, 1966.

91. Mosso, J. A., and Kruger, L.: Spinal trigeminal neurons excited by noxious and thermal stimuli, Brain Res. **38:**206, 1972.

92. Nashold, B. S., and Friedman, H.: Dorsal column stimulation for control of pain; preliminary report on 30 patients, J. Neurosurg. **36:**590, 1972.

93. Nauta, W. J. H.: Hippocampal projections and related neural pathways to the midbrain in the cat, Brain **81:**319, 1958.

94. Noordenbos, W.: Pain: problems pertaining to the transmission of nerve impulses which give rise to pain, Amsterdam, 1959, Elsevier.

95. Oliveras, J. L., Besson, J. M., Guilband, G. and Liebeskind, J. C.: Behavioral and electrophysiological evidence of pain inhibition from midbrain stimulation, Exp. Brain Res. **20:**32, 1974.

96. Orgel, M., Aguayo, A., and Williams, H. B.: Sensory nerve regeneration: an experimental study of skin grafts in the rabbit, J. Anat. **111:**121, 1972.

97. Paine, R.: Vascularfacial pain. In Alling, C. C., editor: Facial pain, Philadelphia, 1968, Lea & Febiger.

98. Pant, S. S., Asbury, A. K., and Richardson, E. P.: The myelopathy of pernicious anemia, Acta Neurol. Scand. **44:**6, 1968.

99. Patman, R. D., Thompson, J. E., and Persson, A. V.: Management of post-traumatic pain syndromes: report of 113 cases. Ann. Surg. **177:**780, 1973.

100. Peet, M. M., and Schneider, R. C.: Trigeminal neuralgia; a review of six hundred and eighty-nine cases with a follow-up study on 65% of the group, J. Neurosurg. **9:**367, 1952.

101. Perl, E. R.: Is pain a specific sensation? J. Psychiatr. Res. **8:**273, 1971.

102. Pert, A., and Yakish, T.: Sites of morphine analgesia in the primate brain: relation to pain pathways, Brain Res. **80:**135, 1974.

103. Pilling, L. F., Brannick, T. L., and Swenson, W. M.: Psychologic characteristics of psychiatric patients having pain as a presenting syndrome, Can. Med. Assoc. J. **97:**387, 1967.

104. Prineas, J.: The pathogenesis of dying-back neuropathies, J. Neuropathol. Exp. Neurol. **28:**571, 1969.

105. Quinn, J. H.: Repetitive peripheral neurectomies for neuralgias of the second and third divisions of the trigeminal nerve, J. Oral Surg. **23:**600, 1965.

106. Raff, M. C., and Asbury, A. K.: Ischemic mononeuropathy and mononeuropathy multiplex in diabetes mellitus, N. Engl. J. Med. **279:**17, 1968.

107. Rasmussen, P., and Riishede, J.: Facial pain treated with carbamazepam (Tegretol), Acta Neurol. Scand. **46:**385, 1970.

108. Rushton, J. G.: Glossopharyngeal neuralgia: a study of 116 cases, Thesis for American Neurological Association, 1966.

109. Rushton, J. G., and Olafson, R. A.: Trigeminal neuralgia associated with multiple sclerosis, Arch. Neurol. **13:**383, 1965.

110. Sacerdote, P.: The place of hypnosis in the relief of severe protracted pain, Am. J. Clin. Hypn. **4:**150, 1962.

111. Sauerland, E. K.: Effect of ethyl alcohol on trigeminal sensory neurons, Bull. Los Angeles Neurol. Soc. **35:**16, 1970.

112. Scott, D. S., and Leonard, C. F.: Modification of pain threshold by the covert reinforcement procedure and a cognitive strategy, Psych. Rec. **28:**49, 1978.

113. Sheldon, H. C., Pudenz, R. H., and Doyle, J.: Electrical control of facial pain, Am. J. Surg. **114:**209, 1967.

114. Simpson, J. A.: Peripheral neuropathy: etiological and clinical aspects, Proc. R. Soc. Med. **64:**291, 1971.

115. Sjoqvist, O.: Ten years' experience with trigeminal tractotomy, Brasil Med. **10:**259, 1948.

116. Snyder, S.: Opiatereceptor in normal and drug altered brain function, Nature **257:**185, 1975.

117. Spielberger, L., and Mazzia, V. D. B.: Anesthesia and Bell's palsy, Anesth. Analg. **50:**77, 1971.

118. Sternbach, R. N.: Pain patients: traits and treatment, New York, 1974, Academic Press, Inc.

119. Stewart, W. A., and King, R. B.: Fiber projections from the nucleus caudalis of the spinal trigeminal nucleus, J. Comp. Neurol. **121:**271, 1963.

120. Stortebecker, T. P.: Dental infectious foci and diseases of the nervous system, Acta Psychiatr. Scand. **36:**1, 1961.

121. Sweet, W. H., and Wepsic, J. G.: Treatment of chronic pain by stimulation of fibers of primary afferent neurone, Trans. Am. Neurol. Assoc. **93:**103, 1968.

122. Sweet, W. H., and Wepsic, J. G.: Controlled thermocoagulation of trigeminal ganglion and rootlets for differential destruction of pain fibers, J. Neurosurg. **39:**143, 1974.

123. Taarnhoj, P.: Decompression of the trigeminal root and the posterior root of the ganglion as a treatment in trigeminal neuralgia; preliminary communication, J. Neurosurg. **9:**288, 1952.

124. Tatlow, W. F. T.: Herpes zoster ophthalmicus and post-herpetic neuralgia, J. Neurol. Neurosurg. Psychiatry **15:**45, 1952.

125. Tatoian, J. A., La Dow, C. S., Jr., Disque, F., and others: Meningitis and temporal lobe abscess of dental origin, J. Oral Surg. **30:**423, 1972.

126. Taub, A.: Relief of postherpetic neuralgia with psychotropic drugs, J. Neurosurg. **39:**235, 1973.

127. Taub, A., and Collins, W. F., Jr.: Observations on the treatment of denervation dysesthesia with psychotropic drugs: post-herpetic neuralgia, anesthesia dolorosa, peripheral neuropathy, Adv. Neurol. **4:**309, 1974.

128. Thomas, P. K.: The morphological basis for alterations in nerve conduction in peripheral neuropathy, Proc. R. Soc. Med. **64:**295, 1971.

129. Tiwari, I. B., and Keane, T.: Hemifacial palsy after inferior dental block for dental treatment, Br. Dent. J. **128:**532, 1970.

130. Tonkin, J. P.: The modern management of Bell's palsy, Med. J. Aust. **2:**824, 1970.

131. Turker, M. N., and Turker, R. K.: A study on the peripheral mediators of pain, Experientia **30:**932, 1974.

132. Victor, M., and Adams, R. D.: On the etiology of the alcoholic neurological diseases with special reference to role of nutrition, Am. J. Clin. Nutr. **9:**379, 1961.

133. Watts, J. W., and Freeman, W.: Frontal lobotomy in the treatment of unbearable pain, Res. Publ. Assoc. Res. Nerv. Ment. Dis. **27:**715, 1948.

134. Westrum, L. E., and Black, R. G.: Changes in the synapses of the spinal trigeminal nucleus after ipsilateral rhizotomy, Brain Res. **11:**706, 1968.

135. White, J. C., and Sweet, W. H.: Pain and the neurosurgeon, Springfield, Ill., 1969, Charles C Thomas, Publisher.

136. Winnie, A. P., and Collins, V. J.: The pain clinic. I. Differential neural blockade in pain syndromes of questionable etiology, Med. Clin. North Am. **52:**123, 1968.

137. Wolff, H. G.: Wolff's headache and other facial pain, ed. 3, New York, 1972, Oxford University Press, Inc.

CHAPTER 27

Care of the hospitalized oral surgery patient

Daniel Gordon Walker

PREOPERATIVE MANAGEMENT

Need, real or imagined, causes the patient to seek care; a working relationship between the patient and the surgeon thus begins. Meyer summarized the basic requirements of this relationship as trust and communication.[25]

Evaluation and selection of patient for surgery. The dynamic emotional tension associated with the oral cavity exceeds that of any other body orifice. Thus the oral surgeon may, even with a most innocuous examination, represent a threat of varying significance to the patient.

It is the responsibility of the surgeon to decide if an operative procedure is justifiable when both the need and the expected results of surgery are considered, and the patients should be advised accordingly. The parents or guardians of the patient who is a minor must be informed also.

An example of a consent form is shown on p. 712. This facsimile is provided *only* to give a general format. The practitioner should use a form provided by the institution in which he or she works or one drawn up by legal counsel based on the concepts of informed consent in the state in which the procedure is to be performed. An operative permit should be used in the office as well as the hospital. The form should be signed in the presence of an adult witness, that is, the nurse or assistant, not the surgeon. It is desirable for the witness to be present during the discussion of the risks involved. After the signatures are attached the surgeon should again ask the patient or responsible party or both if there are any questions about the consent, procedural risks, expected results, or consequences if the operation is not done. A written notation should then be entered on the chart that the risks of the procedure were generally discussed with the patient and others (parents, wife, husband, guardian) and no guarantee of results was implied or given.

The motivations of the disgruntled or litigious patient are complicated by legal advisors, the quest for monetary gain, and the third party intervention of insurance companies. This intervention intimidates the physician-patient relationship directly—it is "the soil on which lawsuits are grown."[27] The surgeon should proceed with caution in evaluating the patient who has one or a combination of the following conditions or dispositions:

1. Multiple surgical experiences inter-

Special consent to operation or other procedure

Name of patient: _____

1   I hereby authorize and direct Dr. _____ and/or the associates or assistants of his choice to perform the following: _____

_____

(Description of operation or procedure)

and such additional therapeutic operations or procedures as his or their judgment may dictate on the basis of said operation or procedure.

2   I have conferred with the said physician and/or other physicians about the nature and purpose of the operation or procedure, the possibility that complications may arise or develop, risks which may be involved and possible alternate methods of treatment.

3   I understand that no warranty or guarantee has been made as to the results or cure.

4   I authorize and direct the above named physician and/or his associates and assistants to provide such additional services as they deem reasonable and necessary including, but not limited to, the administration and maintenance of anesthesia, the administration of blood and blood products and the performance of services involving pathology and radiology.

5   Any tissues or parts surgically removed may be retained or disposed of by this hospital in accordance with its accustomed practice.

6   Having received an explanation and given informed consent, I hereby agree to release this hospital, its employees, agents and Medical Staff from further responsibility with regard to permission for this operation or procedure.

7   Exceptions: _____

(If none, write "none")

I have read this form carefully before signing it and have been given an opportunity to question my physician about this operation or procedure.

_____   _____
Witness (Must be an adult)   Signature*

Date: _____   Time: _____ ☐ AM   ☐ PM

*Where the patient is incapable of signing and another person signs in his stead, complete the following:

State why patient is not able to give consent personally (nor to sign this form).

Explanation:

☐ Minor—any unmarried male or female who has not reached his 21st birthday.
☐ Unconscious
☐ Physical condition
☐ Other _____

Relationship of signer to patient: _____

If patient is a minor, name of parent or legal guardian: _____

Patient identification

spersed with disabling medical illness or multiple procedures on one organ system

2. Multiple complaints out of proportion and not related to clinical findings

3. More concern for improving appearance, real or imagined, than for correcting functional impairment

4. A history of using multiple medications, particularly sedatives, tranquilizers, and mood elevators

5. A domineering family or friends who are coercing the patient into having the procedure

6. Nervous disorders and symptoms of anxiety and depression

7. Intense urgency—a patient who cannot wait to have the procedure done

8. Obsessive distrust in a demanding patient who asks detailed and meticulous questions about techniques

9. Excessive secrecy, particularly in patients who avoid answers to direct or indirect questioning by the surgeon

10. Indecision (the surgeon should not urge the operation to solve the indecision)

The questions "What results do you expect from this operation?" and "Why do *you* want this operation?" should be directed to the patient. The answers to these questions are often revealing. Evaluation of the patient in regards to his or her manifestations of being a positive or negative reactor may be helpful in predicting the response to the procedure.

Patients who appear to be emotionally unstable should have psychiatric consultation before proceeding with elective surgery. "When a surgical procedure is indicated as a result of a threat to the patient's life, a disturbed mental state in the patient is not considered a contraindication to surgery."[27]

Preparation of patient for surgery. High regard for the feelings of the sick person is of utmost importance in the preparation of the patient for a surgical procedure. The surgeon must tread the narrow line between providing enough information to achieve an informed consent and giving information that may cause undue alarm; this responsibility draws deeply on the attending surgeon's wisdom and ability to communicate. A discussion of the risks involved, the anticipated yet not guaranteed outcome, and possible or probable complications of the proposed treatment as well as likely consequences of not treating the condition must be discussed with the patient or the responsible party or both, preferably in the presence of a member of the office staff or hospital staff. Duly warranted notations should be made on the patient's chart or office record. Even in emergency situations, consideration should be given to these matters.

Questions related to the type of anesthesia to be used, the method of administering the anesthetic, and the need for a preoperative medical evaluation and laboratory evaluation should be discussed with the patient and the responsible party before admission whenever possible. Assurance that general anesthesia will keep the patient asleep throughout the surgical procedure, as well as a statement that preoperative enemas are not generally used for oral surgery preparation, will perform a great service in calming the stormy preoperative sea.

Review of past and present medical problems. There is no substitute for the physician's knowledge of the patient. The physician and attendants are required, morally and legally, to be sufficiently acquainted with the physical and emotional status of the patient to be alerted to potentially complicating circumstances. An adequate medical history must be obtained from the patient or some responsible individual. When possible, this may be obtained by having the patient complete a written questionnaire. The patient's or responsible party's signature should be affixed to such a questionnaire with specific acknowledgment that he has read and completed the form. An example of a medical questionnaire is shown

Medical questionnaire

1 Have you been a patient in a hospital in the past two years? If so, for what were you hospitalized? _____ _____.   YES_____ NO_____

2 Are you now, or have you been, under the care of a physician (including a psychiatrist) during the past two years? If so, for what were you treated? _____ _____.   YES_____ NO_____

3 List medicines or drugs you have taken during the past year and for what. _____ _____.   YES_____ NO_____

4 Have you taken cortisone or other hormone medications? Is so, please list. _____ _____.   YES_____ NO_____

5 Have you had any surgical procedures in the past? Describe. _____ _____ _____.   YES_____ NO_____

6 If surgery was performed, name of surgeon: _____

7 Have you had a reaction to any medicine such as penicillin, sulfa, aspirin? Describe. _____ _____.   YES_____ NO_____

8 Do you have hay fever or any allergies? If so, describe. _____ _____.   YES_____ NO_____

9 When you cut yourself, or have a tooth extracted, do you bleed so much that you have to see a doctor to have it stopped?   YES_____ NO_____

10 Have you ever had a reaction during, or following, dental treatment or oral surgery?   YES_____ NO_____

11 Circle the name of any of the following which you have had:

Heart trouble	Rheumatic fever	Congenital heart disease
High blood pressure	Stroke	Diabetes
Asthma	Tuberculosis	Kidney or bladder trouble
Syphilis or venereal disease	Blood disease	Anemia
Hepatitis (yellow jaundice)	Arthritis	Pneumonia
X-ray treatment	Cancer	Nervous disorders
Seizures (epilepsy)	Stomach ulcers	Thyroid disease

12 Do you faint easily?   YES_____ NO_____

13 Do you get short of breath easily?   YES_____ NO_____

14 Have you gained, or lost, more than 15 pounds recently?   YES_____ NO_____

15 Do you smoke? How much? _____.   YES_____ NO_____

16 Do you have any sores or growths in your mouth?   YES_____ NO_____

17 Have you ever had any serious injuries to your face or jaws? Describe.   YES_____ NO_____

_____

_____.

18 WOMEN: Are you pregnant?   YES_____ NO_____

19 Do you have any disease, condition or problem not listed above that   YES_____ NO_____

you think we should know about? _____

_____

_____.

_____

Signature

on p. 714 and above. When time permits, more detailed computerized medical histories often are useful in screening out pertinent from less important information in the medical history. Most computerized questionnaires direct the physician's attention to the areas for which a more detailed medical history is desired. The following questions are considered to be pertinent to a preoperative medical history.[37]

1. Have you ever had a reaction to any specific drug or food?

2. Have you ever had a major allergy such as asthma, hay fever, eczema, or hives?

3. Are you now, or have you recently been, under the care of a physician? (If the answer is "yes," a brief call to that physician is indicated.)

4. Are you now taking _any_ type of medication or have you recently completed a course of medication? (Specific questions should be directed toward the prior usage of adrenocortical hormones, tranquilizers, sedatives, anticoagulants, antimetabolites, and x-ray therapy. Again, it is extremely important that the patient understand why the surgeon is interested in this information, and the questions should be versed in a language that is comprehensible to the patient.)

5. Do you limit your physical activities for any reason? Do you avoid climbing stairs? Are you bothered by shortness of breath or chest pain on exertion?

6. Have you ever had a nervous breakdown?

7. Are you pregnant?

Because of the increasing number of surgical procedures performed on older persons, the trend toward more extensive surgical operations, and the increasing amount of surgical care required for trauma and other emergency surgical problems, every surgeon has an increasing responsibility for the proper evaluation of the patient's preoperative pulmonary status.[21,27] Elective operations in persons with active sinusitis, tonsillitis, acute bronchitis, or a cold should be postponed until the infection has been cleared for 1 to 2 weeks. Cigarette smoking is the most common cause of simple bronchitis, and "anyone who smokes in excess of 20 cigarettes per day can be assumed to have abnormal pulmonary function."[21]

The following positive findings in the preoperative history may be clues to postoperative ventilatory problems: (1) childhood respiratory infections, (2) pneumonia or pleurisy before the discovery of antibiotics, (3) bronchitis often associated with cigarette smoking, (4) the presence of morning sputum, (5) old chest injuries, (6) current physical activity, and (7) asthma. Preoperative thoracic roentgenograms frequently are valuable. However, it must be remembered that x-ray films are not pulmonary function tests but only static photographs of the lung parenchyma and thoracic structures.

Preoperative cardiovascular evaluation is aided greatly by an accurate history in that good exercise tolerance is indicative of a good cardiovascular reserve. A history of orthopnea, paroxysmal nocturnal dyspnea, angina, or dyspnea on mild exertion suggests serious heart disease. Evidence of fluid retention, increased venous pressure, and hepatomegaly indicate low cardiac reserve, and elective surgery should be avoided in those cases. The thoracic roentgenogram is useful in determining cardiac size, and the ECG provides indirect data.

An accurate drug history must be part of the routine history on hospital admission for any reason. If there is any doubt about drug dependence, the patient should be placed on a maintenance dosage of whatever drug he has become habituated to so that postoperative grand mal seizures may be prevented. Abrupt withdrawal in a patient physiologically addicted to barbiturates or nonbarbiturate sedatives such as meprobamate (Miltown, Equanil), glutethimide (Doriden), methyprylon (Noludar), ethchlorvynol (Placidyl), chlordiazepoxide hydrochloride (Librium), diazepam (Valium), and ethinamate (Valmid) can produce delirium or convulsions or both.[12] The phenothiazines are not thought to produce physiological addiction and can usually be stopped abruptly without producing delirium or convulsions, according to Hastings.[18]

The ability of tissue to heal is controlled by many factors, one of the more important being the nutritional status of the patient. Knowledge of the preoperative nutritional condition of the patient is important for this reason. The surgical patient should be maintained or restored to a nutritional balance during all phases of diagnosis, therapy, and convalescence.[10] In the healthy oral surgical patient, an uncomplicated parenteral or oral program or both of alimentation that will maintain adequate circulatory volume, prevent dehydration or electrolyte imbalance, and spare breakdown of body protein often is all that is needed to achieve nutritional balance. This program can be supplied by appropriate amounts of water, glucose, salt, and potassium if parenteral alimentation is indicated. Intravenous administration of 5% dextrose (0.25% saline) solutions within the daily fluid volume tolerance (2,500 to 3,000 ml in the average healthy adult) will supply approximately one third of the caloric requirements (500 to 600 calories) of an average, healthy, resting, afebrile adult. The patient's remaining energy needs are supplied by catabolism of stored glycogen, fat, and protein. Fever, trauma, infection, or need for extensive tissue repair may increase caloric needs as much as fivefold. More careful planning and hyperalimentation is required for the patient who, in the preoperative state, is severely debilitated by chronic disease or malnutrition or who is unwilling or unable to eat properly because of trauma, sepsis, or surgical complications. The need for a vitamin supplement should not be overlooked, and it can be supplied orally or parenterally by any of the several commercial preparations available. In a patient with liver dysfunction or who is taking broad-spectrum antibiotics, vitamin K should be administered to reduce the chance of hypoprothrombinemia. For this reason the adolescent who has been on tetracycline for months or years for control of acne vulgaris may tend to develop more ecchymoses and have poor clot formation when elective surgery is done.

The oral surgery patient requiring a long-term liquid diet can combine imagination with a food blender and maintain an adequate nutritional balance. The new, chemically formulated, bulk-free elemental diets (Vivonex H-N, Codelid 62H) provide nutritional support, although they are somewhat expensive. Patients objecting to the taste of the elemental diet can be fed through a small-gauge, nasogastric feeding tube (No. 8 French transnasal intragastric infant size). When there is intestinal function, this form of hyperalimentation is preferred over parenteral hyperalimentation administered through a subclavian vein catheter into the venae cava.

Preoperative laboratory workup. A complete blood count that includes an evaluation of the hemoglobin and hematocrit indices, a total white blood cell count with a differential count, and an assessment of the circulating platelets, as well as a gross and microscopic urinalysis, should be routine in the preoperative laboratory workup. A carefully recorded history and physical examination usually will direct attention to the presence of any bleeding disorder severe enough to be of consequence. In the event of such a disorder, a hematological consultation can be requested. A partial thromboplastin time (PTT) test and an assessment of the number of circulating platelets are frequently used indices in the preoperative screening for hemorrhagic tendencies. The SMA-12/60 (Sequential Multiple Analyzer) screening battery is processed preoperatively in many progressive hospitals. (It should be done on a fasting blood sample.) Allowable deviations above the normal range, such as an elevated alkaline phosphatase level in growing children, are to be expected and should not cause undue concern.

Preoperative orders. Whenever possible, telephone orders should be avoided. Written or typed orders should be sent with the patient at his admission to the hospital. There are obvious practical and medicolegal implications for this suggestion. Some hospital services are not permitted to accept orders given over the telephone. Typical preoperative orders generally include the following items:

1. *Admitting diagnosis.* Most hospitals require that this be placed on the patient's chart within 24 hours after admission and assume that this is a working diagnosis that may be modified or changed completely by the time of discharge.

2. *Dietary orders.* These should be specific, according to the dietary requirements indicated (for example, nothing by mouth, low salt, mechanical soft, 2,500-calorie high-protein, surgical liquids).

3. *Physical restrictions.* Specificity is desirable (for example, bed rest, ambulatory, bathroom privileges, head elevated, bed rest with bedside commode).

4. *Laboratory requests and special tests.* There should be a specific reason for ordering each of these tests. Many tests performed on one patient are uncomfortable and expensive for the patient. This is a double-edged philosophy, however; it should be remembered that failure to order necessary and indicated laboratory tests simply out of deference to the patient's pocketbook and comfort is not a satisfactory defense before a lay jury.

"Routine lab" in most hospitals usually indicates a complete blood count, gross and microscopic urinalysis, and serology. "Special lab" includes certain definitive testing procedures or perhaps the SMA-12/60 screening battery or other chemistries. Special hematological tests pertaining to clotting factors usually are ordered under this designation. "In this scientific age, physicians need to be reminded that a laboratory test is not a diagnosis. The latter is a judgment based on the patient's history and the results of the physical and epidemiologic examinations. Laboratory tests merely confirm the judgment."[14] If the need for blood is anticipated after such tests have been performed, a type and crossmatch for the desired volume or units is requested.

5. *X-ray requests.* Specificity in ordering the roentgenographic studies and certainty that the radiologist has sufficient clinical information about the patient or his problem is of utmost importance so that an enlightened radiographic diagnosis may be attained.

6. *Medications.* The appropriate use of antibiotics can reduce the incidence of infection and postoperative morbidity in many oral surgical procedures such as im-

pacted third molars, osteotomies, cystectomies, apicoectomies, bone grafts, and others. The need for prophylactic use of antibiotics in the patient with valvular heart disease, with or without a valve prosthesis, has been recommended by the American Heart Association. At the present time, oral or parenteral penicillin therapy or both appears to be the prophylactic method of choice. Some authorities, however, believe that a broader spectrum coverage is indicated to protect the individual from some of the gram-negative and penicillin-resistant organisms that have been cultured from patients with bacterial endocarditis.[29]

The judicious use of appropriate amounts of glucocorticoids to suppress the inflammatory responses of pain and edema after trauma to the head and neck region, iatrogenic or otherwise, is practical in oral surgery. The antipyretic effect of glucocorticoids reduces the diagnostic usefulness of fever as a sign of infection. Massive doses of corticosteroids to reduce cerebral edema secondary to closed head injuries as well as in the shock-lung syndrome and in gram-negative septicemias is now accepted and well documented.[33] Broad-spectrum antibiotic coverage is used in conjunction with this therapy. When surgery involves the removal of impacted third molars, especially if the inferior alveolar neurovascular bundle is involved, the preoperative and immediate postoperative use of corticosteroids and broad-spectrum antibiotics is justified. Corticosteroids are also useful for the reduction of edema and for postoperative discomfort in the surgical correction of jaw deformities. Absolute contraindications for this course of medication are tuberculosis (active or healed), ocular herpes simplex, and acute psychosis. Relative contraindications are diverticulitis, active or latent peptic ulcer, fresh intestinal anastomosis, renal insufficiency, hypertension, thromboembolic tendencies, osteoporosis, diabetes mellitus, acute and chronic infections including fungus and viral diseases (chicken pox), myasthenia gravis, and others.

7. *Sedative drugs.* Drugs to be given the night before surgery should be chosen with care, following an adequate drug history of the patient. Maintenance doses of the sedatives must be used in patients with a heavy drug use history, and barbiturates should be avoided in the very young and the elderly. Cooperation with the hospital's department of anesthesia in prescribing these drugs is beneficial to all concerned.

8. *Special orders.* The administration of intranasal vasoconstrictor agents such as 0.25% phenylephrine hydrochloride (Neo-Synephrine) in the form of nose gels or sprays immediately prior to removing the patient to the operating room is frequently desirable if nasal endotracheal intubation is planned. This maneuver will facilitate respiration through the nose during an oral surgical procedure performed while the patient is under local anesthesia.

Antiembolism stockings may be advisable for the elderly, for women taking oral contraceptives, or for any patient with a history of recent pelvic surgery, deep vein thrombosis, or thrombophlebitis of the lower extremities. These individuals may have their venous flow impeded by bed rest, lengthy operations, or prolonged immobility.

Female patients should be asked to remove all eye makeup before retiring the preceding night.

COMPLICATIONS AND PREVENTIVE MEASURES

Skin and nerve injury. Pressure points on the body, especially on heels, elbows, and hands, must be avoided at the risk of peripheral nerve injury and stasis damage to the skin.

Bacteremia. Complete sterilization of the skin or oral cavity cannot be accomplished. However, the bacterial count can be reduced significantly. Shaving of hair-bearing skin should be done as near to the time of surgery as possible to prevent bacterial colonization of the unavoidable abrasions caused by shaving. Subsequently the operative site can be cleansed vigorously with a suitable detergent. At the present time the iodophors or povidone-iodine preparations are popular for cleansing. Scopp[34] demonstrated in a double-blind study that the povidone-iodine mouthwash reduced bacteremia during exodontics. Of patients treated with the iodine preparation, 28% had bacteremia as compared to 56% of the group receiving placebos. The properly performed intraoral preparation supplemented with appropriate prophylactic antibiotics for patients susceptible to endocarditis is recommended highly. The routine preoperative preparation of the oral cavity, with either a suitable mouthwash for the patient under local anesthesia or with a physical scrubbing and application of one of the iodophors for patients under general anesthesia, is to be highly recommended prior to the extraction of teeth and other intraoral surgical procedures.

Eye protection. Prior to draping, with the patient under general anesthesia, the eyelids should be closed carefully so that no eyelashes are turned under, and the lids should be taped shut with paper tape to protect the cornea and the sclera. The eyes are then covered with sterile ophthalmic pads or some form of metallic eye shields such as the Fox eye shield that is taped from the supraorbital rim to malar eminence. Methylcellulose (artificial tears or Liquifilm) drops or an ophthalmic ointment of low allergenicity may be placed in the conjunctival fold as an additional measure. It is important that female patients be requested to remove all eye makeup the evening prior to surgery.

Pharyngeal protection. After the patient has been anesthetized and intubated either nasoendotracheally or oroendotracheally or if the anesthesia is being administered through tracheostomy tube, it is desirable to insert some form of moistened sterile gauze pack into the oropharynx to screen it from the oral cavity. Most endotracheal tubes are cuffed so that they will prevent the passage of blood, water, or other secretions into the trachea around the endotracheal tube. For various reasons, how-

ever, the cuff may not provide a complete seal. During lengthy procedures, it is wise to deflate the cuff periodically to prevent possible pressure against the tracheal mucosa. The pack should be placed carefully and gently so that unnecessary irritation to the oral and pharyngeal mucosa is avoided. The pack so placed functions as a protective screen, preventing foreign bodies from passing into the pharynx.

Lip protection. In preparation for an intraoral procedure, the lips and oral commissure should be anointed thoroughly with a water-soluble cream, preferably containing one of the corticosteroid agents, to reduce postoperative cheilitis. Petroleum lubricants such as petrolatum (Vaseline) and others are not as satisfactory as the suggested creams because the petroleum base material tends to macerate the skin. Repeated usage of the corticosteroid creams throughout the procedure markedly reduces the incidence of pressure necrosis and cheilitis after oral surgery. This is particularly useful in the patient with dermatographia.[24]

Malignant hyperthermia. Malignant hyperthermia is a serious operative complication and the surgeon must be watchful of it. This complication is described as a syndrome of rapid increase in temperature while the patient is under anesthesia. It occurs usually in apparently healthy children and young adults with an average age of 21 years. There is no sex differential. The syndrome reportedly may follow a familial pattern, indicating a nonsex-linked autosomal dominance. Metabolic causes are believed to be related to the uncoupling of oxidative phosphorylation. Other theories suggest that there is an aberrance in hypothalamic control or that it may be related to a latent or known myotonia, which produces a muscular rigidity subsequent to the administration of succinylcholine. Other causes for the elevation of temperature may be one of the following: (1) loss of cooling mechanisms by radiation, evaporation, conduction, or convection; (2) infection; (3) dehydration; (4) allergic reactions; (5) belladonna derivatives; (6) shivering; and (7) endocrine mechanisms such as thyrotoxicosis or pheochromocytoma. The clinical picture generally develops approximately 2 hours after the anesthesia has started. There is an increased temperature accompanied with flushing and sweating, rising at an approximate rate of 1° F every 10 to 15 minutes. Tachycardia, tachypnea, hypoxia resulting from metabolic uptake, metabolic acidosis (some pHs have been recorded as low as 6.7), a warm soda lime container caused by high carbon dioxide production, hypovolemia caused by extracellular fluid loss, convulsions, sialadenopathy, disseminated intravascular clotting, myoglobinuria are symptoms associated with this usually fatal syndrome.[17,42,43]

The treatment of malignant hyperthermia consists of immediate rapid cooling of the patient. Everything else is incidental unless this is accomplished. This may be done by the following methods:

1. Using water blankets, ice, chilled gastric lavage, iced intravenous solutions of lactated Ringers solution, and a pump bypass with a cooling system if available
2. Hyperventilation with 100% oxygen
3. Correction of acidosis and administration of bicarbonate solution, THAM buffer, or TRIS buffer
4. Administration of calcium ion
5. Diuresis to prevent renal failure produced by myoglobinuria
6. Nondepolarizing muscle relaxants (of questionable effectiveness)
7. Haloperidol to block the uncoupling[43]

POSTOPERATIVE CARE

One of the most critical periods for the surgical patient is the immediate postoperative phase, covering the period of time from the end of the operation until the time when he regains consciousness. It is during this phase that the danger of aspiration, cardiac arrest, and circulatory or respiratory depression is greatest.

Operating room to recovery room. The best method of removing the patient from the operating table to the recovery room bed generally is by placing him on a roller, thus protecting the patient's and the attendants' vertebral columns. The attending surgeon or the responsible assistant should accompany the patient to the recovery room with a recovery room note made on the patient's chart and written postoperative orders. "Many of the physiological disorders which are easily recognized in the fully awake, non-medicated patient are modified, abated, or entirely eliminated by residual anesthesia. In the recovery room, this presents major difficulties in recognizing problems such as hypoxia, hypoventilation, and hypovolemia."[8]

Aldrete method (Apgar). A method of scoring patients recovering from the effects of anesthesia, similar to the Apgar evaluation of the newborn infant, has been described by Aldrete.[1] This rating is based on the repeated evaluation of blood pressure, respiration, color, consciousness, and activity, which are measured every 15 minutes. Unit values of 0 to 2 are given to each of the measured vital signs, thus giving the recovery room personnel more definite guidelines to determine when the patient may safely return to his room or to the intensive care unit, as required. A rating of 10 on this scale indicates that the patient is in the best possible condition. Scores of 8 and 9 are considered safe, but patients given 7 points or less are considered to be in danger.[13]

Recovery room notations. The surgical resident's recovery room note should include a comment regarding the following factors: (1) level of consciousness, (2) pupillary size, (3) airway patency, (4) breathing patterns, (5) pulse rate and volume, (6) skin warmth and color, (7) body temperature, and (8) if the patient is catheterized, a 30 to 50 ml per hour urine output.

Operative notes. The operative notes should describe the operation in specific terms as follows: (1) procedure, (2) surgeon and assistant(s), (3) anesthesia (by type, name, and agents), (4) findings, and (5) estimated blood loss.

Postoperative orders. A review of the patient's known allergies and drug idiosyncrasies should be made; subsequently the orders may be written as follows:

1. Vital signs or "Apgar" rating. These should be evaluated every 15 minutes until stable.

2. Observation of airway for obstruction. Use humidified oxygen by mask, catheter or other appliance, if desired. (See section on complications for special orders.) (A Po_2 of less than 40, Pco_2 greater than 65 with an arterial pH of under 7.25 are absolute indications, in most cases, of the need for respiratory assistance.) A humidified atmosphere provided by a cool mist vaporizer or an ultrasonic vaporizer is desirable. Intermittent positive pressure breathing apparatus with suitable inhalants may be desired to assist in the ventilation of the patient. Some form of acetylcysteine or isoproterenol (Isuprel) may be utilized if indicated, particularly in the treatment of atelectasis or pneumonitis or in the heavy smoker to loosen heavy secretions and thus free them to be brought up spontaneously by coughing.

3. Position. Elevate the head 20 to 30 degrees (bathroom privileges, bedside commode, or bed rest, as indicated).

4. Ice packs or cold compresses to desired areas, if indicated. (The application of bilateral flat ice packs over the sites of osteotomies or third molar extractions, held in place by a 10-cm elastic bandage, is useful in reducing edema and postoperative bleeding.)

5. Parenteral fluid orders. If any are needed, and the type of fluid and volume and rate of the flow (for example, follow present intravenous solution with 1,000 ml 5% dextrose in 0.2% normal saline at 125 ml per hour, intake and output, if indicated, to be recorded). (See section on fluids and electrolytes.)

6. Analgesic. Medication for postoperative pain to be given orally or parenterally, as desired; troche or lozenge if desired for relief of pharyngeal irritation. (This is often useful to reduce postintubation discomfort,

and these analgesics frequently contain topical anesthetics; beware of allergies.) The use of potent narcotics to control severe pain should be of short duration and limited to patients with acute distress or those with inoperable cancer who require long-term relief. The use of antidepressant drugs in the pain regimen has been shown to provide increased relief of pain and often allows the dose of narcotic to be reduced or eliminated.[15]

7. Antibiotic. This is usually a continuation of the drug begun prior to or during surgery or may be chemotherapeutic, added later in light of operative findings.

8. Anti-inflammatory drugs. Continuation of glucocorticosteroids that were given preoperatively or intraoperatively may be indicated. (When the procedure has been short and the trauma minimal, 4 mg of dexamethasone given intravenously before or after the induction of anesthesia generally is adequate. If an oral dose of 4.0 mg dexamethasone was begun the evening before surgery, it is frequently continued into the first postoperative day. The use of glucocorticosteroids is beneficial in the infant child or adult as a means of reducing postintubation laryngitis or tracheitis.)[40]

9. Antiemetic. These usually are given parenterally or by suppository as required. (Meticulous hemostasis on intraoral procedures and the avoidance of oral fluids until the patient has completely regained consciousness will often eliminate the need for an antiemetic.) Selected phenothiazines continue to provide the most desirable results.

10. Sedative medications if indicated or desired, depending on the patient's need

11. Other medications or special orders (For example, resume Doctor Jones' standing orders regarding the patient's insulin therapy.)

12. Diet orders. If the patient has been hydrated adequately prior to and during surgery and gastrointestinal functioning has resumed after general anesthesia, it is deemed advisable to start the patient on clear liquids or surgical liquids and to pro-

Discharge order sheet

1 Diagnosis

2 Medications

3 Diet

4 Activity

5 Follow-up

6 Miscellaneous instructions

7 _____   _____
        Patient discharged this date   Physician signature

I acknowledge and/understand the above instructions that were given to me.

Date: _____ Signature: _____
                                                        Patient and/or responsible party

Discharged: _____

Date: _____ Time: _____

With _____ Signature of discharge nurse: _____

Discharge instructions

White copy—Patient's chart
Yellow copy—Patient
Pink copy—Pharmacy
Gold copy—Physician

gress as tolerated to full liquid or soft diet. These aliments should be delayed until the patient has returned to the full level of consciousness. The best possible diet under the prevailing conditions is essential, that is, a full, nutritious, high-protein diet administered in sufficient amounts to meet the energy requirements of the patient. It is not enough for the surgeon to prescribe a high-protein, high-caloric, high-vitamin diet. Such an order may be a total failure for the following reasons: the diet presented to the patient is not as specified; the diet presented may not be eaten in whole or in part because of anorexia, lack of palatability, or lack of nursing care to encourage eating; the food eaten may be wholly or partially lost because of diarrhea or vomiting. The surgeon should know enough of the details of the fundamental principles of nutrition to apply them and to see that they are properly carried out.[11,19,38] (See form, p. 722.)

Postoperative rounds. All patients in the postoperative state must be evaluated completely for evidence of complications that may jeopardize or protract recovery.[2]

Progress notes during the postoperative phase should include an evaluation of the following factors:

1. Level of consciousness
2. Patency of the airway
3. Evaluation of the patient's cardiopulmonary system
4. Pulse rate and volume, blood pressure, and body temperature
5. Skin warmth and color
6. Intake and output
7. Condition of the wound
8. Survey of the nurses' notes (not necessarily in this order but of utmost importance)
9. Specific patient complaints

POSTOPERATIVE COMPLICATIONS

Acute ventilatory failure. The supply of oxygen to the various tissue cells is probably the most fragile link between man and his environment. Thus *acute ventilatory failure* is the most urgent of all emergency preoperative or postoperative complica-

tions, and common causes are obstructions by secretions, foreign bodies, local trauma, or swelling. Ventilatory failure can be eliminated or bypassed immediately by intubation or tracheostomy. The position of the patient's head and neck may be the subtle cause of a serious obstruction of the upper airway in the unconscious patient. Narcotics and sedatives should be administered with extreme caution in the restless patient until it is certain that the restlessness is not related to cerebral hypoxia rather than pain.[8] The advantages of tracheal intubation, either by endotracheal tube or tracheostomy tube, are obvious when these problems occur. Strict asepsis, particularly in respect to the suction catheter, in any patient with tracheal intubation is absolutely essential. Sterile catheters used by individuals wearing sterile gloves should be mandatory. The sterile, disposable tracheal suction kits help to prevent the entry of pathogenic organisms in the tracheobronchial tree. According to Kinney,[21] tracheal intubation for a period of 4 to 7 days is generally accepted; thus the need for tracheostomy is eliminated in many cases. "Emergency tracheostomy has thus become justifiable only when tracheal intubation is not possible."[21] A consultation from the respiratory therapy division is highly recommended. Pontoppidian[30] recommends intubation or tracheostomy and ventilation in the adult patient whose respiratory rate is greater than 35 per minute with vital capacity of less than 15 ml per kilogram, respiratory force of less than 25 cm of water, alveolar-arterial oxygen gradient greater than 350 mm Hg, and the ratio of dead space to tidal volume while on mask-administered oxygen therapy greater than 0.6. In the patient recovering from respiratory failure, spontaneous respiration requires the ability to produce minimal vital capacity of 10 ml per kilogram. When the vital capacity exceeds 15 to 20 ml per kilogram and the patient is on spontaneous respirations, the removal of the endotracheal or tracheostomy tube is generally possible. When the alveolar-arterial oxygen gradient is greater than 350 mm Hg, weaning the patient from the mechanical ventilator is not successfully accomplished in most instances.[6,30]

Aspiration. The *aspiration of gastric contents or blood* at the time of the injury or during the induction or recovery from anesthesia can lead to significant pulmonary ventilatory problems. Restlessness to the point of belligerency, tachycardia, tachypnea, and occasionally cyanosis should alert the surgeon to this possibility. Physical examination of the chest, auscultation of the breath sounds, and an upright chest film can be used to confirm the diagnosis almost invariably. By early recognition and prompt removal of foreign material from the tracheobronchial tree, secondary sequelae may be reduced or avoided. The prophylactic use of corticosteroids every 6 hours and significant doses of broad-spectrum antibiotic agents supplemented by adequate ventilation therapy are indicated.

Positive end-expiratory pressure (PEEP) appears to be of benefit in improving oxygenation following gastric acid–pulmonary injury as in other instances of pulmonary insufficiency. However, care must be taken to use the lowest level of PEEP required to achieve adequate oxygenation at an acceptable inspired oxygen level. Increased levels of PEEP have been shown to increase the rate of fluid loss from injured pulmonary capillaries.[36]

Aspiration can be avoided often by ascertaining that the stomach is empty prior to surgery. Intubating the patient in the head down position and maintaining the patient on his side or in a head down position during the period of unconsciousness will reduce the incidence of aspiration. The use of cuffed endotracheal tubes is recommended, yet the cuff cannot be relied on entirely because it may be improperly inflated or may leak enough air to permit the passage of blood or gastric contents into the trachea.[39]

Laryngeal edema. Another complication is *edema of the airway* after either oral or nasal intubation. This problem is more likely to occur in infants and children because of the peculiar anatomy of the subglottal trachea. The attending surgeon and others responsible for the care of the patient must be on constant alert for evidence of sudden or gradual obstruction of the airway. The judicious use of glucocorticoids, ultrasonic nebulizers with oxygen therapy, and, reintubation or a tracheostomy are measures that must be available in the postoperative armamentarium. Tracheostomy in the infant is an extremely dangerous procedure and is to be avoided whenever possible because of serious long-term complications. Bag and mask or mouth-to-mouth respiration will force air through a laryngospasm in almost every case.

Epistaxis. Bleeding after nasal intubation may be reduced or controlled with preoperative and postoperative nasal vasoconstrictor agents (0.25% phenylephrine solution), elevation of the patient's head, sedation, and, if necessary, judicious and gentle packing of the bleeding site with well-lubricated ¼- or ½-inch (0.7- or 1.2-cm) gauze. Should these measures fail, it may be necessary to insert a posterior nasal pack.

Sore throat. Pharyngitis is not an uncommon complaint after intubation, and the possibility of this uncomfortable situation occurring should be explained to the patient preoperatively. The early use of a cool mist vaporizer or ultrasonic nebulizer, as well as oral troches containing a topical anesthetic agent (if the patient is not allergic to the topical anesthetic), is successful in reducing postoperative complaints of this type. The uncomfortable symptoms usually disappear within 8 to 12 hours after intubation. If they should worsen, the surgeon should be alerted to the possibility of pharyngeal mucosal tears and infection, which subsequently may extend into the pharyngeal spaces or mediastinum.

Nausea and vomiting. The advent of parenterally administered general anesthetic agents has tended to reduce the incidence of *postoperative nausea and vomiting* as a process of normal recovery from general anesthesia. When protracted nausea and vomiting occur in the postoperative period, the usual indication is that something of a more serious nature has occurred. Unrelieved, *acute gastric dilation* may be lethal within 1 to 2 hours if not relieved. Tachycardia, prostration, and hypotension often are associated with this remarkably painless problem. The dilated and tympanitic epigastrium extends well up into the left thoracic cavity. Elevation of the left diaphragm and roentgenographic evidence of a large gastric bubble are highly suggestive. Moyer[27] recommends that gastric suction be instituted in any case of protracted nausea and vomiting. After lengthy procedures, insertion of a proper-sized nasogastric tube prior to the cessation of general anesthesia and extubation is recommended highly. Once the nasogastric tube is inserted, it should be attached to a low-pressure gastric suction machine. This will facilitate the emptying of the stomach of swallowed blood and thereby reduce the chances of vomiting during and immediately after the patient's emergence from general anesthesia. In the absence of intestinal obstruction and electrolyte imbalance, the maintenance of continuous gastric suction should restore the stomach to functional tone within 36 to 48 hours. Because of the usual loss of potassium and sodium salts during surgery, these elements must be replaced along with the proper fluids to restore the body's chemical balance. Other causes of postoperative nausea and vomiting include ileus, cardiac failure, and infections, as well as the countless number of emetic drugs or drugs that have emetic tendencies. The occurrence of projectile vomiting indicates the need for a neurological evaluation for the presence of increased intracranial pressure. If ileus, uremia, gastric atony, and hypokalemia can be eliminated as possible causes of the nausea and vomiting, then use of a suitable phenothiazine for the control of nausea and vomiting may be indicated. The discontinuance of drugs that have been administered for other reasons may be necessary also.

Generally, it is wise to avoid all oral fluids and medications until the patient is reacting well and bowel sounds are present. Until this status has been reached, medications, fluids, and nutriments may be supplied by the parenteral route. When intraoral surgery has been carried out, good hemostasis to prevent ingestion of blood from the surgical wound is needed. Oral medications usually are tolerated more successfully if taken with foods; this dilutes any irritant effect on the gastric mucosa.

Edema. The oral surgery patient may have edema from many causes, the most common being physical trauma, infection, increased venous pressure, and decreased lymphatic flow. Other less likely causes are decreased arterial blood flow, decreased intravascular oncotic pressure, excessive sodium retention, and cardiac failure and immobility. This undesirable postoperative complication may be reduced by maintaining the operating table in such a position that the field of surgery is elevated above the level of the heart, by maintaining good hemostasis through careful handling of tissues, by the judicious administration of corticosteroids preoperatively and postoperatively, and by the elevation, cooling, and compression of the area of surgery during the immediate postoperative period.

Hyperthermia. The most common causes of *postoperative fever* are wound infection, urinary tract infection, pulmonary complications, thrombophlebitis, and increased osmolarity because of lack of water or salt excess.

The use of estrogen-containing oral contraceptives is now accepted as being associated with six to seven times higher risk of venous thromboembolism, a precursor to pulmonary embolism. The intraoperative fall in antithrombin III activity during exodontics in women taking oral contraceptives has been prevented by a small preoperative dose of subcutaneous heparin.[31]

Bacteremia or septicemia caused by acute thrombophlebitis complicating a continuous intravenous infusion has become a prominent cause of "third-day surgical fever." When it is necessary to administer antibiotic or other irritating solutions intravenously, these should be delivered into the intravenous system by way of a Sol-U-Set type of dilution apparatus rather than by giving the undiluted agent directly into the tubing. The careless use of intravenous catheters is to be criticized, and the tendency to leave them in as long as possible is to be avoided. When possible, the appropriate size scalp vein needle is usually preferred for the administration of parenteral fluids. When continuous intravenous solutions are required over a period of days, a change of the intravenous setup at 24- to 48-hour intervals is recommended with a change in venipuncture site. Routine inspection of the venipuncture site at least every 8 hours is the single most important factor in avoiding the serious sequelae of postinfusion phlebitis. The infusion should be stopped immediately if phlebitis is suspected.[3,4,32] More subtle and less common causes of postoperative fever are drug reactions, recurrent malaria, central neurological disturbances, bacterial enterocolitis, and artificial situations such as the heating of the thermometer with hot liquids or a match and taking the temperature after the ingestion of food or soup or after the patient has just completed smoking.

Needless to say, common sense demands that elective surgery be postponed in a patient who is febrile until recovery has been established. This does not mean that surgery has to be postponed when it may represent a crucial diagnostic maneuver to establish the process causing the fever.

An oral body temperature of 100° F (37° C) in the immediate postoperative period or fever that persists for more than 6 hours, according to Allison,[2] must cause a surgeon to consider certain specific problems that often complicate recovery. In an attempt to determine the cause of the postoperative fever, the following useful procedures should begin immediately:

1. The patient's entire clinical status should be carefully appraised with particular reference to the state of hydration, the relationship of the febrile course to any of the medications being used, and the possibility of a hypersensitivity phenomenon having occurred in the patient's past medical history.

2. Examination of the wounds, surgical and otherwise, and cultures if there is suggestive evidence of infection should be performed.

3. Clinical evaluation of the lungs and urinary tract and appropriate studies of the urine and sputum with cultures when indicated should be done. Gram stain examination of the sputum or urine may also be useful.

4. Blood cultures should be obtained whenever there is the slightest suggestion of sepsis, bacteremia, or peripheral vascular collapse of unexplained cause.

5. Chest radiographs should be taken if pulmonary embolization or infection is suspected. A pulmonary perfusion scan with technetium ^{99m}Tc microspheres is the best screening procedure in suspected cases of pulmonary embolism. An arterial oxygen tension above 90 mm Hg in a patient breathing room air tends to rule out a major pulmonary embolism.[9]

6. Postoperative electrocardiogram, particularly if there has been a preoperative electrocardiographic evaluation, may be useful in localizing the source of the fever.

It should be recalled that fever as a sign of postoperative infection may be absent or markedly depressed if the patient has been placed on corticosteroid drugs.

Hypotension. *Shock* is described by MacLean[23] as "inadequate blood flow to vital organs or failure of the cells of vital organs to utilize oxygen." The precise, expeditious, and successful treatment of shock according to Hardy "depends upon an orderly approach to diagnosis, with recognition of physiologic priorities."[16] Shock in the recovery room or in the postoperative patient may be related to hypoxia, hypercarbia (inadequate ventilation), coronary insufficiency, arrhythmia, or electrolyte imbalance. Other causes may be endotoxic shock, pulmonary embolus, and excessive medication. Miscellaneous causes may be related to drug reactions, transfusion reactions, fat embolism, hepatic failure, and anaphylaxis. According to MacLean,[23] eight measurements should be assayed in the initial assessment and follow-up on all patients in shock:

1. Arterial blood pressure (normal range of adult male, 120/80)
2. Pulse rate (80 per minute)
3. Central venous pressure (5 cm H_2O)
4. Urine flow (50 ml per hour)
5. Cardiac index (3.2 liters per min per m^2)
6. Arterial blood–P_{O_2} (100 mm Hg); P_{CO_2} (40 mm Hg) and pH (7.4)
7. Arterial blood lactate (12 mg per 100 ml)
8. Hematocrit (35% to 45%)

Fat embolism. The *fat embolization syndrome* occurs when fat appears in the circulating blood in droplets that are large enough to obstruct arteries and capillaries. Fat globules may present in the urine and sputum. Serum lipase and tributyrinase levels rise between the third and seventh posttrauma days. The blood gases are abnormal. The classic case is described as a person who is recovering from an accident involving fractures of the long bones, pelvis, or ribs or from an operation or a person in fine health who becomes short of breath, then febrile and disoriented. Hypertension follows with a small fast pulse and oliguria, and finally, the patient becomes comatose. The diagnosis is made certain by the discovery of petechiae over the neck and anterior chest and inner aspects of the thighs. The level of serum lipase is of diagnostic value because the lung parenchyma produces lipase in an attempt to remove the emboli of neutral fat from the lung. The by-products of this fat hydrolysis are the fatty acids, and these cause serious damage to the pulmonary capillary endothelium and reduce the lung surfactant activity.

Because of his or her position on the trauma team, the oral surgeon may occasionally have need to recognize this entity. Present therapy consists of massive doses of corticosteroids given intravenously for 3 days along with positive pressure ventilation supported by rapid-acting diuretics when indicated.[5] Intravenous heparin, alone or with alcohol, is of doubtful value.

Psychological problems. In the immediate postoperative period, transient *emotional upsets* are not uncommon. They usually become manifest about the third postoperative day as an anxiety or depressive reaction that may produce insomnia, poor appetite, fear, apprehension, and decreased pain threshold. Anxiety in rare cases may progress to a point of acute depersonalization, causing the patient to make sudden and unpredictable suicidal or assaultive attempts.[20,25] Most of the postoperative emotional upsets are of a nature that respond to discussion and reassurance by the surgeon as well as discriminating use of sedatives. Often a visit from the dietician or special attention by the nursing service will be of significant help to the patient experiencing this difficult episode.[20]

Hypertension. Occasionally *hypertension* rather than hypotension will be a problem in the postoperative management of the oral surgery patient. If the condition has occurred preoperatively and is of a relatively long-standing duration, the patient probably will be under specific treatment and perhaps a diagnosis is known. A persistent elevation of the diastolic blood pressure above 90 to 95 mm Hg with a corresponding rise of the systolic pressure to 150 to 200 mm Hg is cause for concern in the postoperative patient, unless this has been a pressure to which the patient has been accustomed for some time. Obvious causes of hypertension are postoperative pain, hypercarbia, mechanical errors in taking the measurement or administration of vasopressor or catecholamine agents. If these factors can be eliminated readily and the hypertension continues to mount upward, intramuscular or intravenous administration of one of the *Rauwolfia* derivatives (reserpine, 5 mg) may be useful in preventing a blood pressure elevation to the point at which the patient goes into left heart failure or has a cerebrovascular accident. Titration with sodium nitroprusside drip could be life saving.

An undiagnosed pheochromocytoma or hypercalcemia related to hyperparathyroid activity or the infusion of calcium salts may be implicated.[41] A phenothiazine, such as chlorpromazine administered in amounts from 25 to 50 mg parenterally, may be useful in controlling hypertension if the drug is not contraindicated because of existing central nervous system depression.

Convulsions. *Convulsions* may be one of the most distressing abnormalities of the postoperative period. The most common causes of the occurrence of convulsions, particularly in children, are hyperthermia, anoxia, hypocalcemic tetany, and toxemia resulting from an infection or drug sensitivity. Whatever the cause, it must be investigated and definitive, specific therapy directed toward the correction of the situation. The intravenous administration of diazepam or appropriate barbiturates, such as amobarbital or secobarbital given initially intravenously, generally will control the convulsions. An amount is given sufficient to arrest the convulsions. Attention must be directed toward the adequate respiratory ventilation of the patient.

FLUID AND ELECTROLYTES[28,35]

The management of fluids and electrolytes preoperatively, intraoperatively, and postoperatively is a necessary aspect of surgical care. Certain fundamentals will be reviewed. The subject can be studied in depth in the references.

From a practical standpoint most losses or gains of body fluids come from the extracellular fluid volume, which comprises approximately 20% of the body weight, 5% intravascular (plasma) and 15% extravascular (interstitial).

Preoperative phase. Preoperative extracellular fluid replacement is of great importance because incomplete replacement of fluid may lead to prompt hypotension with the induction of anesthesia. The nonanesthetized patient is able to compensate for a mild volume deficit, and therefore the circulatory collapse may appear to be insidious in the awake patient. The preoperative evaluation of the patient and the replacement of blood loss when indicated cannot be overemphasized.

Intraoperative management of fluids. It is generally recognized that there should be a complete replacement of blood loss plus approximately 450 to 500 ml per operative hour of lactated Ringer's solution, up to a total of 3,000 ml, given intraoperatively. Blood should be replaced as it is lost, with the exception of the first 500 ml.[35]

For the elective surgical procedure requiring blood replacement, autogenous blood can be drawn over a 2-week period prior to surgery and stored for reinfusion at the time of operation. This is the safest type of whole blood transfusion.

Postoperative management of fluids. Once in the recovery room, the patient's fluid status must be assessed. This survey involves the review of the preoperative fluid status, the volume lost and gained during the operation, and a clinical evaluation of the patient's vital signs and urinary output. Orders are written to cover replacement of known existing fluid deficits plus maintenance for the remainder of the day. For the critically ill patient who has received or lost a large volume of fluid, the replacement is ordered a liter at a time and the patient's status is reviewed frequently until it is stable. Postoperative fluid volume management requires accurate measurement of sensible losses, as well as the intake of fluid and electrolytes from all sources, and an estimation of the insensible losses and replacement, if indicated, with the appropriate fluid or electrolytes or both. It is unnecessary and probably unwise to administer potassium during the first 24 hours after surgery unless there is a definite potassium deficit. Shires[35] suggests that in the later postoperative period approximately 1 liter of fluid be given to replace the urinary volume necessary to handle the excretory work load (800 to 1,000 ml); he uses the otherwise healthy 70-kg man as an example. Sensible losses such as gastrointestinal fluids and salivary fistulas are replaced volume for volume, whereas urine volume is not. The insensible loss is estimated at 600 to 900 ml per day, unless fever, hyperventilation, an unhumidified tracheostomy, or hypermetabolism is present; then the volume lost may reach 1,500 ml. In the patient with an uncomplicated postoperative course, the determination of sodium and other electrolytes is generally unnecessary if the parenteral fluid therapy is not continued as the sole source of intake for over 2 to 3 days. The choice of fluid to replace the sensible and insensible losses need not be complicated. Five percent dextrose in 0.2% normal saline solution, administered at the rate of 100 to 125 ml an hour, may be used. After the first 24 hours, if parenteral fluids are maintained, 40 mEq of potassium chloride solution may be added to the volume. Some authorities prefer 2,000 ml of 5% dextrose in water with 40 mEq of potassium and 500 ml of 5% dextrose in normal saline.[21,28,35]

Complications in fluid balance. The most frequent and important problems in fluid balance in the surgical patient are related to changes in extracellular fluid volume. Circulatory instability manifested by hypotension and tachycardia is often the earliest postoperative sign of extracellular fluid volume deficit. Furthermore, the level of consciousness, pupillary size, airway patency, respiratory pattern, body temperature, pulse rate and volume, and skin color must be evaluated. A 30 to 50 ml hourly urine output is minimal. Replacement of the extracellular fluid loss in the postoperative phase reduces the incidence of changes in the composition and concentration of the extracellular water. Attention to the clinical signs of fluid overloads such as weight gain, heavy eyelids, hoarseness, and dyspnea usually will prevent this abnormality of fluid volume from developing or progressing.

Disorders in fluid balance may affect change in the following:
1. Extracellular fluid volume (isotonic salt solution is added or lost)
2. Concentration of osmotically active particles (ion-free water alone is added or lost)
3. Composition when concentration of ions other than sodium are altered
4. Distributional alteration when there is loss of extracellular fluid into a nonfunctional space such as in a burn, ascites, or hemorrhagic shock

Factors affected by acid-base imbalance. As a result of acid-base imbalance, the following four clinical entities can occur.

1. *Respiratory acidosis* may be produced by any condition or combination of conditions that result in inadequate ventilation (atelectasis, pneumonia, airway obstruction). The clinical signs of restlessness, hypertension, and tachycardia in the postoperative patient may indicate the presence of hypercapnia. Treatment consists of providing adequate ventilation and correcting the pulmonary problem when possible.

2. *Respiratory alkalosis* in the surgical patient is caused usually by hyperventilation resulting from apprehension, pain, brain injury, or overventilation by mechanical respirators. If the condition is mild, no therapy is required. When the cause of hyperventilation can be determined and corrected, the problem is eliminated.

3. *Metabolic acidosis* may occur as a result of acute circulatory failure or renal damage, chloride excess, loss of lower gastrointestinal fluids, administration of unbalanced salt solutions, and uncontrolled diabetes mellitus. Correction of protracted metabolic acidosis may require the use of sodium bicarbonate. When cardiopulmonary arrest occurs, restoration of blood flow, pulmonary ventilation, and administration of sodium bicarbonate is required.

4. *Metabolic alkalosis* usually occurs when some degree of hypokalemia exists. It occurs when there is an uncomplicated loss of acids (H ion) or retention of bases. Because of the associated hypokalemia, cardiac arrhythmias, paralytic ilieus, digitalis intoxication, and tetany may develop. Dangerous hyperkalemia (greater than 6 mEq per liter) is unusual if kidney function is normal. Generally, it is unwise to administer potassium during the first 24 hours postoperatively unless there is a definite hypokalemia. These deficits should be replaced after an adequate urine output is obtained. The daily replacement of potassium for renal excretion is 40 mEq plus 20 mEq for gastrointestinal loss if indicated; it should not be administered parenterally in concentrations of more than 40 mEq per liter as potassium chloride.[21,28,35]

BLOOD TRANSFUSION
INDICATIONS[7,21,28]

Blood transfusion is indicated in the following cases:

1. To maintain blood volume and treat or attempt to prevent shock (Measured blood loss is replaced as it occurs; in hypovolemic shock the degree of replacement depends on the clinical findings in regard to the pulse, blood pressure, peripheral circulation, venous pressure, and urine output.)
2. To improve or maintain oxygen-carrying capacity
3. To promote or maintain coagulation
4. For exchange of blood in neonates
5. As a prime for a biomechanical apparatus such as a pump oxygenator

Complications. The possible complications associated with blood transfusions are as follows:

1. Incompatible blood (ABO)—This problem can be prevented in most cases by proper identification of the recipient receiving the proper cross-match.
2. Hemolytic reactions—Simultaneous reactions reportedly occur in from 0.2% to 1% of transfusions and have 36% mortality; delayed hemolytic reactions occur several days after the transfusion with the mortality of 1.8%.
3. Allergic reactions
4. Pyogenic reactions
5. Febrile reactions
6. Air embolism
7. Circulatory overload
8. Cardiac arrests
   a. Hypothermia
   b. Citrate toxicity
   c. Hyperkalemia
9. Thrombophlebitis
10. Delayed transmission of disease
    a. Hepatitis—The instance is 1% for whole blood and 12% for pool plasma.
    b. Postinfusion syndrome
    c. Syphilis
11. Oozing hemorrhage—This occurs in 33% of patients receiving ten or more units of whole blood.

Symptoms of an untoward reaction to a transfusion usually are manifest during the initial 50 to 100 ml of each unit of the infusion.

Rate of infusion. The rate of infusion is begun generally at 2 to 3 ml per minute and increased as follows:

1. For an elective transfusion into a normal circulatory system, infuse 8 to 10 ml per minute with 60 to 80 minutes per transfusion.

2. In the embarrassed cardiovascular system, especially in the elderly, infuse at 4 to 5 ml per minute, 130 minutes per transfusion.

3. In acute hypovolemia, infuse at maximal obtainable rates until systolic blood pressure of 100 mm Hg is attained.

• • •

Careful attention given to preoperative and postoperative care assures the surgical patient optimal conditions for recovery.

REFERENCES

1. Aldrete, A. J., and Kroulik, D.: A postanesthesia recovery score, Anesth. Analg. **40:**924, 1970.
2. Allison, F. J.: Post operative fever. In Hardy, J. D., editor: Critical surgical illness, Philadelphia, 1971, W. B. Saunders Co.
3. Altemeier, W. A., and others: Third day surgical fever, Arch. Surg. **103:**158, 1971.
4. Arnold, R. E., Elliot, E. K., and Holms, B. H.: The importance of frequent examination of infusion sites in post infusion phlebitis, Surg. Gynecol. Obstet. **145:**19-20, 1977.
5. Bivins, B. A., Madauss, W. C., and Griffen, W. O., Jr.: Fat embolism syndrome: a clinical study, J. South. Med. Assoc. **65:**937, 1972.
6. Buckley, J. J.: Airway management in acute trauma. In Najarian, J. S., and Delaney, J. P., editors: Critical surgical care, Miami, 1977, Symposia Specialists.
7. Collins, J. A.: Fluid replacement for extensive blood loss. In Najarian, J. S., and Delaney, J. P., editors: Critical surgical care, Miami, 1977, Symposia Specialists.
8. Cullen, D. J.: Problems encountered in the recovery room, Resident Staff Physician **23**(5):46-55, May 1977.
9. Del Guercio, L. R. M.: Thromboembolic problems associated with the critically injured patient. In Najarian, J. S., and Delaney, J. P., editors: Critical surgical care, Miami, 1977, Symposia Specialists.
10. Dudrick, S. J.: Intravenous hyperalimentation. In Hardy, J. D., editor: Critical surgical illness, Philadelphia, 1971, W. B. Saunders Co.
11. Dudrick, S. J., and Duke, J. H., Jr.: Nutritional complications in the surgical patient. In Artz, C. P., and Hardy, J. D., editors: Management of surgical complications, ed. 3, Philadelphia, 1975, W. B. Saunders Co.
12. Essig, C. F.: Newer sedative drugs that can cause states of intoxication and dependence of barbiturate type, J.A.M.A. **196:**714, 1966.
13. Figueroa, M., Jr.: The postanesthesia recovery score: a second look, J. South. Med. Assoc. **65:**791, 1972.
14. Fiumara, N. J.: A laboratory test is not a diagnosis, J.A.M.A. **217:**71, 1971.
15. Halpern, L. M.: Analgesic drugs in the management of pain, Arch. Surg. **112:**861, 1977.
16. Hardy, J. D.: Shock and cardiac arrest. In Hardy, J. D., editor: Critical surgical illness, Philadelphia, 1971, W. B. Saunders Co.
17. Harpman, J. A.: Anesthetic malignant myopathy hyperthermia, Arch. Otolaryngol. **96:**264, 1972.
18. Hastings, D. W.: Treatment of drug withdrawal, delirium and convulsions, Mod. Med. **40:**58, 1972.
19. Hunt, T. K.: Nutritional requirements of repair. In Ballinger, W. R., editor: Manual of surgical nutrition, Philadelphia, 1975, W. B. Saunders Co.
20. Kahana, R. J., and Bibring, G. L.: Personality types in medical management. In Zinberg, N. E., editor: Psychiatry and medical practice in a general hospital, New York, 1964, International Universities Press.
21. Kinney, J. M., Egdahl, R. H., and Zuidema, G. D.: Ventilation and ventilatory failure. In Kinney, J. M., editor: Manual of pre-operative and post-operative care, ed. 2, Philadelphia, 1971, W. B. Saunders Co.
22. Long, J. M., III, Dudrick, S. J., and Copeland, E. M., III: Update on parenteral hyperalimentation. In Najarian, J. S., and Delaney, J. P., editors: Critical surgical care, Miami, 1977, Symposia Specialists.
23. MacLean, L. D.: The patient in shock. In Kinney, J. M., editor: Manual of pre-operative and post-operative care, ed. 2, Philadelphia, 1971, W. B. Saunders Co.
24. McGovern, J. P., Haywood, T. J., and Walker, D. G.: Allergies of the oral cavity: including delineation of a new symptom-complex of physical allergy about the commissures, J. South. Med. Assoc. **55:**714, 1962.
25. Meyer, E., and Mendelson, M.: Psychiatric consultations with patients on medical and surgical wards: patterns and processes, Psychiatry **24:**197, 1961.
26. Morris, G. K., and Mitchell, J. R. A.: The etiology of acute pulmonary embolism and the identification of high risk groups, Br. J. Med. **18:**6-12, 1977.
27. Moyer, C. A.: The assessment of operative risk and non-operative surgical care. In Rhodes, J. E., editor: Surgery principles and practice, ed. 3, Philadelphia, 1970, J. B. Lippincott.
28. Pestana, C.: Fluids and electrolytes in the surgical patient, 1976, San Antonio, University of Texas Press.
29. Polk, H. C.: Post-operative wound infection: a prospective study of determinant factors and prevention, Surgery **66:**97, 1967.
30. Pontoppidian, H., Laver, M. B., and Geffin, B.: Acute respiratory failure in the surgical patient. In Welch, C. E., editor: Advances in surgery, vol. 4, Chicago, 1971, Year Book Medical Publishers.
31. Sagar, S., Stamatakis, J. D., Thomas, D. P., and Kakkar, V. V.: Oral contraceptives, antithrombin-IV activity, and post operative deep-vein thrombosis, Lancet **1**(7958): 509-511, 1976.
32. Samson, O. D., and Watson, C. L.: A question of safety—the cathether vs. the needle, Am. J. Intravenous Ther. **4**(3):7-12, May 1977.
33. Schumer, W., and Nyhus, L. M.: Corticosteroid effect on biochemical parameters of human oligemic shock, Arch. Surg. **100:**405, 1970.
34. Scopp, I. W., and Orvieto, L. D.: Gingival degerming by povidone-iodine irrigation; bacteremia reduction in extraction procedures, J. Am. Dent. Assoc. **85:**1294, 1971.

35. Shires, T. G.: Fluid and electrolyte therapy. In Kinney, J. M., editor: Manual of pre-operative and post-operative care, ed. 2, Philadelphia, 1971, W. B. Saunders Co.

36. Toung, T., and others: Aspiration pneumonia: beneficial and harmful effects of positive end-expiratory pressure, Surgery **82:**279-283, 1977.

37. Walker, D. G.: Nutrition in oral surgery and its relationship to wound healing and infection, Oral Surg. **7:**797, 1954.

38. Walker, D. G.: Medical emergencies in dental practice. In Goldman, M. M., Forrest, S. P., Byrd, D. L., and McDonald, R. E., editors: Current therapy in dentistry, St. Louis, 1968, The C. V. Mosby Co.

39. Walker, D. G.: Prevention and treatment of post-operative pulmonary complications, J. Oral Surg. **30:**813, 1972.

40. Wassion, W. H., Rosenbluth, B., and Kux, M.: Protective effect of methylprednisone against lung complications in endotoxic shock, J. South. Med. Assoc. **65:**941, 1972.

41. Weidmann, P.: Blood pressure effects of acute hypercalcemia, Ann. Intern. Med. **76:**741, 1972.

42. Wilson, R. D.: Malignant hyperpyrexia with anesthesia, J.A.M.A. **202:**183, 1967.

43. Wilson, R. D.: Biochemical changes in malignant hyperpyrexia, Lancet **1:**1137, 1970.

Index